MW00852210

TREATING ADDICTION

Also Available

Treating Addiction

A Guide for Professionals

SECOND EDITION

William R. Miller
Alyssa A. Forcehimes
Allen Zweben

THE GUILFORD PRESS
New York   London

Copyright © 2019 The Guilford Press
A Division of Guilford Publications, Inc.
370 Seventh Avenue, Suite 1200, New York, NY 10001
www.guilford.com

All rights reserved

No part of this book may be reproduced, translated, stored in a retrieval
system, or transmitted, in any form or by any means, electronic, mechanical,
photocopying, microfilming, recording, or otherwise, without written permission
from the publisher.

Printed in the United States of America

This book is printed on acid-free paper.

Last digit is print number: 9   8   7   6   5   4   3   2   1

The authors have checked with sources believed to be reliable in their efforts to
provide information that is complete and generally in accord with the standards
of practice that are accepted at the time of publication. However, in view of the
possibility of human error or changes in behavioral, mental health, or medical
sciences, neither the authors, nor the editors and publisher, nor any other party
who has been involved in the preparation or publication of this work warrants
that the information contained herein is in every respect accurate or complete,
and they are not responsible for any errors or omissions or the results obtained
from the use of such information. Readers are encouraged to confirm the
information contained in this book with other sources.

Library of Congress Cataloging-in-Publication Data is available
from the publisher.

ISBN 978-1-4625-4044-0 (hardcover)

To Dr. Robert G. Hall, who in 1973
persuaded me that I ought to learn something
about addiction treatment
—W. R. M.

To my sister, who is remarkable,
not because of what she's gone through,
but because of what she's come away with
—A. A. F.

To my grandchildren,
Dylan, Jackson, Harper, and Alexander,
who light up my life
—A. Z.

About the Authors

William R. Miller, PhD, is Emeritus Distinguished Professor of Psychology and Psychiatry at the University of New Mexico. Fundamentally interested in the psychology of change, he is a founder of motivational interviewing and has focused particularly on developing and testing more effective treatments for people with alcohol and drug problems. Dr. Miller has published over 400 scientific articles and chapters and 50 books, including the groundbreaking work for professionals *Motivational Interviewing, Third Edition*, and the self-help resource *Controlling Your Drinking, Second Edition*. He is a recipient of the international Jellinek Memorial Award, two career achievement awards from the American Psychological Association, and an Innovators in Combating Substance Abuse Award from the Robert Wood Johnson Foundation, among many other honors. The Institute for Scientific Information has listed him as one of the world's most highly cited researchers.

Alyssa A. Forcehimes, PhD, is President of The Change Companies and Train for Change. Prior to joining these organizations, she was on the faculty of Psychiatry and Psychology at the University of New Mexico Health Sciences Center. Her research focuses on processes of motivation for change and on effective methods for disseminating and teaching evidence-based behavioral treatments in real-world settings. Dr. Forcehimes works in addiction, mental health, and health care settings to develop, implement, and evaluate behavior change practices.

Allen Zweben, PhD, is Professor and Associate Dean at the Columbia University School of Social Work. His research and publications have focused primarily on innovative assessment and treatment approaches for substance use problems. Dr. Zweben has been a principal investigator on numerous behavioral and medication trials, including two landmark studies funded by the National Institute on Alcohol Abuse and Alcoholism: Project MATCH, a patient–treatment matching study, and the COMBINE study, a project examining the efficacy of combining pharmacotherapy and psychotherapy interventions for alcohol problems.

Preface

Those of us who work in health and social services will regularly encounter substance use disorders (SUDs), no matter what our specialty or setting may be. As discussed in Chapter 1, about one in three North Americans will develop an addictive disorder in the course of their lives, and at any given time the prevalence rate of SUDs is over 15%. In health care and social service populations this percentage is higher still, and many more people are directly affected by a loved one with alcohol/drug problems. The burden of SUDs is similarly high worldwide. If you treat people for health, mental health, or social problems, you will see quite a few whose lives are affected by addictions.

Yet, many professionals still receive relatively little training or encouragement to treat this common family of problems. Although some professionals specialize in addiction treatment, little time is typically devoted to this field in generalist training for social work, psychology, counseling, medicine, or nursing. This lack of professional training is unfortunate, because addictions are intertwined with so many other medical, social, and behavioral problems, and those working in health and social service settings are well positioned to identify and address them. The primary obstacle has been a lack of specific preparation and encouragement to do so.

We have written this book for both generalists and specialists, to provide an up-to-date foundation for helping people with addictive disorders. Together we have over a century of experience in this field, in clinical psychology (W. R. M. and A. A. F.) and social work (A. Z.), and we have had the privilege to work with many dedicated counselors, nurses, physicians, and other professionals over the years who help people escape from the snare of addiction. It is rewarding work and, whether you are a generalist or an addiction specialist, we hope this book will help you gain the knowledge, confidence, and passion to address this common and significant affliction among those you serve.

Throughout this book we have sought to ground our recommendations in the best science available. "Evidence-based treatment" has become a popular phrase in this field, and it is becoming common to require the use of evidence-based practices in order to receive reimbursement. There is a long and fascinating history of evidence here, with well over a thousand published clinical trials of addiction treatment methods. New research appears at a dizzying pace, and we have had the privilege of keeping up with and translating it for clinicians whose days are occupied with providing care. Some findings that we present may be surprising or even disturbing. They certainly were to us when we initially encountered them, sometimes as unexpected results in our own research. We cite both new and old research throughout the book; many important studies and findings were published in the latter half of the 20th century. Blessed with such a large science base, it is time to make good use of it in treating addictions.

That science base also includes many studies showing that *relationship* matters; it makes a difference not just *what* treatment is being delivered, but *who* provides it and *how*. The impact of a therapist's approach is not unique to this field. "Therapeutic rapport," "bedside manner," and "working alliance" are familiar concepts. Yet relationship skills such as empathic understanding seem to be particularly important to success in treating addictions, which have been so stigmatized. It makes a difference when a therapist practices with profound respect, loving compassion, and accurate empathy; some believe that quality of the relationship is the most important and powerful aspect of treatment. Thus, you will find an emphasis on relationship and style interwoven throughout this book.

What we wish to offer you, then, is an updated professional resource that combines both clinical and scientific perspectives. We hope this book will be helpful to professionals who are already treating addictive disorders and also to those who are just learning how to treat addictions. We also encourage health professionals more generally to think of addictions as falling within their own normal scope of work, and we have kept this in mind in our writing. In addiction treatment, it makes a difference what you do and how you do it, and it is far easier to develop evidence-based practice from the outset than to change already established habits.

Changes in the Second Edition

We have strengthened 20 prior chapters with another decade of scientific research on addiction treatment, and we continue to be impressed by the growing volume and quality of research in a field once largely ignored by clinical science. We have also added five more chapters to highlight topics that were not fully addressed in our first edition.

First of these is a new chapter (12) on meditation and mindfulness, which has now joined the menu of evidence-based addiction treatment components. Meditation has an ancient history, and now also has an emerging science of process and outcome research with SUDs.

Our prior edition did not include a separate chapter on contingency management (COM), perhaps because at the time it was rarely used in community treatment programs. That is beginning to change with wider applications, including in U.S. Department of Veterans Affairs hospitals and clinics, and dissemination through the Clinical Trials Network of the National Institute on Drug Abuse. Chapter 13 provides an introduction to the underlying principles of COM, methods of delivery, the efficacy research, and various implementation issues. We also discuss barriers to widespread adoption of COM (e.g., costs, compatibility with treatment principles and practices) and the training of staff in COM procedures.

In addition to updating our chapter on working with couples and families (16), there is a new chapter (15) on working *through* significant others. It highlights in particular the rapidly disseminating community reinforcement and family training (CRAFT) method that has well-replicated success in engaging initially "unmotivated" substance users in treatment by working unilaterally with their loved ones. It is a welcome alternative to waiting for people to suffer sufficiently and "hit bottom."

We struggled with what to call the new Chapter 19, in which we address a variety of practical issues that often arise in addiction treatment, including missed appointments, resumed use, intoxicated clients, and responding to "resistance." It offers practical advice from our clinical experience with thousands of clients, and we settled on the title "Stuff That Comes Up."

Finally, there is a new chapter on implementation of evidence-based treatment methods. Clinicians are unlikely to develop competence in a complex treatment method simply by reading about it or attending a workshop (though we have learned the hard way that doing either can create a mistaken belief that one is now using the new method). Dean Fixsen, a "dean" of implementation science, once quipped that people cannot benefit from a treatment to which they have not been exposed. How does one establish and maintain personal or program fidelity in delivering a new treatment method? That is the focus of Chapter 25.

A Word about Words

In writing this book, we had to make many decisions about terminology. The addiction field has been replete with stigmatizing and moralistic language, such as the terms "clean" and "dirty." Since 1980, the *Diagnostic and Statistical Manual of Mental Disorders* has recommended that diagnostic terms be used to describe disorders ("depression" and "schizophrenia") rather than people ("depressives" and "schizophrenics"). Although language that describes disorders is now the professional norm in most of behavioral health, in the addiction field it is still common to hear labels being applied to people (e.g., "abuser," "addict," "alcoholic"). Terminology makes a difference. When an individual was described in two studies as a "substance abuser," both lay public (Kelly, Dow, & Westerhoff, 2010) and health professionals (Kelly & Westerhoff, 2010) were far more likely to perceive the person as blameworthy, threatening, and deserving of punishment, than when the person had been described as "having an SUD." This detail was the only change in the case description, and the epithet "abuser" yielded significantly more negative perceptions and recommendations. Throughout this book we have been careful to describe conditions rather than labeling people.

A wide variety of terms are applied to those who are under professional care. To our ears the term "patient" suggests a recipient being acted upon by a doctor, with a further unfortunate connotation of passivity: "You must be patient." The clinical approach we describe in this book emphasizes active engagement, responsibility, and empowerment of people for changes in their own lives (which is, of course, important in health care more generally). In the chapters that follow, we have most often used "clients" or "people" as the generic term, and "patients" when the context is explicitly medical.

Similarly, people who treat addictions encompass a wide range of professions and titles. We have used "counselor," "clinician," and "practitioner" as generics for people who provide care. In describing conditions, we have adhered to the current, albeit somewhat awkward, terms "substance use disorder" (SUD) as well as "alcohol/drug problems" or "alcohol and other drug problems," the latter being the traditional reminder that ethyl alcohol is itself a drug. As a shorthand generic, we prefer the term "addiction," which is the title of the oldest scientific journal in the field. We use this term to refer to the full continuum of SUDs, much as Jellinek (1960) used the term "alcoholism."

Another shift in language in this edition is away from the familiar term "detox." Detoxification is literally the elimination from the body of a poison (toxin)—a description that is more accurate for some drugs than for others. Competent withdrawal management, addressed in Chapter 6, is clearly an important component of addiction treatment services, but "detox" itself has taken on fearful connotations of cold turkey and painful suffering that can now be averted through appropriate treatment. The term "detox" also gets associated with a place rather than a process, and can have stigmatizing overtones. We have therefore deemphasized this term in favor of "withdrawal management."

Finally, we have avoided relying on the term "relapse," even though it is still widely used. Our reasoning is that relapse communicates that there are only two possible states: perfection or disaster. Ironically, the term relapse itself implies what Alan Marlatt called the "abstinence violation effect"—that all is lost once the rule has been broken—and thus it can become a self-fulfilling prophecy. Relapse also has rather moralistic overtones and is not commonly used in describing other chronic health conditions. A person with diabetes who comes into the emergency room with hyperglycemia is not typically said to have relapsed. Neither is a person with a recurrence of problems related to asthma, hypertension, or heart disease. Relapse is sometimes used to describe a recurrence of cancer, but not in the sense that the *person* has relapsed. What language, then, might one use instead? Euphemisms retain the assumption of a binary on-or-off state, whereas actual treatment outcomes are much more variable. The clearest solution, we believe, is simply to describe the *behavior* (e.g., drinking, drug use) without adding moralistic baggage. This is the approach that we have taken, using relapse only when necessary to describe the concept. In lieu of "relapse prevention," we focus positively on maintaining change (see Chapter 21). It is a challenging discipline to write in this way, precisely because it requires a new way of thinking, shedding some old habits and assumptions.

Acknowledgments

For me, this book represents a retrospective of what I have learned during five decades working in addiction treatment and research. It is a book I wish I had had while teaching. Now we are pleased to offer this updated second edition. Although particular author names appear on the cover, we are each the product of our relationships through the years with countless mentors, students, colleagues, family, and friends. It is an illusion that an individual writes a book. Like books themselves, we are authored by those with whom we work, live, and love. —W. R. M.

An acknowledgment section is a place to offer thanks to the people who helped make this book a possibility. Here I offer my sincere thanks to the people in my life who shaped this book in one way or another. Some people helped by sharing their knowledge, their wisdom, and their time. Other people helped by offering encouragement, support, and coffee. And then there are people I would like to thank for making the aim of this book a possibility: you, the reader. Thank you for taking the information contained in these pages, offering it to others, and helping one more person move toward change. That is the motivation that led to this second edition, and that is the acknowledgment for which I am most grateful and ever hopeful. —A. A. F.

I am appreciative of the help given to me by Mary Piepmeier, who assisted me with compiling and editing references and copy editing of chapters. —A. Z.

Contents

PART I

AN INVITATION TO ADDICTION TREATMENT

For decades, addiction treatment was an orphan, delivered mostly in specialist settings isolated from mainstream medical and behavioral health care. We begin this second edition with an invitation to this rewarding field in which treatment can and does make a life-or-death difference. In Chapter 1 we consider the very good reasons to make this part of your professional work, as well as a few reasons why this aspect of health care has sometimes been ignored or stigmatized. Chapter 2 offers a broad overview of addiction—what it is, what causes it, and how diagnostic conceptions have changed over the decades. Finally, in Chapter 3 we provide a brief primer on how drugs work, as a context for understanding substance use disorders. Together these three chapters represent a head start on treating the complex and fascinating phenomenon of addiction.

- Is there a difference between treating substance use disorder and addictive personality disorder?

- Do you think there will be a shift in DSM-V to just addictive personality?

CHAPTER 1

Why Treat Addiction?

Treating addiction is not a matter for specialists alone but should be of vital concern for all professionals who work in health care, behavioral health, and social services (Office of the Surgeon General, 2016). The sheer worldwide prevalence of addiction problems and the suffering that they cause would be reason enough (Gowing et al., 2015; Whiteford et al., 2015). Alcohol use disorders alone afflict 14% of the U.S. population in any given year (Grant et al., 2015), with an overlapping 20% of the population addicted to nicotine (Chou et al., 2016) and 4% with other diagnosable drug use disorders (Grant et al., 2016). Lifetime prevalence rates from these same studies are higher still, of course: 29% for alcohol, 28% for nicotine, and 10% for other drug use disorders. These are the most common disorders encountered in behavioral health care, even more prevalent than depression. Other addictive behaviors such as pathological gambling and compulsive buying do not involve a drug, but each afflicts up to 5% of the population (Maraz, Griffiths, & Demetrovics, 2016; Petry & Armentano, 1999). Furthermore, substance use disorders (SUDs)—particularly use of tobacco and alcohol—are by far the leading preventable cause of death in the Western world. Treating addictions is quite literally a matter of life and death. Yet these very common, disabling, and high-mortality conditions often go unnoticed and untreated, a potentially life-threatening clinical error (Degenhardt et al., 2014; Gossop, 2015; Liese & Reis, 2016; Roerecke & Rehm, 2013).

A second reason is that addictions are closely intertwined with the problems that bring people into the offices of medical, mental health, social service, and correctional workers. In most populations seen by such professionals the prevalence of SUDs is even higher than in the general population. In fact, people with addiction problems are far more likely to be seen in health care and mental health services than in specialist treatment programs (Edlund, Booth, & Han, 2012). Thus, aware of it or not, most health and social service professionals are already treating the sequelae of addictions without directly addressing a significant source of the problems.

Why not just refer people with addictions to specialist programs? There is a role, of course, for specialist care, particularly when treatment is closely integrated with other needed services. Yet there is a downside to regarding these disorders as separable, to be treated by unique specialists (Office of the Surgeon General, 2016). Patients are often reluctant to seek care from isolated and stigmatized addiction treatment programs, and may encounter other obstacles such as waiting lists, given the limited supply of specialist treatment. In the United States, only about one in five people with SUDs ever receives *any* help for this condition during their lifetime (Chou et al., 2016; Grant et al., 2015, 2016). Many people with SUDs also have concomitant mental and/or medical disorders that need attention. The presence of concomitant disorders complicates the treatment of addictions, and vice versa. The normal management of chronic medical conditions is not limited to episodes of specialist consultation, but is an ongoing process within a primary care medical home model. For all these reasons, there is movement toward integrating the treatment of addictions within a larger spectrum of health and social services (Compton, Blanco, & Wargo, 2015). In 2010, the U.S. Congress made addiction treatment an expected and fully reimbursable service within U.S. health care, which had already been the norm in Canada and Europe (Humphreys & Frank, 2014).

By the time people are willing to accept specialist addiction treatment or are compelled to do so, their problems have often reached a severe level. Typically they have already been seen repeatedly in health care, mental health, social service, and/or legal and correctional systems for conditions directly or indirectly related to their substance use. Yet their addiction problems were either unrecognized or not effectively addressed. It is clearly possible to identify and treat addiction problems in more general practice settings, and it may even be easier to do so because people tend to turn up in health care and social services at earlier stages of problem development, long before they may accept referral to specialist addiction treatment.

Perhaps the most persuasive reason for addressing addictions, however, is the one that attracted and has held the three of us in this field over the decades: *addictions are highly treatable,* and a range of effective methods are available. When people with addictions recover they *really* get better! You don't need subtle psychological measures to see the change. They look better. They feel better. Their family and social functioning tend to improve. They are healthier and

> Aware of it or not, most health and social service professionals are already treating the sequelae of addictions without directly addressing a significant source of the problems.

happier. They fare better at work, school, and play. And, contrary to public impressions, most people *do* recover. The mistaken impression that addictions are untreatable has been a source of the shunning, negative attitudes toward, and discrimination against, people with SUDs (McGinty, Goldman, Pescosolido, & Barry, 2015). We have quipped that if you must have a chronic illness, addiction would be a good choice because it is so treatable! With the menu of effective methods now available it is rewarding indeed to treat addictions in practice.

Why *Not* Treat Addictions?

So why, then, have so many professionals chosen not to address this very common, life-threatening, and highly treatable class of disorders that are so intertwined with other problems? The answer lies, in part, in several misconceptions.

First, some practitioners believe treating addictions requires a mysterious and highly specialized expertise that is entirely separate from their own. In fact, as will become clear in the chapters that follow, the psychosocial

---

BOX 1.1. Personal Reflection: Why Addictions?

What draws people into the field of addiction treatment? Often it is firsthand experience, and that was certainly the case for me. I departed for college at the same time my younger sister entered an inpatient substance abuse treatment program. The anxious feeling of being on my own for the first time was compounded by the heartache of knowing that my sister was also living away from home and struggling to overcome addiction. When I visited her a few months into treatment, I saw in her a profoundly changed life: her values had shifted and she had found peace with herself.

But *how* did she change, I wondered? When I asked my sister this question, she shrugged and responded that it was hard to explain—something just happened. No one, including my sister, seemed overly concerned with exploring this question, with understanding why. They were content to simply appreciate the results of this change. But I remained curious: What had caused this significant and sudden change that allowed her to overcome addiction?

In my clinical work now, as I hear each client's story and watch changes occur throughout our work together, I continue to wonder how it is that people change. How can I work with people most effectively to help them enact and maintain change? Why is it that some clients like my sister do change profoundly, while others do not, at least during the time in which our lives intersect? It's a privilege to be a companion and witness to such important life changes, and fascinating to continue pondering questions like these along the way.

—A. A. F.

treatment methods with strongest evidence of efficacy are often familiar to behavioral health professionals who treat other disorders, and are commonly part of the ordinary training and practice of many professionals: person-centered listening skills, behavior therapies, relationship counseling, good case management, and motivational interviewing. Effective medications are now available to aid in treatment and long-term management of these chronic conditions. The major professional health disciplines have already contributed and will continue to add much in understanding and treating addiction. To be sure, there are some facts and particular skills that you need to know when addressing SUDs. Providing that background is a primary purpose of this book.

A second challenge is time. Counselors and psychotherapists may have 50-minute hours, but health care appointments are often much briefer, with many other tasks to be accomplished. Those who work in contexts like primary health care, family medicine, and dentistry may understandably see SUDs as "not my job"—falling outside the realm of possibility within time constraints. Yet many other complex chronic conditions are followed and treated within the scope of routine care, and it's possible to do what you can within the time that you have available. Medical professionals may have only a few minutes to address substance use concerns, but it is clear that even this amount of time when used well can make a difference (see Chapter 9). Similarly, those who work in mental health or probation services have other issues to address and may view addictions as beyond their professional responsibility or expertise, but alcohol/drug problems are closely intertwined with mental health and correctional concerns.

A third possible obstacle is the misconception that in order to be effective in treating addictions, one must be in recovery oneself. This is not an expectation in any other area of health care. Although a substantial minority of professionals who treat addictions are themselves in recovery, ample evidence indicates that therapeutic effectiveness is simply unrelated to one's own history of addiction. Those who are in recovery are neither more nor less effective than other professionals in treating addictions, even when delivering 12-step-related treatments (Project MATCH Research Group, 1998e). Rather, effectiveness is related to aspects of counseling style (see Chapter 4).

Then there is, for some, a social stigma associated with addictive disorders, sometimes linked to pessimism about the possibility of change (Schomerus, Corrigan, et al., 2011; Schomerus, Lucht, et al., 2011). This stigma was exacerbated by pejorative writings in the mid-20th century suggesting that people with addictions are pathological liars, sociopaths, "in denial," and highly defended by chronic immature defense mechanisms. One could judge that these disorders are self-inflicted by behavior, but that is also true of many other health problems. In truth, people with SUDs represent a full spectrum of personality, socioeconomic status, intelligence, and character. Research provides no support for the belief that these individuals differ from others in overusing certain defenses, and they surely have no corner on dishonesty. One reason we, the authors, have remained in this field is that we have genuinely enjoyed working with people who are struggling with addictions, and also working with their loved ones. It is rewarding, lifesaving work.

A Continuum of Care

No disease is overcome merely by treating those already suffering from it. Yet care for SUDs has often been limited to identifying and treating those who are the most severely affected. A reservation that we share regarding a "brain disease" model of addiction is that it tends to focus on diseased individuals rather than on the environmental and social influences that can have such large impact on addiction problems (Gartner, Carter, & Partridge, 2012; Heather et al., 2018). Health care for other chronic life-threatening conditions like diabetes, hypertension, and heart disease normally includes universal and selective prevention as well as acute care, addressing the full spectrum of severity. Selective prevention moves upstream a bit to work with people who are particularly at risk of developing problems. A health care example is the identification of "prediabetes" metabolic syndrome, finding people who are likely to develop diabetes within a few years to help them make life changes early before the disease emerges fully or results in organ damage. Universal prevention addresses a whole population in hopes of reducing prevalence.

SUDs are widespread but they are not randomly distributed. Some people are at much higher risk than others. It is abundantly clear, for example, that biological relatives of people with SUDs are at higher risk themselves.

> No disease is overcome merely by treating those already suffering from it.

This is true even when children are adopted at birth and did not know their biological parents. No one or two genes explain hereditary transmission; instead a range of genes contribute to risk and protective factors (Dick & Foroud, 2003). One well-established heritable risk factor for alcohol dependence is tolerance: a relative insensitivity to alcohol, the ability to "hold your liquor" without feeling or appearing to be as affected as others are (Joslyn, Ravindranathan, Busch, Schuckit, & White, 2010; Schuckit & Smith, 2010). There are also particular populations at high risk. A good example is offenders with a history of SUDs who are being released from prison. Release is a key transition point where suddenly restored freedom invites a return to substance use, with increased risk of drug-related death (Merrall et al., 2010), in part due to reduced tolerance and inadvertent overdose.

As with diabetes and other chronic illnesses, different treatment goals and methods are effective for people at different points along the severity continuum (Kiefer, Jimenez-Arriero, Klein, Diehl, & Rubio, 2007). Educational strategies that can be effective in universal prevention of tobacco and alcohol use may be ineffective once nicotine or alcohol dependence is established. One universal prevention strategy has been developmental: to delay the onset of alcohol, tobacco, and other drug use. People who do not begin drinking, smoking, or using illicit drugs before the age of 18 are much less likely to develop disorders related to these drugs. As an example of selective prevention, consider that about 20% of men and 10% of women in the United States drink more than the National Institute on Alcohol Abuse and Alcoholism (NIAAA) recommended limits, placing them at risk for adverse health or other consequences. Helping heavy drinkers to moderate their alcohol use is now recommended as standard practice in health care (National Institute on Alcohol Abuse and Alcoholism, 2005).

To encourage a continuum of care we will describe science and practices appropriate at various levels of problem development. Because SUDs occur all along a continuum of severity it would be ideal to find and intervene with people who are toward the lower end of the spectrum. An important reason for early intervention is to prevent the tragic consequences of heavy drinking or other drug use that require only a single occasion of intoxication, well before dependence sets in (Hingson, Heeren, Winter, & Wechsler, 2005). Even very low blood alcohol levels increase the risk of severe and fatal vehicle crashes (Phillips & Brewer, 2011). SUDs are involved in a substantial proportion if not a majority of deaths from drowning, falls, fire, hypothermia, firearms, cancer, stroke, traumatic injury, suicide, vehicular crashes, pedestrian fatalities, and of course overdose (Laslett, Dietze, Matthews, & Clemens, 2004; Stinson & DeBakey, 1992). Alcohol and other drug-related incidents constitute the leading cause of death before the age of 40. Beyond mortality, intoxication increases incidents of poor judgment that can have lifelong consequences, including injury-related disability, sexually transmitted infections such as HIV, illicit drug use, marital infidelity, child abuse, sexual assault and other violence, felonies, and fetal alcohol effects. Early intervention can shorten the window of vulnerability to such tragedies.

> Alcohol and other drug-related incidents are the leading cause of death before the age of 40.

An Integrative Approach

The approach we describe in this book is integrative in at least four ways. As the chapters to follow reveal, this approach is (1) comprehensive and evidence-based, (2) multidisciplinary, (3) holistic, and (4) collaborative.

Comprehensive and Evidence-Based

Our integrated approach is first of all grounded in clinical science. Professional and public opinions abound regarding addictions. Such opinions, including our own, have often proved inaccurate when carefully examined in well-designed scientific research. In this book we have sought as much as possible to differentiate opinion from science and have given primary emphasis to the substantial base of scientific evidence that is now available to guide practice.

The approach we describe is also comprehensive in that it places treatment within a larger context of scientific knowledge about the nature of addictions, motivation for change, assessment and diagnosis, mutual help groups, case management, and prevention (Miller & Carroll, 2006). We address the full spectrum of addiction treatment, from crucial aspects of the first contact to long-term maintenance, as befits the management of a complex and often chronic condition.

Multidisciplinary

Second, we draw upon a range of professional perspectives including those from counseling and family therapy, medicine and nursing, pastoral care, psychology, and social work. In an ideal world, treatment might be delivered by a collaborative team of professionals representing these differing areas of professional expertise. In reality, treatment often relies upon a single or primary therapist whose role includes providing or serving as liaison with this range of services.

Holistic

Third, we seek in our integrated approach to consider the whole person: biological, psychological, social, and spiritual. Some think that going to a specialist for treatment of addiction is like going to a dentist for care of one's teeth. Yet addictions involve and affect the whole person and those around him or her. They are biological *and* psychological *and* social *and* spiritual. By nature of disciplinary training you may be prepared to deal best with one of these dimensions. Those who treat addictions, however, will meet all of these aspects of the person.

Collaborative

Finally, we advocate the integration and coordination of addiction care with the broader range of health and social services, a trend that has already begun. Sequestering addiction treatment in isolated programs has tended to sustain stigma and discourage treatment. As previously mentioned, we favor involving a broad range of professionals in direct care for people with SUDs. In truth, most health and social service professionals are already seeing people with addiction problems, though they may be unaware of it or regard such problems as someone else's concern. In complex disorders like addictions, where attention is needed in so many spheres, care can begin in almost any area.

Taken together, the chapters of this book represent pieces of a puzzle, the building blocks of an integrative approach to addiction treatment. They describe a system of care that is comprehensive, evidence-based, multidisciplinary, holistic, and collaborative. That's a tall order for us in writing this book, and also for you in practice. Taking the attitude of "My way or the highway" and offering only one brand of treatment is a lot simpler but does a disservice to clients in failing to use the vast amount that has been learned about how to help people with addictions. An integrative approach is a challenging goal, a direction in which you can keep growing throughout your professional career. That has certainly been our ongoing experience, and we are grateful for this opportunity to pass on, for your consideration, what we have learned along the way.

KEY POINTS

🔖 SUDs are prevalent in the general population, and even more so among people seen in health care, social service, and correctional settings.

🔖 Early intervention is possible in the context of ongoing care and can prevent the development of more severe problems and consequences.

🔖 SUDs are highly treatable. A majority of affected people do recover.

🔖 An encouraging menu of effective evidence-based treatment methods is available, no one of which is best for everyone with addiction problems.

🔖 People with SUDs commonly have other significant psychological, medical, and social problems, and coordinated treatment of these problems is best.

🔖 Treating addictions should be a normal part of general health care and social service systems and not be limited to specialist programs.

Reflection Questions

Q Of the people you normally serve (or anticipate serving), what percentage would you estimate have alcohol, tobacco, or other SUDs?

Q What most encourages or motivates you to work with people whose lives are affected by addiction and with their family members?

Q In your community, where are people with alcohol/drug problems most likely to turn up seeking help or services? (Hint: It's not in addiction treatment programs.)

CHAPTER 2

What Is Addiction?

Just about everyone has some notion of what addiction is. In most popular conceptions there are three defining aspects that constitute an addiction, whether to a drug or to compulsive behaviors like buying or Internet gaming (Baggio et al., 2016; Maraz et al., 2016):

1. Is it something done regularly, repeatedly, and habitually?
2. Is there a compulsive quality to it that seems at least partly beyond the individual's volitional control?
3. Does it persist despite potential or actual adverse consequences?

In everyday speech, people are said to be "addicted" when they relentlessly pursue any sensation or activity, be it sex, gambling, alcohol or other drugs, work, food, shopping, or love. Peele (2000) argued that the concept of "addiction" has expanded to describe so many behaviors that it has almost lost its meaning. Something becomes an addiction when it increasingly dominates a person's life and, as a result, harms or detracts from other aspects of life. In this broad colloquial sense, addiction is not unusual.

For purposes of science and health care, however, a more precise meaning is needed. This meaning is usually expressed in the form of a *diagnosis* that is defined by a particular pattern of signs and symptoms. Diagnostic criteria are typically developed by consensus within a professional organization such as the World Health Organization, which is responsible for the *International Classification of Diseases* (ICD). The American Psychiatric Association's *Diagnostic and Statistical Manual of Mental Disorders* (DSM), published for more than half a century, has been a standard for classification by behavioral health professionals in North America. The DSM is revised every decade or so, which means that the names and criteria for diagnosing addictions have evolved over time with some very significant changes.

Understanding Diagnoses

A formal classification system such as the ICD or the DSM is a way to help health professionals mean the same thing when making diagnoses. It is a bit like a biological taxonomy of life forms classified by genus and species. Such classification systems tend to become larger and more complex over time as new species and subspecies are recognized, and this has certainly been the case with the DSM. What was once a single diagnosis of "alcoholism" or "drug addiction" has been differentiated into dozens of more specific categories.

It is also true that formal diagnoses often differ from popular conceptions. For example, schizophrenia is often mistakenly associated with a "split personality." When most people think of depression, they envision someone who is sad. One might imagine a forlorn woman in a housecoat, bent over on the couch with shoulders hunched and her head in her hands. These are the images used in television programming and commercials for prescription medications. Actual clinical presentations often vary widely and can depart substantially from popular stereotypes. For instance, sadness is only one possible dimension that can be present or absent with a diagnosis of depression. Popular conceptions of schizophrenia focus on positive symptoms such as hallucinations and delusions rather than on negative symptoms such as catatonic behavior and flat affect. Part of the skill of a behavioral health diagnostician is recognizing the variability as well as the commonality of individual clinical pictures.

The same is true with addiction, which involves multiple dimensions that are variously present or absent in individuals. Popular conceptions often focus on certain manifestations. Regarding an alcoholic, one might imagine a disheveled man slumped on a sidewalk, surrounded by cans and bottles, having lost his family, job, and home. Such stereotypes envision more severe levels of use and consequences.

Addiction is not currently a diagnosis in itself. For professional purposes within this book, we use *addiction* as the most generic term for SUDs as well as other addictive behaviors, encompassing a broad range of severity. *Addiction* is the title of the oldest scientific journal of this field (founded in 1884) which now covers a range of interrelated clinical problems (Edwards, 2006). As an umbrella concept, addiction encompasses a wide variety of individual presentations such as the following actual cases:

- A 37-year-old man who drinks heavily enough most nights to still be legally intoxicated the next morning, and whose wife is threatening to leave him because of his drinking, but who appears to be in good physical health, has a good job, and has never suffered obvious negative social consequences.
- A skeletal 22-year-old who steals and trades sex to support a daily habit of injecting methamphetamine.
- A successful businesswoman who began taking her daughter's prescribed methylphenidate periodically as a way to be alert and accomplish more during the day, then started needing higher doses, buying stimulants illegally and using them more regularly.
- A college student who drinks 8–12 beers three or four nights a week to feel "buzzed" and has a drink the next morning to calm his nerves.
- A 50-year-old woman who goes to the casino daily to play the quarter slot machines for 6 hours while her husband is at work, and has built up $40,000 in credit card debt.
- A single parent who smokes two packs of cigarettes daily and has unsuccessfully tried several times to quit.

In short, people with addiction look and act in many different ways.

This is one reason why questionnaires that purport to detect the presence or absence of addiction are problematic. Such "dipstick" tests were once popular, an easy list of questions that would yield a yes or no verdict as to whether the person had "a problem." Brief screening questions are useful to indicate whether more evaluation is called for, but do not themselves make a diagnosis (see Chapter 5). For now, we focus on how to think more broadly about addiction and its causes.

Seven Dimensions of Addiction

There are at least seven dimensions of addiction that, though interrelated, are also surprisingly independent of each other. All of them occur along a continuum, and knowing where an individual is on one particular dimension does not reliably tell you his or her location on the others. This is one reason why definitions and diagnostic criteria for addiction are so challenging.

Substance Use

A first dimension to consider is the extent and pattern of the person's use of psychoactive substances. This is most often described in terms of quantity (how much?), frequency (how often?), and variability (steady vs. periodic patterns of use). Other addictive behaviors such as gambling can be measured along similar dimensions.

Problems

Just knowing how much a person is using does not in itself tell you about its effects on the person's life (though there certainly is a relationship). A second dimension to consider is the extent to which substance use or other addictive behavior has resulted in adverse consequences for the individual and those around him or her. The term "problem drinking" historically refers to using alcohol in a way that causes negative psychosocial consequences (Cahalan, 1970). These might include, for example, problems in work, school, family and other relationships, mood, finances, and legal problems. What kinds of consequences is the person experiencing? In what areas specifically?

Physical Adaptation

One characteristic of many psychoactive drugs is that the body adapts as a person uses them. One such adaptation is drug *tolerance:* a reduction in the effect of a particular dose of the drug. Over time a person may require increasingly larger doses to experience the same high as before or even to feel "normal" (*chronic tolerance*). Having even one drink diminishes the additive impact of the next one (*acute tolerance*). Another way in which the body adapts over time is *physiological dependence.* With some drugs, the body gradually becomes accustomed to their presence and adjusts normal functioning accordingly. Then when the drug is withdrawn, there is a physical rebound effect that is usually unpleasant, and opposite to the effects of intoxication. Alcohol intoxication depresses many physical functions, whereas alcohol withdrawal involves heightened arousal and sensitivity to stimuli (ranging in intensity from a hangover to severe and life-threatening withdrawal syndrome). Conversely, stimulant intoxication increases physical arousal whereas withdrawal from stimulants involves a depressing rebound.

Behavioral Dependence

Physical adaptation to a drug is not the only form of dependence. A more general pattern of behavioral dependence is that the drug gradually assumes a more central place in the person's life, displacing other activities, relationships, and social roles that once had greater priority (American Psychiatric Association, 2000; Edwards & Gross, 1976). Increasing amounts of the person's time, energy, and resources are devoted to obtaining, using, and recovering from the effects of the drug. People can also come to rely on a drug for certain coping functions. If the use of a drug is the only or

> Physical adaptation to a drug is not the only form of dependence.

primary way that someone has to cope with a particular feeling or situation, the person is psychologically dependent on the drug for that purpose.

Cognitive Impairment

Psychoactive drugs can also have acute (temporary) or chronic (long-term) effects on cognitive functioning, adaptive abilities, and intelligence. Depressant drugs (like alcohol, tranquilizers, and sedatives) can impair memory, attention, reaction time, and learning abilities during the period of intoxication. This is an important reason why driving under the influence is illegal. With long-term use, alcohol and certain other psychoactive drugs can also produce chronic, even irreversible, mental impairment.

Medical Harm

Many psychoactive drugs also have the potential to damage physical health. Some harm is due to the *acute* effects of intoxication such as risk taking, aggression, and overdose. Other forms of medical harm are related to *chronic* use. There are well-documented links of smoking to heart disease and cancer. Heavy drinking is associated with increased rates of various cancers, heart disease, and damage to the liver and other organ systems. Substance use can also damage health indirectly by diminishing normal self-care, displacing nutrition, and compromising the management of chronic conditions such as diabetes.

Motivation for Change

Finally, motivation for change is commonly recognized as an important dimension of addiction and recovery. Reluctance to recognize the need for change and take action is a common problem in addiction. Historically, it was believed that a person with addiction had to "hit bottom" and experience sufficient suffering before being ready to change, but there are now many tools to help enhance motivation for change much earlier (see Chapter 10).

Each of these, then, is a dimension along which individuals vary. Particular people with diagnosable SUDs can show almost any combination, with different levels of severity across these dimensions. A thorough understanding of a person's addiction, then, would determine the person's current position on each of these dimensions (see Box 2.1).

Studying addiction is in a way like the fabled blind men encountering an elephant. One touches the trunk and concludes that an elephant is like a firehose. Another touching the elephant's side says that it is like a wall. One who holds the tail finds elephants to be like snakes. Another hugs a leg and

BOX 2.1. Applying Your Knowledge: Thinking about the Different Dimensions of Addiction

In the preceding section, we described seven different dimensions of addiction. Consider the following case example and think about where this person might fall on each of the seven dimensions:

Oliver is a 28-year-old male who comes in to your clinic because he tested positive for cocaine on a random drug test at work and is required by his employer to get drug counseling. He reported using cocaine twice in the past 12 months, both times while at parties with old college buddies. He reported that he snorted one line on both occasions and woke up the next morning without any apparent effects of withdrawal. He is a marathon runner and is training for a triathlon, with a "clean bill of health" from his primary care physician. When asked about some of the not so good things about using cocaine, he reported concern about possibly losing his job as a result of this positive drug test and some fears about what cocaine use might do to his body, specifically how it might impact his marathon time. Oliver told you, "I'm done with using cocaine. I won't ever be using it again. This event made me realize that I need to grow up and start acting my age. I'm not some dumb college kid any more, and I want to be successful in my career and continue to improve my times in order to qualify to run in the Boston marathon. I know cocaine isn't going to help me do either of those things."

Where would you say Oliver is on each of the seven dimensions, given what you know so far? What else would you want to know?

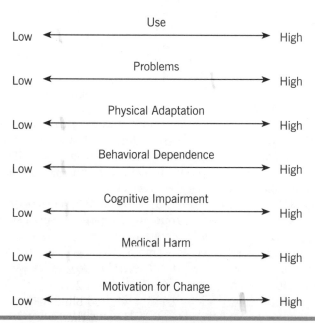

reports that an elephant is much like a tree. An elephant is none of these and all of these. A complete understanding requires combining different perspectives; any one part reveals only a little about other aspects or about the whole elephant.

History of the Diagnostic Conceptions

Technically speaking, there was no alcoholism prior to 1849. That is when the Swedish physician Magnus Huss coined the term "alcoholism" to describe the adverse consequences of excessive drinking (Sournia, 1990). There was drunkenness, inebriety, and intemperance, but no alcoholism. Since then, society has struggled to define what constitutes addiction and to puzzle over its causes.

The history of diagnoses in the DSM illustrates the evolving concept of addiction. Each DSM has offered criteria for deciding whether specific diagnoses fit a particular person's case. The diagnostic decision is binary—present or absent—even though reality may be more of a continuum. To make a yes/no diagnostic decision, then, often means drawing a somewhat arbitrary cutoff point along a continuum of severity. In the DSM this is typically done according to the number of symptoms present.

In the early 1950s, the first edition of the DSM grouped both *alcoholism* and *drug addiction* with sociopathic personality disturbances, indicating that people with addiction suffered from "deep-seated personality disturbance" (DSM-I; American Psychiatric Association, 1952, p. 34). The sociopathic personality category also included sexual deviations and antisocial behavior, suggesting that individuals with addiction were a threat to the societal order. Unlike the detailed lists of criteria that are used to classify disorders today, the first edition contained only a brief paragraph that focused almost entirely on the presumed nature of the disorder. According to DSM-I, addiction was likely a symptom of an underlying brain or personality disorder and was a clear departure from culturally acceptable behavior. The signs and symptoms displayed by someone with an addiction to drugs or alcohol were not clearly described.

In the second edition (DSM-II; American Psychiatric Association, 1968), several new terms were proposed as types of alcoholism, including "episodic excessive drinking," "habitual excessive drinking," and "alcohol addiction." This reflected conceptions from a classic book by E. M. Jellinek (1960), *The Disease Concept of Alcoholism,* that used "alcoholism" as a broad and generic term for alcohol-related disorders (as Magnus Huss had done previously), and hypothesized various subtypes. Similarly, *drug dependence* was expanded in DSM-II to include subcategories by specific drug class. Physiological signs of dependence, such as withdrawal and tolerance, were described as signs and symptoms of these conditions. As in

---

BOX 2.2. Is There an Addictive Personality?

In the mid-20th century it was believed that people with substance use disorders had a particular predisposing personality, with high levels of immature defense mechanisms such as denial. Treatment programs were designed to confront and "break down" these pathological defenses that were seen as a primary cause of addiction. Yet decades of research have revealed few commonalities in the personality of people with addiction problems. People with substance use disorders vary widely on other dimensions, and when their defenses have been measured specifically they appear no different from other people (e.g., Donovan, Hague, & O'Leary, 1975). In other words, many different kinds of people succumb to addiction. There are some developmental factors related to risk of subsequent addiction—difficult temperament, childhood conflicts with the law and authorities, and impaired self-control—but there is no characteristic abnormal personality or defensive structure.

So if people do not walk through the door of addiction treatment programs all with the same personality, what caused counselors to perceive their clients as being in *denial*? Often it came down to disagreement with the counselor over a diagnosis or label, and the client showing (from the counselor's perspective) insufficient distress, acceptance of help, compliance with particular treatment prescriptions, and change—factors that also tend to get clients labeled as "unmotivated." Conversely, treatment providers tended to perceive clients as "motivated" when they agreed with the provider, accepted the provider's diagnosis or label, expressed a desire for help, showed appropriate distress, voiced a need for the provider's assistance, complied with treatment prescriptions, and succeeded in changing. Clients' resistance and defensiveness, which often were attributed to their difficult personalities, are highly responsive to counseling style (see Chapters 10 and 19). A suspicious, authoritarian, confrontational style substantially increases resistance and defensiveness, not only in people with addictions but in most human beings. This creates a self-fulfilling prophecy, with clients who are initially ambivalent digging in their heels and becoming adamant about *not* changing. In contrast, a respectful, listening, and compassionate therapeutic style (see Chapter 4) tends to reduce resistance and promote change.

DSM-I, however, these disorders remained as subcategories of "personality disorders and certain other nonpsychotic mental disorders." The placement of these conditions implied once again that addiction represented a disorder of the personality that caused the individual to use alcohol or other drugs excessively.

During the 1970s, clinical research indicated a need to further differentiate SUDs. The *Feighner criteria* (Feighner et al., 1972) were developed in an effort to diagnose alcoholism on research-based decision rules. This trend toward differential diagnosis was reflected in the third edition of the DSM (DSM-III; American Psychiatric Association, 1980). DSM-III was the first to describe substance abuse and dependence as separate pathological conditions. This differentiation was based, in part, on findings from longitudinal research indicating that many people with a history of alcohol problems never progressed to dependence (Cahalan, 1970; Hasin, Grant, & Endicott, 1990), suggesting the possibility of two separate disorders. As of DSM-III, "alcoholism" was no longer a formal diagnosis. Another significant change in DSM-III was the creation of a separate category for SUDs, removing the prior implication that they represented underlying personality disorders.

DSM-III more generally avoided tying disorders to specific etiologies. With regard to addiction, DSM-III suggested that social and cultural factors were important contributors to the onset and continuation of abuse and dependence. This suggestion further underlined the shift away from thinking of addiction as personality pathology, toward something more akin to a public health model that included environmental factors. *Substance abuse* was defined as problematic use with social or occupational impairment, but with the absence of significant tolerance and/or withdrawal. The DSM-III definition of *substance dependence* emphasized the physiological symptoms of tolerance (needing to take much higher doses of the substance to obtain the same effect) and withdrawal (having a distinct pattern of physiological changes after stopping or reducing use), and required the presence of one or both of these criteria in order to make a dependence diagnosis. In both disorders, impairment in social and occupational function was a prominent aspect of the definitions, creating a significant overlap between the criteria for substance abuse and dependence. In essence, "abuse" was the presence of drug-related problems in the absence of a history of significant physiological adaptation.

Meanwhile, a changing conception of substance dependence was already emerging, a shift away from strictly physiological symptoms toward a broader behavioral syndrome. This shift was strongly influenced by the work of Griffith Edwards (1986; Edwards & Gross, 1976; Marshall, 2015) who conceptualized alcohol dependence as a cluster of interrelated behavioral, psychological, and physiological elements, all varying in severity. Common elements of the dependence syndrome included a narrowing of the drinking repertoire (increasingly patterned and predictable), drink-seeking behavior, tolerance, withdrawal, drinking to relieve or avoid withdrawal symptoms, subjective awareness of the compulsion to drink, and a return to drinking after a period of abstinence. Also contributing to a shift toward emphasis on behavioral aspects of dependence was classic work showing that laboratory animals can be taught to self-administer psychoactive drugs (Brady & Lucas, 1984). Once animals learned to self-administer an addictive substance, most would expend enormous amounts of time and effort to obtain additional doses. This drug-seeking behavior also proved difficult to extinguish, particularly when the administered substance was one with high misuse liability in humans (such as stimulants or opiates).

In 1987, DSM-III was revised (DSM-III-R; American Psychiatric Association, 1987) in a way that gave the behavioral aspects of SUDs equal weight to the physiological components. The DSM-III-R category of *psychoactive substance abuse* was defined as a pattern of use that continues despite knowledge of adverse consequences or by use in situations in which it is physically dangerous. As before, the "abuse" diagnosis was a residual category for people who had never met criteria for dependence. DSM-IV (American Psychiatric Association, 1994) largely continued the definitions of DSM-III, now defining over a hundred different substance-related disorders for 12 different classes of drugs (see Chapter 3). In addition to abuse and dependence, there were diagnoses for drug-related intoxication, withdrawal, delirium, dementia, amnestic disorder, psychotic disorders, mood disorders, anxiety disorders, sexual dysfunction, and sleep disorders. Unlike its predecessors, DSM-IV clearly separated the criteria for dependence from those of abuse. Dependence in DSM-IV was a syndrome involving compulsive use, *with or without* tolerance and withdrawal. *Abuse* was defined as problematic use without compulsive use, tolerance, or withdrawal. A transitional text revision (American Psychiatric Association, 2000) defined substance abuse as meeting any one of four criteria revolving around recurrent problems related to the substance, and dependence as meeting three or more of seven physiological or behavioral criteria. This created a problem of "diagnostic orphans" who, for example, evidenced none of the criteria for abuse and only one or two symptoms in the dependence category.

Underlying these various attempts to differentiate "abuse" from "dependence" was a fundamental problem: Factor analyses showed that the abuse and dependence criteria actually load on a single factor and are interrelated with each other (Martin, Chung, & Langenbucher, 2008; Mewton, Slade, McBride, Grove, & Teesson, 2011). In other words, there was no empirical reason for classifying these as separate disorders. What had been called "abuse" is neither separate from nor necessarily antecedent to "dependence." Attempts to separate these two labels may, in part, have been a vestige of the desire to distinguish "real" alcoholism from problem drinking, despite long-recognized limitations of a binary approach (Jellinek, 1960; Miller, 1986).

The fifth edition of the DSM (DSM-5; American Psychiatric Association, 2013) remedied this problem by removing the distinction between substance abuse and dependence in favor of a single diagnosis of SUD with categories of severity (e.g., mild, moderate, and severe), consistent with the assessment approach described earlier in this chapter. Furthermore, terminology such as "abuse" and "abusers" have always been moralistic and stigmatizing in tone (Broyles et al., 2014; Kelly & Westerhoff, 2010) and we concur with editors who now proscribe the use of such terms. (A wry colleague once quipped that "alcohol abuse" is mixing a single-malt Scotch with root beer!) DSM-5 better represents the actual continuum of severity and removed the implication that those with more severe problems are somehow qualitatively different. It also eliminated the problem of "diagnostic orphans" who did not meet the criteria for prior categories yet still had significant problems related to substance use.

Where Is the Line for Addiction?

Historically, diagnosis has focused on a binary, black-or-white decision: Does the person "have" a particular condition or not? With some conditions it's important to know that. Presence or absence matters with regard to pregnancy or HIV. Many other conditions like diabetes and hypertension, however, involve shades of gray, a gradual continuum of severity, and addiction is one of those. How much is too much? When has a person who drinks or uses other drugs crossed "over the line" to addiction? As illustrated by the evolving DSM, the answers change over time.

The idea that there is a black-or-white line has itself been a source of problems in personal and social response to substance use. At the time of DSM-II, the prevailing belief was that alcoholism was a binary, present-or-absent condition, like pregnancy. One could not be "a little" alcoholic—either you were or you weren't. In this view, alcoholics were constitutionally incapable of handling alcohol and qualitatively different from normal people who could drink with impunity. It thus became a source of significant argument whether a particular person was or wasn't alcoholic. In the common situation where a professional (or relative) diagnosed someone as being over the line, a person who disavowed the diagnosis was then said to be "in denial" (Carr, 2011). Because alcoholism was at that time believed to be a personality disorder, and denial a characteristic defense mechanism of the disorder, this often was seen as confirming the diagnosis. A complementary belief was that only alcoholics had problems with alcohol, a view that discouraged social controls on alcohol or caution in its use by those presumed to be nonalcoholics. Within this perspective, the main approach to prevention would be to identify and educate those unfortunates who have the condition.

The recognition of addiction as a continuum has led to a different approach. Certainly, people with severe dependence deserve humane and effective care. It is also clear that alcohol is a hazardous substance that warrants special social controls (Babor et al., 2010). A majority of those who are harmed or endangered by alcohol use are not dependent drinkers (Institute of Medicine, 1990). Arguing about whether a person is on one side or the other of a diagnostic line misses the point. We find that it is common

> The idea that there is a black-or-white line has itself been a source of problems in personal and social response to substance use.

for clients to balk at a diagnostic label or the idea of "having a problem." Yet if we ask them to tell us about ways in which alcohol or other drugs have caused hassles or harm, there is usually a list and sometimes a long one. The more important issue is to understand how substance use is affecting people's lives, and what (if anything) they need or want to do about it.

How different are individuals diagnosed with mild, moderate, or severe SUD? After all, the cutpoints for these categories in DSM-5 are somewhat arbitrary. Those diagnosed with mild or moderate alcohol use disorder are not very different from each other, and both differ from those diagnosed with severe alcohol use disorder (Rinker & Neighbors, 2015; Suitt, Castro, Caetano, & Field, 2015). As with chronic illnesses in general, people with greater severity may need a higher level of care (see Chapter 7). Likewise, those with less severity may benefit from a different kind of care.

One clear current reflection of this continuum understanding of addiction is the recommendation of "low-risk drinking limits" by the World Health Organization, the NIAAA, and other bodies. Working from epidemiological data, such guidelines inform people about levels of consumption that are linked to increased risk of illness and injury. Regardless of diagnosis, there are levels of alcohol use that are simply risky in terms of short- and long-term health consequences. In a "Rethinking Drinking" website, the NIAAA defined heavy or at-risk drinking as consuming more than four drinks on any day or 14 drinks per week for men, or more than three drinks on any day or seven drinks per week for women (*rethinkingdrinking.niaaa.nih.gov* as of May 2019).

This change in thinking toward a continuum of severity is also occurring in general medicine with regard to chronic illnesses like diabetes, heart disease, and asthma. The arbitrary cutoff points for "normal" versus "elevated" blood pressure, glucose, or cholesterol have been decreasing over the years, with earlier intervention indicated. In the past, diabetes was not treated until the patient became symptomatic. We now recognize a prediabetic metabolic syndrome, and health care professionals can intervene early prior to organ damage. For patients with identified risk factors, such as being overweight or having a family history of diabetes, the routine procedure is to regularly assess fasting glucose or HbA1c levels and encourage lifestyle changes to prevent the development of diabetes.

The idea of intervening prior to someone developing more severe consequences also parallels trends in mental health. For example, there are good reasons to prevent a *first* occurrence of depression. Once a person experiences one episode of major depression, there is an increased likelihood of having another, suggesting the idea of biological *kindling*: the first episode makes that person more vulnerable to future episodes. This finding has increased efforts to intervene early (Muñoz, Le, Clarke, Barrera, & Torres, 2009). For those at high genetic risk of developing depression, there are effective strategies to prevent a first episode. There are also treatment guidelines based on the number of depressive episodes a person has experienced. For example, if someone has had three or more episodes, prophylactic maintenance on antidepressant medication is often recommended.

It is common in health care to use different treatment strategies depending on the level of severity. Treatment varies for hypertension, diabetes, depression, and many other medical and psychological conditions depending on where the individual is on a continuum. The parallels to addiction are straightforward. Yet addiction has often been treated as though it could be cured through acute treatment. If addiction is analogous to chronic illness, then one should not expect the problem to be resolved by an episode of treatment, and ongoing care is as important as it would be with asthma or diabetes (McLellan, Lewis, O'Brien, & Kleber, 2000).

Historically, people seldom received addiction treatment before substantial problems and dependence had developed. In the 21st century, there has been movement toward recognizing, treating, and preventing SUDs at an earlier stage, through screening and intervention within more general health and social service settings (Aldreidge, Dowd, & Bray, 2017; Aldridge, Linford, & Bray, 2017; Miller & Weisner, 2002). The efficacy of relatively brief opportunistic counseling is well documented (see Chapter 9), even with people who were not actively seeking addiction treatment and may not have been thinking about making a change in their substance use.

Another important reason for addressing addiction within primary health care, mental health, and social service settings is the high rate of co-occurrence with other health and social problems (see Chapter 20). Whether or not they know it, professionals working in such settings are likely treating people with addiction problems on a regular basis. In children and adolescents, substance use is a long-recognized common element in clusters of problem behaviors (Jessor & Jessor, 1977). In adults, addiction seldom occurs in isolation. In people with serious mental illnesses, addiction is the most frequently coexisting disorder, occurring at three times the general population rate (Substance Abuse and Mental Health Services Administration, 2009).

Remission

Another important and, at the time, controversial change made in DSM-III-R was the addition of criteria for partial or full remission from substance dependence based on 6 or more months of abstinence or reduced use without symptoms. Remission criteria have remained, and in DSM-5 people who have previously met criteria for an SUD are classified as being in sustained remission if they have met no diagnostic criteria (other than craving) for 12 months or longer. Early remission is defined as not meeting any diagnostic criteria for 3 but less than 12 months. For those with continuing symptoms, current severity is classified as mild, moderate, or severe based on the number of criteria met.

In fact, remission from SUDs is very common; a majority of people do recover within 3 years of seeking treatment (Fleury et al., 2016). In an 11-year follow-up of people with heroin dependence, 75% were in full remission and heroin-free (Teesson et al., 2015). Remission rates are also high with alcohol and cannabis use disorders, often with some continuing use (Feingold, Fox, Rehm, & Lev-Ran, 2015; Kelly, Bergman, Hoeppner, Vilsaint, & White, 2017; Miller, Walters, & Bennett, 2001).

Before moving on to consider causes of addiction, we add a practical recommendation. Don't waste time and effort arguing with people about whether they warrant a diagnostic label. Great emphasis has sometimes been placed on making clients "accept" or "admit" an identity such as "alcoholic" or "addict." There is no scientific evidence that this self-identification is a prerequisite for change. Plenty of people recover without ever accepting a diagnosis or even receiving treatment. Clearly, there are many who readily accept a diagnostic label but continue to struggle. Don't get stuck trying to impose a label. Within the original 12-step philosophy, one never imposes the label "alcoholic" on someone else; it is for each individual to decide whether this identification fits and is helpful (Alcoholics Anonymous World Services, 2001). The writings of Bill W., cofounder of Alcoholics Anonymous (AA), reflect great patience to work with people wherever they are at present (Miller & Kurtz, 1994).

> Plenty of people recover without ever accepting a diagnosis or even receiving treatment.

Etiologies of Addiction

The *etiology* of a condition is its cause or origin. We turn now to consider the etiologies of addiction, those factors that influence its onset, severity, and course. Identifying and understanding these factors is different from diagnosing addiction. Beginning with the third edition in 1980, the DSM has separated diagnosis from etiology.

So what causes addiction? Is it a failure of self-control, a result of poor choices? Can anyone become addicted? Can the blame be placed on the drugs themselves as addictive substances? Is the fault in our genes or personality, with some people more prone to addiction, in the same manner that they are predisposed to diabetes, hypertension, or depression? Should we look to the social environment for causes? To some extent, the answer to all of these questions is "Yes." There is some truth to each.

Personal Responsibility Models

In most societies, problems with alcohol and other drugs have been regarded to some extent as a failure of self-control, a violation of moral, ethical, or religious standards. Most religions have prohibitions regarding the use of certain psychoactive substances. In Jewish and Christian scriptures, for example, alcohol is not proscribed, but drinking in a way that risks or causes harm is described as sinful. The remedies suggested by a personal responsibility model include legislation, education, repentance, punishment, and social sanctions. This perspective is still very much evident in social responses to and sometimes even in treatment of addictions. Underlying these models is the general assumption that substance use is a voluntary, chosen behavior, and that the person could have done otherwise. This is exemplified in social views and practices with regard to driving under the influence. Few would accept a defense that someone just couldn't help but use drugs or drink before driving. Intoxication is rarely a defense or mitigating factor in crime. Substance use is still regarded as a choice for which one is responsible.

Some models place particular emphasis on spiritual factors. Prominent among these is the 12-step approach begun in 1935 for Alcoholics Anonymous (AA) from the experience of its cofounders Bill W. and Dr. Bob. The 12-step programs, which do not endorse any particular model of etiology, nevertheless place considerable emphasis on character flaws as a contributor to addiction. The importance of spirituality is even more central in the 12-step program for recovery. In this perspective, people are powerless to resolve addiction on their own, and the help of a higher power is essential. AA and other 12-step programs (see Chapter 17) provide recommendations for a program of spiritual awakening and personal recovery. This spiritual awakening is understood as the means to move from destructive independence to proper dependence on God and others (Kurtz, 1991). A spiritual path to recovery was also emphasized in Moral Rearmament, another international program that, like AA, had its roots in pastor Frank Buchman's Oxford Groups in the 1930s (Lean, 1985).

Agent Models

Agent models place primary emphasis on the strong effects of the agent (the drug) itself. In this view, anyone who is exposed to the drug is at risk because of its addictive and destructive properties. The U.S. temperance movement, which originally promoted caution and moderation (temperance) in the use of alcohol, evolved into a full prohibition movement, placing primary blame on the drug itself. In 1919, the 18th Amendment to the U.S. Constitution was ratified, making it illegal to manufacture, sell, transport, or import "intoxicating liquor," only to be repealed by the 21st

Amendment in 1933. To be sure, the hazardous qualities of alcohol and tobacco are well documented, and if they were to be introduced as new drugs today, knowing what we know, they would be unlikely to be legalized. An agent model was implicit in the "war on drugs" of the late 20th century. The primary remedy it implies is to rid society of the drug itself.

Dispositional Models

Dispositional models, in contrast, place the primary cause of addiction within the person. They share this emphasis with moral models, but typically construe the cause as a physical condition that is beyond the individual's willful control. Among these is a disease model that regards people with addiction to be constitutionally different from others and incapable of controlling their own use (Campbell, 1903). In part this model served as a transition from prohibition: Rather than being a drug that no one could use safely, alcohol was construed as only dangerous for *certain* people, namely alcoholics. Understandably this view that the cause lay "in the man and not the bottle" was strongly supported and funded by the alcohol industry (Babor, 2017).

A dispositional model diminishes personal responsibility for having the condition and favors humane treatment rather than punishment of addiction. Of relevance to dispositional models, various genetic risk factors have been documented that increase the likelihood of developing addiction to particular substances. Other dispositional models have emphasized changes that occur in the brain with chronic use and that compromise self-control. Most recently this has reemerged in the characterization of addiction as a "brain disease" (Volkow, Koob, & McLellan, 2016), a concept dating from the 19th century (Edwards, 2006). Although a dispositional model may absolve people of blame for their condition, the responsibility for recovery necessarily remains with the individual, who is typically counseled to accept permanent abstinence as the only sure way to prevent further progression and harm.

Social Learning Models

Other models emphasize the role of experience in shaping addiction. The use of alcohol and other psychoactive drugs is clearly responsive to both classical (stimulus–response) and operant conditioning (contingent reinforcement and punishment). Even highly dependent individuals modify their choices and use of substances in response to changes in the social environment. Drinking and drug use practices are also clearly influenced by modeling (learning by observing others), particularly from family and peers. As the psychology of learning embraced human thought processes in the late 20th century, the role of cognition in addiction was also examined.

An important factor highlighted in this research is drug *expectancies,* beliefs and expectations about the likely positive or negative effects of drug use (Brown, Christiansen, & Goldman, 1987; Goldman, Del Boca, & Darkes, 1999). Interventions from a social learning perspective focus on changing the individual's relationship to the social environment: changing patterns of reinforcement for drug use and nonuse (Chapter 14), social support, family interactions, high-risk situations, expectancies, and cognitive-behavioral coping skills (Chapter 11).

Sociocultural Models

A still broader viewpoint emphasizes the influence of societal and cultural factors. The ease of availability and the price of alcohol, tobacco, and other drugs clearly affect the level of use in a community (e.g., Azar et al., 2015). Social environments with high levels of use (such as drinking in the military or in college fraternities) tend to increase consumption in new and continuing members. Advertising and media programming also influence expectancies and perceived norms. Interventions within a sociocultural perspective typically focus on alcohol/drug policy. Examples include the licensing and regulation of sales outlets, training of alcohol servers to prevent intoxication and impaired driving, and taxation to increase the price of legal substances.

A Public Health Perspective

In seeking to prevent, treat, and contain threats to health, the most common approach is a broad one that takes into account all of the above influences. Usually called a *public health* perspective, it groups causal factors into three categories: those involving the *agent* (in this case, the drug itself), the *host* (personal characteristics of an individual), and the *environment.* In containing a flu epidemic, for example, one would consider the particular virus family that is involved (agent), personal factors that increase or decrease an individual's vulnerability to infection (host), and environmental conditions that promote or diminish spread of the disease. The history of addiction treatment has often been characterized by passionate debates about which one of these factors is most important, which model is "correct." This can lead to overinvestment in addressing one particular cause. A public health perspective takes all important factors into account and considers their interactions with each other.

The agent dimension was discussed above, focusing on characteristics of the drugs themselves. Substances have addictive properties, including rapidity of effect, tolerance, and interaction with neurotransmitter systems. The faster a drug reaches the brain, the more reinforcing its use tends to be. (Nicotine from cigarette smoking is a prime example.) Once in the brain, psychoactive drugs mimic or influence neurotransmitters (see Chapter 3). Many, for example, increase the release of dopamine, which is one of the primary neurotransmitters in the experience of pleasure. Dopamine release is one of the reasons substance use can be highly reinforcing. In some cases, dopamine release may produce greater incentive than natural reinforcers like food or sex. It is sensible, then, that drugs can be preferred over natural rewards because of this rapid and intense pleasure. It is possible to classify drugs according to their potential to produce addiction. The toxic side effects of drugs like alcohol and tobacco are well documented. Drug effects also pose particular risks in certain situations (e.g., when driving, during pregnancy). Thus, the drugs themselves deserve attention in social policy.

Much is also known about host factors in addiction, where attention is focused on characteristics of individuals that place them at risk. Propensity for addiction is related to gender, family history of addiction, age, and temperament (Substance Abuse and Mental Heath Services Administration, 2012). Ralph Tarter's construct of neurobehavioral disinhibition comprises a cluster of emotional tendencies, behavioral symptoms, and problems in cognitive function that indicate that a child has not adequately developed psychological self-regulation (Tarter et al., 2003). This construct includes many symptoms that characterize attention-deficit/hyperactivity disorder (ADHD), conduct disorder, and oppositional–defiant disorder. Escalating psychosocial problems in youth, particularly conduct problems, have long been identified as a predictor for later SUDs (Jones, 1968; Sartor, Lynskey, Heath, Jacob, & True, 2007). Temperament is, of course, itself partially inherited. It is estimated that genetic risk factors explain about 50% of the vulnerabilities leading to heavy drinking (Schuckit, 2009), though the picture is less clear for genetic predispositions to other drug addiction (Buckland, 2008).

The environmental dimension includes factors outside of the individual. The environment includes the broader community, such as the legal environment (alcoholic beverage control regulations, laws regarding driving under the influence, minimum purchase age laws, zoning), the economic environment (pricing, tax rate, promotions), and the normative environment (social attitudes and beliefs regarding substances). The environment also includes the physical aspects of the person's environment, such as the setting or context in which drinking and other drug use occurs. Another environmental influence is a person's associates, including their family, friends, coworkers, and other peers, who in turn carry ethnic, religious, and educational influences. Environmental or cultural stress levels may also influence substance use. Certain religious group affiliations may increase or decrease risk for substance use and addiction (Gorsuch, 1995).

These agent, host, and environment factors also interact with each other. A child who inherits a difficult temperament and risk for poor self-regulation may be protected by intensive parenting (Diaz & Fruhauf, 1991).

An individual who lives and works in a hard-drinking environment may be protected by religious affiliation. People differ in the inherited extent to which their brains "light up" in response to particular drugs. Explanations that focus on a single cause or model are clearly too simplistic. Effective treatment and prevention efforts consider the range of factors involved and focus on those most likely to yield benefit for the particular person or community.

KEY POINTS

🔖 Addiction occurs along a continuum of severity, or rather along at least seven continuous dimensions of use, problems, physical adaptation, behavioral dependence, cognitive impairment, medical harm, and motivation for change.

🔖 Knowing where an individual falls on one of these dimensions tells little about the rest of the clinical picture.

🔖 Diagnosis is about classification according to decision rules, which have changed markedly over time.

🔖 Remission from substance use disorders is not only possible but common. A majority of people do recover.

🔖 Explanatory models of addiction have also evolved over time, often emphasizing one causal factor to the neglect of others.

🔖 A public health view of addiction embraces host, agent, and environmental factors and their interactions, providing a more comprehensive perspective for guiding treatment and prevention.

Reflection Questions

🔍 Of the various etiological models described in this chapter, which one(s) have you most strongly emphasized in your own views of addiction? Which one(s) most closely match your current perspective?

🔍 In your own mind, when does a behavior cross the line and become an addiction?

🔍 To what extent do you think that addiction is a "brain disease"?

CHAPTER 3

How Do Drugs Work?

In Chapter 1 we explained why addiction treatment is a matter not only for specialists, but for health and social service professionals in general. The training and experience of behavioral health professionals, for example, provides a good foundation for helping people overcome SUDs and related problems (Miller & Brown, 1997). Yet even in the 21st century, the training of such professionals rarely offers sufficient background and encouragement to treat addictions. Although generalist professional training may provide 80% of the competence needed to help people with SUDs, the remaining 20% of missing information and skills are important. Lacking this preparation, clinicians may overlook addiction problems or refer them elsewhere for treatment. One of our main goals in writing this book is to fill in that remaining 20%.

One important core competence, of course, is at least a basic working knowledge of psychoactive drugs and their effects. That is the primary focus of this chapter. Let us say at the outset, however, that nonmedical practitioners need not have memorized all of the chemical and street names or understand in detail the psychopharmacology of each and every drug. Medical colleagues are available for consultation on such issues, and much of what you don't know about street savvy, your clients can teach you. Compared to clinicians, clients often have more firsthand knowledge about the drugs they use, although street information can also be dangerously inaccurate. Drug users' practical knowledge might be thought of as a disadvantage for the health professional, but it also means that clients are a constant source of learning about lives and cultures that may at first be quite alien to those who have survived the rigors of postgraduate training. We, the authors of this book, have learned much about addictions from our clients. Of course, we also constantly examine such learning, as well as our own hunches and beliefs, in the light of the best science available.

Routes of Administration

A good starting point, before considering major classes of drugs, is to understand the various and sometimes surprising routes by which people self-administer psychoactive drugs. They fall into four major categories, all of which begin with "in": (1) ingestion, (2) inhalation, (3) intranasal, and (4) injection. These do not encompass all possible routes of administration that have been devised (such as placement under the eyelid, insertion into the rectum or vagina, or absorption through the skin as by "patches"), but they do encompass over 99% of drug misuse.

Ingestion

By far the most common way to self-administer a psychoactive drug is by mouth: to eat it, drink it, chew it, swallow it, or let it dissolve under the lips or tongue. Drinking is the exclusive route for the most common problem drug: ethyl alcohol. Prescription and other drugs in pill form are swallowed. Hairspray can be sprayed into a jug of water, shaken, and allowed to settle—a preparation known as *ocean* because of its frothy appearance— that is then drunk. Teas are brewed from various substances including khat and valerian root. The original active ingredient in Coca-Cola was cocaine, from which it derived its name.

Other drugs are chewed, absorbed through the gums, or placed under the tongue in solid or liquid form. Coca leaves, khat root, tobacco, and nicotine gum can be chewed, and their active ingredients absorbed through saliva and the rich supply of blood vessels in the mouth. Some drugs can be introduced through foods that are eaten and then absorbed through the stomach, such as marijuana in brownies, alcohol-injected fruit, or rum-saturated cake.

Psychoactive drugs ingested by mouth pass into the gastrointestinal system, where they are absorbed into the bloodstream through the lining of the stomach and large intestine. Drugs in liquid form (such as alcohol) tend to be absorbed more rapidly. Absorption is usually slowed by the presence of food in the stomach, which is why drinking on an empty stomach yields faster intoxication. It can take from one to several hours to absorb most of a drug dosage taken by mouth.

Inhalation

The second most common way to administer psychoactive drugs is to inhale them as smoke or vapor, absorbing them primarily through the lungs. The lungs have a rich blood supply, and drugs that are inhaled can pass into the bloodstream within seconds. This is, of course, the usual route of administration for tobacco and marijuana. Cocaine in its usual hydrochloride salt form is destroyed by burning, but it can be reduced by various methods to a concentrated base form (such as "crack") that is smokable to deliver very high doses. Other drugs are termed *inhalants* because they are self-administered by breathing them in through the nose or mouth as a gas (such as nitrous oxide) or a vapor (such as "sniffing" glue or "huffing" gasoline).

Vaporization or "vaping" has become a popular alternative to inhaling smoke. This involves inhaling the desired active drug (such as nicotine or cannabinol) in heated water vapor that may also be flavored (Budney, Sargent, & Lee, 2015). A hope is that vaping would reduce the risk of diseases and mortality by removing exposure to carcinogenic and other toxic elements in smoke, though attendant medical risks of short- and long-term use are unknown (Villanti et al., 2018). Vaporization also reduces exposure of others to second-hand smoke. There is concern, however, that vaping may be an attractive and seemingly safer gateway for youth to experiment with flavored psychoactive drugs at a younger age, and there is already evidence of youth transitioning from vaping to cigarette smoking within a year (Watkins, Glantz, & Chaffee, 2018).

> Young people often transition from vaping to cigarette smoking within a year.

Intranasal

A third common route of administration is by snorting a drug into the nose, which also has an extremely rich supply of blood vessels in the mucous membranes. Snuff is a preparation of tobacco that can be drawn up into the nose in this manner. Snorting is a common method for self-administering ketamine and cocaine hydrochloride. Heroin is also sometimes taken intranasally.

Injection

Finally, drugs of abuse can be introduced into the body by shooting them via syringe into a vein (intravenous), muscle (intramuscular), or beneath the skin (subcutaneous). Intravenous injection is the most common route of administration for heroin and certain other opiates. It is also a popular method for taking methamphetamine, which may be combined with heroin. Intravenous injection is, of course, the most rapid method for getting a drug into the bloodstream, producing the fastest and most intense effects. It is also the most dangerous method. When used regularly for injection, veins begin to collapse. As veins in the arms become unusable, injection drug users may make use of blood vessels in the hands, feet, legs, and neck. Bacterial infections and abscesses can occur if sterile procedures are not used. The sharing of syringes by drug users is a major cause of the spread of blood-borne infections such as HIV, methicillin-resistant staphylococcus aureus (MRSA), and the various forms of hepatitis. Containing the spread of such diseases is a principal purpose of *needle exchange programs* where users can obtain new sterile syringes and safely dispose of used needles free of charge (Sawangjit, Khan, & Chaiyakunapruk, 2017). Injection is also the most common route of fatal overdoses of illicit drugs, precisely because the drug effects are so immediate, intense, and often difficult to reverse.

Drug Distribution and Elimination

The brain is the target organ for psychoactive drugs (Volkow, Koob, et al., 2016). Once a drug has been introduced, it moves through the body in more or less predictable ways (*pharmacokinetics*) until finally it is eliminated. A drug first travels from the point of entry into the bloodstream, as by absorption through membranes, unless it has already been placed directly into the circulatory system by intravenous injection. Once a drug enters the bloodstream it is circulated throughout the body within about a minute. To reach its principal site of action in the central nervous system, however, a psychoactive drug must further cross from the bloodstream through the *blood–brain barrier* and into the brain, where it interacts with nerve cells (*neurons*) to produce its effects.

Most psychoactive drugs do not circulate in the bloodstream for long. They are gradually eliminated through the body's filtering systems. They are *metabolized* (broken down) by the liver, excreted through the kidneys in urine, even expelled in air from the lungs, in sweat through the skin, or in breast milk. Drug testing makes use of this elimination process by analyzing expelled air (as in alcohol breath tests) or urine for the presence of psychoactive drugs or their metabolites.

The speed with which a given drug is eliminated from the body is usually expressed in terms of its *half-life,* which is the length of time required for the body to reduce the drug level by half. Within one half-life, the level of a drug would be reduced to 50% of its starting level. It takes two half-life periods to eliminate 75%, and after three half-life periods the amount of drug in the body would be down to about 12% of its original level. Drugs vary dramatically in their half-lives. Ethyl alcohol, for example, is cleared from the body far faster than is methyl alcohol. Methadone has a longer half-life than heroin, making it a better

> Once a drug enters the bloodstream it is circulated throughout the body within about a minute.

substitution drug because its effects are distributed across 1–2 days instead of an hour or two (for heroin). (Substitution medications are used in withdrawal management (Chapter 6) and maintenance (Chapters 18 and 21) to replace drugs that a person has been using.) Speed of elimination can also be influenced by factors including age, gender, health of the liver, interactions with other drugs, and hereditary traits.

Drug Effects

Once they reach the brain, psychoactive drugs interact with particular neural systems to produce their characteristic effects. The brain's communication system relies upon tiny electrical currents transmitted through chains of neurons. Each neuron fires in response to particular chemicals known as *neurotransmitters*. When one of these chemicals comes into contact with a nerve cell to which it is related (by virtue of the cell having receptors for it), the molecule fits like a key into a lock. By fitting into the receptor, it can increase or decrease the cell's ability to transmit electrical signals to other nerve cells farther along in the chain.

A neuron consists of the cell body, *dendrites* that receive chemical messages from previous neurons in the chain, and a tail-like fiber called an *axon* that communicates with subsequent neurons in the chain. Many axons have a *myelin sheath* that speeds up the transmission of information. When a neuron fires, it releases one or more special neurotransmitters from its axon into a *synapse,* the fluid space in between nerve cells. The released chemical comes into contact with the dendrites of other neurons and may cause them to fire. The neurotransmitter is then normally reabsorbed from the synapse by the neurons from which it was released, a process known as *reuptake.*

The human body was not designed by evolution to respond to psychoactive drugs. Some drugs work because they closely resemble molecules that occur naturally within the body. For example, the central nervous system includes a remarkable capacity to reduce pain through the release of natural neurotransmitters known as *endorphins.* Opioid drugs like heroin closely resemble these natural molecules. They stimulate the endorphin (opiate) receptors, artificially activating the body's system for relieving suffering and inducing a pervasive sense of well-being. A drug that can thus mimic the effects of a natural neurotransmitter is called an *agonist* for that system. Most addictive drugs are agonists, activating or amplifying transmitter systems in the brain, usually in a way that is much more intense than normal experience.

One problem with artificial activation, however, is the phenomenon of *drug tolerance,* discussed in Chapter 2. Heroin-dependent people often report that the most intensely pleasant rush of their lives happened during their very first exposure to heroin, and that they have spent the rest of their lives chasing that same high. For a variety of reasons, psychoactive drugs tend to lose their potency with repeated use, so that in order to experience the same high the person must use ever larger doses. The system becomes saturated, and natural neurotransmitter activity is reduced in response to artificial activation. Eventually the person uses the drug trying to feel normal.

Just as some drugs serve as agonists, others serve as *antagonists* for specific neurotransmitters. An antagonist molecule binds to the receptor and blocks it, reducing activation by either the natural neurotransmitter or by its artificial agonists. Some drugs can serve both agonist and antagonist functions; they are *partial agonists* stimulating activity in a specific neurotransmitter system, while also blocking further stimulation by other agonists. We discuss agonists, partial agonists, and antagonists further when we consider therapeutic medications that are used to treat drug dependence (Chapter 18).

Resembling a natural neurotransmitter is not the only way in which drugs can influence the central nervous system. Some drugs exert effects not by mimicking neurotransmitter molecules, but by acting on neurons in other ways. Alcohol is a prime example. Although some of alcohol's many effects do seem to involve activation of receptor systems, alcohol also impacts the entire brain by altering nerve cell membranes in ways that are only partially understood at present. Other drugs exert their effects by blocking reuptake, causing a neurotransmitter to remain longer than normal in the synaptic space and thus continuing to act on postsynaptic neurons.

Major Drug Classes and Their Acute Effects

This section describes major classes of psychoactive drugs that you are likely to encounter, and how they affect the central nervous system. For each drug class we describe the common sought-after effects of intoxication ("the peak") and the rebound period that follows use ("the valley"). These descriptions are necessarily brief. Several classic resources are available that describe in more detail the pharmacokinetics, pharmacodynamics, and specific effects of psychoactive drugs (Advokat, Comaty, & Julian, 2019; Hart & Ksir, 2015; Preston & Johnson, 2016; Stahl, 2017).

Some common street names for major drug classes are listed in Box 3.1. There are hundreds of such street names, which vary among geographic areas, with new slang names appearing regularly. Box 3.2 on page 39 summarizes the neurotransmitter systems particularly affected by the various classes of drugs discussed below.

BOX 3.1. Some Street Names for Drugs

Alcohol	Booze, hooch, juice, sauce
Amphetamine	Speed, crystal, ice, crank, chalk, crystal, glass, meth, uppers, bennies, tweak, truck drivers
Barbiturates	Barbs, reds, ludes, goofballs, phennies, red devils
Benzodiazepines	Benzos, downers, tranqs, candy
Cannabis	Pot, dope, grass, weed, herb, hemp, rope, Mary Jane, hash, ganja, tea, reefer, skunk, joint, blunt
Cocaine	Coke, C, snow, crystal, toot, cola, nose candy, heaven, white, bump
Crack Cocaine	Candy, flake, rock
Fentanyl	China girl, jackpot, apache, friend, TNT
Heroin	Horse, shit, smack, junk, H, skag, fix, China white, whack, brown sugar, dope, tar
Inhalants	Huff, glue, dusters, poppers, rush
Ketamine	K, Ket, Special K, kit kat, vitamin k, purple, cat valium
LSD	Acid, 25, tabs, sugar, blotter, microdots, windowpane, mellow yellow, cubes
Mescaline, peyote	Buttons, mesc, mess, cactus
Phencyclidine	Angel dust, PCP, elephant, hog, love boat
Psilocybin	Mushroom, shroom, sacred mushrooms, magic mushrooms
Steroids	Arnolds, roids, gym candy, juice, pumpers

Stimulants

Stimulants can be ingested, taken intranasally, or injected intravenously. By reducing them to a *base* form, stimulants can also be inhaled in smoke. As a class of drugs, stimulants exert their psychological effects by increasing activity in three key neurotransmitter systems: dopamine, norepinephrine, and serotonin. Cocaine does so by blocking the reuptake of these chemicals from synapses. Amphetamines resemble the neurotransmitter norepinephrine (noradrenalin), and exert their stimulant effect primarily by the dumping of increased amounts of dopamine and norepinephrine into neural synapses. Two other widely used stimulants are nicotine (primarily in tobacco) and caffeine (in coffee, tea, soft drinks, and chocolate). Like other stimulants, both nicotine and caffeine activate reward channels in the brain and increase alertness. Caffeine blockades receptors for the inhibitory neurotransmitter *adenosine,* thereby increasing acetylcholine and dopamine activity. Nicotine directly stimulates one subtype of acetylcholine receptors, releasing adrenalin into the bloodstream and increasing heart rate and blood pressure. Stimulants activate the brain's positive reinforcement system, which normally rewards activities that promote survival and well-being. In essence they directly and intensely trigger the brain system that says "Do that again!" It is no mystery, therefore, why these drugs have such a high capacity for habitual use and dependence.

The Peak

Stimulants have been called "power drugs" because they induce euphoria and a grandiose sense of personal power and achievement. They can be used to remain awake and alert, promote persistence, and suppress fatigue and hunger—effects that historically made these drugs useful to soldiers and to others like students and truck drivers wanting to stay awake and alert. In general they speed up functioning: the person thinks faster, talks faster, moves faster. With higher or repeated doses, the user may develop paranoia or other delusions.

The Valley

As with many drugs of abuse, the stimulant high is followed by a low, a "crash." The rebound from stimulant use is substantial, and not surprisingly involves the opposite of the drug's acute effects. During the postdrug valley the user may experience anxiety, depression, fatigue and drowsiness, increased appetite, and persisting paranoia. Because stimulants suppress appetite, weight gain can occur when the drug is discontinued. Withdrawal symptoms from caffeine are generally mild, characterized by headache and some disruption of concentration, whereas nicotine quickly produces dependence as tenacious as that for cocaine or opiates. Nicotine withdrawal involves a substantial and often prolonged rebound, potentially including depression, anxiousness, agitation, insomnia, increased appetite, and emotional volatility.

Sedatives

Sedative drugs have as their general effect a suppression (and in higher doses, shutting down) of the central nervous system. They all enhance the activity of GABA (gamma-aminobutyric acid), a class of inhibitory neurotransmitters that broadly decrease neural activity. Relatedly, they tend to suppress the NMDA (N-methyl-D-aspartate) subtype of glutamate, which is an activating neurotransmitter. In sum, they enhance neurochemicals that close down the central nervous system and interfere with neurochemicals that activate it. This is true of alcohol, sedative–hypnotic drugs like barbiturates, and tranquilizers such as benzodiazepines.

The Peak

Sedatives are downers and shut-downers. In lower doses they tend to reduce feelings of anxiety and induce mild euphoria. These drugs also interfere with memory and can be quite effective in producing partial or total amnesia ("blackout") for events occurring during a period of intoxication. They progressively slow down nervous system functioning, and are therefore quite dangerous when combined with driving, operating machinery, or engaging in other potentially risky activities that require clear attention and coordination. The sedative "high" is physiologically more like a low and includes dream-like intoxication, damping of distress and memory, loss of inhibitions, and a sense of well-being or at least unconcern. In short, they make the world (especially an unpleasant world) go away.

BOX 3.2. Neurotransmitters Particularly Affected by Psychoactive Drugs

Drug Classes	Receptor Systems Activated	Receptor Systems Suppressed
Alcohol	GABA, endorphin	NMDA glutamate, acetylcholine
Barbiturates	GABA	NMDA glutamate
Benzodiazepines	GABA	
Stimulants	Dopamine, norepinephrine, serotonin	
Caffeine	Dopamine, acetylcholine	Adenosine
Ketamine	Glutamate, dopamine	Acetylcholine
Nicotine	Acetylcholine	
Opioid analgesics	Endorphin	
Marijuana	Cannabinoid	Glutamate
Psychedelics	Serotonin, dopamine	Acetylcholine (PCP suppresses NMDA)
Steroids	Steroid (testosterone)	

The Valley

The rebound (hangover) from sedative intoxication involves agitation and unpleasant arousal. The higher the level of sedative intoxication, the greater the rebound. Sedative hangover can include irritability, anxiety and restlessness, insomnia and nightmares, racing heart, nausea, headache, and sweating. Such symptoms tend to be quickly alleviated by redosing with a sedative ("a bit of the hair of the dog that bit you"), which in turn can encourage cyclic and escalating use. Drug withdrawal with severe alcohol or other sedative dependence can be life-threatening (see Chapter 6 on withdrawal management).

Similar sedative effects result from inhaling solvents (gasoline, nail polish remover) and other volatile substances such as glue and aerosols. The intoxicating effects closely resemble those for alcohol, but most inhalants are far more neurotoxic.

Opiates

The body has a built-in system for *analgesia,* the relief of pain. At the center of it are naturally produced neurotransmitters known as *endorphins* that decrease pain and enhance the sense of well-being. *Opioid analgesics* (or "opiates") mimic endorphins and thereby artificially stimulate the body's analgesic system.

The Peak

Opiates flood the person with a euphoric sense of well-being, combined with drowsiness and relief of pain. Breathing is slowed and in higher doses is suppressed completely—the usual cause of opiate overdose deaths.

The Valley

Unlike withdrawal from sedatives, the discomfort involved in rebound from opiate use is rarely life-threatening, though it can be much feared by users. It has been likened to a very bad case of the flu: sweating, insomnia, aches and pains, agitation, anxiousness and restlessness, a general feeling of being sick—and, of course, a hunger for more of the drug.

Psychedelics

Psychedelic drugs differ in a number of important ways from other drugs of abuse. One of these is that primates and lower mammals will self-administer nearly all psychoactive drugs that humans misuse, but will not use psychedelic drugs (with the exception of phencyclidine [PCP]) when given free access to them. Furthermore, they produce no significant withdrawal syndrome, so that even with prolonged exposure, animals show no inclination to continue the use of psychedelics. Thus, whereas most drugs of abuse produce neural effects that appear to be inherently reinforcing for mammals, the effects of psychedelics are found reinforcing only and uniquely by humans.

The Peak

The experience of loss of control is central to psychedelic experience. Most psychoactive drugs produce effects that are fairly predictable, so that a user knows what to expect and can replicate the experience of prior use (although tolerance often diminishes such effects). One who uses a psychedelic drug, however, does not know what to expect in subjective experience, as illustrated by the "bad trip" events associated with higher doses. Within a dreamlike state, the person experiences sensory and perceptual distortions and hallucinations, often accompanied by disorientation and amnesia. Psychedelic drugs have long been used to evoke or intensify spiritual experiences (Casteneda, 1985; Griffiths, Richards, Johnson, McCann, & Jesse, 2008).

The Valley

There is virtually no withdrawal associated with the use of psychedelics. The person's mental functioning gradually returns to normal within a few hours, without apparent rebound (although it is unclear what would constitute a rebound). *Flashbacks* to distressing subjective experiences sometimes occur in the weeks or months following psychedelic drug use.

Cannabis

Because of some overlapping effects, marijuana has sometimes been classified with the psychedelics, but its effects are quite different. Tetrahydrocannabinol (THC), the active ingredient in cannabis, stimulates particular cannabinoid receptors that are ordinarily activated by the neurotransmitter *anandamide*. Cannabinoids suppress glutamate and thereby exert a general sedating effect like alcohol, slowing reflexes and movement, decreasing attention and concentration, impairing memory and learning, lengthening reaction time, and lowering core body temperature. Unlike alcohol, however, THC appears to decrease aggression.

The Peak

The overlap with psychedelic effects is found in a dream-like state involving time distortion and sensory–perceptual alterations, albeit of a more predictable variety. Food craving ("munchies") can be intensified. Cognitive processes tend to be loosened up by THC, leading to less controlled and more unusual mental associations. Intoxication usually induces a sense of euphoria and well-being, although higher doses can amplify negative emotions.

The Valley

Cessation of regular marijuana use has been associated with various forms of discomfort including insomnia, anxiousness, restlessness, irritability, and nausea, representing a rebound from the sedative effects of THC.

Steroids

Testosterone is a naturally occurring hormone that functions as a neurotransmitter in both men and women (as do many other hormones). When testosterone and related synthetic compounds are taken, they override the body's normal process to self-regulate the circulating level of testosterone. The predictable result of regular use is a substantial increase in masculine characteristics, muscle mass, and aggression.

The Peak

There is little or no acute high from the use of steroids. Typically, they are taken over a span of time to increase muscle mass, enhance athletic performance and aggressiveness, and increase masculine appearance. The payoff is primarily in terms of self-perception and, in the case of female and male athletes, enhanced performance. The effects are quite noticeable and have become increasingly attractive to adolescent boys as well as adults.

The Valley

When steroid use is stopped, unwanted changes usually follow. Besides the gradual loss of muscle mass, people often experience restlessness and depression, decreased self-esteem, insomnia, and decreased appetites including sexual desire.

BOX 3.3 The Eyes Have It

Some drugs of abuse are well known for effects that can be seen by looking into the user's eyes. *Dilated (wide-open) pupils* occur with the use of stimulants and psychedelics. *Constricted (pinpoint) pupils* accompany opiate use. *Bloodshot eyes,* with red streaks in the whites of both eyes, are common soon after marijuana use.

Drug Interactions

SUDs are seldom limited to one drug. Most alcohol-dependent people also smoke tobacco. Those who use marijuana have a much greater likelihood, relative to the general population, of also using alcohol, tobacco, cocaine, heroin, and other drugs.

The effects described above become far more complex when drugs are combined. The use of one drug may sensitize the brain to the reinforcing effects of other drugs (Griffin et al., 2017). Drugs within the same class may produce *cross-tolerance*. People who are dependent on and have a high tolerance to alcohol also have heightened tolerance to other sedatives including barbiturates, benzodiazepines, and general anesthetics. Alcohol-dependent people undergoing surgery may therefore require a significantly higher dose of general anesthetic to induce or maintain unconsciousness and amnesia. However, drugs within the same class when combined tend to *potentiate* each other's effects. For a person already sedated by benzodiazepines, a dose of alcohol will have a much larger effect than it would if taken alone. Furthermore, the potentiation is not merely additive. The total amount of sedation is more than the combined effect of alcohol alone plus benzodiazepines alone. Here is a case where two plus two can equal six. The reason for this is that sedatives also inhibit each other's metabolism: in the presence of benzodiazepines or barbiturates, the body breaks down alcohol more slowly, and vice versa. Thus, each drug remains in the body longer than it would have had it been taken alone. This is one reason why the combination of sedatives with each other or with opiates carries a high risk of lethal overdose.

Similarly, the pharmacological effects of two different drugs can combine in dangerous and unpredictable ways. Even in relatively low doses, either marijuana or alcohol alone significantly impairs the mental and physical functions required to operate a motor vehicle safely. Use of both drugs together multiplies the impairment of driving ability and of judgment regarding one's ability to drive safely (Dubois, Mullen, Weaver, & Bédard, 2015; Hartman et al., 2015). The danger of pharmacological interactions is further complicated by the fact that illicit drug users may not know what drugs they are actually receiving.

SUDs are seldom limited to one drug.

Long-Term Effects

Contrary to lore about denial, by the time people have developed alcohol or other drug dependence they are usually well aware of the dangers and harm related to their drug use. Most smokers, for example, clearly know that they are at increased risk for cancers and heart disease because of their tobacco use. Though they may staunchly reject a label such as "alcoholic" or "problem drinker," most heavy drinkers can readily list ways in which alcohol has put them at risk or created harm and problems. It is no secret that misusing psychoactive drugs is a gamble, risking long-term harm for short-term pleasure.

Certain risks pertain to specific drugs. For example, sudden stroke or heart attack in a young person without a history of heart disease is particularly associated with the use of stimulants, and to a lesser extent with alcohol intoxication. During pregnancy, sedatives (such as alcohol and inhalants) can inflict particularly devastating effects on the unborn child.

Many of the adverse long-term effects of substance abuse, however, are similar across diverse drugs. In this final section we describe several groups of common long-term effects, pointing out as applicable where certain drugs pose particular risks.

Dependence

One of the obvious risks of long-term drug abuse is the development of dependence on the drug. One dimension of dependence is physical addiction, in which withdrawal (abstinence) from the drug produces unpleasant symptoms that are relieved by renewed use of the same or a similar drug. As described in Chapter 2, however, dependence involves much more than physical withdrawal symptoms, and in fact drug dependence can occur without such physiological addiction. Within this larger perspective, becoming dependent involves having one's life increasingly revolve around acquiring, using, and recovering from effects of the drug. Psychoactive drugs vary widely in their potential to produce dependence. For some drugs with very high potential, there are few users who are not dependent. Other drugs have very low potential to produce a dependence syndrome (see Box 3.4).

Acute Events

Some long-term consequences can result from even short-term use. Much of the injury, tragedy, and mortality associated with alcohol and other drugs results from acute events related to drug acquisition, use, and intoxication. Many psychoactive drugs significantly impair human judgment about what is safe, reasonable, or acceptable to do. Consequently, during intoxication, people are more likely to take risks and violate social norms as well as their own values. Intoxication not only affects appraisal of dangerousness, but also tends to impair mental and physical functions that are important to safety (such as reaction time and coordination). The result can be a tragedy that lasts for (or ends) a lifetime. As stated earlier, many deaths by falls, fire, drowning, and other "accidents"; by violence; and of pedestrians and

BOX 3.4. Potential to Produce Drug Dependence

Drugs differ in how likely they are to produce dependence. The following ratings are based on the proportion of users who are drug-dependent.

Potential to Produce Drug Dependence	Drug
Very high	Amphetamine, cocaine, nicotine, heroin, and other opiates
High	Caffeine, PCP
Moderate	Alcohol, marijuana, benzodiazepines, ketamine
Low	Psychedelics, steroids
Very low	Antidepressant, antimanic, and antipsychotic medications

drivers involve victims or participants under the influence of alcohol or other drugs.

Drug intoxication also increases the likelihood of committing acts with long-term or irrevocable consequences. In Western nations, a majority of people in prison are there for crimes committed under the influence of or otherwise related to substance use (particularly alcohol). Stimulants, alcohol, steroids, and psychedelics all significantly increase aggression, particularly in males. Alcohol influences males to misperceive or overestimate hostile intent in the actions of others and to respond more aggressively (Bartholow & Heinz, 2006; Ogle & Miller, 2004). A substantial proportion of people who commit suicide were under the influence of or dependent on drugs (particularly alcohol) at the time.

Toxicity

Beyond these acute events, many drugs of abuse also exert toxic effects on body organs including the brain, liver, lungs, heart, and gastrointestinal system. Heavy use of alcohol or tobacco is associated with greatly increased risk of a variety of cancers. For people who are both drinkers and smokers, cancer risk is not additive but multiplicative. This includes cancers of the lung, breast, mouth, larynx, esophagus, stomach, intestines, and rectum. Alcohol and inhalants are particularly toxic to the central nervous system, and long-term abuse of these drugs is associated with increasing impairment of memory, learning, and cognition.

A *safety index* of drugs is the ratio of a lethal dose (LD-50, or the dose level that is lethal for 50% of humans) to the usual effective dose (ED) that produces desired effects in 50% of people (ED-50). The greater the ratio of LD-50 to ED-50, the wider the margin of safety. High-risk drugs are those with a safety index under 10, including alcohol, nicotine, cocaine, and heroin. The same ratio (called the *therapeutic* index) is used to evaluate prescribed medications, some of which (such as lithium carbonate) have a very narrow safety margin. Of all misused drugs, those that suppress the central nervous system have the highest potential for lethal overdose. These include (1) alcohol, barbiturates, benzodiazepines, and other sedatives; (2) heroin and other opiates; and (3) most inhalants. There has been a major U.S. epidemic of misuse of prescription opioids such as oxycodone and fentanyl, and annual deaths by opiate overdose have far surpassed fatalities from motor vehicle accidents (Rudd, Aleshire, Zibbell, & Gladden, 2016), prompting the revision of clinical guidelines for the use of opioids in pain management (Dowell, Haegerich, & Chou, 2016).

There is increased risk and exacerbation of heart disease associated with certain drugs. The nicotine and carbon monoxide in tobacco smoke increase blood pressure and arterial disease, in turn increasing the risk of coronary disease and heart attack. Heavy drinking clearly increases risk for hypertension and congestive heart disease.

Adverse Consequences

Health Consequences

Beyond toxicity, damage to health also occurs because of poor self-care associated with SUDs. Nutrition may suffer from the use of drugs that suppress appetite and induce anorexia (e.g., stimulants), or from the replacement of dietary calories by ethyl alcohol. Major and enduring dental problems are common with SUDs because of a variety of factors including poor oral hygiene and infrequent dental care. The combination of poor hygiene, injuries, infections, and immune suppression can yield a plethora of skin diseases and lesions.

Interpersonal Consequences

Family, friendship, and intimate relationships often suffer in relation to addictions, which are associated with high rates of divorce, alienation, and loss of child custody. Ties are often broken with people who would encourage sobriety, and replaced by relationships with peers who practice and support drug use.

Intrapersonal Consequences

SUDs also take their toll on personal happiness. Negative emotions increasingly dominate drug-free hours: depression, anxiety, loneliness, anger, and resentment. Stimulant use is linked to other mental disorders, particularly drug-induced paranoia and psychosis.

Social Consequences

The progression of SUDs often involves deterioration in social functioning. As life becomes ever more centered on drug use, people's prior interests, activities, and responsibilities fall away. Impaired work performance, absenteeism, and job loss are common. Illicit drug use, of course, also carries the risk of criminal sanctions and associated long-term social consequences. Financial problems and the decay of relationships contribute to social instability, sometimes leading to cycles of unemployment and homelessness.

Fetal Effects

Virtually all of the commonly misused drugs cross the placental barrier; thus when the pregnant mother uses, so does the unborn child whose body does not have adult capacities to metabolize drugs. Exposure to certain drugs can interfere with normal development and injure the fetus, producing long-term effects on the child's health and behavior. Significant damage can be done during early development, even before the mother realizes that she is pregnant. Nevertheless, stopping drug use at any point in pregnancy is associated with better outcomes.

The use of some drugs can interrupt pregnancy, leading to spontaneous abortion, premature delivery, and stillbirth. These risks are increased by the use of tobacco, stimulants, and alcohol during pregnancy. Drug-using mothers may also neglect self-care in other ways (e.g., nutrition, rest, exercise, and prenatal care) that influence fetal health.

Retardation of fetal growth is another effect of some drug use during pregnancy. Physically smaller babies (e.g., low birth weight, smaller head circumference) may be born to mothers who used tobacco, stimulants, or alcohol during pregnancy. Tobacco use interferes with the delivery of oxygen to the fetus, which can impair development and later intellectual functioning. Amphetamines, cocaine, and other stimulants similarly reduce blood supply to the unborn child. Depending on the particular point in pregnancy, reduced blood flow can disrupt normal development of the brain, heart, or other organs. Babies who have been exposed to regular doses of dependence-producing drugs show withdrawal syndrome in the hours and days after birth. Nicotine and other stimulant use during pregnancy have been linked to increased risk for attention-deficit/hyperactivity disorder (ADHD) when the child reaches school age.

The most devastating effects on unborn children, however, are those associated with maternal use of alcohol or other sedative drugs. A clear fetal alcohol syndrome (FAS) has been described, involving mental and growth retardation, birth defects of the face and limbs, and behavioral problems including ADHD. Alcohol is by far the largest preventable cause of mental retardation. Short of full FAS, a variety of alcohol-related birth defects have been described, mostly lower-level individual components of the syndrome. No safe level of drinking during pregnancy has been established, and women who are seeking to or have already become pregnant are best counseled to abstain from alcohol completely.

The Web of Addiction and Related Problems

All of this information underlines the truth that the treatment of addiction should be closely integrated with a broader spectrum of health and social services. Most people with SUDs also have a daunting array of other life, health, social, and psychological problems. Often the resolution of these other problems is a higher priority for them than addressing their substance use, and not without reason. A mother who is homeless is likely to be more urgently concerned with safety, shelter, and feeding her children than with abstaining from drugs. A man suffering from depression, panic attacks, and posttraumatic stress disorder (PTSD) may not perceive alcohol abstinence as a high priority. To be sure, getting free from alcohol and other drug use often leads to improvement on other dimensions, but it is no longer adequate to treat addiction in isolation from other concerns. As discussed in Chapter 1, people with alcohol/drug problems are most likely to seek help for other, related problems. Often they are seen dozens or even hundreds of times in health care, social service, legal, correctional, welfare, and hospital systems before they seek specialist treatment for addictions, if ever they do. They have not one problem, but many.

> The treatment of addiction should be closely integrated with a broader spectrum of health and social services

Scheduling of Drugs

In the United States, the *Comprehensive Drug Abuse Prevention and Control Act of 1970* established a classification system for controlled substances comprising five "schedules" based on "potential for abuse." Schedule I, the highest level of regulation, is for drugs regarded as having high potential for misuse, no currently accepted medical use, and no "accepted safety" for its use under medical supervision. Schedule I drugs cannot be prescribed. Drugs on Schedule II, which can be prescribed, have currently accepted medical use(s), but still have high potential for misuse in the form of psychological or physical dependence. Schedule III drugs have currently accepted medical use(s), and are regarded as having less potential for misuse and moderate to low risk of psychological or physical dependence. Drugs classified as having low (Schedule IV) or the lowest (Schedule V) potential for misuse or dependence have minimal restrictions on prescription. Alcohol, tobacco, and over-the-counter medicines are excluded from the scheduling system.

BOX 3.5. Examples of Current Drug Classification Schedules	
Schedule I	Heroin, ibogaine, khat, marijuana and cannabinoids, methaqualone, psychedelics (DMT, LSD, MDMA, mescaline, peyote, psilocybin)
Schedule II	Amphetamine, fast-acting barbiturates, cocaine, codeine, fentanyl, hydrocodone, methadone, methamphetamine, methylphenidate, morphine, opium, oxycodone, PCP
Schedule III	Anabolic steroids, buprenorphine, ketamine, intermediate-acting barbiturates, dronabinol (a synthetic THC)
Schedule IV	Benzodiazepines, long-acting barbiturates, modafinil, tramadol
Schedule V	Low-codeine cough suppressants, anticonvulsants

Examples of drugs currently classified at each level of scheduling are shown in Box 3.5. The current assignment of drugs to federal schedules is a political and legislative decision that may not correspond with scientific evidence regarding actual levels of risk for misuse, dependence, and harm. Marijuana (Schedule I), for example, is widely regarded as far less dangerous and dependence-producing than Schedule II drugs such as fentanyl, methamphetamine, and oxycodone.

KEY POINTS

🍃 Drugs can be taken into the body in various ways, but principally by ingestion, inhalation, intranasal, or injection routes of administration.

🍃 A drug is distributed throughout the body via the bloodstream, affecting neurotransmitter systems in the brain until it is ultimately eliminated from the body.

🍃 Acute intoxication (peak) effects vary by drug class, as do withdrawal (valley) effects, which often are mirror opposites of the drug's initial effects.

🍃 Different drugs can interact in the body in various ways such as by cross-tolerance and potentiation.

🍃 Longer-term effects vary according to the drug that is being used and can include dependence, toxicity (also to an unborn child), and adverse consequences resulting from acute or chronic use.

Reflection Questions

Q What implicit messages about drug use are conveyed through the advertising of prescription and over-the-counter medications?

Q What interventions do you think are appropriate to prevent permanent damage to an unborn child from maternal alcohol/drug use?

Q To what extent can drug problems be explained by the biological effects of drugs? What proportion of responsibility for drug dependence might you assign to the drugs themselves? Does your estimate of this proportion vary depending on the drug (e.g., alcohol, tobacco, marijuana, cocaine, heroin)?

PART II

A CONTEXT FOR
ADDICTION TREATMENT

Perhaps the main question that brings you to this book is "What should I do to best help people overcome addiction?" Fair enough, and there is good news ahead. There are not just one or two answers but an encouraging array of evidence-based treatment methods to offer people who are caught in the snare of SUDs. There is no one size that fits all. Rather, there are solid options from which you and your clients can choose. This science-based menu of options is presented in Part III, the largest section of this book.

Before we come to the question of *what* to do, however, there is the equally important subject of *how* to treat people. It turns out that it matters not only *what* treatment is offered, but *who* offers it and *how* they approach the task. This became clear in early research where clients who were given the "same" evidence-based manual-guided treatment had very different outcomes depending on who delivered the treatment (Miller, Taylor, & West, 1980; Najavits & Weiss, 1994). In another early study (Valle, 1981) clients in the same treatment program had up to four times the risk of "relapse" depending on the therapist who treated them. It is not meaningful, therefore, to talk just about "evidence-based" therapies without considering who provides the treatment and the context in which it is provided. Treatment and provider are inseparable (Miller & Moyers, 2015).

In Part II we discuss these important contextual aspects of treatment. Chapter 4 addresses the often-ignored but vital process of *engaging* and offers a person-centered approach to treatment regardless of its particular content. Carl Rogers (1980) described this as the *attitude* with which you treat people, your "way of being" as you help people change. How you relate to your clients is strongly influenced by how you think about them and about the problems that they face. In Chapter 5 we consider screening, assessment, and diagnosis in treating addiction. Physical preparations for treatment—managing withdrawal and addressing health care needs—are the topic of Chapter 6. Chapter 7 completes the contextual picture by exploring how to tailor treatment to the needs of the individual, and finally Chapter 8 offers a framework for ongoing case management.

CHAPTER 4

Engaging

The transtheoretical model of change emphasizes that people enter treatment at very different points of readiness (Norcross, Krebs, & Prochaska, 2011; Prochaska & Velicer, 1997). Yet counselors and treatment systems often seem to assume readiness, skipping over the *whether* and the *why* and charging right into the *how* of change, thus contributing to early client dropout rates. In the past, clients who did not remain, adhere, and succeed in treatment were often blamed for being unmotivated or "in denial." That's simply not good enough anymore because it is now clear that client motivation is highly malleable and influenced by counselor style. We address the practical issue of enhancing client motivation in Chapter 10.

The first order of business in addiction treatment should not be fact gathering, but rather engaging with clients. To be sure, there may be certain facts you need to collect at the outset, though most programs collect far more information at "intake" than they will ever use. Intake should not be a prerequisite to receive care. Treatment should begin with the very first moments of contact, and collecting required bits of data can usually be postponed to the end of an initial session, or done in advance by phone, computer, or on a clipboard in the waiting room. Fact gathering is of minimal value to clients because it's information that they already know! Furthermore, half an hour of good listening will often yield far more important information than asking litanies of questions. Engaging is task number one. Without it clients may not even return.

So what is engaging? Miller and Rollnick (2013) described it as the first of four treatment processes: engaging (forming a working relationship), focusing (negotiating goals of treatment), evoking (eliciting the client's own motivations for change), and planning (choosing and implementing strategies for change). In everyday language these processes can be expressed as four questions:

1. *Engaging:* "Can we walk together?"
2. *Focusing:* "Where are we going?"
3. *Evoking:* "Why is it important to go there?"
4. *Planning:* "How will we get there?"

Jumping straight to "treatment planning" skips over three important processes that provide a foundation for change.

Engaging doesn't need to take a long time. With the skills described in this chapter it can begin within a matter of minutes, and engaging usually flows naturally into subsequent processes. From the client's perspective, engaging addresses what may be unspoken questions:

- "Do I feel comfortable and welcome here?"
- "Will this person (or program) be able to help me?"
- "Do I feel heard and respected?"
- "Can I trust this person (or program)?"
- "Do I want to come back?"

Engaging involves forming enough of a collaborative working relationship to walk together and move forward a few steps. This relationship grows over time and is a vital foundation for everything that follows.

Engaging is a particular way of being with clients, a set of communication skills developed in the person-centered approach described by Carl Rogers and his students (Gordon & Edwards, 1997; Kirschenbaum, 2009; Rogers, 1980; Truax & Carkhuff, 1967). The good news is that this set of skills can be used throughout treatment. It is not something to use at the outset and then set aside. This relational style tends to decrease client "resistance" and dropout, increase adherence, and improve outcome in addiction treatment.

> The first order of business in addiction treatment should not be fact gathering, but rather engaging.

A central theme of this chapter is that effective addiction treatment is not just a matter of *what* you do, but is also strongly influenced by *who* you are and *how* you work with your clients. It is a matter of bringing together the available science with a humane and empathic approach to treatment (Douaihy & Driscoll, 2018). Research documenting the impact of counselor style on treatment outcome has actually been around for a long time, but, as often happens, it has been slow to influence practice (Rogers, 2003). We place this chapter early in the book because counseling *style* has as much or more impact on client outcomes as the particular treatment methods that you use (Imel, Wampold, Miller, & Fleming, 2008; Miller & Moyers, 2015; Wampold & Imel, 2015).

Empathic Understanding

A rather consistent finding in research on the treatment of SUDs is that clients' outcomes differ dramatically depending on the counselor to whom they are assigned (Najavits, Crits-Christoph, & Dierberger, 2000; Najavits & Weiss, 1994). Even when ostensibly delivering the very same manual-guided treatment, therapists differ in their effectiveness (Moyers, Houck, Rice, Longabaugh, & Miller, 2016; Project MATCH Research Group, 1998e). What accounts for such substantial variation among counselors?

One of the strongest predictors of a counselor's effectiveness in treating SUDs is the therapeutic skill of accurate empathy. In one study, among nine therapists, with all delivering the same behavior therapy, clients' successful outcomes varied from 25% to 100% depending on the extent to which the counselor practiced empathic reflective listening during treatment (Miller, Taylor, & West, 1980). Even 2 years later, clients' drinking outcomes were strongly related to how well their counselor had listened to them during treatment (Miller & Baca, 1983). Another early study demonstrated a strong relationship between client "relapse" rates and the counselors' skillfulness in client-centered counseling. The more empathic and client-centered the counselor's style, the better his or her clients fared after counseling (Valle, 1981). Therapist empathy continues to predict better client outcomes even after taking into account client characteristics and the specific treatment methods provided (Moyers et al., 2016). Clients treated by counselors low in empathy tend to have worse outcomes than if they had received no treatment at all (Moyers & Miller, 2013). It's that important!

What is this quality of empathy? Some associate the term with the ability to *identify* with one's clients by virtue of having had similar experiences. In fact, personal recovery status neither increases nor decreases one's success in treating SUDs, even when delivering a 12-step-based treatment (Project MATCH Research Group, 1998e). What *does* make a difference is empathic understanding, which is not the same thing as being able to relate to a client based on your own personal experience. If anything, being too early in one's own recovery can get in the way of effective counseling by fostering overidentification (Manohar, 1973).

Carl Rogers (1959) identified *accurate empathy* as one of the three critical conditions that a counselor can provide to promote growth and change in clients. (The other two were interpersonal warmth, or *unconditional positive regard*, and personal honesty, or *genuineness*.) These "conditions" are measurable as particular counselor skills and practices (Truax & Carkhuff, 1967). What Rogers meant by "empathy" was the ability to listen to your clients and accurately *reflect back to them* the essence and meaning of what they have said. Such reflection, which was termed *active listening* by Rogers's student Thomas Gordon (1970; Gordon & Edwards, 1997), serves at least three purposes. First, it allows you to ensure that you are correctly understanding what your client means. Second, it communicates respect, understanding, and acceptance. Third, and most important in Rogers's theory, it helps clients to clarify their own internal processes—thoughts, feelings, associations—and to experience them in a nonjudgmental atmosphere. It fosters the opposite of defensive "denial." Clients are encouraged to explore their real experiencing, whatever it is, and to do so in the company of someone who continues to regard them with unconditional loving acceptance (Miller, 2017, 2018).

Learning accurate empathy is no quick and easy task. Those who are good at reflective listening make it look simple and natural, but it is actually a skill that is honed over years of practice. Happily, as we will discuss below, your clients can teach you how to do it.

Beneath empathy is an attitude of total interest in and focus on understanding how your client perceives things, on seeing the world through his or her eyes. Empathic listeners suspend, at least for the time being, all of their own material—advice, questions, suggestions, stories, brilliant insights—and focus entirely on the person's own experience. It is a challenging, sacrificial, and much underrated way of being with people (Rogers, 1980).

Why bother to focus so fully on what your client thinks, feels, values, and believes, when you could be conveying your own wisdom? Herein is another of Carl Rogers's assumptions about human nature that we share. He believed that within each person is a seed waiting to grow and blossom. In each client there is wisdom, a desire to be well and whole, a natural tendency to move in a positive direction given the proper conditions, just as a seed grows to its potential if given the right amount of air, water, soil, and sunshine. The counselor's job, Rogers believed, is not so much to plant the seeds as to provide the right conditions for their growth. Like a midwife, you help with the birthing process but don't provide the baby. Rogers trusted his clients' own experiencing, wisdom, and resourcefulness. If you don't share that belief, then it might well seem a waste of time to be listening to what your clients have to say.

The counseling style that we are describing here is one that communicates not "I have what you need," but rather, "*You* have what you need, and together we will find it" (Miller & Rollnick, 2013). That's not to say you never offer any advice, make suggestions, teach new skills, or share personal experiences. There is a time and a way to offer your professional expertise. Here we depart a bit from Rogers, in that we combine the client-centered foundation described in this chapter with other effective treatment methods described in Part III.

One reason why we devote an entire chapter to this counseling style is that it works. Being empathic is itself an evidence-based practice (Elliott, Bohart, Watson, & Greenberg, 2011; Wampold, 2015; Zuroff, Kelly, Leybman, Blatt, & Wampold, 2010). As described above, counselors who have honed their skill in empathic listening are simply more effective in treating people with SUDs. This counseling style meshes well with other treatment methods, including cognitive-behavioral and 12-step approaches (Longabaugh, Zweben, LoCastro, & Miller, 2005; Moyers et al., 2016; Naar & Safren, 2017). In fact, the related client-centered method of *motivational interviewing* (Chapter 10) seems to amplify the effectiveness of treatment approaches with which it is combined (Hettema, Steele, & Miller, 2005). Empathy is also a quality that clients want in their therapist, above and beyond the type of treatment they receive (Swift & Callahan, 2010; Swift, Callahan, & Vollmer, 2011). Reflecting on 40 years of experience with psychodynamic psychotherapy, Khantzian (2012) topped his list of essential elements for clinicians treating addictive disorders in this way:

- Kindness
- Comfort
- Empathy
- Avoid confrontation
- Patience

As stated earlier, there is also evidence that a low level of empathy in addiction treatment can be toxic, that clients whose counselors show low levels of skill in accurate empathy have particularly poor outcomes relative to clients with high-empathy counselors (Valle, 1981), and even relative to self-help alone (Miller et al., 1980). In Valle's (1981) study, clients whose counselors showed low levels of the critical skills described by Carl Rogers were two to four times more likely to be drinking across 2 years of follow-up, relative to high-skill counselors' clients. Studies have illustrated that certain counselors are outliers in having outstandingly poor outcomes (Luborsky, McLellan, Woody, O'Brien, & Auerbach, 1985; McLellan, Woody, Luborsky, & Goehl, 1988; Project MATCH Research Group, 1998e). Screening for empathic skill when hiring addiction treatment personnel is not only possible (Miller, Moyers, Arciniega, Ernst, & Force-himes, 2005), but well justified as an evidence-based practice to improve client outcomes (Moyers & Miller, 2013). First, do no harm!

> Being empathic is itself an evidence-based practice.

In sum, empathy is not something that you *have* so much as something that you *do*. It is a learnable skill. Most counselors already think of themselves as empathic and "good listeners," but accurate empathy is a particular kind of listening that does not come naturally to most. Once you learn

> **BOX 4.1.** Personal Reflection: Learning to Listen
>
> The main emphasis in my own graduate training was on fairly directive behavior therapy, but along the way we were also exposed to the humanistic client-centered approach of Carl Rogers and the particular skill of accurate empathy. I found this kind of listening to be challenging and awkward at first, but something about it just felt right to me. I also found that clients responded very well even to my stumbling early efforts to listen well. When subsequently on internship, I found myself working on a ward for people with alcohol use disorders, and I fell back on these listening skills, mostly because I knew almost nothing about addictions. I let the clients be the experts on their own lives and problems and educate me. It turned out to be a helpful and enjoyable approach for both of us. I quickly developed both a real respect and appreciation for these people and their struggles and a curiosity that led me to the primary focus of my professional career. I have always enjoyed talking with people with addiction problems. The ability to listen in this way has also greatly enriched my personal as well as my professional life.
>
> What really surprised me, though, was how important empathy turned out to be in my subsequent treatment outcome research. I taught my own students both behavioral and client-centered treatment methods, as I had been trained, and it turned out that this ability to listen empathically was a very strong predictor of successful outcomes, even within a highly structured behavioral approach. That finding ultimately led me to the development of motivational interviewing, and to focus on the quality of counselor–client relationships.
>
> —W. R. M.

it, however, you have a remarkable gift to give not only to your clients, but to others around you (Miller, 2018).

Reflective Listening

It sounds easy enough. Just repeat back what the client says. It is the substance of parodies of Carl Rogers and of counselor characters in situation comedies.

Skillful reflective listening actually does far more than repeat what a client says. Simple repetition just tends to go around in circles. Try it for a while and you'll probably feel like you are getting nowhere. Instead, skillful reflective listening moves ahead, if only just a little at a time. It considers what the person has *not* quite spoken, but may mean. Instead of merely repeating whatever the client has just said, complex reflections offer what *might* be the next, as yet unspoken, sentence of the person's paragraph.

How do you know what a client *hasn't* said? There are many ways. Sometimes you pick it up from the person's nonverbal cues. Sometimes you're trying out a hypothesis about what the client might mean by a word or phrase that you heard. Perhaps you are voicing what, based on your own clinical experience, the person may be feeling in relation to what was said, or perhaps you remember something that your client told you two sessions ago and you make a connection. Not all reflections make brilliant leaps to the unspoken. Sometimes you do mostly summarize what the client said, or just substitute a synonym, particularly when you're not clear what is meant. If the person keeps on talking, keeps exploring, tells you something more, then you know you did it right.

In fact, that's how you learn this skill. What you are really doing when you offer a reflection is making a guess. Based on your own experience and what you heard, you're stating to the best of your ability what you think the person may have meant. It is a hypothesis, and you are testing it. When you state your hypothesis in the form of a good reflection, the client will either confirm or revise it. If you hit it on the head, the person is likely in some form to say "Yes . . . " and will continue to elaborate. If you missed it, the person will probably in some form say "No. . . ." and will continue to elaborate. Thus there is no penalty for missing. Either way you learn more about your client's experiencing, and so does the client. When your client continues to elaborate, that's your signal that you reflected well.

Sometimes, though, a person does not respond with a yes or no followed by elaboration. Sometimes what you see instead is a kind of defensiveness—a backing off, closing down, taking back, or arguing. That's usually a sign that your reflection was not accurate, or perhaps that you jumped too far ahead of your client. Psychoanalysts call it a "premature interpretation." It might also have something to do with your tone of voice. (The simple reflective statement "So you don't see any problems with your drinking" is quite different when adding a hint of sarcasm: "So *you* don't see *any* problems with your drinking!"). When you reflect well, the person accepts (even if correcting) what you said, and moves ahead. Once you know what to look for, you will continue for the rest of your counseling career to receive accurate feedback from your clients that helps you improve your skillfulness in reflective listening. That also, by the way, is how you get to be more accurate in your empathy. After listening reflectively to people for years and receiving immediate feedback about whether you got it right or not, you simply get better at guessing what people mean. You're more likely to get it right, and sometimes your clients regard you as a kind of wizard. "How did you know that?" It's not magic. It's practice with constant feedback.

Reflective listening is not a simple skill to learn. Be patient with yourself at first. This is a complex and demanding skill, but one that is very worth the time it requires. It is also something at which you can become increasingly adept through all the years of your life (Miller, 2018).

So what is a good reflection? First of all, it is a *statement* and not a question. The natural tendency is to ask your client if this is what he or she means. After all, you're not sure. Your reflection is just a guess. You might be wrong. Wouldn't it be better to *ask* your client if you're right? Here is one place where the natural instinct is misleading. Even though your intention in asking a question (rather than making a statement) is respectful, the actual *effect* of questioning is often to cause the person to step back. Questions demand something of the person, whereas statements do not. Consider the difference between these two counselor responses:

- "You're angry with me?"
- "You're angry with me."

Say them out loud. The first one is subtly different from the second. If your clinical antennae are like ours, the first one is more likely to cause the person to back away from the feeling, to deny it or qualify it. A simple statement, on the other hand, gives permission to continue exploring and experiencing. Until you get used to this, it can feel unnatural. The worry is that you are "putting words in the person's mouth," dictating what he or she means. Very rarely do people perceive good reflective listening in this way. They just keep going.

So a good reflection is a statement. It doesn't need any fancy words at the front. Stereotypic counselor responses such as "What I hear you saying is that you . . ." are unnecessary window dressing, and can be annoying after a few times. The only thing you need in most cases in order to begin a good reflection is the word "You." Consider this snippet from an initial session with a 33-year-old woman:

CLIENT: I'm not really sure why I'm even here, actually. There is so much going on in my life right now, I don't know if this is what I should be doing.

THERAPIST: You're feeling confused right now, and pretty over-whelmed.

CLIENT: Well, I'm just about to be kicked out of my apartment, and my ex says he's not going to pay child support any more. I already owe my lawyer a lot of money and I can't run up any more attorney fees.

THERAPIST: You're feeling at the end of your rope. So you wonder if you should even be here.

CLIENT: I just don't know what to do, and I know drinking is part of the problem, but is that what I should be focusing on right now?

THERAPIST: Seems like there might be more important things for you to worry about.

CLIENT: Like my kids. How am I going to feed them?

THERAPIST: You care a lot about your kids.

CLIENT: They're all I have! I just want them to grow up and be happy.

THERAPIST: And that, in part, is why you're here.

CLIENT: I guess so. I don't want them to have a drunk for a mother.

All of the therapist responses above are reflective listening statements. None of them is a straight parroting of what the client said. Also, all of them are statements rather than questions. Consider the potentially different impact if the counselor had instead asked:

- "Are you feeling overwhelmed?"

  or

- "So, do you think there are more important things to talk about than your drinking?"

  or

- "Do you care about your kids?"

  or

- "So is that why you're here?"

The difference may not seem very large, but the tone is changed if you turn it from a statement into a question just by inflecting your voice upward rather than downward at the end, or adding question words like "Do you . . . ?" It puts the person on the defensive, if only just a little, even though you didn't have that intention. Good reflections are better as statements rather than questions.

When you're listening with accurate empathy, there are also a lot of things that you're not doing. You're not giving advice, offering solutions, or asking probing questions. Neither are you warning, educating, persuading, or sympathizing. You're not agreeing or disagreeing, analyzing or diagnosing. Your whole attention is focused on following and accurately understanding the person's own perspectives, and that's work enough in itself.

Of course, reflection is not everything that you do, even at the outset of counseling. While it is an interesting and challenging exercise to try 100% reflective listening for even 10 minutes, counseling normally involves a dance back and forth between reflection and other types of communication.

> A good reflection is a statement, not a question.

We emphasize accurate empathy first, both because it appears to be a key to effective counseling and because other responses (like asking questions) are so much easier that it's tempting to overuse them when it might be better to listen.

OARS: Fundamental Counseling Skills

Reflection is one of four fundamental skills that form a client-centered foundation and safety net in counseling. When you're just getting started, or whenever you're feeling lost and unsure what to do next, you can always fall back to these fundamental four and be reasonably sure that you are helping and not harming your client. These four skills are summarized by the acronym OARS: Open questions, Affirmation, Reflection, and Summaries.

O: Open Questions

The first of these is asking open questions, with an emphasis on the O (open) rather than the Q (questions). Many counselors, we find, ask far too many questions, a majority of which are closed questions, ones that require a short answer. Open questions, in contrast, are not easily answered with a yes or no, or with short-answer information. They leave the client some room to move, to think, to explore. They invite the client's own reflection. Box 4.2 provides examples of closed and open questions.

A reasonably good rule of thumb is *never ask three questions in a row*. After an open question you should usually be listening and reflecting. Asking a question is not listening; rather, it creates an opportunity for you to listen. Another simple rule of thumb is to offer about two reflections for each question that you ask: a two-to-one ratio. Give it a try! Listen to a tape of an ordinary counseling session and count up the number of questions that you asked and the number of times you offered a reflective listening statement. We find that it's not uncommon for counselors to ask 10 or more questions per reflection.

There are times, to be sure, when you need to ask more questions. Some treatment programs require a structured intake interview, such as the Addiction Severity Index (see Chapter 5), that involve asking a preset series of questions. Here we offer two suggestions. First, try not to start off your counseling with a slew of questions. Asking a number of questions in a row, particularly closed questions, tends to create a mind-set of passivity in the client. If possible, just sit down and listen to your client for a while, even just for 15 minutes, before you start questioning. Ask an open question like "What brings you here today?" and then listen with curiosity and reflect.

Second, put a frame around the questions so that your client does not confuse them with the normal course of treatment. "In a little while I have a series of specific questions that we ask everyone [the frame], but before I do, I just want to hear in your own words what brings you here today [open question and opportunity for you to reflect]."

A final working rule of thumb that we recommend is to ask more open than closed questions. Of the questions that you do ask, try to make more than half of them be open questions that give you an opportunity to listen to something more than a short answer, and to reflect.

BOX 4.2. Closed and Open Questions

CLOSED QUESTIONS

- "How old are you?"
- "Do you live with your parents?"
- "When did you last use marijuana?"
- "Do you want to quit drinking?"
- "How many drinks did you have yesterday?"
- "Have you ever had a blackout?"
- "Isn't it time to do something different?"
- "Do you think you're an alcoholic?"
- "What do you want to do about cocaine—keep using, cut down, or quit?"
- "Whose idea was it to call us?"
- "How long has it been since you went for a few days without drinking?"
- "Do you belong to a church?"

OPEN QUESTIONS

- "What brings you here today?"
- "Tell me about your family."
- "What do you like about marijuana?"
- "And what's the other side . . . in what ways has drinking not been so good to you?"
- "How does alcohol affect you?"
- "So what are you thinking about your drinking at this point?"
- "What do you want to do about cocaine?"
- "How have you been feeling this week?"
- "How did you happen to call us?"
- "Tell me about the last time you felt really good without drugs or beer."
- "How, if at all, is religion or spirituality important in your life?"

So when it comes to using questions in counseling:

- Try listening before you ask a lot of questions.
- Avoid asking three questions in a row.
- Shoot for more than half of your questions to be open questions.
- Offer about two reflections for each question that you ask.

If you listen to recordings of some of your counseling sessions you can literally count reflections, open and closed questions, and see how you're doing.

A: Affirm

The second of the four OARS skills is to *affirm* your client. This sounds easy enough. Look for opportunities to comment positively. Thank your client for being on time or for coming in at all, even if late. Find things that you can genuinely appreciate, admire, respect. Reframe client experiences as laudable strengths.

> CLIENT: I've been on the street for 3 years, and I've had to do some bad stuff to get drugs. I've been beaten, busted, OD'd, hungry, cold—you name it.
>
> COUNSELOR: You've been through an awful lot. You're a real survivor. I don't know if I could handle what you've been through.

Look for successes, even small ones, in the client's past or present and affirm them. Here's the familiar choice of half-full or half-empty. After years of having between 8 and 12 drinks every night, and some initial success in cutting back, a client wanted to make it through a whole week without drinking at all. On Monday she came back to the clinic looking dejected and defeated. She had had six alcohol-free days, but then on the weekend she had two drinks on Saturday. You could shame her: "I thought you said that you weren't going to drink this week! What happened?" Why not instead congratulate her on her first 6 days of sobriety in years, be impressed that she somehow managed to go from about 70 drinks a week down to two, and ask her how she did it?

Where did the crazy idea come from that if you can just make people feel bad enough, then they will change? Most clients, we find, have already been rather thoroughly shamed, humiliated, and blamed in their lives before coming to see us, and more of the same is unlikely to help. One of the many insights of Carl Rogers was that when people feel unacceptable, they are immobilized and unable to change. It is, paradoxically, when people experience acceptance that they are freed to change.

R: Reflect

This one we have already discussed. Reflective listening is perhaps the most important of the four OARS skills.

S: Summarize

Beyond immediate reflections, it is helpful to pull together in short summaries what your clients say. This shows and requires that you have been listening carefully, which is an important message in itself. Summaries also allow you to emphasize and integrate what a client has offered. At least three kinds of summaries can be helpful.

First, there are *collecting* summaries. These happen in the midst of a counseling session, and pull together several related things that the person has said. If, for example, you have asked about ways in which drinking has had negative effects in the person's life, you begin collecting those mentally, and in addition to reflecting them as you go, you also periodically give them back to the client like a small bouquet. Then you continue the process by asking, "What else?"

> "So far you've told me that you don't like how you feel in the morning when you get up, and you know that your work has suffered some from being hung over. Your daughter has also been worried about you, and has told you she thinks that you drink too much—which kind of annoys you. You've also noticed that sometimes you don't remember things that happened. What else?"

Second, there are *linking* summaries, which make a connection between something that the person has just said and material that was offered earlier, perhaps in a prior session. Again you are communicating that you remember and regard as important what your client tells you. Beyond this, the point of a linking summary is to suggest a connection, to test a hypothesis that two things you've learned might be related.

> "I wonder if this feeling of panic that you're talking about is somewhat like how you felt when your husband suddenly announced that he wanted a divorce. Both of them seem to involve a feeling of being out of control, which really upsets you."

There is some similarity here to analytic interpretations, where the therapist does not want to be too far ahead of the person's current awareness. The primary purpose of a linking summary is to increase understanding (both your own and the client's) of what the person is experiencing.

Finally, there are *transitional summaries*. These tend to be a bit longer, and are used to end a session or to shift from one task or topic to another within a session. They draw together what has already transpired, and point toward something new.

> "OK—here's what I understand about your situation from what you've told me today, and let me know if I've missed something important. You came here primarily because your probation officer sent you, and you understand now that you could get treatment somewhere else if you're not happy here. What got you in trouble was the misfortune of having cocaine in your car when you were pulled over, and it also turned up in the drug test they gave you. It seems to you that it's really nobody's business what you do, and that you were just unlucky, but now you have this probation officer watching over you. There have

been some times when you used quite a bit more than you meant to, and felt scared and paranoid. And you've spent a lot of money on drugs, which has created some financial problems for you. You really don't like having to be here, but as you've said, you might as well make the best of it. Did I miss anything?"

With these four fundamental OARS skills, you can often make substantial progress. This client-centered style can be quite helpful in itself. It's a good way to begin a counseling session, and as we've said, you can always fall back on the OARS when you're not sure what to do. Confident skillfulness in this way of being with people is an excellent foundation for further counseling interventions.

> When people experience acceptance they are freed to change.

Staying Focused

A simple but important principle in effective treatment is to be professional and focused in your counseling. That may sound self-evident, but a surprising amount of time in addiction treatment can be spent in informal "chat" that is unrelated to clients' treatment needs (Martino, Ball, Nich, Frankforter, & Carroll, 2009). In one study with Hispanic clients, the amount of such off-topic chat was *inversely* related to client motivation for change and retention in addiction treatment (Bamatter et al., 2010). This is consistent with the more general finding in psychotherapy research that better outcomes are associated with the therapist's adherence to an organized, coherent theoretical approach (Beutler, Machado, & Neufeldt, 1994).

Taking an Active Interest in Your Client

It is important for clients to be actively involved in their own recovery. That is one reason for a client-centered foundation in counseling, rather than leaving clients in a passive role. A good predictor of successful behavior change is the extent to which a person is actively involved, doing things that are steps toward change.

At the same time, active involvement in counseling is a two-way street. It should be clear to clients that you are actively engaged and interested in working with them. Don't hesitate to take steps that can facilitate change. Consider how you might make a referral for other services (see Chapter 8). Is it best just to give your client the phone number, leaving the responsibility to him or her to make the call, or might it be better to place the call while the person is still in your office? Some favor the former, thinking that it is vital for clients to take personal responsibility (which it is). Consider, however, that clients are about three times more likely to actually complete the referral if you place the call together while they are still in your office (Kogan, 1957). Perhaps they can get there first, and then work on personal responsibility! Similarly, it has been known for a long time that people are about twice as likely to return after an initial visit or after a missed appointment if you send them a short handwritten note of encouragement (not a form letter) or give them a simple telephone call to say that you look forward to working with them (Gottheil, Sterling, & Weinstein, 1997a; Koumans & Muller, 1967; Koumans, Muller, & Miller, 1967; Nirenberg, Sobell, & Sobell, 1980; Panepinto & Higgins, 1969). Such simple messages of caring and active interest require little time, but can make a big difference.

Menschenbild

The client-centered counseling style described in this chapter has been shown to improve client outcomes in the treatment of addictions, and it can meld well with other counseling methods. It is unclear exactly why this particular therapeutic style works so well, but we suspect that it has something to do with one's underlying assumptions about people. Each therapeutic approach, at least when put into practice, includes an implicit picture of human nature. A useful noun for this is the German *Menschenbild*—literally, one's picture of people. A similar noun, *Weltanschauung,* may be more familiar to psychotherapists, referring to one's broad assumptions about the nature of the world and reality. *Menschenbild* is more specific: it's how we think about people.

Within the context of counseling, your *Menschenbild* can make a great difference. One important dimension has to do with your belief in people's potential to change. In a classic study, researchers conducted psychological testing with clients in three alcoholism treatment programs, and in appreciation for the staff's cooperation they identified those clients who had particularly high alcoholism recovery potential according to the tests. Sure enough, the staff did find that those clients were more motivated, attended sessions on time, and worked harder in treatment. Indeed, a year after discharge, these clients were more likely to be abstinent and employed, and had had fewer slips and longer spans of sobriety. The secret of the study was that these "high potential" clients had actually been chosen at random, and were in no way different from others in the same treatment programs, *except* that their counselors had been told that they would do particularly well (Leake & King, 1977). Belief in your clients' potential (or lack thereof) is a self-fulfilling prophecy. In a still older study, researchers listened to doctors' tone of voice when interviewed about people with alcoholism, having filtered out the content so that raters could not understand what was being said, only *how* it was being said. Voice tone strongly predicted whether patients would complete a referral: the more anger and irritation in the doctor's voice, the less likely it was that the person would go to treatment (Milmoe, Rosenthal, Blane, Chafetz, & Wolf, 1967).

The person-centered approach that we advocate focuses primarily on the client's own strengths, motivations, and potential for change. An opposite perspective focuses on *deficits,* that which clients are assumed to lack. As discussed earlier, a deficit model communicates to the client "I have what you need, and I'll give it to you," whereas a client-centered approach implies that "*You* have what you need, and together we'll find it." It communicates *potential*: hope, empowerment, and responsibility. Being a deficit detective is easy enough. Finding clients' own strengths and resources takes some intentional effort.

Another important dimension of *Menschenbild* has to do with the counselor's degree of support for client autonomy (Deci & Ryan, 2008). At one extreme pole of this dimension is the assumption that people (in this case, people with addictions) are fundamentally flawed and require external controls. They cannot be given choice, allowed to think for themselves, or trusted to make good decisions. They simply lack the necessary insight, honesty, maturity, skills, character, or self-control. This view, of course, suggests the need for a no-nonsense, authoritarian approach. At the opposite pole is the *Menschenbild* of Carl Rogers and the human potential movement: that people have within them an inherent tendency and potential to grow in a positive direction, given the proper therapeutic conditions. Each person has a natural and positive self that can be realized or suppressed. Somewhere in between these extremes is a tabula rasa view that people have no inherent nature at all, but are simply shaped by their environment. Depending on which view of human nature they affirm, counselors might be more trustful or less inclined to honor the client's autonomy and choice.

There is a sense, however, in which client autonomy is just a reality. Short of extreme restriction of freedom (as in imprisonment), people do in fact determine their own goals and make their own decisions. To tell someone, "You can't drink," does not acknowledge the truth. In one early and somewhat naïve study, we randomly assigned problem drinkers to either an abstinence or a moderation goal (Graber & Miller, 1988). People in both groups felt equally free to ignore the goal that we had set for them. A belief that "You can't let clients choose" implies an impossible level of counselor power. The ability to choose cannot be taken away. Viktor Frankl (1969) observed that even under the extreme privations of a Nazi concentration camp, people still made life-shaping choices about how they would think and be. Suicide crisis counselors know that people in distress do ultimately retain autonomous choice, and yet there is much that can be done to help them. We find it helpful to acknowledge, honor, and work within the client's autonomy.

Finally, we commend thinking of your client as your partner, as a collaborator or co-counselor (Gordon & Edwards, 1997; Miller & Rollnick, 2013). No one knows more about clients than they do themselves, and it is vital to draw on their own expertise and wisdom. After all, recovery is a long-term process, and the hours you share with clients represent but a tiny part of their lives. A collaborative partnership allows you to move together toward change.

But I Don't Have *Time* for Listening!

Many professionals don't have the luxury of 50-minute hours for counseling and feel the pressure of heavy caseloads with short visits. The temptation is to fall back on a director role and just tell people what to do. Yet empathic listening is a valuable skill that can be practiced in just a few minutes if that's all you have, and even brief spans of good listening can make a difference (see Chapter 9). Empathic listening also turns out to be a good tool even for collecting information and making sure that you're not missing something important. Just a few minutes of good listening can help the people you serve feel cared for and understood. If you have a lot to do—information to collect and convey, multiple problems to address, dual roles to fulfill—it may be all the more important to listen well in the short time you have. There is a paradox here: slow is fast and fast is slow. If you act like you only have a few minutes, it seems to take a long time to get a task done. If you act (and feel) like you have all day, it may only take a few minutes (Roberts, 2001). Don't be afraid that if you open the door to listening, you'll never be able to close it again. Sometimes people keep talking and repeating themselves precisely because they're not sure that you are hearing them.

KEY POINTS

❧ Engaging is task number one, a vital first process that lays the foundation for all that follows.

❧ Treatment providers vary widely in their effectiveness. A significant determinant of clients' outcomes is the person who treats them.

❧ It matters not only what treatment you provide, but also how you provide it. Therapeutic relationship matters.

❧ Accurate empathy—the learnable skill of reflective listening—has a particularly positive impact on addiction treatment retention and outcomes, and its absence can be harmful.

🦙 Think of your clients as partners in the change process. No one knows more about them, and they do get to make their own choices about whether and how they will change.

🦙 Counselor perceptions of clients can be self-fulfilling prophecies. To some extent in counseling, what you expect is what you get.

Reflection Questions

Q Given your life experience thus far, how optimistic or pessimistic do you feel about the likelihood that people will recover from addiction?

Q Listen to a recording of your own counseling and count the OARS.

Q After treating people with addictions, do you feel more like you've been dancing or wrestling with them?

CHAPTER 5

Screening, Evaluation, and Diagnosis

In this chapter we consider three assessment tasks—screening, evaluation, and diagnosis—and how they inform addiction treatment. As discussed in the preceding chapter, we don't think of assessment as a prelude to but rather an ongoing part of treatment. "What do I really *need* to know at this point in order to proceed with helping this person? How will this information be useful?" These three assessment tasks are interrelated and serve different purposes.

Screening for SUDs

People with SUDs and their family members turn up in many different settings including emergency rooms, primary care and mental health clinics, correctional systems, and social service agencies (Rose & Zweben, 2003; Rose, Zweben, Ockert, & Baier, 2014; Rose, Zweben, & Stoffel, 1999). Some examples might include a pregnant woman who is seen in a mental health clinic for intimate partner violence, a professional coming to an employee assistance program for poor job performance, a 24-year-old treated in an emergency room after a motor vehicle accident, and a 75-year-old seen for depression in a social service agency. In such settings, staff may be less familiar with symptoms of addiction that present as injuries, family conflict, or mental health problems. Thus, despite the high incidence of SUDs in health and social service settings, they are often missed (Weisner, 2002), with only the more debilitated individuals being recognized. This means that many people who could benefit from addiction treatment do not receive it (Dawson, Grant, Stinson, & Chou, 2006). Routine screening in such settings helps to prevent this.

Screening is sometimes confused with diagnosis (confirming the presence of a disorder) and evaluation (doing a more thorough assessment in order to understand a problem). By definition, screening procedures are meant to be overinclusive, to detect the *possible* presence of a problem and the need for further evaluation.

There are two kinds of possible mistakes that can occur in screening: a *false positive* and a *false negative*. Think of a drug screen. A false positive occurs if the screen says that a drug is present (e.g., in breath or urine) when in fact it is not. A false negative happens if the test says that a drug is not present when in fact it is. The relative frequency of these mistakes is determined by where one sets the test's "cutoff point": the sensitivity threshold at which the test says "yes" versus "no" (Cherpitel, 1995). A false negative indicates no need for further evaluation, which means that a potentially important condition is missed. A false positive results in unnecessary additional evaluation to confirm the absence of a condition. In the case of drug screens, a positive finding typically results in a different (usually more expensive) test to confirm or disconfirm the presence of the drug. Ideally a screen would give no false negatives or false positives, but in reality this is rarely achievable. In order to have a lower false negative rate, it is necessary to accept a larger number of false positives. A test's *sensitivity* is its ability to accurately detect true positives and avoid false negative errors. A test's *specificity* is its accuracy detecting true negatives and avoiding false positive errors. The cutoff point of a screening test is meant to offer the right balance between sensitivity and specificity.

Consider a situation in which many people are seen for health or social services, and the goal is to identify which people also have addiction problems that may complicate outcomes and that need to be addressed. The service is already busy, so ideally a screening procedure would be fairly simple and not require much time. It should also be fairly sensitive in case finding (to avoid false negatives) but also reasonably specific (so as not to yield false positives that trigger unnecessary additional evaluation). Add to this the complexity that addiction problems occur all along a continuum of severity, as well as the desire to detect problems early instead of waiting for them to become severe and entrenched, and screening can be quite a complex task (Cooney, Zweben, & Fleming, 1995).

> Screening is sometimes confused with diagnosis and evaluation.

People seeking help in specialist addiction treatment settings are more likely to be aware of and open about their substance use problems. Frequently they have already experienced significant consequences of addictive behaviors (e.g., loss of job, family conflict, and incarceration) as well as pressure from family and friends to seek help. In a way, just walking through the door of an addiction treatment setting is a positive screen indicating a need for further evaluation.

In contrast, people seen in general health and social service settings may not have yet experienced severe consequences or pressures resulting from their substance use. Consequently, they often do not think of themselves as having "a problem," let alone a need for addiction treatment. They come for help with other concerns such as medical or emotional problems, and may or may not have made a connection between their concerns and their substance use (Cooney et al., 1995). Reluctance may also be related to stigma attached to addiction treatment. Thus, people seeking health and social services are sometimes surprised, even defensive, about being screened for SUDs. In particular settings (such as child welfare services, employee assistance, and criminal justice) there may be formidable obstacles to honesty about substance use (Zweben, Rose, Stout, & Zywiak, 2003).

A few guidelines can be helpful in presenting screening questions to clients, particularly when used outside specialist addiction services:

- Give clear instructions for how to complete the screening task.
- Provide accurate assurances about privacy and confidentiality.
- Explain (as appropriate) that this is a routine procedure used with all clients.
- Listen to and reflect any concerns that are raised (see Chapter 4)— for example, "You're wondering why we're asking about your alcohol/drug use when you came into the emergency room to be treated for your injury."
- Answer the person's questions clearly and honestly.

Screening Tools

A variety of screening tools are available, many of them in the public domain and thus free of charge. (Links to screening and assessment measures relevant to addiction treatment are available in Box 5.4, on pp. 89–90.) Considerations in selecting an appropriate screener include the instrument's demonstrated sensitivity and specificity, its feasibility in your setting (e.g., length, ease of administration, and cost), and the particular populations with whom it is to be used (e.g., language and reading level).

Clinical Questions

Perhaps the most common screening approach is to ask one or more carefully worded questions during the course of conversation. Substance-focused items can be intermixed with questions about other health or social issues to reduce defensiveness. A simple screening question can be employed to identify unhealthy alcohol or drug use such as:

- "How many times in the past year have you had five or more drinks (men) or four or more drinks (women) in a day?"

  or

- "How many times in the past year have you used illegal drugs or prescription medication for nonmedical reasons?"

In one study, this single question identified 86% of individuals with an alcohol use disorder (Williams & Vinson, 2001). Similarly, a simple single question yielded good results (100% sensitivity, 74% specificity) in screening for SUDs in primary care (Smith, Schmidt, Allensworth-Davies, & Saitz, 2010). A good single screening question can be just as effective as longer, more complicated screening devices for identifying unhealthy alcohol or drug use (Saitz, Cheng, Allensworth-Davies, Winter, & Smith, 2014). A major advantage of single questions is that they can be readily used in health care settings where large numbers of people with SUDs are seen.

Other screening questions probe for problematic patterns and effects. An early four-question screener for alcohol problems was the CAGE (Ewing, 1984). The usual cutoff point indicating a need for further evaluation is two "Yes" answers. It is sensible to precede these questions by asking "Do you sometimes drink beer, wine, or other alcohol beverages?" because the "Have you ever" format of these questions can produce false positives for people who have quit drinking.

Various modifications of the CAGE have been developed and tested. A modification based on the four-item Rapid Alcohol Problems Screen (RAPS4) further improved on the sensitivity of the CAGE (Cherpitel, 2006). The CAGE-AID (Brown & Rounds, 1995) changed the wording of questions to address alcohol and other drugs simultaneously. Other modifications of the CAGE have been developed specifically for use with pregnant women (Russell et al., 1994) and older adults (Fleming, 2002).

A single screening question is sufficient in many settings.

Questionnaires

The Alcohol Use Disorders Identification Test (AUDIT) is a state-of-the-art screening instrument developed by the World Health Organization (Babor & Grant, 1989; Babor, Higgins-Biddle, Saunders, & Monteiro, 2001). It has been validated cross-culturally in various nations and languages. Its 10 items deal with amount and frequency of drinking, alcohol dependence symptoms, personal problems, and social problems. Scores of 0–7 are indicative of low problem severity, while those of 26–40 suggest high problem severity. The AUDIT has a consistent time reference for items (i.e., the last 12 months), and its specificity remains strong for people with other behavioral health problems (Hulse & Tait, 2003). The AUDIT has also been adapted as a screening tool for detecting both alcohol and drug problems called the AUDIT-ID (Includes other Drugs; Campbell, Hoffmann, Madson, & Melchert, 2003).

Concern with gender differences led to a female-specific version of the AUDIT termed the AUDIT-C, which has been tested with women veterans and college students (Chavez, Williams, Lapham, & Bradley, 2012; DeMartini & Carey, 2012). In this version, the frequency of drinking is reduced to "four" or more drinks on occasion" rather than "six or more drinks" as in the original questionnaire. Also, lower cutoff points for alcohol use are used to categorize women as positive for AUD. The AUDIT-C has been shown to be more sensitive than the original AUDIT in detecting AUDs with women (DeMartini & Carey, 2012). In one study with female veterans, nearly half of women with positive scores on the AUDIT-C reported lifetime domestic violence, in contrast to 30% prevalence in the overall sample (Chavez et al., 2012).

There is a parallel Drug Use Disorders Identification Test (DUDIT) focused on illicit drugs (Berman, Bergman, Palmstierna, & Schlyter, 2005; Durbeej et al., 2010; Dwyer & Fraser, 2017; Hildebrand, 2015). The DUDIT is relatively easy to administer, and has been successful in identifying SUDs with diverse client populations in outpatient, inpatient, and criminal justice settings (Hildebrand, 2015). As with the AUDIT-C, different DUDIT threshold scores for harmful use have been set for men and women (Dwyer & Fraser, 2017).

The National Institute on Drug Abuse (2010) encourages screening and brief intervention in general medical settings and produced an instrument for this purpose, the NIDA-Modified Alcohol, Smoking and Substance Involvement Screening Test (NM-ASSIST) based on a World Health Organization instrument (WHO ASSIST Working Group, 2002). A longer interview, it first queries lifetime and then recent use in 12 drug classes, and level of risk to determine the kinds of interventions that may be needed for various patient subgroups. The ASSIST has been used in medical and correctional settings with adolescent and adult patient populations (Gryczynski et al., 2014; McNeely, Strauss, Rotrosen, Ramautar, & Gourevitch, 2016; McNeely et al., 2014; Wolff & Shi, 2015).

The audio-guided computer-assisted self-interview (ACASI) version of the ASSIST is a valuable alternative to interviewer-administered ASSIST in screening for SUDs in clinical settings (McNeely et al., 2016, 2014; Wolff & Shi, 2015). The ACASI-ASSIST has comparable rates of sensitivity and specificity with the interviewer-administered version. The audio helps in gathering accurate data with clients who have reading difficulties (text is read aloud), reduces sensitivity to stigmatized questions, and can be translated into multiple languages (McNeely et al., 2016). What is noteworthy is that the ACASI-ASSIST requires less time than the interviewer-administered

ASSIST to administer and can be completed either at home or in a waiting room with data directly entered in electronic health records (McNeely et al., 2016). All these factors are helpful for case finding in busy medical settings.

Biological Markers

In some cases it might be helpful to include biological measures such as lab tests along with self-reports to obtain accurate screening data, particularly when the honesty of a self-report is in question. Such might be the case for people whose employment or legal status is at risk due to drinking or drug use. One advantage of biological measures is that, unlike self-report measures, they cannot be influenced by motivational or cognitive issues (Babor & Higgins-Biddle, 2000). Biological measures may also increase the accuracy of self-report by serving as a "bogus pipeline;" that is, individuals are more likely to provide accurate self-reports if they believe that the information will be corroborated by other measures such as laboratory tests.

TOBACCO USE

Plasma samples of cotinine (a by-product of nicotine metabolism) are widely used in smoking cessation studies (Heatherton, Kozlowski, Frecker, & Fagerstrom, 1991). Cotinine concentrations are considered a reliable device to detect the presence and intensity of smoking and to measure changes in tobacco use across time (SRNT Subcommittee on Biochemical Verification of Tobacco Use and Cessation, 2002).

HEAVY DRINKING

Three markers of recent heavy drinking are gamma-glutamyltranspeptidase (GGT), carbohydrate-deficient transferrin (CDT), and ethyl glucuronide (ETG). Such tests are not a replacement for self-report. They are assayed to *confirm* self-reports of abstinence or no heavy drinking. GGT and CDT tests have low sensitivity (high false negatives), identifying only 10–30% of problem drinkers (Anton, Lieber, Tabakoff, & CDTect Study Group, 2002; Babor & Higgins-Biddle, 2000). Further, GGT and CDT levels are significantly affected by age, gender, and smoking status, and GGT is heavily influenced by liver disease and medication use. ETG provides a sensitive and reliable biomarker of recent alcohol consumption and is detectable in urine for up to 3 days after drinking depending on the amount of alcohol consumed (Jatlow & O'Malley, 2010; Sarkola, Dahl, Eriksson, & Helander, 2003; Wurst et al., 2006; Wurst, Wiesbeck, Metzger, & Weinmann, 2004). Hair analysis is also a useful means for verifying self-report, even for heavy drinking (Morini & Polettini, 2009).

DRUG USE

Similar challenges are found in assessing drug use. Urine screens for cocaine, opiates, and amphetamines have only a 2- to 3-day window for detection, and more than a week window for heavy marijuana use (Anton, Litten, & Allen, 1995). The urine screen is strongly influenced by the individual's metabolism, use of legally prescribed drugs, route of administration (injection or orally), and its potency (Connors, Donovan, & DiClemente, 2001). False negatives are common. Alternative biological markers have been developed and tested. One such approach is an exhaled breath test for detecting drug use (Skoglund, Hermansson, & Beck, 2015). Clients' breath is collected by having them blow into a plastic bag which is then sealed and stored for later analysis. Preliminary study found breath tests to be superior to both plasma and urine samples in detecting self-reported recent (1–2 days) cannabis use (Skoglund et al., 2015).

Based on research findings, we recommend that lab tests serve mainly as adjunctive aids in screening for SUDs; that they be used in combination with standardized screening devices, clinical interviews, and collateral reports; and that they be used mainly when self-reports are considered to be suspect (Anton et al., 2002; Babor & Higgins-Biddle, 2000).

Subtle Tests

In response to concerns about honesty, many attempts have been made since the 1950s to develop subtle or indirect screening instruments to detect possible SUDs despite respondents' denial and fabrication. Such indirect scales have typically included items that bear no obvious relationship to alcohol/drug problems, but are purported to have high sensitivity and specificity even in the face of intentional dishonesty. A short summary of six decades of research on indirect scales is that they have no better sensitivity and specificity than simpler, more direct, and free public domain scales that ask about alcohol/drug use, such as those described above (Feldstein & Miller, 2007; Miller, 1976). Therefore, we do not recommend using "subtle" scales, and certainly not relying on them to make important decisions about clients.

Evaluating Addiction Problems

Screening casts a wide net to identify a broad range of people with possible SUDs. Diagnosis, as discussed later in this chapter, identifies a subset of these people who fall above a certain level of severity. Neither screening nor diagnosis, however, provides much information about what is actually happening in a particular person's life and substance use, why problems are emerging, and what treatment options would be most appropriate to try. These tasks—to understand the nature and causes of the individual's particular situation and to consider possible routes to change—lie at the heart of evaluation. A more comprehensive evaluation of this kind generates working hypotheses about what could be most likely to help, and what concerns may need priority attention. This in turn yields information to formulate change goals and treatment plans (see Chapter 7).

Conducting a Multidimensional Evaluation

Addictions, like diamonds, have multiple facets. As discussed in Chapter 2, knowing about one dimension tells you surprisingly little about the others. For example, the amount and pattern of substance use is only modestly correlated with the extent of negative health and social consequences or

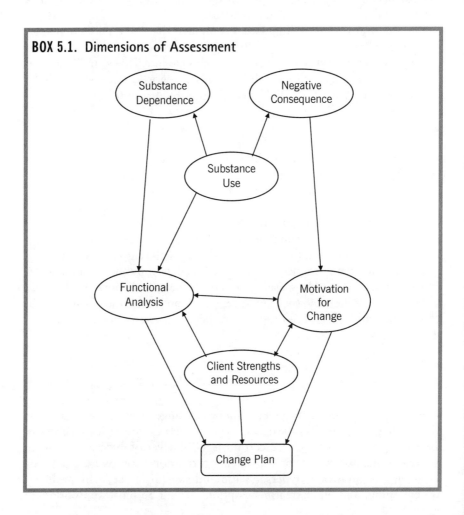

BOX 5.1. Dimensions of Assessment

the person's level of substance dependence. There are also important contextual factors to consider. What events or conditions are most likely to interfere with recovery? How does the person's substance use relate to and affect his or her employment, family, social networks, emotional states, and stressors? What resources does the person have in terms of coping skills, personal strengths, and social support? What motivates this person; what does he or she care about?

Obviously, such a thorough evaluation can take some time, and we do not encourage delaying treatment for extensive evaluation. Think of treatment as beginning with the very first contact, and of evaluation as an ongoing process interwoven with treatment (Poston & Hanson, 2010). Evaluation can be done sequentially, and indeed as treatment proceeds it becomes clearer what you need to know next.

With that said, we discuss four broad domains for evaluation that encompass the seven dimensions of addiction discussed in Chapter 2, areas in which to gather information over time during the process of treatment: (1) nature and severity of substance use and problems, (2) motivation for change, (3) client strengths and resources, and (4) functional analysis (see Box 5.1).

> Think of treatment as beginning with the very first contact.

Nature and Severity of Substance Use and Problems

SUBSTANCE USE

One obvious domain to assess in addiction treatment is substance use. What drug(s) has the person been using during the past few months? How were the drugs taken (orally, intravenously, etc.), how much, how often, and what is the pattern (e.g., steady maintenance, periodic binge use)? This can quickly devolve into a very long series of closed questions, which is not an optimal way to establish rapport and engage clients (see Chapter 4). A simple start is to ask clients to tell you about what they have been using, how, and how often (an open question), and then listen.

If more detail is truly needed, there are some structured interview formats to make sure you cover all the possibilities. These include the above-mentioned ASSIST instruments and the Form 90 interview (Miller, 1996a; Tonigan, Miller, & Brown, 1994; Westerberg, Tonigan, & Miller, 1998), both available free of charge in the public domain. They survey patterns of use for a dozen drug categories. The Form 90 includes a modified time line follow-back method (L. C. Sobell & Sobell, 1992, 1996), reconstructing drug use across a 90-day calendar. A reliable measure of nicotine dependence is the Fagerstrom scale, also a good predictor of smoking cessation (Heatherton et al., 1991). Changes in cigarette smoking over time can be reliably captured on the Fagerstrom scale (Baker et al., 2007).

NEGATIVE CONSEQUENCES

One indication of the severity of SUDs is the extent to which substance use has caused adverse consequences in the person's life and family. The Drinker Inventory of Consequences (DrInC; Forcehimes, Tonigan, Miller, Kenna, & Baer, 2007; Miller, Tonigan, & Longabaugh, 1995) was designed as a relatively pure measure of alcohol-related problems. It is in the public domain, easily administered in paper-and-pencil form, and covers five problems areas: physical, social responsibility, intrapersonal, impulse control, and interpersonal. Scores derived on this measure can be placed along a continuum of severity. The parallel Inventory of Drug Use Consequences (InDUC; Tonigan & Miller, 2002) assesses negative consequences of alcohol/drug use more generally. These instruments can be motivationally useful as well, because they connect substance use with current problems and hassles that the client might want to change (Maisto & McKay, 1995).

The Addiction Severity Index (ASI; McLellan et al., 1992, 1990) is a psychometrically sound, multidimensional public domain interview examining severity of problems in five different areas that may be affected by SUDs: medical, employment, legal, family relations, and psychological. It assesses both client's and interviewer's perceptions of problems. Interviewers require special training in the ASI to obtain valid information. A commercial computer-administered version of the ASI is also available (Butler et al., 2001). Along with motivational feedback, the ASI can be useful to develop a treatment plan specifically targeting problem areas that abstinence alone may not resolve. Clients who receive additional services to address these troublesome areas fare better than those who do not (McLellan et al., 1997, 1999).

DEPENDENCE

Another indication of severity is the extent to which clients have developed behavioral or physiological dependence on their preferred drugs. The potential for withdrawal syndrome and need for supervised withdrawal management is one important issue in addiction treatment (see Chapter 6). The broader behavioral spectrum of SUDs outlined in DSM-5 (American Psychiatric Association, 2013) can also be used to rate severity, and is reliably measurable (Grant et al., 2003, 2014).

Motivation for Change

A second important domain is the client's current motivation for change in substance use. Motivation is one of the more consistent predictors of how clients will fare in addiction treatment. Higher levels of motivation have been associated with better adherence and more favorable outcomes in

---

BOX 5.2. Personal Reflection: How Useful Is Assessment?

I must admit that I am rather ambivalent about assessment. I have personally devoted countless hours to developing and evaluating clinical assessment scales for the addiction treatment field. I know well how challenging it is to measure things reliably, even substance use itself. And there is something satisfying about having clear objective numbers that allow us to compare a unique individual with broader norms or to measure a degree of change. When I go for a health checkup, my vital signs and lab tests are checked against norms and my past values to see if any of my aging functions are going astray. Somehow that feels more solid than my doctor just looking me over and pronouncing me healthy or not. Reliable measures are also among the tools of clinical science, without which most of the research on which this book is based would not have been possible.

But I also share Carl Rogers's healthy skepticism about the value of all this measuring of human beings. When we have asked a lot of questions and taken some measures, we can feel like we have *done* something, although our clients may not share that confidence. Questions can get in the way of listening, of understanding, of really engaging with our clients. In a treatment program that I directed, the intake process had consisted of about 4 hours of questions before a person ever got to see a counselor. I asked how much we really needed to know in order to get paid for a first session, and it turned out to be about 20 minutes' worth of information. So I had our most senior counselors, rather than clerks, be the first people a new client would see, and I told them to start with this statement: "After a while I'm going to ask you some questions that we need to ask everyone, but right now I just want to know why you're here, what's happening in your life, and what you hope we might be able to do for you." They spent 30 minutes hearing the client's story, using good reflective listening skills, and when the half hour came and it was time to ask our standard questions, they found that they already knew the answers to most of them. Our retention rate went way up; we didn't have so many people drop out during those first visits; and the clients often wanted very much to stay with the counselor who did their intake. They had engaged from the very first session because someone listened to them. Relatively simple systemic changes like this can significantly decrease no-shows and dropouts, reduce waiting lists, and enhance engagement in treatment (Rukowski et al., 2010).

—W. R. M.

---

several addiction treatment trials (Burke, Arkowitz, & Dunn, 2002; Donovan & Rosengren, 1999; Litt, Kadden, Cooney, & Kabela, 2003; Zweben & Zuckoff, 2002).

Public domain questionnaires assessing motivation are available for clients to complete in or between sessions. Some of these are open-ended, and can be applied to any particular behavior change. The original "stages of change" measure is the University of Rhode Island Change Assessment (URICA; Abellanas & McLellan, 1993; DiClemente & Hughes, 1990).

The URICA has good reliability and predictive validity with alcohol clients (Carbonari & DiClemente, 2000; DiClemente, Doyle, & Donovan, 2009; Prochaska & DiClemente, 1992). Items refer to problems generically but can be focused specifically toward substance use. Various subscales were developed by clustering items reflecting the four stages of change (i.e., pre-contemplation, contemplation, action, and maintenance; Connors et al., 2001; Donovan, 1995, 2013). Individuals are categorized as being in a particular stage of change based on the scale where they score highest. With time constraints, a shorter 12-item form of the URICA is also available (Connors et al., 2001; downloadable from *www.umbc.edu/psyc/habits/content/ttm_measures/index.html*).

Simple rating scale "rulers" can be used to assess motivation for change in a clinical interview. For example:

- *"On a 0–10 scale, how important would you say it is for you to change your _____ use?"*
- *"On a 0–10 scale, how confident are you that you could make a change in your _____ use?"*

Similarly, the 12-item Change Questionnaire was based on the natural language of motivation for change (Miller & Johnson, 2008). A factor analysis pointed to three items (on a 0–10 disagree–agree scale) that accounted for 81% of variance, and that can be incorporated in a clinical interview:

- Importance: "It is important for me to _____."
- Ability: "I could _____."
- Commitment: "I am trying to _____."

Other public domain instruments specifically measure motivation for change in substance use. These include the 12-item Readiness to Change Questionnaire (Rollnick, Heather, Gold, & Hall, 1992) and the 19-item Stages of Change Readiness and Treatment Eagerness Scale (SOCRATES; Miller & Tonigan, 1996). The 10-point rating items like those above do converge well with longer motivation measures such as the SOCRATES and are easier to administer (Maisto et al., 2011).

Another important aspect of motivation is the client's reasons for continuing drug use, which essentially work against change (S. A. Brown, Goldman, Inn, & Anderson, 1980; Goldman et al., 1999). In a clinical interview you can simply ask a client, "What do you like about using _____? What does it do for you?" (Miller & Pechacek, 1987). There are also psychometrically sound questionnaires to measure expectancies, particularly regarding alcohol use. The original of these is the Alcohol Expectancy Questionnaire (AEQ; Brown et al., 1987). It contains 90 items designed to assess several dimensions of alcohol-related expectancies. The AEQ has been used with both help-seeking and non-help-seeking populations and has good psychometric properties (Donovan, 2013). Several adaptations of the scale have added negative as well as positive expectancies (Connors & Maisto, 1988; Fromme, Stroot, & Kaplan, 1993; George et al., 1995; Jones, Corbin, & Fromme, 2001; Rohsenow, 1983). Positive and negative expectancies may have a different impact on treatment outcomes and therefore both outcome expectancies should be included in the assessment (Donovan, 2013).

The Commitment to Sobriety Scale (CSS) is a clinically useful measure to assess motivation for abstinence (Kelly & Greene, 2014). The measure is a stronger predictor of future abstinence than the widely used SOCRATES; Kelly & Greene, 2014). The CSS measures the extent to which the individual remains committed to sobriety regardless of his or her situation or condition at the time. The question of interest is whether clients' circumstances interfere with or reduce their commitment to sobriety. The individual is asked to rate the level of agreement on a 6-point Likert scale (i.e., strongly agree to strongly disagree) to the following statements:

- "Staying sober is the most important thing in my life."
- "I am totally committed to staying off alcohol/drugs."
- " I will do whatever it takes to recover from my addiction."
- "I never want to return to alcohol/drugs again."
- "I have had enough alcohol and drug."

Low commitment scores suggest a need for further intervention to strengthen motivation for recovery.

The Theory of Planned Behavior scale (TPB; Ajzen, 2002) is a motivation measure intended to prevent premature dropout from treatment. It focuses on specific components (listed below) that can interfere with or delay treatment completion:

- "It would be extremely valuable to complete treatment" (attitudes).
- "Most people who are important to me think that I should attend treatment" (subjective norms).
- "If I wanted to, I could easily complete my treatment program" (perceived control).
- "I intend to complete my treatment program" (intentions).

Each item is rated on a 7-point response scale ranging from 1 (disagree very strongly) to 7 (agree very strongly). The *attitude* and *control factors* seem to be the most salient components associated with treatment completion (Zemore & Ajzen, 2014). Information from the TPB has been used to develop interventions specifically targeting attitudes and beliefs that threaten treatment completion (Stecker, McGovern, & Herr, 2012). Using cognitive therapy principles, clients are asked to consider the accuracy of the belief (0–100% truth), whether they have thoughts that question the accuracy of the belief, and how these thoughts impact on their initial attitude toward treatment. In other words, the client is asked about thoughts that dispute the reported attitudes and beliefs about treatment. To illustrate:

> CLIENT: I strongly disagree with the statement that it is valuable to complete treatment.
>
> THERAPIST: Is there anything that might happen to cause you to change this belief?
>
> CLIENT: Yes, if my wife decides to leave me. I love my wife and kids. You know, I really don't want to risk my marriage by leaving the program. This would be terrible for me.

The overall aim is to modify current beliefs or discover alternatives that lead to remaining in treatment.

Client Strengths and Resources

The context of addiction treatment easily lends itself to assessing people's deficits and shortcomings, but there are good reasons also to assess and affirm clients' strengths and the social supports that favor change (Corcoran, 2004; Lawrence & Sovik-Johnston, 2010; Rapp, 2002). After all, most people who recover from addictions do so on their own, without ever seeking formal treatment. Whatever time you spend with a client is but a small sliver of that person's life. Mobilizing clients' own strengths and social supports is important not only in rehabilitation, but in maintenance as well. Exploring strengths can also bolster clients' self-efficacy, which is a predictor of successful change, and helps to build a working therapeutic alliance.

PERSONAL STRENGTHS

As with all of the topics in this chapter, you can explore clients' strengths as part of normal conversation in clinical sessions. What does the client have going for him or her that can be an asset in changing? What successful changes has the client made in the past? What social support and resources are there to accompany the client on the road to sobriety? What are the values that guide the client's life? What does the client most want, hope for, and/or envision for the future?

If a little structure helps here, consider using "Some Characteristics of Successful Changers" (see Box 5.3; Miller, 2004). It is an arbitrary list of 100 positive traits that people may have. Showing this list to a client, ask, "Which of these words best describe you? Which ones are most true

BOX 5.3. Some Characteristics of Successful Changers

Accepting	Committed	Flexible	Persevering	Stubborn
Active	Competent	Focused	Persistent	Thankful
Adaptable	Concerned	Forgiving	Positive	Thorough
Adventuresome	Confident	Forward-looking	Powerful	Thoughtful
Affectionate	Considerate	Free	Prayerful	Tough
Affirmative	Courageous	Happy	Quick	Trusting
Alert	Creative	Healthy	Reasonable	Trustworthy
Alive	Decisive	Hopeful	Receptive	Truthful
Ambitious	Dedicated	Imaginative	Relaxed	Understanding
Anchored	Determined	Ingenious	Reliable	Unique
Assertive	Diehard	Intelligent	Resourceful	Unstoppable
Assured	Diligent	Knowledgeable	Responsible	Vigorous
Attentive	Doer	Loving	Sensible	Visionary
Bold	Eager	Mature	Skillful	Whole
Brave	Earnest	Open	Solid	Willing
Bright	Effective	Optimistic	Spiritual	Winning
Capable	Energetic	Orderly	Stable	Wise
Careful	Experienced	Organized	Steady	Worthy
Cheerful	Faithful	Patient	Straight	Zealous
Clever	Fearless	Perceptive	Strong	Zestful

From Miller (2004). This material is in the public domain and may be reproduced without further permission.

of you?"; When the client chooses several adjectives, you can explore "In what way does this describe you?"; "Give me an example of when you have been _____"; and so on. Listen, reflect, and affirm (Chapter 4).

A clinical assessment aimed at measuring an individual's capacities, coping, and social resources can be useful in developing goals and interventions in a strengths-based approach Rapp & Goscha, 2006; C. A. Rapp, Kelliher, Fisher, & Hall, 1996). Two instruments with good potential for use in strengths-based treatment are the Client Assessment of Strengths, Interest and Goals (CASIG) and the Strengths Assessment Worksheet (SAW). The CASIG has been used primarily in mental health services, but can be adapted for use in addiction treatment programs (Bird et al., 2012; Wallace, Lecomte, Wilde, & Liberman, 2001). It is administered as a structured interview examining the individual's goals for improvement in independent living skills in such areas as financial/vocational resources, social and familial relationships, and physical and mental health. The client is asked about expectations for improvement, how it might be accomplished, and the type of support that is needed to achieve these goals. The CASIG has good psychometric properties with regard to internal consistency, interrater reliability, and construct validity.

The SAW is a semistructured interview examining the current status of an array of domains pertaining to personal attributes, relationship skills, resilience, spirituality, and community/social supports (C. A. Rapp & Goscha, 2006; R. C. Rapp et al., 1996, 2006). The individual's desires and aspirations are linked with each of these domains. For example, an individual may determine that strengthening ties with family members can help avoid certain high-risk situations. The SAW has been positively associated with outcomes such as increased enrollment and retention in SUD treatment programs, improved education, and reduced hospitalizations (Bird et al., 2012).

Another strength asset is self-efficacy, a client's belief that he or she is capable of making a particular change (Bandura, 1997). One common way to strengthen this sense of self-efficacy is to explore changes that clients have made successfully in the past. What was the change? How did they do it? What obstacles did they encounter and how did they overcome those? You can tie these into characteristic strengths identified in the "successful changers" method described above. The Abstinence Self-Efficacy scale (ASE; DiClemente, Carbonari, Montgomery, & Hughes, 1994), describes a variety of situations in which clients may feel able (or less able) to abstain, based on factors originally identified by Marlatt (1996; Marlatt & Donovan, 2005). Closely related to the ASE is the Coping Resources Inventory (CRI; Moos, 1993), which assesses how the person handles stress. It takes about 10 minutes to complete and includes cognitive, emotional, social, spiritual, and physical components of stress reduction.

SOCIAL SUPPORT

Another potentially important strength to explore is a client's social support system. As discussed in Chapter 16, including a supportive significant other in treatment tends to improve outcome. Who is there in the client's social networks—family, friends, coworkers, support from religious communities and mutual help groups (Zweben et al., 2003)? The extent to which these people actively support the client's sobriety (vs. favoring continued use) predicts stability of sobriety (Longabaugh, Wirtz, Zweben, & Stout, 1998, 2001). The support system can play a valuable role in enhancing treatment engagement and adherence, buttressing motivation and, more importantly, offering alternatives to a lifestyle of drinking or drug use. If evaluation reveals that a client's current support system strongly favors continued substance use, it is reason to construct an alternative support system such as that found in the 12-step fellowships (Tonigan, 2001; Tonigan, Connors, & Miller, 2003; Zweben et al., 2003).

The Important People and Activities interview (IPA; Longabaugh, Beattie, Noel, Stout, & Malloy, 1993) was constructed specifically to measure network support for drinking (in contrast to general social support). The IPA includes two important dimensions that predict treatment outcomes: (1) network drinking and (2) opposition to client drinking. Clients are asked to identify people in their social network and rate them on the following: (1) their response to the client's drinking (e.g., opposition) and (2) their own drinking behavior (network drinking). Higher frequency of network drinking predicted more client drinking during treatment, whereas greater network opposition to drinking predicted less heavy drinking during follow-up (Longabaugh, Wirtz, Zywiak, & O'Malley, 2010).

Functional Analysis of Substance Use

People use alcohol and other drugs for good reasons. It is not for naught that substance use persists despite adverse consequences. Functional analysis, a classic behavior therapy component, seeks to understand what roles or functions substance use is playing in the person's life (Meyers & Smith, 1995; Miller & Pechacek, 1987). It focuses both on *antecedents* (triggers or stimuli that increase the likelihood of use) and *consequences* of substance use (which may reinforce it). These can be explored in a structured interview (Miller & Pechacek, 1987; see Chapter 14), by having clients keep self-monitoring records of use (Miller & Muñoz, 2013), or via self-report questionnaires.

Several questionnaires have been used to identify situations that pose particular risk of return to substance use. The Inventory of Drinking Situations (IDS; Annis, Graham, & Davis, 1987) and the Inventory of Drug Taking Situations (IDTS; Annis & Graham, 1991) cover eight types of potential high-risk situations, again based on the work of Alan Marlatt: unpleasant emotions, pleasant emotions, physical discomfort, testing personal control, urges and temptations, conflict with others, social pressure, and pleasant times. Clients rate the frequency of their drinking or drug use in these situations. A client profile is created identifying areas that pose the greatest and least risk for substance use. A simpler scale (12 or 20 items) that is available free of charge is the Situational Temptation Scale that has three subscales: negative affect, social/positive use, and cravings/habitual use (Maddock, Laforge, & Rossi, 2000). The underlying assumption with these scales is that past substance use in these situations increases risk of future use in the same circumstances. Individualized risk profiles can inform treatment plans to identify and address high-risk situations (Kadden et al., 1992; Monti, Abrams, Kadden, & Cooney, 1989; Monti, Kadden,

Rohsenow, Cooney, & Abrams, 2002; see Chapter 11), particularly when risk level varies across situations (Annis & Graham, 1991).

The Situational Confidence Questionnaire (SCQ; Annis & Graham, 1988) is a companion instrument querying clients' perceptions of their ability to deal with high-risk situations without resorting to substance use (i.e., level of self-efficacy). The situations parallel those contained in the IDS. A client profile is again generated based on levels of client self-efficacy in potential high-risk situations. As with the IDS, profiles on the SCQ can inform treatment goals and strategies. The underlying strategy here is that increased levels of self-efficacy lead to better outcomes, and situations with low self-efficacy warrant targeted intervention (Solomon & Annis, 1990).

The risk or coping situations identified on the aforementioned instruments will not always be pertinent to a particular client's circumstances or "slippery slopes." It is therefore useful to invite clients completing these measures to also choose their own high-risk/coping situations (Connors et al., 2001): "What situations were most problematic for you during the past year? How confident are you now in handling these same events?" This can increase the clinical relevance of the process to individual clients.

Assessing all four areas (nature and severity of substance use and problems, motivation for change, personal strengths and resources, and functional analysis of substance use) can help you understand the interrelationships between these different areas and form working hypotheses about what action steps are needed for the client to accomplish and sustain change. Such assessment can also be used to provide feedback for your clients to promote motivation for change, increase awareness of risk situations that pose the obstacles to sobriety, and identify targeted strategies for reaching identified change goals. Assessment along with feedback, if done collaboratively, can greatly benefit clients (Poston & Hanson, 2010).

The development of a change plan is a negotiated process, of course, informed by what clients expect, prefer, need, and are willing to do. Box 5.4 lists instruments we recommended above for screening and for each of the four evaluation areas, along with current website sources. Recognizing practical obstacles (such as heavy caseloads and cost) when conducting evaluations in real-world clinical settings, we have emphasized shorter instruments and those available free of charge.

Diagnosing Addiction Problems

The purpose of screening is to determine whether further evaluation is warranted. Evaluation is an ongoing process that begins with the first contact, to provide whatever information is needed as treatment proceeds. Diagnosis has a different purpose from both screening and evaluation (Miller, Westerberg, & Waldron, 2003). In etymology, *diagnosis* literally means to

BOX 5.4. Some Recommended Instruments for Screening and Multidimensional Evaluation

Purpose	Recommended Instruments (Choose those most appropriate to your setting.)
Screening	• Alcohol Use Disorders Identification Test (AUDIT)[a] *www.drugabuse.gov/sites/default/files/files/AUDIT.pdf* • NM-ASSIST[a] *www.nida.nih/nidamed/screening/nmassist.pdf* • Drug Use Disorders Identification Test (DUDIT)[a] *www.paihdelinkki.fi/sites/default/files/duditmanual.pdf* • RAPS4[a] *alcoholism.about.com/od/tests/a/raps.htm*
Nature and severity of substance use and problems	• Addiction Severity Index (ASI)[a] *http://adai.washington.edu/instruments/pdf/Addiction_severity_index_baseline_followup_4.pdf* • Alcohol Dependence Scale *www.emcdda.europa.eu/attachements.cfm/Att_4075_EN_tads.pdf* • Drinker Inventory of Consequences (DrInC)[a] *casaa.unm.edu/inst.html* • Inventory of Drug Use Consequences (InDUC)[a] *casaa.unm.edu/inst.html* • Severity of Alcohol Dependence Questionnaire (SADQ)[a] *www.drinksafely.soton.ac.uk/SADO*
Clients' personal strengths and resources	• Abstinence Self--Efficacy Scale[a] *adai.washington.edu/instruments/pdf/Alcohol_Abstinence_Self_Efficacy_Scale_17.pdf* • Important People Interview (IPI)[a] *casaa.unm.edu/inst/Important%20People%20Initial%20Interview.pdf* • Coping Responses Inventory (CRI) *www4.parinc.com/Products/Product.aspx?ProductID=CRI* • Strengths Association Worksheet (SAW)[b] • Client Assessment of Strengths, Interests and Goals (CASIG)[c]

(continued)

BOX 5.4. *(continued)*

Purpose	Recommended Instruments (Choose those most appropriate to your setting.)
Functional analysis of substance use (and high-risk situations)	• Alcohol Expectancy Questionnaire[d] • Situational Temptation Scales[a] *https://habitslab.umbc.edu/situation-temptation-scales/* • Desired Effects of Drinking[a] *casaa.unm.edu/inst/Desired%20Effects%20of%20Drinking.pdf*
Motivation for change	• University of Rhode Island Change Assessment (URICA)[a] *https://habitslab.umbc.edu/urica* • Stages of Change Readiness and Treatment Eagerness Scale (SOCRATES)[a] *casaa.unm.edu/inst.html* • Change Questionnaire[a] *casaa.unm.edu/inst.html* • Readiness to Change Questionnaire[a] *www.ncbi.nlm.nih.gov/books/NBK64976/Table/A62295* • Commitment to Sobriety Scale (CSS)[e] • Treatment of Planned Behavior (TPB) questionnaire *www.webcitation.org/66zom97zq*

[a]Instruments available free of charge.
[b]See Rapp and Goscha (2006) and Rapp et al. (1994). [c]See Wallace et al. (2001).
[d]Request in writing to Sandra Brown, PhD, 9500 Gilman Drive (0109), San Diego, CA 92093-0109.
[e]Request in writing to John Kelly, Massachusetts General Hospital and Harvard Medical School, Boston, MA 02114.

know the difference, to recognize patterns that constitute identifiable diseases or conditions. In current practice, as discussed in Chapter 2, diagnosis involves determining whether a person currently meets predetermined criteria for having a particular condition, which in turn may influence eligibility for treatment. Third-party payers often require a diagnosis as a precondition for reimbursement. A diagnosis is meant to establish the seriousness of a condition and, ideally, suggest what treatments might be most appropriate. However, because most behavioral health diagnoses are not linked to particular etiology, diagnosis alone does not determine how to proceed with treatment.

As described in Chapter 2, two similar classification systems have been most commonly used for diagnosing SUDs (Hasin et al., 2013): the DSM and the ICD. The most common approach to diagnosis is through a clinical interview comparing an individual's current symptoms with the specified criteria (Hersen & Turner, 2003). Where greater precision and reliability are required, structured interview procedures have been developed to assess initial severity level (based on symptomatic status) to monitor treatment progress, and to evaluate treatment outcomes. The most common of these instruments is the Structured Clinical Interview for DSM-5 (First, Williams, Karg, & Spitzer, 2015). There is also a website (*www.psychiatry.org/psychiatrists/practice/dsm/educational-resources/assessment-measure*) listing "emerging measures" for assessing initial symptomatic status, monitoring treatment progress, and interpreting scoring information within DSM-5. Professionals need to have specialized training for reliable use of these structured diagnostic interviews.

KEY POINTS

- Screening for addictions is appropriate when working with a diverse client population, to identify those for whom additional evaluation is warranted.

- Screening instruments do not establish a diagnosis. Diagnosis determines whether an individual meets certain pre-established criteria for a disorder.

- Evaluation is a process that occurs over time, not merely a prelude to treatment.

- Four broad domains for evaluation are (1) the nature and severity of substance use and problems, (2) motivation for change, (3) client strengths and resources, and (4) a functional analysis of substance use.

- There is a wide array of instruments with documented reliability and validity, many of which are available free of charge in the public domain. It is unwise to develop homemade assessment instruments when evidence-based options are available.

Reflection Questions

- If you work in a setting where a wide variety of people seek services, how might routine screening for alcohol/drug problems be implemented? What assessment measures do you currently use in your own practice, and why? What do you know about their reliability and validity?

- What information do you really need in order to begin treatment?

CHAPTER 6

Withdrawal Management
and Health Care Needs

The process of physiological dependence involves the body adjusting to drug use so that it can function more normally while the drug is present. Discontinuation of the drug then triggers a complementary adjustment process known as *withdrawal* or *abstinence syndrome*. In Chapter 3 we described this rebound effect, which is opposite to the effects of intoxication, as the "valley."

Withdrawal is the physical elimination of a drug and readjustment of the body to normal functioning in its absence. *Withdrawal management* addresses a client's biopsychosocial needs while drugs are being cleared from the body, in preparation for recovery-oriented treatment.

Depending where you work, helping individuals through withdrawal management may be something you do a lot or a little. Intoxicated people may be seen in an emergency department or medical clinic seeking palliative care. However, even if you aren't working in a medical or withdrawal management setting, it is still a good idea to understand drug withdrawal and know what it looks like. For instance, clients in outpatient treatment might describe symptoms such as insomnia, anxiety, depression, paranoia, or sweating, which they may attribute (correctly or not) to withdrawal. Clients might be fearful of what withdrawal will be like, wanting to know what to expect. Withdrawal from some drugs can be medically hazardous, even life-threatening. For these reasons, it is good to have a working knowledge of what people should anticipate during the process and be able to assess the potential seriousness of the withdrawal.

The particular interventions used in withdrawal management are determined by the type(s) and amount of drugs people have been using, their history of withdrawal, and their other current psychosocial and medical needs. The goal of withdrawal management is to alleviate symptoms and minimize physical risk or harm while drugs are being cleared from the body. Management of withdrawal does not constitute recovery-oriented addiction treatment in itself; rather, it is a preparation for ongoing treatment and continuing care. Three main tasks in managing withdrawal are evaluation, stabilization, and transition into treatment (Miller & Kipnis, 2006).

> Withdrawal can be hazardous, even life-threatening.

Evaluation

A first step in managing withdrawal is evaluating what drugs are in the person's body and screening for possible medical and behavioral health conditions that could complicate the process. The focus is to learn what substances were taken and when, determine the appropriate level of care, and understand what may help the person through the withdrawal process, considering that the client's immediate concerns may differ from yours. In addition to the person's self-report, lab tests of blood, breath, or urine are useful to identify drugs that are present. It can be tempting to fire pressing closed questions: "What did you take? I know you took something. Tell me right now! We can't help you unless you tell us right now what you took." You are likely to get more cooperation and more

> Take some time to listen and engage.

meaningful and accurate information if you take some time to listen and engage. Without the client's participation in decision making, it is difficult to move forward in managing withdrawal and facilitating transition into recovery-oriented treatment services.

Several important decisions are made during the evaluation process and, as with health care more broadly, it is a shared decision-making process regarding options and possible outcomes (Barry & Edgman-Levitan, 2012). One is the appropriate level of care. The vast majority of withdrawal management can be done safely in ambulatory care (Abbott, Quinn, & Knox, 1995; Day & Strang, 2011). However, other factors such as homelessness, suicidality, or medical complications may increase the need for residential care and medical supervision. Another decision is whether to use medications to help patients through the withdrawal process. This is determined in part by the person's presenting symptoms, history of past withdrawal, and the substance(s) the person has been using. For example, there are particular medical safety issues involved in withdrawal from alcohol and sedative–hypnotic drugs depending on severity of dependence, requiring medically assisted withdrawal management (Merkx et al., 2014; Stein et al., 2017).

BOX 6.1. Personal Reflection: Necessity Breeds Discovery

In the early 1980s, the Reagan administration developed the "block grants" program that transferred funding of addiction treatment programs from the federal to the state level. This seemed a good idea, in that individual states would be more likely to understand local needs, and of course there was excitement to have this new stream of funding under state control. What was not so immediately evident, however, was that the total amount of funding was being reduced by half. The result was a sudden shortage of resources for public programs.

The University of New Mexico at the time was operating two large public treatment programs for SUDs. One was a residential 28-day detoxification and rehabilitation center that treated a few hundred people per year. The other was an outpatient treatment facility that served a few thousand people annually. The two programs had similar budgets, and funding was being cut in half. Which one would we close? The answer seemed fairly clear, particularly in that research was already showing similar overall outcomes from inpatient and outpatient treatment (W. R. Miller & Hester, 1986).

We were concerned, though, because we had been accustomed to handling withdrawal management through the inpatient unit, and there were now no beds for this purpose except for emergency hospital beds. How would we handle severe alcohol and complex multidrug withdrawal? Could more severely dependent people really be treated on an ambulatory basis? For all but the affluent, we really had no choice but to find out. What we found was the same thing being discovered across the country: that withdrawal management (in our case, with good on-site medical supervision) was safe and effective on an outpatient day treatment basis for 99% of our patients, and we had no untoward outcomes (Day & Strang, 2011). In fact, we tended to hospitalize only those patients who required inpatient treatment for some *other* reason in addition to withdrawal (such as suicidality or severe medical illness). People who would otherwise be sitting in an inpatient bed instead came to the clinic each day for observation and medication as needed, until they were safely through the withdrawal process. This also eased their transition into treatment at the same clinic. We changed procedures because we had to, and in the process discovered that we could serve more people at lower cost without compromising quality of care.

—W. R. M.

Some practical guidelines have been proposed by the American Society of Addiction Medicine (ASAM; Mee-Lee, Shulman, Fishman, Gastfriend, & Miller, 2013) for choosing an appropriate level of care during withdrawal. Individuals are evaluated on six dimensions, corresponding to needs and strengths in behavioral health services: (1) acute intoxication or withdrawal potential; (2) biomedical conditions and complications; (3) emotional, behavioral, or cognitive conditions and complications; (4) readiness to change; (5) continued use, or continued problem potential;

and (6) recovery environment. The ASAM criteria include five different contexts for withdrawal management:

- *Level 1-WM:* Ambulatory withdrawal management without extended on-site monitoring.
- *Level 2-WM:* Ambulatory withdrawal management with extended on-site monitoring.
- *Level 3.2-WM:* Clinically managed residential withdrawal management.
- *Level 3.7-WM:* Medically monitored inpatient withdrawal management.
- *Level 4-WM:* Medically managed inpatient withdrawal management.

Some practical questions to help guide this decision include:

- What is the person's history regarding the amount and duration of substance use?
- How long ago was the last use of each substance?
- When was the last time the person went for a few days without using? What happened?
- Does the person have a history of delirium tremens or withdrawal seizures?
- Is the person taking anything else that might affect his or her withdrawal symptoms?
- Are there any co-occurring medical or behavioral health problems (hallucinations, traumatic brain injury)?
- Is there any risk of harm to self or others?
- Is there any risk of violence at home?
- Can the person understand and carry out routine medical instructions?
- Does the person have reliable transportation?
- Does the person have a supportive person to assist with withdrawal management?

Screening for Likelihood of Complicated Withdrawal

There are several instruments helpful in screening for the probability of complicated withdrawal. If you are not a medical professional, your main role in this part of evaluation may be to refer people for appropriate medical consultation. Nevertheless, it is important to know some basic information about the withdrawal process, what to expect, and the potential seriousness of withdrawal and complications. Monitoring for signs of withdrawal, such as changes in mental status, hallucinations, seizures, fever,

---

BOX 6.2. Applying the ASAM Criteria

Josephine is a 23-year-old female brought into the emergency department (ED) at 7:00 P.M. after her mother called the police. Earlier in the evening, Josephine had gotten into an argument with her father and threw a knife at him. The incident did not injure either Josephine or her father, and appeared to be an isolated event in direct relation to her acute intoxication. Josephine's parents report that their daughter's life is "spiraling out of control," and that they "don't know what she is going to do next." Josephine has not been in addiction treatment in the past, and told the psychiatric team that she has used opioids "daily" for the past 3 years, including using alcohol "on occasion." She told the team that she uses because her family life is stressful and her parents expect too much from her, reporting that opioid use makes her feel less stressed and she is better able to cope with their criticism of her. When she attempts to cut down on the opioids or can't get any, she begins to feel anxious and shaky. While waiting in the emergency department to be seen, she vomited and said it was because she needs to take a pill every 4 hours to feel normal and that she hadn't taken anything since 11:00 A.M. One year ago she attempted to "go cold turkey" by attending a family reunion out of state and not bringing any pills. By the end of the first day she was shaking uncontrollably, and excused herself from all activities by saying she had the flu. By the second day into the week-long vacation, she had a friend come to pick her up so that she could get back home because the withdrawal was too much and she felt like she was "going to die." She immediately returned to using. She said she wants to get over this and is disgusted with her daily use and feels like it has been out of control, but lacks confidence that she will be successful, particularly since almost everyone in her group of friends uses opioids. Both of Josephine's parents are present in the ED, but Josephine is refusing to speak with them even though she acknowledges that they "support anything that would help me get better." One of her friends who has successfully maintained more than a year of abstinence from opioids called her during her stay in the ED and offered to take her to an Narcotics Anonymous (NA) meeting sometime during the next week.

Josephine is evaluated on the following six clinical dimensions:

1. *Acute intoxication or withdrawal potential:* Substantial. She is reporting several symptoms of acute opioid withdrawal. She has been unable to maintain more than 2 days of abstinence over the past 3 years.

2. *Biomedical conditions and complications:* No problem. There are no issues in this dimension that would impact the level of service needed.

3. *Emotional, behavioral, or cognitive conditions and complications:* Mild. The knife throwing appears to be an isolated incident related to her intoxication. This emotional lability, anger, and impulsivity in her behavior are factors that should be considered in developing a treatment plan. At this time, however, emotional or behavioral factors do not appear to be an issue that will impact the intensity or type of services needed.

(continued)

BOX 6.2. *(continued)*

4. *Readiness to change:* Mild. She described her disgust with her daily use and reported it's "gotten out of control." She also has had a prior attempt to abstain.

5. *Relapse, continued use, or continued problem potential:* Substantial. The likelihood of her return to use is substantial because of her previous attempt at withdrawal and her history of profound physical discomfort and cravings. She has used opioids daily for almost 3 years. She views family problems as reasons to use. She uses opioids to minimize her stress and does not currently have other ways of coping with negative events.

6. *Recovery/living environment:* Moderate. Her parents are very supportive of any type of treatment that will help. Her good friend is also aware of the problem and verbally supportive. This friend attends NA regularly and they are planning on attending a meeting together. However, many of her other friends are regular opioid users.

PLACEMENT AND DISCUSSION

Based on the dimensional assessment, what type of withdrawal management care do you think would be the best fit for Josephine? Why? What additional information or evaluation might be useful?

---

and abdominal pain (Kosten & O'Connor, 2003; Mirijello et al., 2015) can also be part of a multidisciplinary approach to patient care. Such signs and symptoms require immediate medical attention.

Alcohol

There is an advantage to using a validated instrument such as the Clinical Institute Withdrawal Assessment for Alcohol Scale, Revised (CIWA-Ar; J. T. Sullivan, Sykora, Schneiderman, Naranjo, & Sellers, 1989). It takes just a few minutes to administer and helps to make the decision about the person's level of need for medical supervision. The CIWA-Ar (Box 6.3) is a public domain instrument that measures 10 subjective signs and symptoms of alcohol withdrawal: nausea, tremor, autonomic hyperactivity, anxiety, agitation, tactile disturbances, visual disturbances, auditory disturbances, headache, and disorientation. The CIWA-Ar should be repeated at regular intervals (every 1–2 hours initially) to monitor the client's progress and changes in withdrawal symptoms. People who score less than 10 usually do not need medication for withdrawal.

BOX 6.3. Clinical Institute Withdrawal Assessment for Alcohol Scale, Revised (CIWA-Ar)

Patient:_____ Date:_____ Time:_____

Pulse or heart rate, taken for one minute:_____ **Blood pressure:**_____

NAUSEA AND VOMITING—Ask "Do you feel sick to your stomach? Have you vomited?" Observation.

0 no nausea and no vomiting
1 mild nausea with no vomiting
2
3
4 intermittent nausea with dry heaves
5
6
7 constant nausea, frequent dry heaves, and vomiting

TACTILE DISTURBANCES—Ask "Have you any itching, pins-and-needles sensations, any burning, any numbness, or do you feel bugs crawling on or under your skin?" Observation.

0 none
1 very mild itching, pins and needles, burning or numbness
2 mild itching, pins and needles, burning or numbness
3 moderate itching, pins and needles, burning or numbness
4 moderately severe hallucinations
5 severe hallucinations
6 extremely severe hallucinations
7 continuous hallucinations

TREMOR—Arms extended and fingers spread apart.
Observation.

0 no tremor
1 not visible, but can be felt fingertip to fingertip
2
3
4 moderate, with patient's arms extended
5
6
7 severe, even with arms not extended

AUDITORY DISTURBANCES—Ask "Are you more aware of sounds around you? Are they harsh? Do they frighten you? Are you hearing anything that is disturbing to you? Are you hearing things you know are not there?" Observation.

0 not present
1 very mild harshness or ability to frighten
2 mild harshness or ability to frighten
3 moderate harshness or ability to frighten
4 moderately severe hallucinations
5 severe hallucinations
6 extremely severe hallucinations
7 continuous hallucinations

PAROXYSMAL SWEATS—Observation.

0 no sweat visible
1 barely perceptible sweating, palms moist

(continued)

From Sullivan, Sykora, Schneiderman, Naranjo, and Sellers (1989). This scale is in the public domain and may be reproduced without further permission.

BOX 6.3. *(continued)*

2
3
4 beads of sweat obvious on forehead
5
6
7 drenching sweats

VISUAL DISTURBANCES—Ask "Does the light appear to be too bright? Is its color different? Does it hurt your eyes? Are you seeing anything that is disturbing to you? Are you seeing things you know are not there?" Observation.

0 not present
1 very mild sensitivity
2 mild sensitivity
3 moderate sensitivity
4 moderately severe hallucinations
5 severe hallucinations
6 extremely severe hallucinations
7 continuous hallucinations

ANXIETY—Ask "Do you feel nervous?" Observation.

0 no anxiety, at ease
1 mildly anxious
2
3
4 moderately anxious, or guarded, so anxiety is inferred
5
6
7 equivalent to acute panic states as seen in severe delirium or acute schizophrenic reactions

HEADACHE, FULLNESS IN HEAD—Ask "Does your head feel different? Does it feel like there is a band around your head?" Do not rate for dizziness or lightheadedness. Otherwise, rate severity.

0 not present
1 very mild
2 mild
3 moderate
4 moderately severe
5 severe
6 very severe
7 extremely severe

AGITATION—Observation.

0 normal activity
1 somewhat more than normal activity
2
3
4 moderately fidgety and restless
5
6
7 paces back and forth during most of the interview, or constantly thrashes about

ORIENTATION AND CLOUDING OF SENSORIUM—Ask "What day is this? Where are you? Who am I?"

0 oriented and can do serial additions
1 cannot do serial additions or is uncertain about date
2 disoriented for date by no more than 2 calendar days
3 disoriented for date by more than 2 calendar days
4 disoriented for place/or person

Total **CIWA-Ar** Score
Maximum Possible Score 67

This assessment for monitoring withdrawal symptoms requires approximately 5 minutes to administer. The maximum score is 67. Patients scoring less than 10 do not usually need additional medication for withdrawal.

Cocaine

The Cocaine Selective Severity Assessment (CSSA; Kampman et al., 1998) is an 18-item scale that reliably measures cocaine withdrawal signs and symptoms (see Box 6.4). The scale is designed to be administered at each withdrawal management visit and measures withdrawal over the past 24 hours. High scores on the CSSA are correlated with treatment dropout and return to cocaine use.

Opioids

Three rating scales that are reliable indicators of the severity of the opioid withdrawal syndrome are the Subjective Opiate Withdrawal Scale (SOWS), the Objective Opiate Withdrawal Scale (OOWS), and the Clinical Opiate Withdrawal Scale (COWS). A difference among these instruments is whether the assessment is based on client self-report (SOWS) or professional observation of withdrawal signs (COWS, OOWS).

The COWS is a clinician-administered, pen-and-paper instrument that rates 11 common opiate withdrawal signs or symptoms. The summed score of the 11 items can be used to assess a patient's level of opiate withdrawal and to make inferences about his or her level of physical dependence on opioids (Wesson & Ling, 2003).

The SOWS (Handelsman et al., 1987) is a 16-item questionnaire assessing common motoric, autonomic, gastrointestinal, musculoskeletal, and psychic symptoms of opioid withdrawal. Clients can rate their own symptom severity on a scale of 0 to 4. The sum of the scores on each item is the total SOWS score, which can range from 0 to 64, with higher scores indicating more severe withdrawal. The items are shown in Box 6.5.

To administer OOWS (Handelsman et al., 1987), you would observe a client for about 10 minutes and indicate if any of the 10 signs of withdrawal are present. The OOWS consists of observable signs that reflect common motoric and autonomic manifestations of withdrawal. Scores range from 0 to 13, with higher scores again indicating more severe withdrawal.

Transitioning from Evaluation to Stabilization

The goal of evaluation is to collaboratively develop a withdrawal plan that meets the physical and psychological needs of the person. When evaluation is complete, a determination has been made regarding the withdrawal management model (social or medical) and setting (inpatient or outpatient). Because paths into withdrawal management can pass through an emergency department, correctional system, or primary care, some of the evaluation may already have been completed by the referring agency.

BOX 6.4. Cocaine Selective Severity Assessment (CSSA)

Symptom   **SCORE**

1. HYPERPHAGIA: [ ]
  0 = normal appetite
3–4 = eats a lot more than usual
  7 = eats more than twice usual amount of food

2. HYPOPHAGIA: [ ]
  0 = normal appetite
3–4 = eats less than normal amount
  7 = no appetite at all

3. CARBOHYDRATE CRAVING: [ ]
  0 = no craving
3–4 = strong craving for sweets half the time
  7 = strong craving for sweets all the time

4. COCAINE CRAVING: (Please rate intensity) 0–7   [ ]
Please rate the highest intensity of the desire for cocaine you have felt in
the last 24 hours:
  0   1   2   3   4   5   6   7
No desire at all   Unable to resist

5. CRAVING FREQUENCY: (Please have subject rate intensity) 0–7   [ ]
Please identify on the line below how often you have felt the urge to use
cocaine in the last 24 hours:
  0   1   2   3   4   5   6   7
Never   All the time

6. BRADYCARDIA   [ ]
              0   1   2   3   4   5   6   7
Apical Pulse > 64   64–63   62–61   60–59   58–57   56–55   54–53   < 53

7. SLEEP 1:   [ ]
  0 = normal amount of sleep
3–4 = half of normal amount
  7 = no sleep at all

(continued)

From Kampman et al. (1998). This scale is in the public domain and may be reproduced without further permission.

BOX 6.4. *(continued)*

8. SLEEP II: [ ]
    0 = normal amount of sleep
3–4 = could sleep or do sleep half the day
    7 = sleep or could sleep all the time

9. ANXIETY: [ ]
    0 = usually does not feel anxious
3–4 = feels anxious half the time
    7 = feels anxious all the time

10. ENERGY LEVEL: [ ]
    0 = feels alert and has usual amount of energy
3–4 = feels tired half the time
    7 = feels tired all the time

11. ACTIVITY LEVEL: [ ]
    0 = no change in usual activities
3–4 = participates in half of usual activities
    7 = no participation in usual activities

12. TENSION: [ ]
    0 = rarely feels tense
3–4 = feels tense half the time
    7 = feels tense most of the time

13. ATTENTION: [ ]
    0 = able to concentrate on reading, conversation, tasks, and make
         plans without difficulty
3–4 = has difficulty with the above half the time
    7 = has difficulty with the above all the time

14. PARANOID IDEATION   [ ]
    0 = no evidence of paranoid thoughts
3–4 = unable to trust anyone
    7 = feels people are out to get him/her
    8 = feels a specific person/group is plotting against him/her

15. ANHEDONIA   [ ]
    0 = ability to enjoy themselves remains unchanged
3–4 = able to enjoy themselves half the time
    7 = unable to enjoy themselves at all

(continued)

BOX 6.4. *(continued)*

16. DEPRESSION   [ ]
  0   = no feelings related to sadness or depression
 3–4 = feels sad or depressed half the time
  7   = feels depressed all of the time

17. SUICIDALITY   [ ]
  0   = does not think about being dead
 3–4 = feels like life is not worth living
  7   = feels like actually ending life

18. IRRITABILITY   [ ]
  0   = feels that most things are not irritating
 3–4 = feels that many things are irritating
  7   = feels that mostly everything is irritating and upsetting

Total Score: _____

Stabilization

During the stabilization phase, the person is assisted safely through acute intoxication and withdrawal. Previously used drugs are cleared from the body, and withdrawal symptoms are managed to minimize risk and discomfort.

There are two broad models for stabilization in withdrawal management: a social model and a medical model. There are also mixed-model social programs that have some on-site or on-call medical staff. Social model or "drug-free" withdrawal management programs provide nonmedical services to manage withdrawal without medication, drawing on off-site medical facilities as needed. The types of psychosocial services offered by social model programs vary widely. Medical model programs are directed by a physician and staffed by health care personnel. They may be hospital-based inpatient programs, residential programs, or ambulatory facilities in the community. Medically supervised programs may be particularly important when there is risk of severe life threatening withdrawal from drugs like alcohol or benzodiazepines. Therapeutic medications can be used during stabilization is to help clients achieve an initial period of abstinence. It is not necessary or helpful for people to suffer severe withdrawal in order to be motivated for change. Reducing withdrawal symptoms through pharmacological means can actually improve subsequent treatment outcomes (Mannelli et al., 2011; Merkx et al., 2014).

BOX 6.5. Subjective Opiate Withdrawal Scale (SOWS)

Symptom	Not at all	A little	Moderately	Quite a bit	Extremely
1. I feel anxious.	0	1	2	3	4
2. I feel like yawning.	0	1	2	3	4
3. I'm perspiring.	0	1	2	3	4
4. My eyes are tearing.	0	1	2	3	4
5. My nose is running.	0	1	2	3	4
6. I have goose flesh.	0	1	2	3	4
7. I am shaking.	0	1	2	3	4
8. I have hot flashes.	0	1	2	3	4
9. I have cold flashes.	0	1	2	3	4
10. My bones and muscles ache.	0	1	2	3	4
11. I feel restless.	0	1	2	3	4
12. I feel nauseous.	0	1	2	3	4
13. I feel like vomiting.	0	1	2	3	4
14. My muscles twitch.	0	1	2	3	4
15. I have cramps in my stomach.	0	1	2	3	4
16. I feel like shooting up now.	0	1	2	3	4

From Handelsman, Cochrane, Aronson, and Ness (1987). This scale is in the public domain and may be reproduced without further permission.

Managing Withdrawal

Pharmacological withdrawal management typically involves substituting a longer-acting agent for the drug the person has been using, then gradually tapering the dose. Though there is no single best way to manage withdrawal and stabilization, there are some common guidelines. For example, using medication for opioid withdrawal management (and beyond) is generally recommended over abrupt cessation of opioids. Systematic reviews have provided strong evidence that, when used as indicated, these medications are effective in reducing opioid-related withdrawal and craving, increasing retention in treatment, and minimizing the risk of subsequent fatal overdose that can occur with decreased opioid tolerance reviews (American Society of Addiction Medicine, 2013). So-called "ultrarapid" opiate withdrawal—administering intravenous naltrexone under general anesthesia—received much public attention, but is not recommended because of increased risk for adverse events or death (Kampman & Jarvis, 2015). In Chapter 18 we provide more specific information on some types of medication used to manage withdrawal and facilitate rehabilitation and maintenance.

Withdrawal syndromes vary depending on the drugs people have been using. In this regard, it is good to know what may occur during the withdrawal process, information that you may also share with clients (although they may already have considerable knowledge and experience in this regard). Clients often feel more comfortable when they know what to expect and can prepare themselves. There are often disproportionate fears about opioid withdrawal. While opioid withdrawal can certainly be protracted and intensely symptomatic—even with the use of pharmacologic agents—there is virtually no risk of mortality. It's important to be empathic with these concerns, while also providing realistic assurance and information to assuage fears and reduce ambivalence. Box 6.6 describes the signs and symptoms of intoxication from specific drugs as well as the characteristics, duration, onset, length, and complications of withdrawal.

It is common for people to have been simultaneously or serially using several drugs before entering treatment. Individual effects of the various drugs can interact, amplify, and complicate each other. Similarly, the body's adjustments to simultaneous withdrawal of several drugs can interact in complex ways. Withdrawal time curves for individual drugs can overlap or prolong each other. Priority is usually given to determining which of the used drugs poses the most serious withdrawal risks (Miller & Kipnis, 2006). Alcohol and sedative–hypnotics typically get priority of attention because their withdrawal syndromes can be fatal.

Addressing Other Health Care Needs

Another important task during the stabilization process is to identify and address acute health and social problems that need imminent attention. Even if you are not a medical professional, it is important to be aware of health problems that are often encountered in addiction treatment in order to protect your clients' and your own health. Here are some common issues related to physical health.

Nutritional Needs

Malnutrition is a common concern with people in withdrawal management. Alcohol is calorie-dense, and tends to displace food intake. People who are using alcohol or other drugs may also have irregular eating habits and poor

BOX 6.6. Examples of Drug Withdrawal Symptoms

	Cocaine	Alcohol	Heroin	Cannabis (marijuana)
Onset	Depends upon type of cocaine used: for crack will begin within hours of last use	24–48 hours after blood alcohol level drops	Within 24 hours of last use	Some debate about this, may be a few days
Duration	3–4 days	5–7 days	4–7 days	May last up to several weeks
Characteristics	Sleeplessness or excessive restless sleep, appetite increase, depression, paranoia, decreased energy	↑ blood pressure, ↑ heart rate, ↑ temperature, nausea/vomiting/ diarrhea, seizures, delirium, death	Nausea, vomiting, diarrhea, goose bumps, runny nose, teary eyes, yawning	Irritability, appetite disturbance, sleep disturbance, nausea, concentration problems, nystagmus, diarrhea
Medical/ Psychiatric Issues	Stroke, cardiovascular collapse, myocardial and other organ infarction, paranoia, violence, severe depression, suicide	Virtually every organ system is affected (e.g., cardiomyopathy, liver disease, esophageal and rectal varices); fetal alcohol syndrome and other problems with fetus	During withdrawal individual may become dehydrated	

Based on N. S. Miller and Kipnis (2006).

dietary intake. Alcohol and other drugs can also interfere with nutrient utilization and storage. For example, opioids tend to decrease calcium absorption (Cardenas & Ross, 1976) and alcohol can cause thiamine deficiencies (Singleton & Martin, 2001). Thus, a nutritional evaluation is often warranted during stabilization, accompanied by appropriate dietary counseling. When poverty contributes to malnutrition, stabilization includes connecting people with community food supplementation resources.

Behavioral Health Needs

Diagnosing co-occurring disorders is tricky during acute intoxication and withdrawal because SUDs can often mimic other behavioral health disorders (see Chapter 20). Nevertheless, as withdrawal symptoms abate, co-occurring disorders may become more apparent. Professional consensus is increasingly to address addiction and co-occurring disorders concurrently, rather than waiting for one to resolve before treating the other (Mueser & Drake, 2007; Mueser & Gingerich, 2013; Sacks & Ries, 2005). In one study with clients presenting for withdrawal management, mental health problems were among their greatest concerns (Stein et al., 2016). It is important to link clients with the appropriate treatment services during the stabilization process.

Urgent mental health needs may require more rapid attention. Suicidal ideation is common among clients in withdrawal management. Suicide risk can be exacerbated by intoxication and withdrawal symptoms that cloud a person's reasoning. Emotional lability is also common, and protocols for staff and client safety should be in place to manage angry clients who act aggressively toward others.

> Suicidal ideation is common in the course of withdrawal.

Infectious Diseases

Drug use is associated with risk behaviors such as sharing of contaminated needles and unsafe sexual practices that contribute to the transmission of infectious diseases. There are elevated rates of tuberculosis (TB), hepatitis, HIV, and sexually transmitted diseases (STDs). Identifying at-risk clients is the first line of defense, and the stabilization period provides an opportunity to assess and address these concerns. Elevated risk of infectious diseases crosses the SUDs and is definitely not limited to injection drug users (Rehm et al., 2010; Walker, Pratt, Schoenborn, & Druss, 2017). Beyond needle sharing, infection risk is also increased by poor nutrition, poor hygiene, unprotected sex, contact with other substance users, incarceration, and institutionalization.

Screening for infections such as STDs, TB, HIV, and hepatitis is an important health care function during stabilization. In addition to curing or managing the infection itself, interventions should seek to reduce the risk of future infections, and to locate and test others who may have been exposed (Semaan, Neumann, Hutchins, D'Anna, & Kamb, 2010). Needle and syringe exchange programs are effective in reducing HIV transmission (Aspinall et al., 2014).

TUBERCULOSIS

TB is a contagious bacterial infection that mainly involves the lungs, but may spread to other organs. The primary stage of the disease is usually asymptomatic. Symptoms of the active disease include fatigue, cough, fever, coughing up blood, chest pains, excessive sweating, and unintentional weight loss. All clients entering treatment programs (and those who treat them) should receive a skin test for TB (Mulligan, 1995). Due to immuno-suppression, HIV-positive people are at particular risk for developing TB. Effective treatment requires taking medications for about 6–9 months, and close adherence to the prescribed regimen is important. This is a challenge with substance use and associated lifestyles, but failure to adhere can result in medication-resistant TB that is still more difficult to treat. Medications for TB may interact with pharmacotherapies used for people with addictions such as methadone and disulfiram, so medical monitoring is obviously important.

HEPATITIS B

The hepatitis B virus (HBV) spreads through blood, semen, vaginal secretions, and other body fluids. Infection can also occur when people have blood transfusions, are stuck with a contaminated needle, or have unprotected sex with an infected person. Many people with HBV initially have few or no symptoms and may not feel sick, even though they are infectious. Again, routine screening for HBV is indicated. A vaccine is available, and all at-risk individuals (including those who regularly treat patients with addiction) should be vaccinated. Early symptoms may not appear for up to 6 months after the time of infection and can include appetite loss, low-grade fever, muscle and joint aches, nausea and vomiting, yellow skin and dark urine due to jaundice, and fatigue. Certain medications such as methadone and disulfiram may be contraindicated for people who have ongoing liver disease due to hepatitis infection.

HEPATITIS C

There is a high prevalence of hepatitis C virus (HCV) among substance users, especially injection drug users. HCV most often spreads through direct contact with blood and contaminated needles, but can also be sexually transmitted. As with HBV, many people with HCV do not have symptoms. All people born between 1945 and 1965 and those with risk factors including current or prior IV drug use or nasal cocaine use should be screened for HCV. If the infection has been present for many years, the liver may be permanently scarred, a condition called cirrhosis. Symptoms that can emerge with HCV infection include abdominal pain, fatigue, jaundice, nausea, vomiting, and loss of appetite. Whereas curing HCV once required 6–12 months of chemotherapy with interferon or related medications, current treatment typically involves only oral direct-acting antiviral medications for as little as 8 weeks. Again, close adherence to medication regimens is important. Because HCV affects liver function, other medications such as methadone and disulfiram may be contraindicated during treatment.

HIV AND AIDS

Infection with HIV is associated with a progressive disease process. HIV is a chronic medical condition that can be treated, but not yet cured. Most cases are transmitted sexually through intimate sexual contact where there is exposure to body fluids such as semen, blood, and vaginal secretions. HIV can also be spread by the use of contaminated needles and syringes. Once someone has contracted HIV, there are effective ways to prevent complications and to delay progression to AIDS. Symptoms related to HIV are usually due to an opportunistic infection in some part of the body and include diarrhea, fatigue, fever, headache, mouth sores, rashes, sore throat, and swollen lymph glands.

STDs

People under the influence of alcohol and other drugs are more likely to engage in risky sexual practices, and routine screening for STDs is warranted in addiction treatment services. In addition to screening, effective counseling methods are available to reduce rates of unprotected sex for both men (Calsyn et al., 2009) and women (Tross et al., 2008). These treatment modules include information about HIV transmission, self-risk assessment, discussion of safe sex options, assertive communication and negotiation skills, and exploration of ways to have enjoyable sex without drugs. Therapist guidelines for these (and many other) evidence-based modules are available for free download at *www.ctndisseminationlibrary.org*.

More than 30 organisms can cause STDs. Four of the most common among people seeking addiction treatment are syphilis, gonorrhea, chlamydia, and genital herpes. Transmission of *syphilis* infection can occur by needle sharing, though in most cases it is sexually transmitted. The bacteria that cause it spread through broken skin or mucous membranes. If left untreated, syphilis progresses through several phases. Initial symptoms of syphilis may include painless sores and swollen lymph nodes. These usually occur within 3 weeks of infection and may go unnoticed. In the second stage, symptoms can include fever, fatigue, rash, aches and pains, and loss of appetite. Tertiary syphilis damages the heart, brain, and nervous system. Syphilis is responsive to treatment with antibiotics. Encourage HIV testing in people who have syphilis, since the presence of syphilis increases the risk of acquiring HIV.

Symptoms of *gonorrhea* usually appear 2–5 days after infection. In women, these symptoms can be very mild and nonspecific, but may include vaginal discharge, burning and pain while urinating, increased urination, painful sexual intercourse, severe pain in the lower abdomen, and fever. In men, symptoms may take up to a month to appear and can include burning and pain while urinating, increased urinary frequency or urgency, discharge from the penis, red or swollen opening of the penis, and tender or swollen testicles. About half of women diagnosed with gonorrhea are also infected with chlamydia, another very common sexually transmitted disease that can result in sterility. Immediately treating a gonorrhea infection helps prevent permanent scarring and infertility.

Chlamydia is a bacterial infection transmitted mainly through sexual intercourse with an infected person. Chlamydia has a high prevalence, is easily transmitted, and is associated with gonorrhea. It is very common for both men and women to experience no symptoms of chlamydia. In men, symptoms of chlamydia are similar to those of gonorrhea and may include a burning sensation during urination, discharge from the penis, testicular tenderness or pain, and rectal discharge or pain. Symptoms that may occur in women include a burning sensation during urination, painful sexual intercourse, vaginal discharge, rectal pain or discharge, and symptoms of pelvic inflammatory disease. Screening is strongly encouraged, particularly for high-risk pregnant women, adolescents, and people with multiple sexual partners. Asymptomatic infection can lead to infertility if untreated. Chlamydia can be treated with an antibiotic regimen, and clients should refrain from sexual intercourse until treatment is completed.

Genital herpes is a viral infection that can be treated but currently cannot be cured. It is easily transmitted through genital contact. Initial symptoms in the first week after exposure can be mild and vague, such as fatigue, malaise, headache, or fever. A first outbreak usually occurs during 1 month after exposure and can include genital pain, blisters, sensitivity and itching, swollen lymph nodes, fever, and fatigue. Outbreaks typically last for about 2 weeks, and often recur for months or years. Even in the general U.S. population, about one in four adults have been infected. The virus can be passed from mother to newborn baby during vaginal delivery, which can be fatal due to the infant's undeveloped immune system.

Routine medical screening for STDs is an important service to link with addiction treatment. As described above, initial symptoms of STDs are often unnoticed or ignored. The presence of one STD increases risk for other STDs including HIV. Screening is particularly important with pregnant women because of risks for transmission to the child. Bacterial STDs are curable and viral STDs are treatable. Counseling for safe sex practices should also be routine with sexually active clients to reduce the spread of infections (Calsyn et al., 2009; Tross et al., 2008).

VACCINE-PREVENTABLE ILLNESSES

People in (as well as providers of) addiction treatment may be eligible for various vaccines to prevent future illness. Hepatitis B vaccine involves a series of three doses over 6 months and should be given to anyone who injects drugs, has HIV or hepatitis C, is in a correctional facility, or seeks care in a drug treatment facility. Hepatitis A vaccine is given in a series of two doses over 6 months and should be given to anyone who uses illicit drugs of any kind or has HIV or hepatitis C. Pneumococcal vaccine prevents diseases such as pneumonia that are caused by the bacteria streptococcus pneumoniae. There are two pneumococcal vaccines available, PPSV-23 (Pneumovax) and PCV-13 (Prevnar). PPSV-23 should be given to anyone who smokes, has an alcohol use disorder, or has hepatitis C or HIV. Those with HIV should also receive PCV-13.

CONTRACEPTION COUNSELING

Substance use during pregnancy is associated with multiple adverse outcomes for both the mother and the fetus. These include low birth weight, hypertensive disease of pregnancy including pre-eclampsia, preterm labor, and even miscarriage. Pregnant women actively using substances should be referred to an appropriate medical facility for ongoing prenatal care and careful monitoring. Women of childbearing age who are not pregnant and being treated for addiction should be offered contraception counseling. There are many safe, reliable, and long-term contraceptive options available. There are estrogen and progesterone methods such as "the pill," patches or a vaginal ring, progesterone-only methods such as the DepoProvera shot and Nexplanon implant that can last 3 months to 3 years, and intrauterine devices that can last 3–10 years.

OTHER HEALTH CARE NEEDS

People presenting for addiction treatment often have other untreated health problems. These may be related to injuries, nutritional and hygiene practices, and the toxic effects of alcohol and other drugs. As part of case management, it is important to ensure and facilitate each client's linkage with a primary care provider. Oral health is also a common problem related to SUDs, and one that can impact health more generally. Ask whether clients are receiving routine dental care and, if not, help them to do so. Such coordination is facilitated when addiction and health care services are located together or nearby.

It is indeed unfortunate that specialist treatment programs for SUDs have so often been isolated and located away from medical and behavioral health care facilities, even from the hospitals and medical clinics that own and operate them. This often reflects a spoken or unspoken prejudice that "we don't want *those* people around our hospital or clinic." In truth, people with SUDs are already being seen far more often in hospitals, medical settings, and behavioral health facilities than in specialist addiction treatment.

We hope that in the future addiction treatment programs will be co-located with other health care services, thus facilitating integrated care. At the very least, free and convenient shuttle service can be provided between addiction treatment facilities and the other health services that are so often needed.

Transition from Stabilization to Treatment

Stabilization has often been the only treatment phase that people receive. There are several reasons for this. Sometimes clients become discouraged and distressed during stabilization and leave against medical advice. On the other hand, stabilization may give them the relief they wanted, and feeling better they see no immediate need for further treatment. Geographic separation of withdrawal management and treatment facilities also hinders transition, as do waiting lists and other barriers to receiving treatment services. The result is the familiar "revolving door" phenomenon whereby people turn up repeatedly in withdrawal management, hospital, social service, and correctional systems. For this reason, motivation for and transition to rehabilitation is a third important function in withdrawal management, along with evaluation and stabilization. Withdrawal management in itself is insufficient treatment, and very unlikely to change substance use.

Timing is an issue. When the withdrawal process is particularly severe, it is wise to wait for mental functions to clear and physical distress to subside. It's somewhat like working in an emergency department: if someone is coding and in imminent danger of death, that is not the moment for a substance use consult! Yet there is also a risk in waiting too long. The stabilization period is a window of opportunity during which need for treatment may be more salient, and people are sometimes discharged prematurely, thus losing this opportunity. As soon as feasible, begin discussing and enhancing motivation for the next phase of treatment. Doing so and attending to clients' other needs can also decrease the likelihood of their leaving withdrawal management prematurely.

Enhancing Motivation for Change

Motivation for change is not a client trait, but rather a state that emerges and fluctuates through interpersonal interactions. You do not have to wait for people to become "ready" for change. Motivation for treatment is heavily influenced by what you do and how you interact with clients (Miller & Rollnick, 2013; Walitzer, Dermen, & Connors, 1999). In Chapter 10 we discuss in detail some strategies for strengthening client motivation, so here we will mention just a few key aspects.

Compassion

First and foremost, offer a welcoming atmosphere of acceptance, respect, and compassion (see Chapter 4). Someone entering the service should feel cared for from the outset. A good model of this is found in AA, where people are always welcomed back. A program is there to serve the clients, not vice versa. Motivation for change is promoted by therapeutic acceptance, not rejection; by compassion, not judgment; and by hope, not shame. In numerous studies just a brief, compassionate, client-centered conversation in the emergency room significantly increased motivation for and initiation of SUD treatment (Bernstein, Bernstein, & Levenson, 1997; Bernstein et al., 2009; Bernstein et al., 2005; Bernstein et al., 2015; Chafetz, 1961; Chafetz et al., 1962; Monti, Colby, & O'Leary, 2001).

Discrepancy

Although you might like to install motivation in a client, what really matters is the client's *own* motivation for change. One way to think about this internal motivation is as a discrepancy between the current reality and goals that are important to the client (Miller & Rollnick, 2013). Help clients to voice their own goals and values, and how changing their substance use could help to achieve them (see Chapter 10).

> You do not have to wait for people to become "ready" for change.

Hope

Clients are not the only people who can become discouraged. It's common for clinical staff to feel disheartened or annoyed to see the same person coming back repeatedly for withdrawal management and to wonder, "What makes this time any different from the last?" It is a good question to ask, in part because it suggests that perhaps it is time to try something different from the last time. It's important to treat clients, even "frequent fliers," with hope and optimism that this visit will bring the change the client hopes to achieve. Because the consequences of substance use are often so readily apparent during withdrawal management, this is a useful window of opportunity to try different strategies to enhance motivation for change (see Chapter 10). Most people do ultimately escape from the cycle of addiction, and one reframe is that each turn around the circle brings the person one step closer to change. During the withdrawal management process, clients may feel very little hope of their own as a result of both the immediate physical discomfort and awareness of the long road ahead, so you may need to lend them some of yours (Yahne & Miller, 1999).

Case Management

Addressing barriers to treatment such as housing, child care, transportation, and career assistance can facilitate engagement in treatment. There are basic needs clients may have during the withdrawal management process, including food and clothing, financial assistance, and access to a safe living environment. If these needs are not met, it is harder for the person to commit to a course of treatment. It is important to begin assertive case management during withdrawal management to link the person with needed services or resources, including peer support specialists (see Chapter 8).

Linkages to Treatment

Once clients have progressed past the most severe withdrawal symptoms and are medically stable, it is appropriate to prepare them for the transition to rehabilitation and continuing care (see Chapter 7). Whether they will take this next step is influenced by a number of factors including:

- *Motivation.* The client's level of motivation, as mentioned above, is malleable and can be increased by specific clinical strategies. People are more likely to initiate and remain in treatment if they believe the services will help them with specific life problems (Fiorentine, Nakashima, & Anglin, 1999). Find out what clients want, need, and prefer from treatment and actively assist them in finding a good fit.
- *Direct linkage.* Making a specific appointment with a treatment service while the person is still in withdrawal management can roughly double the chances of completing the referral, compared to just giving the information to clients and asking them to make the contact. It is better still if clients can meet and connect with treatment providers while still in withdrawal management.
- *Convenience.* The farther clients have to travel in order to get to continuing care, the less likely it is that they will persist (Prue, Keane, Cornell, & Foy, 1979).
- *Transportation.* Even among those who make an appointment for addiction treatment, a substantial proportion may not show up (Gottheil, Sterling, & Weinstein, 1997b). Scheduling a staff member, volunteer, or significant other to transport and accompany the client to the appointment will increase arrival. It can also be helpful for the client to have such an advocate along in order to persist through any frustrations or administrative hurdles.
- *Minimal wait.* The longer clients have to wait for treatment services, the less likely it is that they will engage (Carroll, 1997).

KEY POINTS

🔖 Withdrawal management represents preparation for ongoing addiction treatment and continuing care and can usually be accomplished without hospitalization.

🔖 Stabilization involves identifying and addressing urgent needs including nutritional and other health care problems, infectious diseases, and pressing behavioral health or psychosocial needs.

🔖 It is important in addiction treatment to assess the likelihood of withdrawal, which can range from minimal to severe.

🔖 Withdrawal management is offered in both residential and ambulatory settings, and within each there are both medical and social (drug-free) programs.

🔖 Withdrawal management is just the beginning of addiction treatment. It is rarely sufficient in itself. A primary task during stabilization is to facilitate motivation for and transition to rehabilitation and maintenance.

Reflection Questions

❓ How do you help or refer patients who need medical evaluation during the stabilization process? Is such medical consultation available within your setting?

❓ What experience(s) would help you be more comfortable and competent to recognize, evaluate, and/or manage drug withdrawal?

❓ What types of attitudes, beliefs, and problems could be obstacles to engaging clients in withdrawal management and subsequent recovery services?

❓ Dropout after management of withdrawal is a common problem. How can you assess, prioritize, and consider additional needs to help ensure that patients make the transition into further treatment?

CHAPTER 7

Individualizing Treatment

What does it mean to individualize treatment for each client's needs? "We customize treatment" has become a common claim among treatment providers, but how is that to be accomplished in practice?

The opposite of custom-tailored treatment is plain enough: a "one-size-fits-all" approach whereby clients must accept and accommodate to standard treatment. Such an approach is sometimes called "Procrustean" after Procrustes, the inhospitable character of Greek mythology who had only one iron bed and adjusted every guest to fit it by stretching or amputating. An analogy in golf is to have only one club and then blame the ball for not going into the cup.

One conception of individualizing treatment is to match clients to a treatment that is most likely to help them, a familiar scenario in medicine. Medical providers are expected to keep up with research on which treatments are most effective (or ineffective) for particular conditions, and failure to deliver an appropriate treatment can constitute malpractice. The emerging field of precision medicine involves matching people to the treatment that is most likely to be effective for their disease, taking into account individual variation in genes, environment, and lifestyle (Collins & Varmus, 2015). For example, surgery, radiation, chemotherapy, immunological, and hormonal treatments are available for specific cancers, and sometimes the most appropriate approach is just to "watch and wait." Ideally providers do not advocate just for their own specialized form of treatment (with surgeons recommending surgery and radiologists advising radiation). Instead good practice is to offer patients an informed choice among the available options, along with an accurate account of what is known scientifically about their relative efficacy. In this chapter we

> Offer patients an informed choice.

begin by considering four phases of care, explore the process of choosing among treatment approaches, and then offer a broader perspective on individualizing addiction treatment.

Four Phases of Treatment: A Continuum of Care

Within the bigger picture of managing a chronic condition over time, it is helpful to think about phases of care. Where is this person in the process of recovery? What does he or she need at present? This is part of individualizing care, in that the goals and processes of treatment vary depending on where clients are in their journey. There are various stage models of treatment for addiction, and we think in terms of four phases: palliative care, stabilization, rehabilitation, and maintenance (see Box 7.1).

Phase 1: Palliative Care

Phase 1 actually precedes what many people would think of as "treatment" for addiction. Palliative care for people with addictions is what normally happens when they seek health care. They may see no need at all to be treated for alcohol/drug problems; they may not even think of their drinking or drug use as problematic. A provider may encourage the person to seek formal help (Phase 2 or 3), but it is common for such referral attempts to fail. What then? Should providers ignore or give up on their patients' addiction problems? People still deserve to be cared for, and there is concern to protect not only them, but their families and society from harm.

Some general goals in Phase 1 are to keep the person in contact with systems of care; reduce risks of illness, harm, or death; enhance motivation for change in substance use; and facilitate access and entry to Phase 2 or 3 services. The person may be willing to consider options short of formal treatment, such as self-help materials (Apodaca & Miller, 2003; Miller, 2014) or referral to a mutual help resource such as 12-step groups (Chapter 17). Although most addiction treatment programs do not see people during Phase 1, this is an important phase of care. Most people with diagnosable SUDs are not receiving Phase 2 or 3 treatment, and many *never* seek such treatment. Though our primary focus in this book is on Phases 2–4, palliative care remains the most commonly sought form of treatment for people with SUDs.

Phase 2: Stabilization

Given the range and severity of addiction's possible effects on people's health, social, and psychological functioning, it is sometimes necessary to stabilize them in preparation for Phase 3 treatment. This can include

BOX 7.1. Four Phases of Care

Phase of Care	Specific Tasks
Phase 1: Palliative care	• Prevent drug-related death. • Maintain user's contact with care systems. • Enhance self-care to reduce health risks and harm for the user. • Decrease risks and harm to society. • Identify and support family members, as appropriate. • Strengthen motivation for change in substance use. • Facilitate access and entry to Phase 2 or 3 services.
Phase 2: Stabilization	• Detoxify—safely eliminate drugs from the body. • Enhance retention in and completion of Phase 2. • Stabilize—address acute health and welfare needs. • Initiate case management. • Increase motivation for treatment/rehabilitation (Phase 3). • Facilitate access and entry to Phase 3 services.
Phase 3: Rehabilitation	• Establish an empathic therapeutic relationship. • Enhance retention in Phase 3. • Negotiate and clarify goals for change. • Develop a clear and realistic change plan (including treatment plan). • Implement change plan to stabilize initial change in substance use. • Assess client strengths and resources. • Identify and involve family/support network, as feasible. • Initiate sampling of and participation in mutual help groups, as appropriate. • Address the most pressing concomitant problems and disorders. • Increase motivation for continuation of changes and personal growth (Phase 4). • Initiate a maintenance plan to prevent recurrence. • Facilitate access and entry to Phase 4 services.
Phase 4: Maintenance	• Support motivation for maintenance of change. • Negotiate and clarify goals and plan for maintenance of change. • Implement maintenance plan to prevent recurrence. • Continue case management, facilitate access to needed services. • Continue monitoring and treatment contact as appropriate and desired. • Establish and maintain rewarding drug-free activities and relationships. • Facilitate spiritual development. • Maintain mutual help group involvement, as appropriate.

withdrawal management and attention to basic health care needs, as discussed in Chapter 6. There may be pressing social problems that require attention, such as a need for housing, food, or child safety. A person may also be in acute distress or suicidal, and need crisis and case management (see Chapter 8). All of these issues may need to be addressed before a person is sufficiently stabilized to begin Phase 3 treatment.

The transition to Phase 3 is also by no means automatic. As mentioned in the preceding chapter there is a familiar revolving door phenomenon of people with addictions returning repeatedly for Phase 1 (e.g., emergency room) or Phase 2 (e.g., withdrawal management) services without changing their substance use. A vital function in Phase 2, then, is to strengthen the person's motivation to change his or her substance use and, as appropriate, to seek help in doing so. Methods for enhancing motivation for change will be discussed in Chapter 10.

Phase 3: Rehabilitation

Historically, Phase 3 services are what most addiction treatment programs have provided. For this phase of care we prefer the term *rehabilitation*—literally, to make fit and able again.

Phase 3 has its own unique goals. One of these, of course, involves changing prior substance use, but most people have a much broader range of problems and needs. In fact, changing substance use may be well down the person's own list of priorities. The beginning of Phase 3 is the time to develop a problem list, negotiate and clarify goals for change, and agree upon a clear and realistic change plan. Strengthening motivation to achieve the negotiated goals is another important up-front task (see Chapter 10), and early attention to factors that promote retention in treatment is wise. Phase 3 then proceeds into implementation of the initial change plan, all the while strengthening motivation and skills to maintain the gains that are made (Phase 4). All of this relies upon the establishment and maintenance of an empathic working relationship (Chapter 4).

One reason why we are so enthusiastic in encouraging behavioral health professionals to treat addictions is that SUDs and other addictive behaviors seldom occur in isolation (Chapter 20). Those who treat people experiencing addiction encounter the entire DSM, as well as a host of employment, family, legal, medical, and social life problems. Counselors who are prepared only to treat addictions face the challenge of what to do about this host of concomitant problems and disorders: ignore them, put them on hold, assume they are secondary to the addiction and will clear up, try to treat them without adequate professional preparation, or refer out for other services? Professionals who are also competent to treat a broader panoply of health and psychosocial problems are, we believe, better prepared to help people with SUDs.

Phase 4: Maintenance

The real challenge with addictions is not making the initial change so much as maintaining it. Mark Twain quipped that quitting smoking is easy—he had done it dozens of times. As with chronic medical illnesses, there is a need for ongoing care and monitoring. Treatment is not over when a Phase 3 episode has ended. People with asthma, diabetes, or heart disease normally receive ongoing monitoring and treatment from a primary care provider, with occasional acute care visits (e.g., to an emergency room) to deal with recurrences. Addiction has been, arguably, the only chronic disease for which there is typically only acute and specialist care with no primary care (McLellan at al., 2000). We discuss Phase 4 care in Chapter 21.

Choosing among Treatments

As will become evident in Part III of this book, there is already an encouraging array of evidence-supported methods for treating SUDs, with more than a thousand randomized clinical trials published to evaluate their efficacy. It is a sensible idea that people do not all respond the same or best to any one particular treatment approach. One size does not fit all. A method that works very well for one person may be ineffective, unacceptable, or culturally inappropriate for another. It is reasonable to ask which of an array of potentially effective methods might be best for a particular person. Matching patients to optimal treatment is an idea that can be traced right back to the very beginning of systematic treatment for addictions (Bowman & Jellinek, 1941). How then does such matching occur?

Natural Matching

Wherever treatment options are available, some degree of natural matching is already happening. People vote with their feet. If they try a treatment program and it doesn't feel right, they are less likely to come back for a second visit. When they find a place or approach that suits them, they are more likely to stay. It's a bit like how churchgoers choose their home congregation and AA members find their home group. They shop around, in person or by telephone or online, until they find one that they perceive to meet their needs, and where they feel at home. Being coerced into a particular program (e.g., by the courts) narrows the options, but even then there is a substantial degree of variation in attendance and adherence.

There are many important influences on natural matching, one of which is word of mouth. Deserved or undeserved, programs develop different reputations in the community, and people talk to each other about the options. ("Go there! It's a place where they *listen* to addicts," a newcomer to our center had been told. We were pleased.) There are practical considerations such as relative cost, ease of access, length and type of commitment required, geographic accessibility, waiting lists, safety, and past experience. In a managed care context, only one or a few options may be covered by a particular health plan. Then there is the experience that people have during initial sessions. Early dropout is quite common in addiction treatment, and dropout rates vary widely across providers. Clients quickly develop a sense of the quality of the working alliance they would have with a counselor or program, and this perception affects the course and outcome of therapy. All of these factors influence the treatment options that people choose for themselves.

Clinical Judgment

A second potential source of matching is the clinical judgment of professionals. Again, many different factors might influence such decisions including client characteristics and preferences, one's training and theoretical orientation, past experience, personal recovery history, program reputation and marketing, cost, location, health plan coverage, and interprofessional relationships and agreements. In one disconcerting study, however, there was little variability in treatment recommendations (Hanson & Emrick, 1983). Actors who presented with very different alcohol problem histories went to various treatment programs asking for advice as to what approach would be best for them. The study was intended to discern what criteria were being used to match people to programs. They found instead that programs almost always recommended themselves regardless of a client's problems or severity.

A prerequisite for matching is the availability of different treatment options. When there is only one option available, there is no need for matching. Where different options are available, matching depends on knowing about the alternatives and who is most likely to benefit from each of them.

So how good are expert clinicians at knowing which addiction treatment approach will be best for different kinds of people? The largest controlled trial ever conducted for alcohol treatment methods was designed to answer this very question (Project MATCH Research Group, 1993). Three treatment methods were selected, representing conceptually different approaches: 12 sessions of 12-step facilitation therapy (TSF; Nowinski, Baker, & Carroll, 1992), four sessions of motivational enhancement therapy (MET; Miller, Zweben, DiClimente, & Rychtarik, 1992), or 12 sessions of cognitive-behavioral therapy (CBT; Kadden et al., 1992). Because it was unclear which personal characteristics would prove most important, the 1,726 participants completed extensive pretreatment assessment. Clients were then randomly assigned to one of the three treatment methods, and a priori matching hypotheses were formulated and tested (Longabaugh

& Wirtz, 2001). The full story of Project MATCH is recounted in a single volume (Babor & Del Boca, 2003), summarizing findings from a series of more detailed published reports (Project MATCH Research Group, 1997a, 1997b, 1998a, 1998b, 1998c, 1998d).

As hoped, the three therapeutic methods produced, on average, excellent and equivalent outcomes, whether offered as outpatient treatment or as aftercare following residential treatment. Furthermore, clients' outcomes were reasonably stable across 3 years of follow-up, with relatively little loss of posttreatment improvement. On one outcome measure—the percentage of clients who remained totally abstinent—the TSF group showed about a 10% advantage throughout follow-up.

> A prerequisite for matching is the availability of different treatment options.

Project MATCH was not primarily a horse race, however; the central interest was in matches between clients and therapies. The study revealed surprisingly few robust matches. Nearly all previously reported matching effects from single studies were not confirmed in this multisite trial. A few reliable matches were found, however, suggesting some clinical guidelines for choosing among these three treatment approaches:

• As predicted, clients whose social networks supported continued drinking rather than abstinence fared best in the long run with TSF, presumably because the fellowship of AA provided them with a strong social support network for sobriety. The key for such clients appears to be to get them involved in AA or another recovery-supporting network *during treatment*. When clients' own social support networks favored abstinence, they fared at least as well in the other two treatments as in TSF.

• Some people did better with MET. The clinical method of motivational interviewing (see Chapter 10) was designed to reduce client resistance and elicit internal motivation for change. As predicted, more angry clients fared best with MET (Waldron, Miller, & Tonigan, 2001). Angry clients are more likely to offer resistance when directed to change, and resistance in turn predicts poorer outcomes. Clients with lower initial motivation for change also had better 1-year outcomes in MET (Witkiewitz, Hartzler, & Donovan, 2010).

• Clients with less concomitant psychopathology (whose problems centered mainly on alcohol) fared better in TSF than in CBT. This was an unpredicted and unexplained finding—that the advantages of this AA-focused approach were clearest for clients with relatively few psychological problems.

• In aftercare, clients with more severe alcohol dependence also fared better in TSF than in CBT, whereas the opposite was true for clients with less alcohol dependence. This is consistent with the more severe conception of alcoholism that is often presented in AA, with which more severely impaired individuals might be expected to identify.

• Subsequent analyses of the MATCH data have revealed matching effects not tested in the original trial. In one study, regardless of the form of treatment they received (CBT, MET, or TSF), clients with concomitant depression fared significantly worse when treated by therapists with a high focus on negative emotional issues (Karno & Longabaugh, 2003).

• In another analysis, Native American clients were found to fare significantly better in MET than with CBT or TSF, whereas such differences were not found for Caucasian and Hispanic clients (Villanueva, Tonigan, & Miller, 2007).

Triage into different kinds of psychotherapy is only one kind of matching. Far less is known about how to match clients at other decision points such as group versus individual therapy or behavioral versus pharmacotherapies. Guidelines for knowing when clients are likely to require withdrawal management are provided in Chapter 6.

Decision Rules

One way to reduce the arbitrariness of individual clinical judgment is to use a consistent set of decision rules. For example, research-based criteria have been suggested for advising people as to the likelihood of success with abstinence or moderate drinking goals in their particular case (Miller & Muñoz, 2013; Miller et al., 1992). The advantage of matching by such systems, of course, depends on the scientific validity of the decision rules.

Another approach is to develop decision rules that are based on the professional consensus of experts in the field. The most common example of this in the United States is the *Patient Placement Criteria* of the American Society of Addiction Medicine (Gastfriend, 2003). In the 1970s and 1980s, a majority of funds for addiction treatment in the United States were being spent on inpatient and residential treatment, typically of 28 days' duration (which was the maximum duration that most insurers would reimburse). As it became clear that the outcomes of inpatient programs were on average no different from those in less costly outpatient options (Institute of Medicine, 1990; Miller & Hester, 1986), third-party reimbursement for inpatient treatment was dramatically curtailed. In this managed care environment, a group of treatment program directors convened to develop a professional consensus set of decision rules, called the Cleveland Criteria (Hoffman, Halikas, & Mee-Lee, 1987), to guide and justify placing people into various levels of care. These were adopted and published by ASAM in 1991 (Hoffman, Halikas, Mee-Lee, & Weedman, 1991) and have been subsequently revised in increasingly complex systems (American Society of

Addiction Medicine, 1996, 2001). Six levels of care are now recognized, of increasing intensity and cost: early intervention (Level 0.5), opioid maintenance treatment (OMT), outpatient treatment (Level I), intensive outpatient or "partial hospitalization" (Level II), residential/inpatient treatment (Level III), and medically managed intensive inpatient treatment (Level IV). Decision rules for placement are based on assessment of two medical and four psychosocial dimensions. These data are combined by prescribed decision rules to arrive at a recommended level of care based on this consensus clinical judgment system, including sublevels of care and attention to concomitant mental health diagnoses.

A single basic prediction underlies the scientific validity of any such system for matching people to different treatments: that those who are correctly matched to recommendations should have better outcomes than do people who are mismatched according to the criteria. Research on matching came of age when this hypothesis began to be tested directly. Fortunately, it is not necessary to randomly assign people to be matched or mismatched to treatments in order to test this hypothesis. Such a design is logically equivalent to a normal clinical trial in which people are randomly assigned to different treatments (Miller & Cooney, 1994). As long as the criteria for matching are specified ahead of time before looking at the outcome data, and the appropriate measures of client characteristics are obtained, virtually any matching hypothesis can be tested retrospectively within a clinical trial (Longabaugh & Wirtz, 2001).

Matching to Levels of Treatment Intensity

The ASAM criteria for assigning people to levels of treatment intensity provide an example of the matching hypothesis. If these decision rules are valid, then patients who are correctly matched to the recommended level of treatment should show better outcomes than those who are given a different intensity of treatment. Cases are "matched" when the assessed level of need is the same as the level of treatment received. With six levels of care this creates six possible matched conditions and 30 possible mismatches. (These possibilities are multiplied when more than one outcome measure is used.) If a person received a *higher* level of care than recommended by the criteria, the case is said to be *overmatched*. Conversely, when the level of care provided is *lower* than that recommended by the placement criteria, the case is said to be *undermatched*.

Studies of the predictive validity of the ASAM criteria have yielded mixed findings. An early study of the Cleveland criteria (McKay, McLellan, & Alterman, 1992)—a precursor of the ASAM criteria—found no significant differences in 6-month outcomes between matched and undermatched cases receiving outpatient treatment (Level II). In a complementary study of inpatient treatment (Sharon et al., 2004), only one outcome difference was reported between matched and mismatched groups: under-matched people at the highest level of severity (Level IV) had more days of subsequent rehospitalization.

Potentially more informative are studies with clients in more than one level of care. One such study (Magura et al., 2003) followed people who were naturalistically (nonrandomly) assigned to Levels I, II, or III. Of the nine potential mismatches, only one affected outcomes ($p < .018$): People assessed at Level II fared better when receiving intensive outpatient (II) than regular outpatient treatment (I). In a controlled clinical trial (McKay, Cacciola, McLellan, Alterman, & Wirtz, 1997), no significant matching effects were found for medically stable people randomly assigned to Level II (day hospital) or Level III (inpatient) treatment for cocaine or alcohol dependence. A similar randomized trial (Angarita et al., 2007) reported only one significant effect: among overmatched patients (assessed at Level II but given inpatient treatment), those with co-occurring mental disorders were more likely to be no-shows for treatment.

There are numerous methodological challenges with such studies. Typically, there are multiple potential mismatches, and a variety of outcome measures are assessed. When one outcome variable is related to one possible match, its "significance" is dubious if there is no correction for the number of tests run. In most studies, the match that was found had not been predicted *a priori* but was found among multiple a posteriori tests, and the outcome variable showing a match differs across studies. None of the observed matches described above would be statistically significant if corrected for these factors. Another complexity is that the decision rules have evolved from the original criteria through subsequent ASAM versions.

More encouraging findings were reported from one naturalistic study in Norway (Stallvik, Gastfriend, & Nordahl, 2015). Comparing only two naturalistically assigned levels of care (I and III), undermatched cases showed higher attrition, less improvement in severity, and no significant reduction in substance use when compared with matched cases who were offered the recommended level of care.

In sum, scientific evidence for the validity of ASAM's placement criteria is weak thus far. No consistent outcome differences have been found or replicated for cases matched versus mismatched according to ASAM criteria.

Classification software for a computer-assisted structured interview has recently become available with a bank of over 1,000 questions administered in branching fashion so that any given client is likely to answer 100 to 200 questions. Naturalistic convergent validity studies in Norway (Stallvik & Nordahl, 2014) examined cases assigned by clinicians to three types of treatment programs varying in the extent to which they addressed concomitant mental health diagnoses. The ASAM software made similar recommendations to those of the clinicians. This could automate and improve the reliability of placement recommendations, although their predictive validity remains questionable.

Stepped Care

A simpler alternative to clinician or decision-rule matching is to follow the stepped care approach commonly used in medicine in the treatment of chronic diseases (e.g., Baker, Turner, Kay-Lambkin, & Lewin, 2009; Sobell & Sobell, 2000). The logic of stepped care is to offer the least intensive and intrusive level of care that is likely to help. If one level of care is not sufficient to resolve the problem, then the client is stepped up to the next higher level of intensity. With type 2 diabetes, for example, one might try first to control blood glucose by combinations of diet, exercise, and oral medication. If this is insufficient, medication might be changed or dosage increased. Insulin could be initiated next, with hospitalization used only when there is a need for acute stabilization of medically ill individuals.

There are several advantages in this approach. One is a cost advantage, in that less expensive options are the first line of defense. If these are sufficient, then the more expensive level of care is unneeded (and is more available for those who do need it). It is common for clients to surprise us—to respond to lower levels of care than a clinician might expect to work (Miller, 2000). It is easy to overestimate the amount of help that clients will require. Another advantage is that lower levels of care are often more readily available. When clients are placed on a waiting list, the window of motivation for change may have closed by the time a space opens up. Offering something immediate, albeit less intensive, can foster improvement. When space opens in the higher intensity care setting, the client can be transitioned if that level of care is still needed. In the meantime you've been doing something helpful and supportive.

It is by no means a foregone conclusion that if one level of care fails, only a higher level of care will work. There is no guarantee that more intensive care will succeed. Indeed, there is no overall relationship of the planned or actual duration of treatment to client outcomes (Schmidt, Bojesen, Nielsen & Andersen, 2018). Another option is to try a different approach at the same level of intensity, particularly if higher level options are not available. A client who has not responded to a 12-step-oriented outpatient program, for example, might be referred to a cognitive-behavioral outpatient approach. A more general principle is that if one approach hasn't been working, *try something else*. In a clinical trial (Liddle et al., 2018), adolescents with co-occurring SUDs and mental health issues, most of whom had had prior residential treatment, were randomly assigned to outpatient family therapy or residential treatment. For the first 2 months both groups showed similar reductions in substance use and delinquency, but thereafter the outpatient group was more significantly effective in maintaining these gains through 18 months of follow-up.

Expert Systems

It is a nearly universal finding in psychological research that as clinicians we place unwarranted trust in our own clinical judgment. Give accurate information for about 100 cases to a computer and also to a clinician and then ask each to make predictions about 100 new cases. It has been known for a long time that the computer is usually far more accurate in predicting diagnoses or outcomes in the new cases (Wiggins, 1973). But what if the computer were given only a particular clinician's own judgments, rather than the actual truth about the 100 cases? In this case, the computer develops a mathematical model of the clinician's judgment, and armed only with that model it *still* outperforms the clinician in accuracy on the next 100 cases. It has, in essence, abstracted the rules by which the clinician makes reasonably good judgments, and then applies them with perfect reliability (Goldberg, 1970).

Computer algorithms known as "expert systems" have been developed to improve the accuracy of many decision processes, from making medical diagnoses to flying spacecraft. When your judgment tells you one thing and the computer tells you another, which should you trust? In most situations the computer is more likely to be right, but as clinicians we do overwhelmingly prefer to trust our own judgment.

Suppose that the outcome to be predicted is the risk that a driving-while-intoxicated (DWI) offender will repeat the offense. Computer algorithms can do a reasonably good job of predicting recidivism, given accurate data about the characteristics and outcomes of past cases (C'de Baca, Miller, & Lapham, 2001). The accuracy of such actuarial prediction programs is very likely to exceed that of nearly all clinicians, and yet these important public safety decisions continue to be made largely by clinical judgment.

As long as both predictor and outcome data are available, expert systems can be developed to assist in decision making. An automated client assessment system such as that mentioned above (Stallvik & Nordahl, 2014) need not be limited to implementing decision rules developed by clinical judgment. The same data can be used to derive predictive equations that can then be tested for validity with a future or hold-out sample. This was the original vision behind the "core-shell" system for improving client–treatment matching (Martin, 1995; Weisner, 1995).

Informed Choice

Yet another option is to involve clients in selecting and designing their own treatment. There are at least two possible advantages in doing so. First, people know something about which approaches are likely to be helpful, acceptable, and attractive for them. In oncology medicine it is normal good practice to give patients a fair description of the treatment options that are available to them and the most likely outcomes and side effects of each, and allow them to make an informed choice as to what treatment they prefer. The same could surely be done with regard to addiction treatment options. The self-referral biases of treatment programs suggest that such matching ought to be done by an independent professional or agency not invested in particular choices (Martin, 1995), but the implementation of such a system can be both complex and expensive, as illustrated by the "core-shell" system experiment in Ontario (Weisner, 1995), and it still might be no better than clients choosing for themselves.

A second reason for informed self-matching is the motivational advantage of having chosen. When people perceive that they have freely selected a

---

BOX 7.2. Personal Reflection: On Giving People What They Want

I once worked with a hospital's psychiatry consultation liaison service. We would receive consult requests from the medical teams for patients who had been admitted to the hospital, and go to see them.

This particular consult request read, "Patient interested in abstinence from alcohol." I met with this middle-aged man for a little while, discussing what led him to this point and what types of help he might prefer on his path to recovery. After a long discussion, he decided that inpatient treatment was his preference. He liked the idea of being away from people who might encourage him to drink and from places where he would feel tempted. Access to residential treatment programs was very difficult, though, particularly for public programs. While he was still in the hospital we were able to get his name on a waiting list, but he wasn't able to transition directly into an inpatient program from the hospital. I was frustrated by this, knowing that he was ready and willing to make a change, and that the barrier was the unavailability of treatment.

A few days later, I was walking through the emergency department when I heard him call out my name from behind one of the curtains. I turned around and peeked in, wondering why he was back in the hospital. He had seemed to be one of the most highly motivated people I had talked to while on this rotation, and yet here he was back for an alcohol-related hospital admission. A few days after his prior discharge, he had gone sober to a local treatment program, where he was told that immediate admissions were only for people who were acutely intoxicated. "Basically," he explained, "they were telling me to come back when I was good and drunk!" Even though he had stayed sober during the days since he left the hospital, what he really wanted was the structure of a residential program. So he did what seemed logical: in order to show up at the treatment program drunk and thus get into treatment, he went to the liquor store and bought two fifths of vodka.

"So what happened?" I asked with interest.

"Well, I drank so much that I forgot to go back!" he replied.

—A. A. F.

particular product or course of action from among options, they are likely to be more satisfied with and committed to it. There is evidence that taking active steps toward change increases the likelihood of successful change, no matter what the action happens to be. If what matters is for the client to do *something* and stick with it, then it makes sense to allow clients to select that to which they will be most committed.

Imagine this. Clients who come seeking treatment are offered a menu of available services with good evidence of efficacy and are invited to say what they would like from the menu. In one study we did exactly that (Brown & Miller, 1993). Inpatients were given at admission a list of possible services (see Box 7.3 later in this chapter) and asked which ones they wanted as part of their treatment. Then at discharge they were asked again, via a parallel questionnaire, which services they had actually received. Sobriety at 3 months after discharge was predictable from the extent to which they received the services they had wanted. The extent to which they had been given other services (that they had not asked for) was unrelated to treatment outcomes.

And the menu need not be limited to addiction-focused services. People who present for treatment of SUDs often come with a host of additional problems. Because health and social service systems have often been fragmented into specialty clinics, there is a tendency to focus addiction treatment solely on substance use. It is now clear that clients will be more successful in recovering from addiction when their other needs are being addressed as well (McLellan et al., 1998, 1999). This is not to say that clinicians who treat addictions must also handle every other problem that clients present. What it does imply is the need to make sure clients are at least referred to other services they need, and do connect with those services. If those additional services are provided at the same location (one-stop treatment), so much the better, but if not there are effective ways to help people get to the services they need. These case management functions are discussed more fully in Chapter 8.

Developing a Change Plan

Helping people to develop a change plan is a useful step in treatment. A change plan is broader than a treatment plan, though related. A good change plan lists the client's specific goals for change, and for each the particular steps or strategies to move toward that goal. Not all of these will involve additional treatment, and sometimes none of them do. Getting professional help is but one possible strategy to pursue a change goal. A treatment plan therefore represents a subset of the change plan: those parts of the change plan for which additional treatment is anticipated.

Setting Goals

A first step in developing a change plan is to clarify the client's goals. What changes would your client welcome? This is a process of negotiation. Although your aspiration for someone might be that he or she would stop all drug use immediately and permanently, what change is the person interested in and willing to pursue? The "miracle question" from solution-focused therapy (de Shazer et al., 2007) is one way to get at this: "If a miracle happened, if you woke up tomorrow and all of the problems that you have described were magically gone, how would you know? How would things be different?"

Often there is a need to move from broad or vague desires to more specific goals. A good change goal is one you can get your "ARMS" around (Miller & Mee-Lee, 2012):

- A—It is *Achievable*. It's fine for a goal to be challenging, but it should be realistic, something that is actually possible for the person to accomplish.
- R—It should be *Rewarding*. A good goal is one that the person wants and is willing to work toward achieving.
- M—It is *Measurable*. How will you know that progress is being made toward this goal? What observable changes will there be?
- S—It is *Specific*. Vague and general goals are harder to achieve. If there is a bigger long-term goal, one way to be more specific is to identify a next step to take toward it.

One broad approach is to offer your client a menu of possible goals or topics. An advantage of a menu over open-ended discussion of needs is that you can quickly survey a range of possible goals that might not otherwise be considered. One simple format is a "What I Want from Treatment" questionnaire (see Box 7.3). The menu can be as long or short as you choose, and the items can be tailored to your own particular setting and population. What we provide in Box 7.3 is just one example.

But to back up a step: Why ask at all about what clients want? Why not just prescribe the goals of treatment or announce what the program's goals are for everyone? One obvious reason is that people's needs differ, even if a program happens to treat them all the same. If you personally or programmatically cannot address some of the client's goals, you can at least link the client with other resources to help achieve them (see Chapter 8). There is also the pragmatic point that when it comes right down to it, no one but clients themselves *can* set their own goals. There is also the advantage mentioned earlier that when people choose their own goals, they tend to be more motivated to pursue them.

There are different ways to present a finite list of goals. What I Want from Treatment items could be placed instead on small cards, one per card.

BOX 7.3. What I Want from Treatment

William R. Miller, PhD, and Janice M. Brown, PhD

People have different ideas about what they want, need, and expect from treatment. Please tell us what you hope to happen in your treatment here.

1. I want to receive detoxification, to ease my withdrawal from alcohol or other drugs.   Yes   No

2. I want to find out whether I have a problem with alcohol or other drugs.   Yes   No

3. I want to stop drinking alcohol completely.   Yes   No

4. I want to decrease my drinking.   Yes   No

5. I want to take medication that would help me to avoid drinking.   Yes   No

6. I want to quit smoking (tobacco).   Yes   No

7. I want to stop using other drugs.   Yes   No

8. I want to decrease my use of other drugs.   Yes   No

9. I want to learn more about alcohol/drug problems.   Yes   No

10. I want to learn how to keep from returning to alcohol or other drugs.   Yes   No

11. I want help in dealing with cravings or urges to drink or use drugs.   Yes   No

12. I want to know more about 12-step groups like Alcoholics Anonymous (AA)   Yes   No

13. I want to know more about mutual help groups other than the 12-step groups.   Yes   No

14. I need to fulfill a requirement of the courts.   Yes   No

15. I want to learn how to resist social pressure to drink or use drugs.   Yes   No

16. I want to find enjoyable ways to spend my free time without drinking/using.   Yes   No

17. I want to decrease the level of stress, tension, or anxiety in my life.   Yes   No

18. I want to improve my physical health and fitness.   Yes   No

19. I want help in managing my depression or moods.   Yes   No

(continued)

This questionnaire is in the public domain and may be reproduced without further permission.

BOX 7.3. *(continued)*

20. I want help in managing my anger.	Yes	No
21. I want to have healthier relationships.	Yes	No
22. I want to discuss sexual problems.	Yes	No
23. I want to learn better ways to express my feelings.	Yes	No
24. I want to learn how to deal with boredom or loneliness.	Yes	No
25. I want to decrease or prevent violence at home.	Yes	No
26. I want to find a job (or a better job).	Yes	No
27. I want to find a better place to live.	Yes	No
28. I want help with legal problems.	Yes	No
29. I want to feel better about myself, to have more self-esteem.	Yes	No
30. I want to discuss my thoughts about suicide.	Yes	No
31. I want information about or testing for HIV/AIDS.	Yes	No
32. I want information about or testing for other infections (like hepatitis, TB, STDs)	Yes	No
33. I want someone to listen to me.	Yes	No
34. I want to learn to have fun without drugs or alcohol.	Yes	No
35. I want someone to tell me what to do.	Yes	No
36. I want help in setting goals or priorities for my life.	Yes	No
37. I want to learn how to use my time better.	Yes	No
38. I want to talk about my past.	Yes	No
39. I want to learn how to use my time better.	Yes	No
40. I want help in getting more motivated to change.	Yes	No
41. I want my spouse (or someone close to me) to come to treatment with me.	Yes	No
42. I want my treatment to be short.	Yes	No

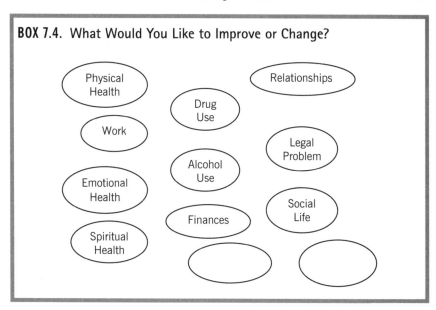

BOX 7.4. What Would You Like to Improve or Change?

- Physical Health
- Relationships
- Drug Use
- Work
- Legal Problem
- Alcohol Use
- Emotional Health
- Social Life
- Finances
- Spiritual Health

The client then sorts these cards into stacks—like Yes, Maybe, and No piles. For shorter menus, another approach is to use a single sheet of paper with a number of bubbles (circles or ovals) on it. Each bubble contains a possible topic for discussion, which in turn could lead toward change goals (see Box 7.4). Note that there are also several empty bubbles on the page, and you can say something like this:

> "Here are some things that people sometimes want to improve or change in their lives. Or perhaps there are priorities on your mind that are not here at all. That's why there are some empty bubbles. Which of these (if any) are important to you, as things you might choose to work on?"

The same approach can be used to set the agenda for a particular session:

> "Here are some things that we could talk about today, but maybe what's most on your mind is something that's not listed here. That's why there are some empty bubbles, for anything else you might want to talk about. Where would you like to start?"

Abstinence and Moderation Goals

An enduring and often controversial issue in addiction treatment, particularly in the United States, regards what to do with clients who do not embrace a goal of total lifelong abstinence, but do want to reduce their use (Witkiewitz, Hallgren, et al., 2017). For the sake of simplicity, imagine that there is only one drug involved. You favor complete abstention and the client says absolutely not, but does want to cut down to a moderate, problem-free level. What would you choose to do?

1. Tell the client to try out moderation on his or her own and come back when he or she is ready to abstain (Mann, 1950).
2. Explain why the client's goal is unrealistic, unachievable, and ill-advised, and push him or her to commit to abstinence (Milam & Ketcham, 1984).
3. Indicate that you are willing to work with the client to reduce his or her use and see how it goes (Sanchez-Craig, 1996).
4. Say that you are willing to help him or her to taper down toward an ultimate goal of abstinence, quitting "warm turkey" (Miller & Page, 1991).
5. Encourage the client to at least try out a period of abstinence and negotiate an agreeable trial period (Meyers & Smith, 1995).
6. Explore the reasons for the client's preferences.

There are practitioners who do each of these things, and there is no one right answer for all situations. It depends in part on your own level of comfort with each of these options. One historic conception of addiction (discussed in Chapter 2) is that it involves a permanent loss of the ability to control one's own use, except via abstinence. Even within this view, however, there are many other people who, for example, drink too much and suffer adverse consequences. Few professionals object to screening for alcohol use in primary health care and counseling heavier drinkers to reduce their consumption (National Institute on Alcohol Abuse and Alcoholism, 1996, 2005). Some evidence-based methods for doing so are described in Chapter 11.

Choosing Strategies

The next step in developing a change plan is to discuss possible steps or strategies to move toward each goal. These also should meet ARMS criteria, and it's usually good to have a time line attached to them. "By next week I will make an appointment to see my doctor." Considering the available options to move toward each goal, what is the person most ready, willing, and able to do? People who receive the treatment they prefer are more likely to stick with it and have better outcomes (Swift et al., 2011).

The change plan is a living document. A strategy is simply a next step to try in the direction of a change goal. As steps are accomplished, new ones take their place until a goal is reached. New goals may be added and others modified. Involve your clients directly in preparing their own change plans, and gradually turn the whole process over to them to make the plan fully their own. It can be useful to prepare and provide a written change plan that can be easily modified. Erasable writing on heavy paper works; so do electronic documents.

Getting to "Yes"

Because the change plan is developed with and belongs to your client, he or she should be willing and able to say "yes" to it. The basic question for the overall plan is "Is this what you choose to do?" For a more specific piece of the plan (like a task to be completed before next session), a better question is "Is this what you're *going* to do?" If you sense reluctance, there is more work to do. What is the reluctance about? The importance and confidence rulers might be helpful here:

> "On a scale from 0 to 10, how *important* would you say it is for you to reach this goal, if 0 means not at all important and 10 means very important?
>
> "And on the same scale from 0 to 10, how *confident* are you that you can reach it, if 0 is 'I'm sure that I can't' and 10 is 'I'm sure that I can'?"

Sometimes reluctance reflects doubt about how important a goal really is, and sometimes it signals low self-efficacy to achieve it (Miller & Rollnick, 2013).

Person-Centered Treatment

Thus far in this chapter we have focused on identifying particular goals and strategies that match each client's needs. There is a broader sense, however, in which the process of treatment is itself person-centered, focused on the particular individual. This is the approach described in Chapter 4 on engaging, and can be practiced throughout the course of treatment. In a person-centered approach the counselor is attending, responding, and adapting to clients in the moment, not just following a prescribed set of procedures. This compassionate attention to the client's own experience transcends particular treatment strategies. It is in essence a way of being while providing treatment (Rogers, 1980).

A person-centered approach can be particularly important when working with clients who are quite different from yourself, be it with regard to race, ethnicity, gender and sexual identity, religion, social class, or culture. Individual variability within such broad categories is often larger than average between-group differences, so just knowing someone's identified category may tell you little about the person. To be sure, cultural competence includes understanding group differences that may be particularly important or sensitive in treatment, but individual differences within a cultural group are large. For example, advice to *always* treat people from a particular racial group in a unique way is in itself racist, assuming uniformity. An advantage of a person-centered approach is that clients are always the experts on themselves, and uniformity is not assumed. Ideally, services should always be delivered in a manner focused on the person and free from stereotypes that may be conscious or unconscious.

> In a person-centered approach the counselor is attending, responding, and adapting to clients in the moment.

Feedback-Informed Treatment

Individualizing treatment for clients at the "front end" is just a beginning. The process of treatment should be adjusted and tailored over time to meet clients' changing needs. One well-developed method for doing this is feedback-informed treatment (FIT) whereby clients are asked to offer their perceptions of how things are going after every session (Schuckard, Miller, & Hubble, 2017). There is good evidence that doing so significantly reduces client deterioration and dropout and improves treatment outcome (S. D. Miller, Bargmann, Chow, Seidel, & Maeschalck, 2016; Prescott, Maeschalck, & Miller, 2017). Like a person-centered counseling style, this relatively simple and structured method for obtaining client feedback can be used regardless of the particular treatment methods being offered. Immediate feedback is also an important component of learning that allows you to improve your own practice over time.

Happily, practical clinical support tools have been developed to help you collect and use immediate client feedback (S. D. Miller, Duncan, Brown, Sorrell, & Chalk, 2006; Whipple et al., 2003). Two brief four-item measures can be administered to clients after each visit: the *Outcome Rating Scale*, which measures client progress, and the *Session Rating Scale*, which assesses the therapeutic relationship; both are available free of charge to individual practitioners (*www.scottdmiller.com*). Each of these scales can be administered and scored in less than a minute, providing reliable information about clients who are doing well or at risk of deterioration or dropout. The usefulness of such feedback depends on two obvious factors: whether you pay attention to it promptly, and how you respond to it (de Jong, van Sluis, Nugter, Heiser, & Spinhoven, 2012).

Good Practice Guidelines

Given the findings of research to date, what are some practical implications for matching clients to optimal treatments?

1. *Put client welfare first.* In essence, match treatments to people, rather than trying to make people fit into particular programs. The purpose here is to find the approach that is best for this particular person, a goal that can conflict with a desire to fill certain beds or treatment slots.

2. *Offer a menu.* Provide clients with a variety of options, and also supply the information they need to make informed choices. Make use of clients' own wisdom and preferences about what will work for them.

3. *Try something different.* If the person has tried a particular approach in the past without success, consider other options rather than more of the same.

4. *Attend to the person's larger needs.* Look beyond SUDs, and connect the person with needed services.

5. *Practice appropriate humility.* Research clearly supports modesty regarding clinical judgment in knowing what is best for clients. Consider the possibility that like customers, "the client knows best."

6. *Make use of available knowledge.* There are findings to inform the matching process. As described above, for example, if the person has very little family and other social support for abstinence, consider mutual help programs as an enduring social support network (see Chapter 17). If motivation seems low and resistance high, consider a treatment approach to enhance motivation for change (Chapter 10).

7. *Consider collecting your own data.* While matching guidelines from other settings can be informative, consider the possibility of developing your own. If you have reliable information about what treatment people have received and about their outcome (such as recidivism data), you have the basics for developing data-based decision rules that may work for your own client population (e.g., C'de Baca et al., 2001; Martin, 1995).

8. *Remember general factors.* There is considerable evidence that therapist and client factors have a greater impact on outcome than the particular treatment procedures used (Imel et al., 2008; Miller & Moyers, 2015). Empathic listening, hope and optimism, treating clients with respect, and honoring their autonomy will go a long way beyond whatever specific treatment methods you use. Similarly, there is much you can do to activate the client factors that promote change: hope, self-efficacy, motivation, and taking small steps. Don't get too invested in clients taking a particular path that you favor. It may be more important for them to do

something to move in the right direction than to take the particular route that you have in mind.

KEY POINTS

🦶 A change plan involves negotiation of a client's goals and strategies for reaching them. A treatment plan is a subset of a change plan.

🦶 Goals and methods of care vary across four phases of treatment: palliative care, stabilization, rehabilitation, and maintenance.

🦶 A menu of evidence-based treatment approaches is available from which to choose what best meets each person's needs.

🦶 There is a modest research base on what treatment approaches work best for whom.

🦶 People should be active participants in designing their own treatment, based on informed choice.

Reflection Questions

🗨 How do you currently go about selecting the most appropriate treatments for the people you serve?

🗨 In developing change plans, to what extent do you rely on clients' own wisdom and preferences about how to proceed?

🗨 In the setting where you work, how might a stepped-care approach be implemented, starting with briefer interventions and stepping up level of care as needed?

CHAPTER 8

Case Management

People seeking treatment for SUDs often have problems beyond their substance use in areas such as employment, finances and legal issues, family relationships, health and emotional concerns (Siegal et al., 1995). Individuals with co-occurring disorders and life problems are not a minority subpopulation, but the norm in addiction treatment (see Chapter 20).

Historically, many treatment providers have not responded adequately to such concomitant problems (Benshoff & Janikowski, 2000; Rose et al., 2014; Willenbring, 1996). This may stem in part from a belief that SUDs represent the "primary" disease, the resolution of which will naturally result in improvement in extended problem areas (Siegal et al., 1995). Within this belief, it would be considered irrelevant to focus on issues beyond substance use because they are only secondary consequences of a primary disorder. In fact, efforts to alleviate other problems have sometimes been construed as "enabling," interfering with the recovery process by not allowing clients to experience natural negative consequences of substance use that could enhance their motivation for change.

This is, in our view, a strangely punitive perspective. With what chronic illness would one refuse treatment for related conditions in order to sustain suffering in hopes of increasing motivation for change? Substantial evidence seriously questions the validity of this perspective. Research indicates instead a complex or reciprocal relationship between substance use and sundry social, legal, and economic problems (Rose & Zweben, 2003; Rose et al., 2014). People often have diminished capacities to cope with everyday hardships during the process of recovery (J. M. Brown, 1998). Failing to address such concomitant problems during treatment may actually increase risk for continuing or recurring substance use (Morgenstern,

Hogue, Dauber, Dasaro, & McKay, 2009; Substance Abuse and Mental Health Services Administration, 1998; Willenbring, 1996). Some of the most strongly evidence-based treatment methods, in fact, do not focus primarily or exclusively on addiction itself but on improving the individual's coping capacities and social relationships (Berglund et al., 2003; Miller & Carroll, 2006; Miller, Wilbourne, & Hettema, 2003; Office of the Surgeon General, 2016).

Ancillary services can yield positive changes for people with addictive disorders. Clients who are also involved with medical and social services are more likely to remain longer in treatment and tend to have better posttreatment outcomes on social and psychological well-being as well as reduced substance use, relative to those not receiving such services (Hesse, Vanderplasschen, Rapp, Broekaert, & Fridell, 2007; Kuerbis, Neighbors, & Morgenstern, 2011; McLellan, et al., 1999; Rapp, Van Den Noortgate, Broekaert, & Vanderplasschen, 2014; Siegal et al., 1996; Siegal, Li, & Rapp, 2002; Siegal, Rapp, Li, Saha, & Kirk, 1997; Sullivan, Wolk, & Hartmann, 1992).

These findings underscore the importance of good case management (CAM) in addiction treatment. First, CAM can help clarify for clients the relationships of their social, legal, economic, medical, and psychosocial problems to substance use. Second, CAM can avert setbacks that may result in premature withdrawal from treatment.

In this chapter we examine different CAM models, identify active ingredients of CAM, and review current research evidence. We give particular emphasis to practical issues and discuss the importance of embedding CAM within an interdisciplinary team.

What Is CAM?

The overall aim of CAM is to help clients acquire resources to resolve their life problems while providing strong support to reduce the stress of everyday hardships and improve coping resources (Zweben, 2012). This is in contrast to treatment where the focus is on producing interpersonal and intrapersonal change (Alexander, Pollack, Nahra, Wells, & Lemak, 2007; Rothman, 2003). CAM is not an alternative to or substitute for treatment, but rather is an important complement that attends to matters *not* routinely dealt with in therapy (Hesse et al., 2007). Linking clients with needed services such as housing, economic, employment, and legal assistance facilitates rehabilitation (Rapp et al., 2008; Tiderington, Stanhope, & Henwood, 2013). Although a few treatment methods such as the community reinforcement approach (Chapter 14) do give substantial attention to ancillary issues, CAM services are often provided by nonclinical staff with particular expertise in CAM. There are also peer-delivered CAM models (e.g., "recovery coach") that emphasize mutual assistance in recovery (Office of the Surgeon General, 2016). Finally, CAM can be incorporated within hospital, residential, and other health service settings or as a stand-alone service offered by individual providers or a team (Vanderplasschen, Rapp, Wolf, & Broekaert, 2004).

There are various approaches to CAM, including a traditional broker/ generalist model as well as more intensive interventions such as strengths-based assertive community treatment (ACT) and clinical/rehabilitation approaches (Rapp, 2002; Rothman, 2003; Substance Abuse and Mental Health Services Administration, 1998; Test, 2003; Walsh, 2003). Differences among these models pertain mainly to the number and kinds of services provided and the amount of emphasis placed on particular components. Some models focus primarily on assessment, information, and referral activities, whereas others (e.g., strengths-based models) place more emphasis on therapeutic skill and building a working alliance, providing information, and linking clients with suitable services. Nondegreed paraprofessionals are more likely to be employed as case managers in programs that are based on broker/generalist models than in a therapeutic strengths-based model of CAM.

The ACT model is more comprehensive than a broker-generalist approach (Inciardi, Martin, & Scarpitti, 1996; Substance Abuse and Mental Health Services Administration, 1998; Test, 2003) and pursues a larger number and variety of goals. Unlike other CAM models, ACT also advocates proactively for developing new community resources as a response to the needs of clients in coping with the problems of everyday living. ACT programs most often serve clients with both SUDs and concomitant serious mental health conditions. Such vulnerable groups often flounder if left alone to deal with fragmented service systems, and can particularly benefit from intensive, wraparound CAM that offers a wide variety of concrete resources and unlimited contacts to improve their functioning in the community (Rapp et al., 2014; Ridgely, 1994; Shavelson, 2001).

Research on CAM

The evidence for including CAM in addiction treatment is convincing. Outcome studies on CAM have been conducted with diverse populations including welfare recipients, homeless persons, dually diagnosed individuals, people in methadone treatment, and HIV-infected opiate users, many of whom were not seeking treatment for substance use problems (Rapp et al., 2014). Data show that people who are given CAM are more likely to enter and remain in addiction treatment, are less likely to be readmitted, and show greater improvement across a number of life areas including substance use, employment, physical and mental health, HIV risk behaviors, parenting skills, criminal justice/legal problems, housing, and family functioning compared to those not receiving CAM (Conrad et al., 1998; Cox,

1998; M. W. Kirby et al., 1999; Morandi, Silva, Golay, & Bonsack, 2017; Najavits, Weiss, Shaw, & Muenz, 1998; R. C. Rapp et al., 2014; Robles et al., 2004; Siegal et al., 1995, 1996, 1997, 2002).

Which components of CAM are particularly associated with these positive outcomes? CAM appears to be more effective when there is a strong working relationship between client and manager, when needed services are more readily available and accessible, and when the case manager follows a more structured approach. In addition, the more time that is spent on CAM core functions—goal setting, case monitoring, client advocacy, and service coordination (especially when setbacks occur)—the greater likelihood that positive outcomes will emerge (Alexander et al., 2007; Morgenstern et al., 2008; Noel, 2006; Rapp et al., 2014; Vanderplasschen et al., 2004). There are also some basic core competencies (such as motivational interviewing; see Chapter 10) for case managers. As with treatment services (Miller, Sorensen, Selzer, & Brigham, 2006), the quality in delivering CAM services is enhanced by more thorough training, coaching, and supervision, and by strong administrative support (Vanderplasschen, Wolf, Rapp, & Broekaert, 2007). Successful CAM, of course, does depend on having available community resources for helping clients deal with their various problems (J. Walsh, 2003). Case managers are in a good position to notice significant gaps in care, and so to advocate for needed services.

Outcome evaluations of CAM are challenging to conduct in real-life systems. The typical design compares usual care with or without additional CAM services, and thus far it is not possible to conclude whether it was specifically the CAM and/or additional time and attention that contributed to better outcomes. Another limitation is the lack of monitoring and quality assurance to ensure the fidelity of CAM services delivered.

Illustrating this complexity, McLellan and colleagues (1999) studied the impact of CAM services on client outcomes in eight addiction treatment programs. Because of the large volume of clients seeking services from these programs, not all could be given CAM, and whether or not they received it was essentially due to chance. This permitted a natural experiment of CAM. Clients who had been given CAM were compared with non-CAM clients on a variety of outcomes such as medical status, employment, family relations, and legal status. Two waves of clients were evaluated in this study: one at 12 months and the other at 26 months after CAM was initiated in the treatment system. In Wave 1 few benefits of CAM were found, but in Wave 2 CAM clients fared significantly better with CAM in regard to drinking, drug use, behavioral health problems, and legal and employment issues. Differences on the Addiction Severity Index (see Chapter 5) were particularly large. The difference in outcomes might be explained by the fact that CAM clients in Wave 2 made greater use of services than did their counterparts in Wave 1. For example, in Wave 1 only 25% of the CAM clients became involved with an employment specialist, whereas in

Wave 2 the comparable figure was 52%. This was in turn attributable to the fact that more community services such as drug-free housing, employment, and training opportunities became available between the two waves. The case managers may also have become more skilled with experience (McLellan et al., 1999).

Another concern is the lack of information on the relative efficacy of stand-alone CAM models. An exception is a randomized trial comparing CAM, motivational enhancement therapy, and the community reinforcement approach (CRA) for non-help-seeking homeless adolescents seen in a drop-in center (Slesnick, Guo, Brakenhoff, & Bantchevska, 2015). All three groups showed significant and similar improvements in the frequency of alcohol use, mental health, stress reduction, and coping responses. CRA yielded greater reduction in the frequency of drug use, which nevertheless remained high in all groups (40–50% of days in the 90 days of follow-up). Given these modest differences, the authors expressed support for CAM as stand-alone harm reduction intervention for homeless adolescents.

Client Readiness for Change

An important consideration in developing and implementing CAM plans is client *readiness* to seek services. How willing clients are to undertake various CAM tasks depends on at least two factors: (1) their perceived *importance* of or need for the service, and (2) their perceived *ability* to use the service (Zweben & Zuckoff, 2002). In other words, clients are more likely to use a service if they perceive it to be both relevant to their personal goals and possible for them to access (Siegal et al., 1996). Suppose you wanted to refer a woman who is in addiction treatment to a free shelter for victims of domestic violence. The woman is most likely to accept and complete the referral if (1) she believes that her violent partner has been a barrier to the changes she wants to make and it is important for her to be protected; and (2) she believes that it is possible for her and her children to get to the shelter safely.

What might stand in the way of the first of these factors, perceived *importance*?

- *Need.* Clients may perceive that they do not really need the services.
- *Efficacy.* They may not believe that the services would help or work for them.
- *Relevance.* They may not perceive a relationship between the services and their problems.
- *Priority.* They may see a need, believe the services would be helpful, and understand their relevance, but just have higher priorities right now.

And what might interfere with the second factor, perceived *ability?*

- *Practical obstacles.* Clients may feel obstructed by real-life factors (e.g., child care, safety, transportation, and cost) that prevent them from seeking services.
- *Self-efficacy.* They may perceive that they are personally unable to do what is needed (e.g., don't have the skills, time, or education).
- *Feeling overwhelmed.* They may generally be too demoralized to do it (resulting from depression, medical problems, everyday hardships, confusion, and low self-esteem).

As in treatment (see Chapter 10), enhancing clients' readiness for change is part of the case manager's task and skill. With appropriate clinical strategies, it is possible to increase clients' acceptance of and engagement in services (Conrad et al., 1998). This is particularly important for individuals with serious addiction problems, who may not benefit from conventional CAM approaches in a broker-generalist model (Substance Abuse and Mental Health Services Administration, 1998).

> Enhancing clients' readiness for change is part of the case manager's task.

Assessing CAM Needs of Clients

A useful tool is a services request form (see example in Box 8.1) on which clients can quickly indicate areas where they would like help. The form covers such life matters as finances, child care, living arrangements, employment, medical health care, and behavioral health care. On this form clients assign a priority rating (1–10) for each service. Having clients complete a services request form helps acquaint them with community resources that are available and could support their efforts to change addictive behaviors. It also provides information for completing a CAM plan with specific goals and tasks.

A first step in CAM is to identify broader goals and specific objectives. This in turn leads to a list of particular tasks to be completed by the client or case manager. What specific manageable steps could be taken to fulfill CAM goals? Accomplishing small, practical steps enhances self-efficacy, which is an important component in building commitment to change. To illustrate, improving physical health could be identified as a broad goal, having a medical exam as a more specific objective, with component tasks that are steps in that direction; such steps could include locating a physician in the resource directory, making an appointment, arranging transportation, and keeping the appointment. Box 8.2 offers a case example of how CAM can be used in ongoing practice.

BOX 8.1. Services Request Form

Would you like assistance in any of these areas? If YES, mark with an X and indicate how important it is for you on a scale from 1 (least important) to 10 (most important).	If YES, mark X	How important? (1–10)
1. Housing (place to live, landlord, etc.)		
2. Employment (finding a job, better job, etc.)		
3. Legal problems or advice		
4. Health care or medical problems		
5. Medications or managing medications		
6. Self-help or support groups		
7. Child care (or other dependent care)		
8. Parenting and family issues		
9. Obtaining or keeping benefits or insurance (disability, Medicaid, SSI, VA, etc.)		
10. Financial assistance (debt, budgeting, food stamps, welfare, etc.)		
11. Work or employment training		
12. School, education, GED, etc.		
13. Personal or family safety		
14. Mental health or psychological problems		
15. How I spend my free time		
16. Advocacy with another system		
17. Utilities (telephone, heat, water, etc.)		
18. Food		
19. Clothing and household needs		
20. Transportation		
Are there other areas (not listed) in which you need assistance? *Please write these below.*		
21.		
22.		
23.		

This instrument is in the public domain and may be reproduced without further permission.

BOX 8.2. CAM in Addiction Treatment: A Case Example

Sondra listed "job training" as a major priority on her services request form. Asked what her concerns were in this area, Sondra revealed that she had been haphazardly employed and that with better training, she hoped she might find steady employment. To understand and enhance Sondra's motivation for change, the case manager asked how getting assistance with this might help her, and specifically might support her intention to be free from drug dependence. She said that having stable employment would improve her financial situation, which in turn would allow her to move away from her current neighborhood which was "infested" with drug dealers and users. Living in this environment made it particularly difficult for her to remain drug-free. Because Sondra did not have specific ideas about a direction to pursue, the case manager suggested some career testing and counseling to discover where her skills and interests might best fit. She agreed, and accepted the referral. The case manager called the career counseling service while she was still in the office, and gave the phone to Sondra to make the appointment. Later, they met again to discuss what she had learned and to explore options for further education and training.

Facilitating the Referral Process

It is common in addiction treatment that clients need ongoing encouragement, contact, and support to complete the tasks within a CAM plan. This usually involves taking quite a proactive and assertive role to help clients follow through with the steps they need. Sometimes counselors worry that their clients should "take responsibility" and do it on their own, but the plain fact is that proactive CAM substantially increases the likelihood of getting there. Our inclination is to help clients get there as a first step. What will it take to do that? Sometimes what may be needed is meeting them in the community and accompanying them to social service agencies to obtain the needed resources (Willenbring, 1994). It is also possible to enhance clients' own personal motivation to follow through, using some of the methods described in Chapter 10. For example, identifying areas of past successes, affirming strengths and current steps in the right direction, and generally supporting self-efficacy can be important in sustaining motivation (Najavits, 2002; Najavits et al., 1998).

Forging a Consensus

Honoring client autonomy is vital in facilitating adherence with CAM plans. This involves negotiating a change plan that your client will endorse, own, and commit to follow. Clients tend to become disengaged from the change process when counselors push their own agenda rather than listening to and understanding clients' own goals (Cooney et al., 1995; Rapp, Kelliher, Fisher, & Hall, 1996). An important task, therefore, is to establish a consensus with your client concerning which life domains (e.g., medical care, employment, leisure time, or permanent housing) need to be addressed, and in what order of priority. In one study using this consensus approach, two-thirds of CAM objectives were completed across nine life domains (Siegal et al., 2002). The more clients were involved and participating in planning, the more improvement occurred in their family, employment, and overall psychosocial functioning along with a reduction in cocaine and marijuana use.

An interesting way to assess discrepancies between the client's perceptions and your own is for *both* of you to complete the services request form for the client, including priority ratings. This lets you identify differences in perceptions of what is needed and how important each issue is to reaching a specific goal. You can then discuss these differences in priorities. Do they arise, for example, from different perceptions of how these areas impact alcohol/drug use? You can explore this in more detail using an assessment instrument such as the Inventory of Drinking Situations (IDS; Annis et al., 1987) or the Desired Effects of Drinking (DED) scale (Doyle, Donovan, & Simpson, 2011) that can help to further clarify CAM needs (see Box 20.1 in Chapter 20 for the DED scale). These instruments provide relevant data on various events (e.g., mood disorder) that might serve as high-risk situations for drinking or other drug use.

Just sharing relevant information may not be enough to resolve counselor and client differences regarding CAM needs (Zweben & Zuckoff, 2002). Clients' reluctance about agreeing to or following through on a referral may be more related to underlying concerns about the consequences of change rather than unawareness of their CAM needs. For example, gaining steady employment may estrange clients from their familiar pastimes and companions, or enable separation for a spouse who had been previously unable to leave due to financial instability. Clients may also have real doubts about their own abilities to succeed with certain goals and the tasks that they require, and this can interfere with willingness to proceed.

Failing to understand and address such underlying motivational issues can increase the chances of treatment dropout (Zweben & Zuckoff, 2002). The following section describes several motivational strategies that can be helpful.

Motivational Strategies to Strengthen Adherence

Motivational Interviewing

Skillful motivational interviewing (see Chapter 10) can help develop a consensus on a CAM plan. Empathic listening (Miller, 2018; see Chapter 4) can help both you and your clients clarify their misgivings or reluctance about pursuing particular goals or tasks. It can also be useful to normalize counselor/client differences in perception, explaining that this is quite common and arises from differences in perspectives and interpretations. It is important here to recognize, acknowledge, and honor clients' own perspectives and autonomy, their right and ability to make their own choices.

Developing Proximal Goals

Accomplishing even a minor goal can help build confidence, which is important for improving motivation. Break down a broader goal into more specific short-term component tasks that can be accomplished. What would be a first step in the right direction? Perhaps it is asking to use a friend's phone to arrange a baby-sitter for a medical appointment. If the client does not seem confident, it can be helpful to role-play a conversation to practice the skills needed for completing the task (Rapp, 2002; Sullivan, 2003). You might, for example, first model how to call a social service agency to ask for an immediate appointment. Then have the client try it out and give positive feedback on what he or she is doing right. In some situations, merely providing a safe space so that clients feel comfortable in expressing ambivalence about changing can become an important first step in facilitating the change process (Tiderington et al., 2013).

> Break down goals into specific short-term component tasks.

Problem-Solving Obstacles

In preparing a client to undertake a referral or other task, consider possible obstacles that might occur after leaving your session. You could ask, "What might happen to prevent you from doing this?" If the client is uncertain or unable to identify potential obstacles, you might suggest some possibilities (e.g., transportation, waiting lists, lack of child care, unexpected illness) and ask how he or she might respond to those if they arise. Also normalize such setbacks so that there is no shame should the client not succeed in carrying out a task (Zweben & Zuckoff, 2002). Respond to nonadherence or setbacks with problem solving. What went wrong? What can you and the client do to make it work next time? Again, emphasize personal choice. If they find one referral source unsatisfactory, explore together other options to try (Siegal et al., 1996). In this way you can reduce the danger of clients avoiding you or dropping out if they are unable to complete a specific task.

Use of Written Materials

Written materials can also be useful in helping clients to understand and think further about CAM needs and tasks (Najavits, 2002). These might be brochures or downloads from possible referral agencies that describe location, services, contact person, fees, insurance coverage, and the waiting period for an initial appointment. You can review such material with clients to clarify misunderstandings, alleviate concerns, and support intentions to take specific action steps. Sending written materials home also allows clients to share the information with and obtain support from significant others. Some written materials are interactive, asking clients to respond to and personalize the material being presented (Miller, 2014; Proctor, Hoffman, & Allison, 2012).

The Importance of Follow-Up

A vital component of CAM is proactive, assertive follow-up of your clients' progress at subsequent sessions, or via other contacts between sessions. This communicates that you care and are available and willing to help and support them. Checking in during or between sessions allows you to intercede if there are obstacles to progress. You can initiate these follow-up contacts, or arrange for your clients to contact you with progress reports by telephone or electronic messages. If the client is to contact you, set up a reminder system for yourself so that you will notice if you don't hear back as expected. The objectives of follow-up are to provide support, monitor progress toward CAM goals, and, if needed, modify current goals/plans or develop new ones.

At follow-up, ask what has happened since your last contact in terms of completing agreed-upon tasks toward CAM goals. For some clients, it is helpful to have them keep a log of particular tasks (e.g., job interviews) completed. Affirm all efforts that are made toward CAM goals, even if they did not have the intended outcome (Sullivan, 2003). Some clients enjoy planning for a particular reward after completing an agreed-upon task. Remain supportive and nonjudgmental even if the client has not finished the task (Zweben & Zuckoff, 2002). If a particular task was not completed, ask the client to take you through the step-by-step process of what prevented it (e.g., logistics, low self-efficacy or motivation, unclear assignment, or poor social support). This can help you and the client learn how to anticipate and plan together to respond to such obstacles in the future. For example, for one client an obstacle to attending AA meetings might be arranging child care (logistics). Another may lack the confidence to attend AA sessions (low self-efficacy). A third client might be unclear about the location of meetings (unclear assignment).

When client motivation or confidence is shaky, it can be helpful to involve a significant other (Meyers & Smith, 1995; Zweben & Barrett, 1997). This can be useful not only in bolstering the clients' confidence but in providing constructive feedback on the task assignment as well. When breaking down goals into component tasks, follow up as each successive task is completed and agree on a next step, staying engaged until the goals have been met. It is possible for CAM follow-up to continue after formal treatment has been completed. This helps not only in pursuing CAM goals, but in detecting early a need to resume treatment (see Chapter 21).

BOX 8.3. Personal Reflection: Is There a Role for the Significant Other in CAM?

As head of social work at a large agency in the 1980s I often advised practitioners to involve the significant other (SO) in helping clients address everyday problems associated with their substance use such as managing finances or inadequate housing. My advice was met with mixed results. Some social workers preferred to work with the client alone (in part, because it's easier!). Not unexpectedly, most practitioners chose the spouse as the SO, many of whom were overwhelmed with the stress and hardships of living with a partner who is drinking excessively or using drugs. As a result, many of these SOs were not very supportive and helpful in the planning process.

As I gained experience in addiction treatment, I realized that involving an SO could be more beneficial if you choose the appropriate person. The SO you are looking for does not have to be a spouse or live-in partner, but an individual who is strongly committed to the relationship, is interested in promoting positive change, and whose support is highly valued by the client. This could certainly mean involving the spouse if she or he meets these criteria, but it might also be a friend, employer, sponsor, clergy, or relative.

How do you go about finding such a person? Take some time early on to consider whether there is a supportive SO in the client's social network. Ask clients whether there is anyone around whom they see often, has an interest in their sobriety, and might be willing to attend sessions with them. When there is doubt as to whether the proposed SO is actually supportive of sobriety, my experience is that it's best not to invite that person, since he or she could even undermine the client's efforts to change (Zweben, 1991).

If you identify such a person and the client agrees, you can invite the SO to join in some or all of the sessions. How many sessions SOs attend will depend on their availability and how helpful they prove to be in the CAM process. Depending on the person selected, SOs can be helpful in a variety of ways. Based on their knowledge of and relationship with the client, SOs can offer constructive feedback on the client's plans, identify potential obstacles, suggest options to facilitate sobriety, and provide practical and moral support.

It is important to coach the SO about how best to participate in sessions—for example, how to make suggestions without the client feeling ganged up on or controlled. Ultimately it is the client who decides what to change, no matter how much the SO (or you) might like to make that choice. Help SOs to understand that change does not always come quickly and that it is normal for the client to experience "ups and downs" before positive change is sustained. This can help keep the SO from jumping in and eliciting resistance when the client appears reluctant to change.

—A. Z.

Refocusing

Despite your best efforts, some clients may continue to have strong reluctance about accepting or carrying out a particular CAM task or referral. Rather than continuing to press, shift the focus to a goal or task that is more acceptable (Zweben, 2012). What *is* the client willing and interested to do? Success with some less ambivalent tasks can pave the way later to discuss other goals and tasks.

Delaying a Decision

Remember and acknowledge that a decision about a CAM goal or plan doesn't have to be made right away. When clients seem to be reluctant to commit, invite them *not* to decide now, but to continue talking about it in future visits. This is better than pressuring clients to make a premature decision or agreement to please you, and then later save face by not returning for future appointments (Zweben, Bonner, Chaim, & Santon, 1988). Clients who are confronted with decisions that conflict with their own current beliefs and attitudes may be better prepared to act favorably on them at a later time. Pressing for an immediate commitment is more likely to engender resistance. Another advantage of this approach is that it allows the client time to gain additional information and support from significant others about undertaking the various tasks (Cooney et al., 1995).

> What is the client willing and interested to do?

Integrating CAM in an Interdisciplinary Team

Many SUDs are chronic problems that require different aspects to be addressed concurrently over an extended period of time (McKay, 2005; Saitz, Larson, LaBelle, Richardson, & Samet, 2008). In such circumstances, a variety of providers may be involved in managing the care of vulnerable clients. For example, individuals with co-occurring disorders may involve a medical provider to prescribe and manage medication and a therapist to address the individual's intrapersonal and interpersonal problems (Zweben, 2012). In some cases, the client may be treated in group therapy, with CAM as a valuable individual adjunct. The case manager can play a vital role in working with a multidisciplinary team, particularly when team members are located in different settings. Having a case manager embedded or integrated into the multidisciplinary team can avert fragmented or disjointed services (Zweben, 2012). For example, a counselor may need to confer with a psychiatrist if the side effects from a prescribed medication are interfering with a client's participation and retention in treatment. Team members might advise the case manager to increase CAM visits to alleviate a client's discouragement or depression (Kuerbis et al., 2011). The case manager might help to extend the benefits of psychotherapy by engaging an individual in a mutual help group (Chapter 17), particularly for clients who are embedded in a heavy drinking or drug-using social network (Zarkin, Bravy, Hinde, & Saitz, 2015). In short, case managers play a vital role in interdisciplinary teams. They may obtain ongoing feedback of clients' perceptions of care (Chapter 7), and alert the team to potential dropout or other problems. With a broader picture of clients' lives, case managers can help to modify treatment goals and plans, provide linkage with needed resources, and support clients' ongoing participation in treatment.

KEY POINTS

🔖 CAM helps clients access resources for resolving the practical problems that often accompany addiction.

🔖 Psychosocial problems may be a precipitant, consequence, and/ or maintaining factor in SUDs that, if unaddressed, compromise treatment retention and outcome.

🔖 Addressing these concomitant problems *during* addiction treatment facilitates recovery.

🔖 Therefore, CAM is a vital component in addiction treatment, helping clients find, gain access to, and use supplemental services that will support their recovery.

🔖 Beyond a traditional broker/generalist model, there are also more intensive CAM models that integrate a higher level of therapeutic skills.

Reflection Questions

❓ Within the population you serve what are the most common co-occurring problems?

❓ How can the people you serve gain access to a case manager?

❓ If specialist CAM is not accessible to your clients, how might you include this service in the care you provide?

❓ Why is it important to embed a case manager in an interdisciplinary treatment team?

PART III

A MENU OF EVIDENCE-BASED OPTIONS IN TREATING ADDICTION

As noted in Chapter 7, one reason for optimism is the range of different methods with good evidence of effectiveness in treating addiction. Just as there is no single treatment for all cancers, there is no one superior approach indicated for all addictive disorders. The following chapters describe 10 different options, each of which has a solid evidence base. If one approach isn't working, there are others to try. As is common in medicine, you can describe for clients the "menu" of different approaches that are available and engage in a process of shared decision making. No single provider will be skilled in all of these options, but ideally any system of care can offer competent practice in a range of these alternatives.

CHAPTER 9

Brief Interventions

Throughout this book we describe people with addiction problems as a diverse population with widely varying levels of severity, and we advocate a continuum of services to meet clients' needs. From the menu of available treatment options, this chapter addresses relatively brief and low-cost interventions. Brief intervention was originally opportunistic: people receiving health care in medical settings were screened for heavy drinking and alcohol-related problems. A positive screen triggered a brief intervention, even if the client was not seeking consultation regarding his or her alcohol use (Bien, Miller, & Tonigan, 1993; Dunn, Deroo, & Rivara, 2001; Fleming & Manwell, 1999). Early studies of brief intervention showed significant reduction in alcohol use, improved mental health, and increased utilization of health services (McCambridge & Cunningham, 2014). A review of treatment approaches for alcohol problems found brief interventions to be among the most strongly supported methods (Miller & Wilbourne, 2002).

Consequently, it became clear that brief interventions can be effectively implemented in a wide range of settings including primary care clinics, social service agencies, emergency and trauma units, employee assistance programs, public schools, child protection services, criminal justice facilities, and college health services (Miller & Weisner, 2002; Moyer, Finney, Swearingen, & Vergun, 2002; Rollnick, Miller, & Butler, 2008). In 1980, the World Health Organization initiated an international screening and brief intervention project that was aimed at identifying and intervening with people with harmful and hazardous alcohol use, followed in 2003 by a nationwide U.S. demonstration project for Screening, Brief Intervention, and Referral to Treatment (SBIRT). The latter project more broadly targeted alcohol, illicit and prescription drugs, tobacco, and mental health (Bray, Del Boca, McRee, Hayashi, & Babor, 2017). Referral to treatment was included to establish linkages between general and specialty care settings so that those needing more intensive treatment could access a full spectrum of services (Bray et al., 2017; Jonas et al., 2012).

This evolution of brief intervention mirrored changing perceptions of alcohol and drug problems as public health issues that could be addressed beyond the bounds of specialist addiction treatment. Most people with SUDs never enter specialist treatment, but many of them regularly contact health care, social service, employee assistance, and correctional systems, where brief on-site interventions can be used alone or to facilitate referral to specialist care (Babor & Higgins-Biddle, 2000; Institute of Medicine, 1990; National Institute on Alcohol Abuse and Alcoholism, 2005; National Institute on Drug Abuse, 2010).

Brief interventions should be included in any continuum of addiction services. Many people complete only one or a few visits in specialist care (Urbanoski, Kenaszchuk, Inglis, Rotondi, & Rush, 2018), and front-loading brief interventions ensures that even those who do not return have been offered potentially effective services. Providing early brief intervention is ethically preferable to placing people on a waiting list (Miller, 2015a), and may improve retention and activate intrinsic change resources (McHugh et al., 2001). Many people respond relatively quickly to treatment (Anton et al., 2006; Project MATCH Research Group, 1997a, 1998c), and brief intervention can serve as the entry point of stepped care, whereby short-term treatment is provided initially and then followed by additional treatment as needed (Bischof et al., 2008; Smith et al., 2001). Because brief interventions can be implemented in various contexts for different purposes, this chapter considers both generalist and specialist settings.

> Many people respond quickly to treatment.

What Is Brief Intervention?

Brief interventions may range from a few minutes of counseling and advice, to blends of various components in one or more sessions of 15–60 minutes. Case management may also be included (Chapter 8). Brief intervention can be a freestanding event intended to enhance motivation for change, embedded within nonspecialty programs that focus primarily on other concerns such as injuries (emergency departments), medical concerns (primary care clinics), and academic performance (student advising). The usual aims are to detect and address substance use problems early, and facilitate further treatment if needed. Brief intervention can also be a service offered within a spectrum of specialist addiction care.

Six components of effective intervention have been summarized by the mnemonic acronym FRAMES (Bien, Miller, & Tonigan, 1993; Miller & Sanchez, 1994):

- F: *Feedback* to the client of personally relevant information about his or her substance use and its consequences.
- R: An emphasis on the client's personal *Responsibility* for change— that it is up to the individual to decide and choose what, if anything, to change.
- A: Some clear *Advice* from the provider recommending behavior change.
- M: A *Menu* of options from which to choose, if the client should decide to pursue change.
- E: An *Empathic* counseling style (Chapter 4) that is respectful and supportive, listening to the client's own concerns and perspectives.
- S: Encouragement of *Self-efficacy*, that the client could be successful in changing.

These elements facilitate change by honoring the client's autonomy and personal choice while offering advice, options, feedback, and encouragement to evoke the client's own motivations for change (Chapter 10). The essential goal is to activate the person's own self-regulation processes (Baumeister, Heatherton, & Tice, 1994; Brown, 1998; Vohs & Baumeister, 2011), typically by enhancing motivation and mobilizing their own resources for change (de Shazer et al., 2007; Viner, Christie, Taylor, & Hey, 2003). When the primary obstacle is client ambivalence (rather than a lack of resources or skills), motivational interviewing may be particularly useful to help the person move from contemplation to preparation and action (DiClemente & Velasquez, 2002; Tomlin & Richardson, 2004).

Why Would Brief Intervention Work?

The brevity and content of brief FRAMES interventions don't correspond well to popular notions of what is required for successful treatment. There is no skills training, contingency management, personality or cognitive restructuring, confrontation, induction to mutual help networks, or working through transference. How is it that brief counseling can trigger a change in addictive behavior that may have persisted for years or decades despite adverse consequences? Brief interventions don't always work, of course, but why do they work at all?

One plausible explanation is that they activate normal self-regulation processes (Brown, 1998; Miller & Brown, 1991). Like a thermostat, behavioral self-regulation systems assess whether current conditions are within a desirable range. During waking hours, and even to some extent while asleep, these systems continuously monitor the stream of sensory and perceptual input available (Vohs & Baumeister, 2011). This information (the current state) is compared to norms or expectations (the desired state) to identify discrepancies that may signal a need for a change. When no discrepancies are detected, the system maintains the status quo—no problem, no change. Indeed, a commonly stated reason for not having changed addictive behavior is that "I didn't think I had a problem" or "I didn't think I needed to change."

When a significant discrepancy is detected, however, there can be instigation to change and a search for acceptable options. If an option appears reasonable and feasible, the person may try out new behaviors, which in turn provides new information for evaluating: "Is it better now?" This loop continues until the discrepancy is satisfactorily resolved. The elements of FRAMES correspond to this process and provide support where needed. Providing feedback (sometimes in comparison to norms) in an empathic counseling style can decrease defensiveness and facilitate acceptance of new and potentially threatening information. Emphasizing personal responsibility and freedom of choice while supporting self-efficacy encourages initiative. Presenting a variety of options and offering gentle advice supports a vision for accessible means to achieve change.

If the triggering of self-regulatory processes is a key step in changing addictive behaviors, then the evidence regarding brief intervention begins to make sense. Without perceiving a need for change, protective self-regulation efforts are unlikely to occur. (To describe this condition as "denial" just means that someone else perceives a problem.) However, when a discrepancy is recognized (the current state is undesirable), then behavior change is more likely. Activating self-regulatory processes may be enough to trigger change without further intervention. This may also explain why substantial behavior change is often observed very early in the course of addiction treatment. It is worth noting, however, that people with SUDs often show significant impairment of normal self-regulation processes and may thus need additional strategies to maintain change (Baumeister et al., 1994; Brown & Miller, 1993).

Evidence for the Effectiveness of Brief Intervention for SUDs

The research literature on brief interventions for SUDs has been growing rapidly. As described in the introduction to this chapter, early studies of brief intervention focused primarily on alcohol use. The consistent finding that brief interventions delivered opportunistically in primary care settings reduced drinking and facilitated openness to additional services led to more widespread adoption of this strategy (McCambridge & Cunningham, 2014). Subsequent studies have found that brief intervention can reduce drinking in postpartum women seen in obstetrical practices (Fleming, Lund, Wilton, Landry, & Scheets, 2008; Velasquez, von Sternberg, & Parrish, 2013), diminish illicit drug use among patients seen in medical clinics (Bernstein et al., 2005; Madras et al., 2009), reduce heavy drinking and marijuana use among young adults seen in emergency departments and military settings (Gmel, Gaume, Bertholet, Fluckiger, & Daeppen, 2013; Magill, Barnett, Apodaca, Rohsenow, & Monti, 2009), decrease pathological gambling (Petry, Weinstock, Ledgerwood, & Morasco, 2008), diminish antisocial behavior and family conflict (Van Ryzin, Stormshak, & Dishion, 2012), and reduce problem drinking among college students (Baer, Kivlahan, Blume, McKnight, & Marlatt, 2001; Jonas et al., 2012; Walters, Bennett, & Miller, 2000). In short, there is substantial evidence that brief interventions can influence addictive behaviors in diverse populations and across an international array of settings (Elzerbi, Donoghue, & Drummond, 2015). When offered as a freestanding "check-up," brief interventions can also engage people who would not otherwise seek traditional behavioral health services (Miller & Sovereign, 1989; Morrill et al., 2011).

This is not to say that a single brief intervention alone will suffice. Repeated sessions of brief intervention combined with case monitoring can yield good outcomes more quickly, reducing the period of risky use (Glass et al., 2017; Jonas et al., 2012; Moyer et al., 2002; O'Malley et al., 2003; Project MATCH Research Group, 1998a; Saitz et al., 2014). Better long-term outcomes have sometimes been associated with more extended or intensive treatment (Alterman et al., 1994, 1996; Burke, Dunn, Atkins, & Phelps, 2004). Two studies aimed at reducing HIV risk-taking behaviors among injection drug users showed that more intensive cognitive-behavioral intervention yielded greater benefits than a brief motivational intervention (Baker, Heather, Wodak, Dixon, & Holt, 1993; Baker, Kochan, Dixon, Heather, & Woadk, 1994). In a rigorously designed multisite trial (Babor, 2004), multiple sessions were more effective for reducing marijuana use. Multiple-session treatment included motivational interviewing, cognitive-behavioral therapy, and case management, and additional sessions were associated with greater long-term reductions in marijuana use.

Overall, the literature on brief interventions offers two important lessons in service delivery. First, it is possible to overestimate clients' level of need for clinical services. There is a natural tendency for behavioral health professionals to assume that more treatment is better treatment. In an environment where need far exceeds availability of services, the good news is that we may be able to serve more people well by building in effective brief intervention at the front end of treatment, which has often been occupied with administrative tasks and assessment.

Second, it is necessary to adjust service delivery to clients' capacities, resources, and needs (Chapter 7). A single session of FRAMES is likely to yield significantly better results than no treatment at all (Barnett et al., 2010; Bien, Miller, & Tonigan, 1993; Dunn et al., 2001; Landy, Davey, Quintero, Pecora, & McShane, 2016; Moyer et al., 2002) and for some clients may be sufficient to yield outcomes comparable to more extended treatment (Babor, 2004; Chapman & Huygens, 1988; Edwards et al., 1977; Project MATCH Research Group, 1997a, 1998a; UKATT Research Team, 2005). As we discuss later in this chapter, front-end brief intervention can also serve to enhance retention and outcomes in subsequent treatment (Aubrey, 1998; Dench & Bennett, 2000; Zweben, Bonner, Chaim, & Santon, 1988).

For other clients, brief intervention will be insufficient to produce behavior change (Aldridge et al., 2017). This may be particularly true for those who have yet to experience negative consequences related to their substance use or who do not recognize risks and harms associated with their use. For such individuals, providing information and advice alone may engender a defensive reaction creating discord in the counseling relationship and withdrawal from services. In such cases, motivational interviewing may enhance clients' acceptance of and commitment to change (Lee et al., 2010), which in turn contributes to improved treatment outcomes.

As an illustration, Barnett and colleagues (2010) studied brief interventions with individuals being treated for injuries in an emergency department. Clients were randomly assigned to receive either (1) a written personal feedback report describing their alcohol severity status with minimal counselor contact or (2) a counselor-involved session where they also received the same written feedback along with motivational interviewing intended to build rapport, increase awareness of substance use problems, reduce ambivalence, and enhance self-efficacy. All clients also received two telephone booster sessions at 1 and 3 months after the initial interview. Individuals who had been drinking just prior to their injury benefitted from simple personal feedback; the emergency visit was sufficient to confirm the connection between their drinking and injury without additional services beyond standard care. In contrast, individuals who had not been drinking immediately prior to their injury benefited more from motivational interviewing. The link between alcohol and consequences was less apparent to them, and the additional brief intervention was more effective than feedback alone. Thus, individuals with higher initial readiness to change may need less intensive services than those with low pretreatment readiness to change. Feedback alone may provide the necessary nudge to change, whereas those with lower readiness for change may benefit more from motivational interviewing (Witkiewitz et al., 2010).

> Brief interventions can engage people who would not otherwise seek traditional services.

BOX 9.1. Personal Reflection: Evidence-Based Treatment

When I go to my primary care doctor or other health care providers, I expect them to be keeping up with new research in their field and to provide me with current science-based advice and treatment. I certainly experienced this in facing a life-threatening illness. One of the earliest things I did after diagnosis was to read the clinical trial literature on the outcomes of the various treatments that were available to me. None of my doctors found this threatening; in fact they encouraged me to do so. To my eyes as a patient, a 5% difference in outcomes looked pretty large, whether or not it was statistically significant.

How odd it is that this same standard has only recently been applied to the treatment of addiction, which is definitely a life-threatening condition! There is a long history of "one approach fits all" in this field, that approach being whatever the provider happened to have learned or experienced. Impassioned debates have raged between different "schools" of thought as to which is the one correct (or at least superior) perspective. These generate more heat than light.

I am just as concerned about the cynical view that it doesn't really matter what treatment method is used—that all treatments are equally effective. (Imagine being told this if you went for cancer treatment!) To be sure, the specific treatment method used is not the *only* thing that influences outcome. Client characteristics and efforts matter, and as emphasized in prior chapters, counseling *style* (such as empathy and basic kindness) can have a larger impact than specific treatment techniques. Nevertheless, having for three decades reviewed all clinical trials for alcohol problems, I simply cannot agree that one treatment method is as good as any other (Miller, Wilbourne, et al., 2003). We really ought to be using what research tells us is most effective.

Yet implementing and monitoring evidence-based treatment is no simple matter (Miller, Zweben, et al., 2005). As most states have begun to *require* the use of science-based treatments, the tendency has been to develop a list of treatments that are "in" versus "out." The criteria for and selection of which treatments are "in" can be a highly political process, and there is pressure to approve a relatively long list of alternatives that meet some minimum standard, rather than focusing on those with strongest evidence.

Quality control in the delivery of evidence-based counseling methods is also challenging. I once gave a talk at a regional conference in Albuquerque on the current state of outcome research, concluding with a list of treatment methods having the strongest evidence of efficacy. A week later one of the local residential treatment programs ran a newspaper ad claiming that they were offering everything on my list, even though to my knowledge no one on their staff had received specific training in any of them. Without quality control, the requirement to use a specific list of methods may change only the self-report of what is being provided. Yet how does one audit the quality of talk therapy that occurs behind closed doors?

Furthermore, retraining in new evidence-based treatment methods requires significant time and resources. It is a reasonable question to ask whether the cost of retraining staff will be offset by a significant improvement in outcomes. Just

(continued)

BOX 9.1. *(continued)*

attending a continuing professional education workshop is unlikely to yield much real change in practice, although it may convince participants that they now are delivering this new method (Miller & Mount, 2001; Miller, Yahne, Moyers, Martinez, & Pirritano, 2004). The requirement to use new methods should be accompanied by resources to learn them.

The key, I think, is to find a middle way between simple-minded unfunded mandates of brand-name therapies and giving up on evidence-based treatment. Clearly we ought to be teaching the most effective treatment approaches to the next generation of providers from the very beginning. There have been experiments with paying for good outcomes, and leaving it up to the providers to figure out how best to do that—a situation that tends to create sudden interest in evidence-based treatment methods. We also need to pay attention to who is providing treatment and how, since there is clear evidence that this strongly influences client outcomes. The best path is unlikely to be simple, but we owe it to our clients to get it right.

—W. R. M.

Brief Intervention and Treatment Adherence

Brief Intervention as a Referral Adherence Strategy

Various clinical guidelines have recommended that individuals with higher severity of SUDs should receive more intensive specialty treatment (American Society of Addiction Medicine, 2001; National Institute on Alcohol Abuse and Alcoholism, 2005). In this regard, brief intervention might be used to facilitate referral completion (Sterling et al., 2017). A rigorously designed meta-analysis of alcohol treatment utilization following brief intervention (Glass et al., 2015, 2016) focused on health care settings including emergency departments and medical inpatient units. Disappointingly, alcohol treatment utilization was no higher for clients who had received a brief intervention during health care. Further outreach efforts may thus be needed to help people follow-through with a referral (Elvy, Wells, & Baird, 1988; Kogan, 1957; Sisson & Mallams, 1981). Repeated reminders, same-day appointments, and improved training of staff in motivational interviewing skills may improve referral completion after brief intervention (Glass, et al., 2017; McCambridge & Rollnick, 2014; Simioni, Rolland, & Cottencin, 2015; Turner et al., 2017).

Brief Intervention as a Medication Adherence Strategy

The efficacy of pharmacotherapies for SUDs (see Chapter 18) is inextricably linked with medication adherence. Individuals who faithfully take their prescribed medication are more likely to reduce their substance use than are those who do not (Baros, Latham, Moak, Voronin, & Anton, 2007; Chick, Anton, et al., 2000; Gueorguieva, Wu, Krystal, Donovan, & O'Malley, 2013; Pettinati, 2006; Weiss, 2004; Zweben et al., 2008). In addition to compromising full potential benefits of a medication, poor adherence can also affect safety issues such as hazards of prematurely withdrawing from treatment (Farmer, 1999; Rohsenow et al., 2000; Serebruany et al., 2005).

A medication management protocol was created as a multicontact brief intervention to facilitate adherence to medication and treatment, provide support for abstinence, and improve clinical outcomes with alcohol use disorders, including those encountered in primary care and other non-specialty settings (Anton et al., 2006; Pettinati & Mattson, 2010). Medication management has been effective in identifying and managing medication nonadherence and improving treatment outcomes (Anton et al., 2006; Mason & Goodman, 1997; O'Malley et al., 2003; Zweben et al., 2008; Zweben, Piepmeier, Fucito, & O'Malley, 2017).

Medication management typically involves orienting the person to the purposes of the medication, potential side effects, and details of the medication regime. More recently, based on encouraging findings (Glass et al., 2017; McCambridge & Rollnick, 2014; Zomahoun et al., 2016; Zweben et al., 2008, 2017), motivational interviewing has been integrated in medication management when adherence issues compromise client response to a medication. Techniques such as reflective listening, normalizing, promoting optimism, and evoking change talk have been used to reduce uncertainties or resolve ambivalence about medication and to bolster commitment to the medication regime (see Chapter 10).

Moving from Preparation to Action in Brief Intervention

Opportunities for renewed brief interventions arise when people come for health and social services, though in this context they may be initially reluctant to discuss their drinking or other drug use. After all, they came for help with other health and social issues, and although substance use may play a salient role in these presenting concerns, they may not think of themselves as having "a problem" or needing a change in this area. They may not yet have experienced serious adverse consequences, and thus may feel little external pressure to change. Attempts to pressure or persuade such people to curtail their substance use are likely to engender resistance (see Chapters 10 and 19) and can jeopardize one's professional relationship with and retention of clients.

Over time it is often possible to help clients see the connection between their substance use and the concerns that bring them in for services. Windows of opportunity open up to evoke people's own motivations for change. Also, it is not necessary to wait for people to express a willingness to change before you provide them with some options. Offering opportunities for steps in the right direction may be effective regardless of the individual's initial intentions (Aveyard, Begh, Parsons, & West, 2012; McCambridge & Rollnick, 2014; Richter & Ellerbeck, 2015). There is a parallel here to stepped care, offering help with whatever steps the person is willing to take. It places greater control in the hands of clients and underscores your commitment to the individual's capacity to change.

Technological Resources in Brief Intervention

Computer-Based Interventions

Recent evidence demonstrating the efficacy of computer-based brief interventions (CBIs) has stimulated interest in developing and implementing such interventions in health care settings (Blow et al., 2017; Cucciare, Weingardt, Ghaus, Boden, & Frayne, 2013; McCormack, 2017; Nilsen, 2010; Ondersma, Svikis, Thacker, Beatty, & Lockhart, 2014; Pemberton et al., 2011; Rosenblum, 2012; Schwartz et al., 2014). CBIs offer several advantages:

1. Less professional time is needed to deliver them
2. They can be provided anonymously and privately, thus reducing stigma
3. CBIs can contain the same content as in-person brief interventions and are delivered consistently, thus improving quality assurance.

Given these advantages, CBIs have been applied to address treatment needs of college students (Neighbors et al., 2010), postpartum women (Ondersma et al., 2014), veterans (Cucciare et al., 2013), active-duty military personnel (Pemberton et al., 2011), primary care clients (Gryczynski et al., 2015; Schwartz et al., 2014), emergency department patients (Blow et al., 2017), and Internet help-seekers (Bertholet et al., 2015; Sinadinovic, Wennberg, & Berman, 2014).

CBIs can also adapt to individual differences and needs. For example, after completing an online screening and assessment, users can receive a tailor-made feedback report that includes frequency and quantity of alcohol and other substances and a summary of financial/health/social consequences of substance use (Hartzler et al., 2017; Hester, Squires, & Delaney, 2005; Ondersma et al., 2014; Schwartz et al., 2014). Normative feedback can be provided where the individual's substance use is compared with that of people of the same gender and age group. Programmed decision trees can adjust content to individual differences and needs. In interactive formats, users may be involved in synchronous exercises with an animated narrator targeting goals, choosing strategies, and developing future plans. Potential options for change can be offered, with emphasis on personal choice.

It should be noted that components of these sessions can vary depending on the type of drugs used, severity of the problems and dependence, and level of commitment to change. Other programs may include skill building such as coping with urges, avoiding high-risk situations, and drink refusal strategies. Informational print resources can be made available, and booster sessions may be offered if needed or wanted (Blow et al., 2006).

How Effective Are CBIs?

Initial results from controlled trials of Internet-based interventions have been encouraging (White et al., 2010). CBIs have been found to be at least equally effective on average as counselor-delivered brief interventions in reducing substance use (Bertholet et al., 2015; Blow et al., 2017; Gryczynski et al., 2015; Nilsen, 2010; Ondersma et al., 2014; Pemberton et al., 2011; Riordan et al., 2015; Schwartz et al., 2014). These outcomes have been observed with a broad range of individuals (e.g., young adults, postpartum women, and military personnel) seen in diverse settings (such as colleges, primary care facilities, and emergency departments).

As an example, Blow and colleagues (2017) compared the effectiveness of three different modalities of brief intervention targeting drug use in an emergency department setting: (1) CBI plus an adapted motivational enhancement therapy booster (AMET), (2) therapist brief intervention (TBI) plus AMET, and (3) enhanced usual care. Both CBI and TBI incorporated motivational interviewing in the screening, assessment, and intervention procedures used with clients, and both interventions yielded significantly fewer days of marijuana use, relative to usual care. At 3 months, however, these gains were sustained only in the TBI group. Nonetheless, the authors argued that the relative savings in staff time and cost warrant the implementation of CBIs in emergency department settings. CBI might be improved by adding text messaging during the months after initial intervention. Adding individual self-monitoring, prompting, and option-giving via smartphone may extend the effect of an initial CBI (Ondersma et al., 2014; Riordan et al., 2015).

Technological advances in responding to addictive behaviors have been favorably received by providers and consumers alike, who have been willing to use them (Nilsen, 2010). Clearly such technological advances can expand the reach of brief intervention to at risk and underserved populations (Muñoz et al., 2006).

> Computerized and counselor-delivered brief interventions are equally effective on average.

Print Resources

Self-help books are abundant, but as with CBIs, there are some print resources that have been well evaluated as interventions (Apodaca &

Miller, 2003). Providing self-help information (sometimes called *biblio-therapy*) shares some of the same advantages of privacy, confidentiality, and proceeding at one's own pace, and does not require computer use (though it does, of course, assume reading ability). Self-help resources are readily available for alcohol use disorders (Fletcher, 2009; Miller & Muñoz, 2013; National Institute on Alcohol Abuse and Alcoholism, 1996; Sanchez-Craig, 1995), and some studies have found similar average outcomes when the same intervention is delivered via bibliotherapy versus in-person counseling (Apodaca & Miller, 2003; Miller & Baca, 1983; Miller, Gribskov, & Mortell, 1981). Interactive journals have also been developed to engage the reader in responding to presented material (Miller, 2014; Miller & Mee-Lee, 2010). Of course, materials available in print format can also be adapted for delivery via computer and the Internet (Ahmed, 2007; Boß et al., 2018; Hester & Delaney, 1997; Hester, Delaney, & Campbell, 2011; Hester, Delaney, Campbell, & Handmaker, 2009).

Text Messaging

Technologically enhanced brief intervention may also involve text messaging. In this approach, clients use a smart phone to report on drug or alcohol use in real time in their own environment (Blow et al., 2006; Gonzalez & Dulin, 2015; Riordan, Conner, Flett, & Scarf, 2015). Users receive prompts, reminders, and advice about what to do to handle particular challenges related to their substance use. Periodic messages can also be sent to reinforce awareness of adverse consequences of substance use. Data gleaned from an earlier assessment can be used to tailor the timing, frequency, and content of individual messages—for example, a reminder of a personal commitment to specific goals.

Final Thoughts

Throughout this book we have encouraged treating addiction well beyond specialist care contexts where the barriers to access are often high (McLellan, 2006). Brief interventions increase opportunities for delivering effective services to a wider range of people (Willenbring & Olson, 1999). Addressing addictions through broader health care and social service systems is a way to provide care to those who cannot or will not access specialist treatment (Miller & Weisner, 2002; Weisner, Mertens, Parthasarathy, Moore, & Lu, 2001). SUDs are already overrepresented among health care and social service consumers, contributing to and exacerbating treatment of the issues addressed in these contexts. Given the already busy workloads of physicians, it may be more feasible for brief interventions to be provided by nurses or behavioral health specialists working in health care clinics

(Ernst, Miller, & Rollnick, 2007), using medical management protocols that have been developed and tested in clinical trials (Pettinati, 2006). Onsite provision of addiction counseling in primary care and family practice settings seems a sensible way to treat substance use as a health behavior, address client reluctance to seek specialist care, and assist medical staff with concerns about prescription drug misuse and related problems (Christian, Krall, Hulkower, & Stigleman, 2018).

KEY POINTS

🪧 Brief intervention for substance use is often effective and is a reasonable first step within a stepped-care approach.

🪧 Immediate brief counseling is preferable to placing people on a waiting list and should be included in any continuum of care for SUDs.

🪧 Brief intervention can be freestanding, an initial session, or embedded within treatment being offered for other issues.

🪧 There is an opportunity for brief intervention whenever people with SUDs seek health or social services for other concerns.

🪧 Computer-based interventions can expand the reach of brief interventions to underserved at-risk populations seen in health care facilities.

Reflection Questions

Q Where in your community are people with SUDs already receiving health or psychosocial services? How might brief interventions be integrated into these services?

Q Sometimes providers believe that if you only have a short time, you just have to tell people what to do. Suppose that you had only 10 minutes to counsel someone regarding his or her drinking, smoking, or other drug use. How would you use the time?

Q How do you explain the fact that such brief interventions are often effective in changing substance use patterns that have been ongoing for a long time? What do you think is happening?

CHAPTER 10

Motivational Interviewing

Once upon a time it was believed that if clients weren't sufficiently motivated for change, then there was nothing you could do. "Come back when you're ready to change" was common advice. When people didn't respond well to treatment, it was often chalked up to their poor motivation.

We now know that's not good enough. It is clear that client motivation, while a good predictor of change, is not a stable trait that people carry around with them but rather a dynamic process that has everything to do with interpersonal interactions. That makes it part of our clinical task to enhance clients' motivation for change instead of blaming them for not having enough of it.

One of the earliest clues for this perspective came from studies in the 1950s and 1960s searching for a client dropout profile (Miller, 1985). Personality measures were administered to predict which people were going to drop out of treatment early. If those likely to drop out could be identified, then programs could either not waste time with them or take extra steps to prevent attrition. It turned out, however, that there was no dropout personality. Instead, it appeared that the best predictor of dropout was the counselor to whom the client had been assigned. Some counselors had very low dropout rates, whereas others lost many clients early on.

Subsequent research has confirmed that regardless of the type of treatment for addiction, it makes a difference *who* delivers it. The particular clinician to whom people are assigned can be the difference between getting better or worse (McLellan et al., 1988; Valle, 1981). Even when treatment is manual-guided and standardized, client outcomes are significantly and sometimes substantially linked to the therapist who delivers them (Miller & Moyers, 2015; Moyers et al., 2016).

To be sure, clients do begin with a wide range of readiness for change. The transtheoretical model's stages of change offer a way of understanding how far along a person is at any given point with regard to making a particular change (Heather & Hönekopp, 2013; Prochaska & Norcross, 2013). The transtheoretical model, in fact, was a significant factor in the addiction field's change of heart and mind regarding client motivation. Once it became clear that clients are at different starting points of readiness, then it followed naturally that they need different kinds of help in order to move along toward change. Just helping people to advance one stage (e.g., from precontemplation to contemplation) increases the likelihood of eventual behavior change (Heather, Hönekopp, Smailes, & UKATT Research Team, 2009).

> It is part of our job to enhance clients' motivation for change instead of blaming them for not having enough of it.

The Dynamics of Ambivalence

Ambivalence, feeling two ways about something, is a normal response when facing potential change. People newly diagnosed with type 2 diabetes, for example, need to make a panoply of behavior changes in order to maintain their health and quality of life, and are usually unenthusiastic about doing so (Steinberg & Miller, 2015). In some ways they don't want to change, and in other ways they do. They have mixed motives. Such ambivalence is also very common, even normative, with SUDs.

What happens when someone (including a counselor) points out to ambivalent people that they have a problem and need to do something about it? Most likely they will respond with the other side of their own ambivalence, sometimes vehemently. An angry defensive response suggests that you have touched a sensitive nerve connected to underlying ambivalence. People are, after all, most stung by those accusations that contain some grain of truth. Argue for change, and it is natural for an ambivalent person to argue against it. It's human nature. In a way, you are acting out the person's ambivalence, which might be harmless enough except for the fact that people tend to believe and get committed to whatever they themselves say. When clients are caused to argue against change, they become more committed to the status quo and are less likely to change. They literally talk themselves out of changing.

Decisional Balance

So how can you help people resolve ambivalence without making the arguments for change yourself? One approach has been to help clients voice all of the pros and cons of each alternative that they are considering.

This is actually a very old approach dating at least to Benjamin Franklin (1904/1772) if not ancient Greece. Janis and Mann (1977) refined it as a way to help people make and be at peace with difficult decisions when you mean to maintain neutrality and *not* influence the direction of choice, and it is an ethical approach for doing so (Miller & Rollnick, 2013). Somewhere along the line, however, decisional balance became popular as a technique for promoting a decision to change, particularly in smoking cessation.

There never was any theoretical reason to expect that doing a decisional balance would increase the likelihood of making a particular change. In fact, unless the perceived benefits already far outweigh the disadvantages, the expected outcome of having a client thoroughly voice all the pros and cons of change would be ambivalence or status quo. Of more concern, a review of outcome research (Miller & Rose, 2015) found that when done with ambivalent people, the actual result of a decisional balance was to *decrease* commitment to change. In contrast, once people had already made the decision to change, a decisional balance only served to reinforce it. When your hope is to encourage change with clients who are undecided, a decisional balance can be harmful rather than helpful, and we do not recommend it. There is neither theoretical nor empirical reason to use a decisional balance for this purpose.

> A decisional balance can be harmful rather than helpful.

The Method of Motivational Interviewing

If doing a decisional balance or arguing for change yourself are unhelpful, then what can you do to increase clients' motivation for change? That is a central aim of motivational interviewing (MI; Miller & Rollnick, 2013; Naar & Safren, 2017), which was originally developed for working with alcohol use disorders (Miller, 1983) but is now used to facilitate change in a wide range of contexts, cultures, and professions (Miller & Moyers, 2017).

MI is fundamentally a particular way of having a conversation about change that strengthens people's own motivations and commitment. Its foundation is the person-centered relational skills discussed in Chapter 4. Miller and Rollnick (2013) described an underlying mindset or "spirit" of MI comprising four broad themes. First, MI is *collaborative,* a partnership in which clients are recognized as experts on themselves. Second, it is *evocative,* calling forth people's own insights, motivations, and resources, rather than trying to install things that clients are presumed to lack. As discussed in Chapter 4, the basic assumption is not that "I have what you need," but rather "You have what you need, and together we will find it." Third, MI spirit communicates *acceptance,* respecting and supporting clients' *autonomy,* their power and right to make decisions about their own lives and behavior. In this way, MI is consistent with *self-determination theory* (Deci & Ryan, 2008) and its emphasis on transforming external into autonomous motivation (Markland, Ryan, Tobin, & Rollnick, 2005). Fourth, the final component of MI spirit is *compassion,* a fundamental commitment to the clients' best interests and well-being as prime priority.

MI involves four processes among which counselors move flexibly. First is the *engaging* process, listening to and developing a working alliance with clients. A metaphoric question underlying this process is "Can we walk together?" Next is the process of *focusing,* developing shared goals for the journey: "Where are we going?" A third process, relatively unique to MI, is *evoking* the person's own motivations for change: "Why do you want to go there?" Finally, there is the *planning* process: "How will we get there?" Too often addiction treatment ignores the first three processes and jumps right to planning, a prime example of which is requiring a "treatment plan" within the first session or two. It's not a shared goal (focus) or plan until the client has participated in developing it and is on board with it.

One might think of these four processes as linear: first you engage, then you focus, then you evoke, and finally you plan. Actual practice is more like moving flexibly back and forth among the processes, with the engaging skills being foundational throughout. One visual representation of the processes is as stair steps toward change, with the counselor moving up and down in response to a client's immediate experience (see Box 10.1).

MI was originally conceived as a preparation for treatment, and in several early studies, providing even a single MI session at the outset of addiction treatment doubled the rate of abstinence at follow-up (Aubrey, 1998; Bien, Miller, & Boroughs, 1993a; Brown & Miller, 1993). An initial surprise, however, was that an MI intervention alone was often sufficient to trigger change in longstanding substance use patterns (Miller, Benefield, & Tonigan, 1993; Miller, Sovereign, & Krege, 1988), a finding now widely

---

BOX 10.1. Processes in Motivational Interviewing

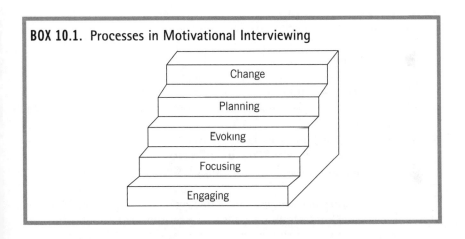

Change

Planning

Evoking

Focusing

Engaging

replicated (Heckman, Egleston, & Hofmann, 2010; Hettema et al., 2005; Jensen et al., 2011; Lindson-Hawley, Thompson, & Begh, 2015; Lundahl, Kunz, Brownell, Tollefson, & Burke, 2010; Samson & Tanner-Smith, 2015).

MI may be of differential benefit to clients with more serious levels of substance use and problems. A region of response analysis revealed that among pregnant drinkers, MI benefitted the heavier drinkers, where clinical concern would be greatest (Handmaker, Miller, & Manicke, 1999). Similarly, in a study of MI with cannabis users, it was the heavier users who benefitted from MI (Mason, Sabo, & Zaharakis, 2017).

MI pays particular attention to certain aspects of client language. Counselors seek to evoke and explore client *change talk*—speech that favors change. Four linguistic forms of preparatory change talk are *desire* ("I want," "I wish," "I would like to"), *ability* ("I can," "I could," "I am able"), *reasons* ("If I did, then . . ."), and *need* ("I have to," "I need to," "I must"). Three additional linguistic forms exemplify mobilizing change talk: *commitment* ("I will," "I am going to," "I promise"), *activation* ("I'm willing," "I plan to," "I'm considering"), and *taking steps* (specific actions toward change). The same forms of speech can be uttered on behalf of not changing (*sustain talk*), and the balance of change talk to sustain talk during an MI session predicts the likelihood that subsequent behavior change will occur (Campbell, Adamson, & Carter, 2010; Gaume, Bertholet, Faouzi, Gmel, & Daeppen, 2013; Hodgins, Ching, & McEwen, 2009; Morgenstern et al., 2012; Moyers, Martin, Houck, Christopher, & Tonigan, 2009; Walker, Stephens, Rowland, & Roffman, 2011). Importantly, this balance can be influenced by counselor skill in MI (Gaume, Bertholet, Faouzi, Gmel, & Daeppen, 2010; Glynn & Moyers, 2010; Moyers, Houck, Glynn, Hallgren, & Manual, 2017).

Remember the OARS from Chapter 4? Here's where you can use OARS to get moving in a particular direction. In MI these skills are applied in a consciously strategic manner to steer toward change. For example, open questions can be used to elicit different forms of change talk:

- "How might you *like* for things to be different?" (desire)
- "If you did decide to quit, how *could* you do it?" (ability)
- "What *reasons* might there be for you to make a change?" (reasons)
- "How *important* is it for you to do something about your cocaine use?" (need)
- "What do you think you'll *do*?" (commitment)
- "What would you be *willing* to do?" (activation)
- "What have you already done to work toward change?" (taking steps)

When you hear such change talk—the person's own expressed motivations for change—reflect and affirm it. Each time the client expresses a desire, ability, reason, or need for change, it is as if they are offering you a flower. Collect the flowers, and periodically offer them back to the client in short summaries, like a bouquet:

"So you don't like having the courts and your probation officer butting into your life, and drug use has caused some troubles with your girlfriend. In fact, you're worried she might leave you if things don't change. You also think you waste too much money and time on drugs. What else?"

When MI is going well, clients hear themselves expressing their own motivation for change, then hear you reflect it back to them, then later hear it all again drawn together in your summaries. This is a process that people often have difficulty doing on their own. Ambivalent people tend to think of one reason for change, then a reason for not changing, then feel stuck and stop thinking about it. In MI you help people keep moving in the same direction and thus find their way out of the forest (Miller & Rollnick, 2004).

In MI, "resistance" is differentiated into *sustain talk* (the status quo side of ambivalence) and *discord,* a signal of tension in the working alliance (Miller & Rollnick, 2013). Both are highly responsive to counselor style (Glynn & Moyers, 2010; Moyers & Rollnick, 2002) and MI includes a variety of strategies to diminish them. In essence the counselor does not push against perceived resistance but rolls with it.

> When you hear change talk, reflect and affirm it.

Over 1,000 controlled clinical trials of MI have been published, many reporting significant beneficial effects across a broad range of problem behaviors, with some of the strongest evidence being in the area of addictive behaviors. MI has also been successfully applied to reduce drug-related risk from perceived peer norms (Doumas, Esp, Johnson, Trull, & Shearer, 2016; Magill et al., 2017), injection practices (Bertrand et al., 2015), and overdose (Bohnert et al., 2016).

It is also clear, however, that the effectiveness of MI varies widely across programs and clinicians providing it (Ball et al., 2007; Project MATCH Research Group, 1998d; Winhusen et al., 2008). This suggests that MI is sensitive to the manner and context in which it is delivered. In this regard, it is important to understand the "active ingredients" of MI and what aspects of it are most important in delivery. Closer counselor adherence to and skillfulness in the prescribed style of MI predict greater client change in addictive behaviors (Barnett et al., 2014; Gaume et al., 2010; Moyers et al., 2009; Pirlott, Kisbu-Sakarya, Defrancesco, Elliot, & Mackinnon, 2012; Vader, Walters, Prabhu, Houck, & Field, 2010).

MI may be a particularly good approach for cross-cultural counseling with people who are quite different from yourself, precisely because clients are the experts on themselves (Miller et al., 2008). In a secondary analysis of Project MATCH data, Native American clients responded significantly better to an MI-based approach than to cognitive-behavior therapy or a 12-step approach (Villanueva et al., 2007). A meta-analysis revealed that the effect size of MI was double when clients were from minority groups (primarily African American and Hispanic American) rather than Caucasian non-Hispanics (Hettema et al., 2005), even though the providers themselves were primarily Caucasian. When your own background is very different from that of your client, quality listening is a good idea!

Motivational Enhancement Therapy

When clients appear to be in "precontemplation" and change talk is scarce or absent, it may be useful to obtain and discuss some objective assessment results. It can be interesting and motivating to receive credible, accurate information about oneself. Why are bathroom scales found in so many homes? Feedback lets people know how they're doing, and whether they may need to make a change.

In a large clinical trial (Project MATCH Research Group, 1993) MI was expanded to a four-session format by adding personal feedback of clients' assessment results (Miller, Zweben, et al., 1992). The resulting combination of MI with assessment feedback was termed *motivational enhancement therapy* (MET). Earlier trials of a similar "drinker's checkup" had found this combination to be effective in changing alcohol use (Miller & Sovereign, 1989; Miller et al., 1988) and it was subsequently extended to marijuana use (Martin, Copeland, & Swift, 2005; Stephens, Roffman, Fearer, Williams, & Burke, 2007; Walker, Stephens, Towe, Banes, & Roffman, 2015), other drug use (Miller, Yahne, & Tonigan, 2003), and family functioning (Van Ryzin et al., 2012). In the MATCH study, the MET intervention yielded similar improvement to that from 12 sessions of cognitive-behavior therapy or 12-step facilitation therapy (Project MATCH Research Group, 1997a).

Characteristic of MET is the collaborative way in which such feedback is provided, an informational and nonconfrontational manner that does not evoke defensiveness. Assessment findings are often offered in relation to norms from a general or clinical population. Where does the client stand on this measure, relative to other people? The dimensions might include level of use, severity of problems and dependence, physical health, and risk factors. Information is provided in small bites, checking in regularly to ask with curiosity how the person understands and responds to the feedback and then following with reflective listening.

It is also possible to offer an evaluation checkup for people who are not seeking treatment, which was actually the format of the original drinker's checkup. We advertised to the community a free checkup for people who would like to find out whether their alcohol use was harming them (Miller & Sovereign, 1989; Miller et al., 1988). The advertisement specified that it was not part of any treatment program, that participants would not be labeled, and that they were free to use the information (or not) as they saw fit. This approach attracted drinkers who were 3–5 years earlier in the development of alcohol problems, relative to people entering treatment programs. Most of them had never sought any form of help for their drinking, but the checkup caught their attention. Why had they not sought help before? In essence they didn't think that they needed it. They didn't view themselves as alcoholics or problem drinkers, and thought that their drinking wasn't all that serious. Why, then, did they come in for a checkup? They suspected that they might have problems with alcohol, might be alcoholic, might be harming their health, and were concerned about some of the things happening in their lives with regard to alcohol. In short, they were ambivalent enough to come for a checkup, but not (yet) considering formal treatment. After their checkup and feedback we offered participants a list of local treatment agencies. A few sought formal treatment, but most did not. Nearly all, however, significantly changed their drinking, on average cutting their alcohol use in half (Miller et al., 1993).

MI is more than just "being nice" and practicing empathic listening. In a controlled comparison, MET yielded substantial changes in substance use whereas client-centered counseling did not (Sellman, Sullivan, Dore, Adamson, & MacEwan, 2001). The person-centered skills described in Chapter 4 are, we believe, necessary but not sufficient for delivering effective MI-based interventions.

> MI is more than just "being nice" and listening.

Learning MI

MI is sometimes described as simple but not easy. It soon became apparent that attending a 2-day workshop did not significantly improve clinical skill in MI, certainly not enough to make any difference to clients, although it did incorrectly convince participants that they had now learned and were practicing it (Miller & Mount, 2001). As with any complex skill like a sport or musical instrument, developing proficiency in MI is improved with some feedback and coaching based on observed practice (Madson, Loignon, & Lane, 2009; Miller, Yahne, Moyers, Martinez, & Pirritano, 2004; Mitcheson, Bhavsar, & McCambridge, 2009). As few as three or four feedback/coaching follow-up sessions can sustain or extend competence in practice (Schwalbe, Oh, & Zweben, 2014). A variety of resources are available to support learning of this clinical method (see *www.motivationalinterview.org*; Miller, Rollnick, & Moyers, 2013; Rosengren, 2018). Happily, once you know what signals to look for, your clients also become your teachers. When a client expresses change talk, you know that you're headed in the right direction. Persistent sustain talk and discord, in contrast, signal a need to change how you are responding.

Combining MI with Other Treatment Methods

Although MI alone can lead to change, it has become common to combine the clinical style of MI with other treatment methods (Miller, 2004; Naar & Safren, 2017). In this sense MI is a way of doing whatever else you do. In a meta-analysis, combining MI with another active treatment yielded more sustained effects over a year of follow-up (Hettema et al., 2005). The result can be synergistic. Increased adherence boosts the efficacy of the other active treatment, which in turn adds to the effect of MI itself. Virtually every other treatment described in this volume, including pharmacotherapies, can be delivered in an MI style.

MI has often been combined with contingency management (see Chapter 13), bringing together two different motivational boosts. Adding MI appears to prolong effects on substance use beyond the initial impact of contingent reinforcement (Sayegh, Huey, Zara, & Jhaveri, 2017).

KEY POINTS

🕯 Client motivation for change is a good predictor of behavior change and is highly responsive to counseling style.

🕯 Depending on their initial level of readiness for change, clients need different kinds of help.

🕯 Doing a decisional balance tends to undermine commitment to change with clients who are still ambivalent.

🕯 MI is a collaborative and evocative counseling approach helpful in promoting motivation for change.

🕯 Motivational enhancement therapy is a combination of MI with assessment feedback.

Reflection Questions

❓ What do you believe is most important to help people who are experiencing addiction become more motivated for change?

❓ Among the clients with whom you work, what would you say is their most common motivational stage of readiness for change on first contact: precontemplation, contemplation, preparation, action, or maintenance?

❓ If you have been applying MI in your own work, what have you already done to learn and develop proficiency in it?

CHAPTER 11

Behavioral Coping Skills

One way to make sense of addictive behavior is to view it as a coping strategy. Someone using a particular drug may be seeking, for example, to relax, reduce pain, get to sleep, or feel better. This is not an uncommon use of medications. Public airwaves, print, online, and social media are filled with advertisements for over-the-counter or prescription medications to alleviate all manner of symptoms and improve life quality. An implicit message is that one need not tolerate discomfort even for brief periods: Don't suffer! Take something!

The "self-medication" hypothesis of addiction posits that people are "taking something" in order to feel better by treating symptoms and discomfort. The original self-medication hypothesis suggested that a person's drug of choice was related to his or her particular behavioral health symptoms. Someone suffering from anxiety might use a drug with depressant properties to reduce arousal. While the diagnosis-specific self-medication hypothesis has been challenged (Lembke, 2012), many studies have supported the broader hypothesis that people use drugs or other addictive behaviors to cope with negative affect (Bolton, Robinson, & Sareen, 2009; Leeies, Pagura, Sareen, & Bolton, 2010; Robinson, Sareen, Cox, & Boulton, 2011; Takamatsu, Martens, & Arterberry, 2016). Some people use drugs to cope with or avoid everyday emotions, frustrations, and challenges. Others may consciously or unconsciously seek to self-treat a condition such as attention deficit disorder or an affective disorder. Most of the research on drug use to cope with specific symptoms is correlational, but in a longitudinal study with over 34,000 adults, baseline mood and anxiety disorders significantly predicted the incidence of nonmedical opioid use and opioid use disorders several years later (Martins et al., 2012). A woman who gets in a fight with her spouse and drinks a bottle of wine, the man who begins relying on more and more opioids to reduce feelings of depression, the person whose anxiety is alleviated by going to a casino and playing cards—each of these behaviors becomes a road—a known pathway to turn onto when difficulties emerge. After time, this road can become well traveled.

A common theme in cognitive-behavioral treatment of addictions has been to teach clients coping skills that they presumably lack, so that they need not rely on chemicals or addictive behaviors in order to handle the expected and unexpected challenges of life. Alan Marlatt placed particular emphasis on this skill-building approach in his original "relapse prevention" model for treating addiction (Cummings, Gordon, & Marlatt, 1980; Marlatt & Donovan, 2005). With new skills in place, the person is presumably better able to adjust to life's challenges and is no longer psychologically dependent on addictive behaviors for coping.

There is good reason for focusing on clients' coping skills. A return to using alcohol or other drugs often occurs in situations where other coping skills were needed (Hendershot, Witkiewitz, George, & Marlatt, 2011; Marlatt, 1996; Witkiewitz & Marlatt, 2004). It is not exposure to high-risk situations per se that threatens recovery, because virtually everyone treated for addiction problems will encounter many such situations. Rather what predicts sustained recovery is the person's capacity for dealing with life's continuous challenges, particularly with coping strategies that do not involve avoidance (Miller, Westerberg, Harris, & Tonigan, 1996). Avoidance of high-risk situations can be useful in early sobriety, but in the longer run one needs more positive coping skills (Monti et al., 2002). Developing and maintaining longer term coping skills is also consistent with the self-management perspective emphasized throughout this book.

> Cognitive-behavioral treatment teaches clients coping skills.

The Evidence Base

Clinical research has provided strong support for the value of a skill-enhancing approach. Most trials have evaluated skill training as an add-on to treatment as usual, which is a fairly rigorous test of efficacy. In this value-added design, the new method that is being tested has to produce improvement above and beyond that resulting from normal treatment practices. In essence, this kind of clinical trial answers the practical question, "Is it worth my time and effort to add this new method onto what I'm already doing for my clients?" From studies of coping skill training, the answer has rather consistently been "Yes"—that there is significant added benefit above counseling as usual (Kiluk, Nich, Babuscio, & Carroll, 2010; Miller, Wilbourne, & Hettema, 2003; Miller, Zweben, & Johnson, 2005).

In Project MATCH (see Chapter 7), however, cognitive-behavioral skill training (CBT; Kadden et al., 1992) was compared head-to-head with two other well-supported treatment methods: 12-step facilitation (TSF) and motivational enhancement therapy (MET). During the 12-week treatment phase, clients receiving CBT or TSF showed quicker reductions in their drinking as compared to those in MET (Project MATCH Research Group, 1998c). Once treatment had ended, however, all three therapies yielded similar (and substantial) benefit through 3 years of follow-up on the study's main outcome measures (Babor & Del Boca, 2003; Project MATCH Research Group, 1998a).

A skill-enhancing approach is not incompatible with other treatment methods like TSF and MET. In the subsequent COMBINE study, CBT and MET were merged with encouragement to attend mutual help groups, forming a "combined behavioral intervention" (Longabaugh et al., 2005; Miller, 2004) that significantly improved client outcomes (Anton et al., 2006; Donovan et al., 2008; Moyers et al., 2016). Enhancing clients' coping skills is not the whole picture in treating SUDs, but it is one very useful tool to have on hand.

Skill training is a treatment method that can be offered quite well in group format. Clients can benefit from each other's range of skills and ideas, and also learn vicariously as each group member develops new ways for coping with challenges. There is economy of scale in teaching new material to a group, rather than to one individual at a time (see Chapter 22). Furthermore, groups offer more opportunities to practice new skills with a variety of individuals in a supportive atmosphere.

Advances in technology have yielded diverse ways to learn coping skills in real time and individualize skill training to address those immediate needs. Ecological momentary assessment, for example, measures clients' cravings, urges, and coping behaviors in real time to minimize recall bias. Technology-based treatment delivery platforms are being evaluated as stand-alone treatment, as an adjunct to treatment, and as a tool for ongoing self-management following more intensive treatment. These formats can improve access to and reduce cost of services, reaching a broader population (Marsch & Dallery, 2012; Muñoz et al., 2016; Sugarman, Campbell, Iles, & Greenfield, 2017). People are able to use the web (Chebli, Blaszczynski, & Gainsbury, 2016; Hester et al., 2009; Hester, Lenberg, Campbell, & Delaney, 2013), a computer (Kiluk et al., 2017), or mobile phone (Keoleian, Polcin, & Galloway, 2015; Moore et al., 2017) to receive on-demand access to skill-building strategies.

What Skills?

What skills, then, should one focus on in treatment? It makes little sense to have the same standard skill-training package for all clients because people enter treatment with very different sets of skills. This is the main drawback of manual-based approaches with a one-size-fits-all approach to skill building. Some clients already have sufficient ability in managing their own mood states, for example, whereas for others this skill is underdeveloped. Some already have good jobs, whereas others need skills for finding and keeping employment. We therefore recommend having a menu of skill-learning options available, from which clients can choose the areas that are most likely to benefit them.

The general strategy is to strengthen the client's skills for coping with expected and unexpected situations that could trigger resumed use and problems. Part of the clinical challenge here is in identifying skills that need to be strengthened in order to help your clients live fulfilling lives without relying on drugs or other addictive behaviors. Sometimes these are rudimentary but important life skills: how to use public transportation, prepare meals at home, or open a bank account. This is an area where peer support specialists or case managers can be meaningfully involved in helping clients to learn basic life skills in the everyday world (see Chapter 8).

Nevertheless, there are a few major psychosocial skill areas that often need strengthening among people entering addiction treatment. Five in particular have been well researched: job finding, social skills, emotion regulation, behavioral self-control, and coping with urges and craving. In each of these areas there are also specialized training resources for clinicians and clients.

Job Finding

Employment is a strong predictor of sobriety. Despite seemingly positive response during a treatment episode, clients who are unemployed are much less likely to refrain from substance use. Discharging a client to unemployment is an invitation to failure.

Helping people to find a job may not seem like it is part of addiction treatment and should be someone else's responsibility. Yet there is sufficient evidence that helping people acquire the skills needed to obtain employment can be done as part of treatment (Hamdi, Levy, Jaffee, Chisholm, & Weiss, 2011; Liu, Huang, & Wang, 2014; Svikis et al., 2012). Indeed, it was part of the original community reinforcement approach (Chapter 14). Referring out to an employment agency always runs the risk of clients not getting there or having insufficient patience to get through the bureaucracy. Getting (and keeping) a job involves particular strategies and social skills that may or may not be offered in traditional employment agencies.

Help with job-finding skills can be included in individual or group counseling and in case management. Some common and effective components to include are help in preparing an effective résumé, advice on how to dress and present oneself for interviews, teaching job-searching skills, asking friends and relatives to be alert for and pass on job leads, taking the initiative to contact potential places of employment, rehearsing job interviews, and completing applications for available positions. Treatment programs can also set up an ongoing "job club" program, usually operated each morning. The basic idea here is that finding a job is itself a full-time job that requires substantial devoted effort. Unemployed clients come to the job club daily to learn some of the above-described skills and to devote time to contacting potential employers, calling friends and relatives for leads, and completing applications. The job club facilitator coaches clients on interviewing skills, listens in on cold contact calls, and provides resources. Then in the afternoon each day, clients visit potential employers and go for interviews. Clients keep coming to the job club daily until they get a job.

Social Skills

Perhaps the strongest evidence for enhancing coping skills comes from studies of social skill training. The emphasis here is on strengthening clients' abilities to form and maintain rewarding drug-free social relationships (Monti et al., 2002).

Like employment, the client's social support network is a strong predictor of posttreatment sobriety. Those who have a strong social network in support of sobriety are significantly more likely to achieve it. Those whose friends and family support continued drinking or drug use are at much higher risk, and in essence need to develop new social networks (Hunter-Reel, McCrady, & Hildebrandt, 2009; Longabaugh, Wirtz, Zweben, & Stout, 1998, 2001; Owens & McCrady, 2014). As we will discuss in Chapter 14, some of this change involves engaging the client in new networks that support sobriety, such as mutual help groups or religious communities.

Some clients, however, may not have developed the social skills they need to enter and succeed in ordinary social networks. If their family and current friends support substance use, they are also likely to benefit from preparation to respond in new ways to social temptations, particularly when old networks cannot be completely avoided.

Regarding the first of these tasks—preparing clients to develop new positive social relationships—research and clinical resources have focused mainly on communication skills. The concept of *assertive communication* represents a middle ground between two extremes: passivity and aggression (see Box 11.1). When operating in a passive mode, people sacrifice their own needs by acquiescing, not expressing themselves, and suppressing their feelings and reactions. Giving other people what they want does tend

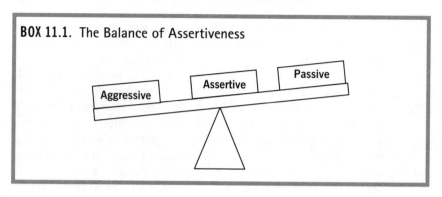

BOX 11.1. The Balance of Assertiveness

to please them, but it comes at a cost if this is someone's consistent coping style. In essence, the person's own needs are not met, and there is little genuine two-way communication and negotiation. At the other extreme of aggression, people demand and coerce in order to meet their own needs at the expense of others. This tends to yield some immediate gratification but sacrifices relationship, engendering resentment and hostility.

Assertive communication honors and balances one's own needs with those of others. Feelings, requests, and feedback are not suppressed, but rather are expressed in a way that respects others, thus inviting and fostering relationship. This is a delicate balance, and one that varies substantially across cultures. An appropriately assertive response within one culture or subculture, for example, may constitute an aggressive and socially inappropriate response in another, or passive and ineffectual behavior in yet another. The point is to help clients recognize this search for middle ground in communicating, and to differentiate effective assertiveness from passive and aggressive responses in their own social contexts. This is a process in which group counseling can be particularly useful. Some basic tips for assertive communication are offered in Box 11.2.

Other basic social skills can also be strengthened. The ability to listen to others and reflect back the meaning that one heard (Chapter 4) is useful not only for clinicians, but in social relationships more generally (Miller, 2018). Sometimes nonverbal communication skills, such as maintaining an appropriate level of eye contact, also need strengthening.

When it comes to dealing with old relationships that support substance use and afford temptation, assertive communication skills can also be quite useful. Drink- or drug-refusal skills may need bolstering. "Just say no" is simple advice, but it can be useful to actually practice specific ways in which to do so in order to build a client's self-efficacy (Kadden et al., 1992; Monti et al., 2002; Witkiewitz, Donovan, & Hartzler, 2012).

> Assertive communication honors and balances one's own needs with those of others.

BOX 11.2. Basic Tips for Assertive Communication

1. **Use an "I" message.** When you are expressing yourself—your thoughts, feelings, opinions, requests—begin with the word "I" rather than "You." By starting with "I," you take responsibility for what you say. Statements that start with "You" tend to come out as more aggressive—blaming, threatening, and so on.

2. **Be specific.** Address a specific behavior or situation and not general "personality" traits or "character." A specific request, for example, is more likely to result in a change, whereas general criticism is unlikely to improve things.

3. **Be clear.** Say what you mean. Don't expect the other person to read your mind, to just "know" what you want or mean. When you make a request, make it clear and specific. When you respond to a request, be direct and definite. "No, I don't want to do that" is clearer than "Well, maybe . . . I don't know." Your facial expression and body language should support your message. Speak loudly enough to be easily heard and use a firm (but not threatening) tone. Look the person in the eye (not at the floor). Don't leave long silences.

4. **Be respectful.** Don't seek to intimidate, win over, or control the other person. Speak to the person at least as respectfully as you would like to be spoken to. If you have something negative or critical to say, balance it with a positive statement before and after. Recognize that people have different needs and hear in different ways. In conflict situations, take partial responsibility for what has happened and is happening.

ASSERTIVE COMMUNICATION IN CONFLICT SITUATIONS

Three Parts of an Assertive Message

1. Describe the behavior.
2. Describe your own feelings or reactions.
3. Describe what you want to happen.

When Receiving Criticism

1. Keep cool; avoid escalation.
2. Listen carefully; show that you understand the other's perspective.
3. Correct any misunderstandings.
4. Take partial responsibility and apologize when appropriate.

When Giving Negative Feedback (Constructive Criticism)

1. Keep calm; don't speak in anger or hostility.
2. Choose the right time and place.

(continued)

From Miller (2004). This material is in the public domain and may be reproduced without further permission.

BOX 11.2. *(continued)*

3. Be specific; describe behavior and don't blame.
4. Check out misunderstandings.
5. Use "I" language.
6. Take partial responsibility and offer to help, as appropriate.

When Asking for Change

1. Describe what the person is doing—the specific behavior that you would like to change.
2. Describe your own feelings or reactions using an "I" message.
3. Describe what you would like to happen.
4. Take partial responsibility or offer to help, as appropriate.

Emotion Regulation

People who have difficulty with self-regulation of emotions are also at higher risk for SUDs. Their mood may shift quickly among fear, anger, and despair. Their skills in self-soothing, in calming oneself down when emotions flare, may also be shaky. Alcohol and other drugs are sometimes used in an attempt to regulate or soothe emotions.

A good first step is to help clients understand what emotions are and how they occur. One useful heuristic for this is the STORC model that describes a cycle:

- *Situation*—the stimuli or antecedents in the person's environment
- *Thoughts*—how the person interprets and thinks about the situation
- *Organism*—what happens physically in the body
- *Response*—what the person does
- *Consequences*—what happens as a result, which in turn changes the situation.

An optimistic aspect of this STORC model is that it places experienced emotion in the context of the environment and the person's behavior, and it suggests multiple points in the chain where changes are possible (Miller & Mee-Lee, 2010). People can change aspects of their situation (e.g., by avoiding certain places or people), modify how they think about and interpret it (a focus of cognitive therapies), alter how they react physically (by learning relaxation and mindfulness skills or adjusting medication), change how they respond behaviorally, or take steps to affect the consequences they experience.

Self-monitoring is a common step in learning emotion regulation skills. A STORC diary (see Box 11.3) can be used to analyze situations in which significant emotions arise. When a significant feeling occurs (usually recorded in the organism column), what was the situation in which it occurred, what were the person's thoughts and interpretation, what did he or she do (response), and what were the results (consequences)? Making a change at any step in the STORC chain is likely to affect other parts of the cycle.

Managing moods is a common issue in addiction treatment, perhaps especially so for women, who have a higher incidence of concomitant depression. What is it about the person's situation that might be contributing to depression (e.g., very little positive reinforcement)? Does the person have thinking patterns that are often associated with depression, and might these be changed via cognitive therapy (Beck, Wright, Newman, & Liese, 2001)? Might meditation, which we discuss in more depth in Chapter 12 (Bowen et al., 2014; Witkiewitz, Bowen, et al., 2014; Witkiewitz, Lustyk, & Bowen, 2013) or a medication (see Chapter 18) be appropriate to alter the underlying physiology (organism)? How is the person responding that might exacerbate depression (e.g., excessive sleeping and isolation)? Behavioral activation, an effective treatment for major depression, also increases abstinence in people with concomitant SUD and depression (Daughters et al., 2018). Is depression being reinforced in some way (consequences) in the person's social environment?

Similarly, anger management is a common addiction treatment issue, more often for men than for women. What are the situational factors, the stimuli that seem to trigger an individual's anger? What are the thought patterns that exacerbate and maintain anger and resentment? (Anger is an emotion that needs constant cognitive fueling.) What is going on in the person's organism, his or her body, when anger flares? Might relaxation skills or breathing exercises interrupt this, and might an evaluation for medication be appropriate? Is the person using stimulants (like caffeine, nicotine) that are likely to increase autonomic arousal? How does the person respond when angry, and what alternative responses are available? Are there payoff consequences for the person's aggression (like he gets what he wants)? Again, making changes at any of these links in the STORC chain may affect the whole cycle. You can help clients to learn these skills in individual or group counseling (Nay, 2012, 2014).

Behavioral Self-Control

Impaired self-control, including the inability to restrain impulses and modulate emotions, is associated with elevated risk for addiction. Deficiencies in self-regulation that are observable in childhood and adolescence predict later SUDs (Brown, 1998; Moffitt et al., 2011). *Behavioral self-control training* (BSCT) interventions are designed to strengthen self-regulation skills. This method generally involves teaching people how to apply principles of learning

BOX 11.3. STORC Self-Monitoring

Situation	Thoughts	Organism	Response	Consequences
Where was I? Whom was I with? What was going on?	What was I thinking? Or what *must* I have been thinking?	What was I feeling? What was happening in my body?	What did I do? How did I respond?	What happened? What was the result?

to manage their own behavior. The most common use of BSCT in the addiction field has been in helping people with alcohol problems to moderate or stop drinking (Miller & Muñoz, 2013; Sanchez-Craig, 1995; Sanchez-Craig, Davila, & Cooper, 1996). BSCT strategies have also been applied to help clients learn how to cope with cravings and urges, and more generally to maintain treatment gains and prevent a return to prior substance use (Kadden, et al., 1992; Marlatt & Donovan, 2005; Miller, 2004; Monti et al., 2002). People seem to be able to learn and use such skills not only with the help of a clinician, but also working on their own with self-help guidelines in book form (Apodaca & Miller, 2003) or computer-based formats (Bickel, Christensen, & Marsch, 2011; Hester & Delaney, 1997; Hester et al., 2009).

Common components of BSCT (Hester, 2003) include:

- Setting specific individualized goals such as upper limits for drinking.
- Self-monitoring alcohol use.
- Implementing specific strategies for slowing down and limiting consumption.
- Self-reinforcing progressive attainment of goals.
- Identifying high-risk situations for overdrinking.
- Developing specific coping strategies for high-risk situations.
- Learning alternative coping skills to replace drinking.

Change is often broken down into small steps in the right direction, and the principle of reinforcing successive approximations applies here. Small changes may be made in the target behavior, and alternative responses learned and practiced. Both client (Levy, 2007; Miller & Muñoz, 2013) and therapist guidelines are available (Hester, 2003; Sanchez-Craig, 1996). The usual course of outpatient counselor-facilitated BSCT is six to 10 sessions.

Coping with Urges and Cravings

Another element in skill training focuses on coping with cravings and urges to use alcohol or other drugs (Elwafi, Witkiewitz, Mallik, Thornhill, & Brewer, 2013; Kadden et al., 1992; Miller, 2004; Monti et al., 2002; Navidian, Kermansaravi, Tabas, & Saeedinezhad, 2016). A few basic perspectives can be helpful to clients who are troubled by urges to use:

- Urges are common during recovery and are not reason for alarm or an indication of failure. You are not helpless when they occur, and need not respond by using.
- Urges are not random or mysterious; they tend to occur in particular circumstances. It is possible to learn from them.

- Urges are temporary. The common fear is that craving will grow steadily until it becomes unbearable, but in fact it usually peaks after a few minutes and then dies down like a wave on the ocean. "Urge surfing" (Harris, Stewart, & Stanton, 2016; Marlatt & Donovan, 2005) is riding it out until it subsides rather than falling into the wave.
- Giving in to urges strengthens them; riding them out weakens them.

Keeping records of urges and the circumstances in which they occur can help to demystify them, and may also suggest additional coping strategies. This can be done on an index card or sheet of paper with four columns:

1. The date and time the urge occurred.
2. The situation in which it occurred: where, with whom, what was happening, and so on.
3. The strength of urge, rated on a 0–10 or 0–100 scale.
4. How you responded to the urge.

This is essentially a functional analysis of urges and cravings: what happened just before and after they occurred. Remember that the "situation" need not be something happening in the environment. It can be an internal event like a memory, emotion, or physical sensation.

As the circumstances associated with urges become clearer, a next step is to develop coping strategies. There are four basic alternatives (Miller, 2004):

1. *Avoid.* Reduce exposure to the situations that trigger urges to use. If seeing other people use triggers cravings, avoid such situations. If having alcohol around the house increases urges to drink, get rid of it. Avoidance of high-risk situations is particularly useful early in the recovery process.

2. *Escape.* It is not possible to avoid all problematic situations. A second strategy, when encountering an urge-exacerbating situation is to leave it, to get out of the situation as soon as possible. Brainstorm with clients what situations might occur and how they could remove themselves from the risk.

3. *Distract.* Remember that urges are time-limited and tend to subside if they aren't indulged. When avoidance or escape isn't feasible, find an enjoyable distraction to surf through the urge. What could your client do in this situation that would take his or her attention away from the urge?

4. *Endure.* Then there are some situations that can't be avoided or escaped, and where distraction isn't feasible or helpful. Here people need strategies to get through until the urge subsides. Some possibilities are

talking it through with someone, mindfully observing the urge until it passes, calling someone for help in getting through it, and taking along a reminder of the importance of sobriety (e.g., a photograph or an AA coin).

> Urges are temporary.

Do Clients Really Learn New Coping Skills?

The usual rationale for coping skill training is straightforward: that clients will learn new skills that they did not previously have, and subsequently will apply them in their lives to successfully manage their own behavior. Does this actually happen? There has been slow progress in understanding the role of coping skills as a mechanism of change in behavioral treatments for addiction (Roos & Witkiewitz, 2016). Morgenstern and Longabaugh (2000) reviewed research studying the extent to which clients had actually acquired the intended skills, and the relationship of such learning to treatment outcome. Their findings were surprising. In some studies, clients did not learn the intended coping skills, but the treatment nevertheless worked. In other studies, clients did acquire some coping skills, but the extent to which they had done so was unrelated to outcome. In another study, although client coping skills did predict better outcomes, clients had not learned them in treatment (Litt et al., 2003). In other words, although coping skill training is a treatment approach with good evidence of efficacy, it does not necessarily work for the presumed reason, by teaching clients new skills! There is also reason to doubt whether CBT is any more effective than other bona fide treatment methods with which it has been compared (Imel et al., 2008; Project MATCH Research Group, 1997a; UKATT Research Team, 2005).

Research continues to emerge on how and why CBT helps. One study found that improvement in clients' coping skills after CBT did predict longer posttreatment abstinence (Kiluk et al., 2010). Other research found that the quality of coping skill acquisition mediated the effect of treatment on duration of cocaine abstinence (Decker et al., 2016). Another possibility is that simply focusing on coping skills may increase self-efficacy; that

> Belief that a client will succeed has a way of becoming a self-fulfilling prophecy.

is, the clients' belief that he or she is capable of making the intended change (Bandura, 1997). This may mobilize skills that they already possess, which they then use to move toward change. The same optimism regarding the client's capability for change is also being communicated by the counselor who is teaching coping skills, and that belief is contagious. The therapist's belief that a client will succeed in recovery has a way of becoming a self-fulfilling prophecy (Leake & King, 1977).

KEY POINTS

🖈 Alcohol and other drugs are sometimes used for coping and to get from one (usually undesirable) state to another.

🖈 CBTs are generally designed to teach self-management skills for successful living without substance use.

🖈 Job finding, emotion regulation, social skills, behavioral self-control, and coping with urges and craving are among those topics commonly addressed in addiction treatment.

🖈 Increased self-efficacy may also underlie the well-supported efficacy of CBTs.

Reflection Questions

💬 In your experience, what are some of the most common ways in which people use alcohol, drugs, and other addictive behaviors for coping?

💬 What life skills do you think are most helpful for people in moving from addiction to recovery?

💬 If someone needs to develop a particular social skill for drug-free living, how might you best help him or her to strengthen it?

CHAPTER 12

Meditation and Mindfulness

Meditation has been around for a long time. It is a mainstay of 2,500-year-old Buddhism (Salzberg, 2010), and the subject of a Christian mysticism classic dating to 1375 (Anonymous, 1957). In various forms it has been called meditation (Dalai Lama & Hopkins, 2017), contemplative or centering prayer (Keating, 2009a, 2009b), mindfulness (Kabat-Zinn, 2016; Thich Nhat Hanh, 2015), and the relaxation response (Benson & Klipper, 2000). Although meditative practice has been a historical part of several major world religions, it can be taught and practiced in either spiritual or secular contexts.

What is a chapter on meditation doing in a book on addiction treatment? To start with, there is a long-observed inverse relationship between meditation and addiction. People with a regular meditative practice are less likely to use, overuse, or develop problems or dependence with psychoactive substances now or in the future (Aron & Aron, 1980; Shafil, Lavely, & Jaffe, 1975). When measured as a trait, mindfulness is also inversely related to substance use (Karyadi, VanderVeen, & Cyders, 2014). More recently, clinical trials have shown reduced resumption and frequency of substance use after treatment when mindfulness training has been added (e.g., Bowen et al., 2014; Witkiewitz, Warner, et al., 2014). Although no specific form of meditation is prescribed in AA (Alcoholics Anonymous; 1976), Step 11 of the 12-step program involves seeking "through prayer and meditation to improve our conscious contact with God, as we understood Him, praying only for knowledge of His will for us and the power to carry that out."

> There is an inverse relationship between meditation and addiction.

There are many different forms as well as some common elements in disciplines that have been called meditation, contemplation, mindfulness, and the relaxation response. Typically, one practices in a quiet setting in order to minimize distractions, and centers attention in some way: perhaps on one's own breath, a fixed object like a candle flame, or a *mantra*—a repeated sound or word. Practice in silence involves observing and accepting thoughts or feelings that arise without following, judging, or attaching to them, and instead returning to the center of attention. Some images for this are to let thoughts and feeling pass by like:

• Watching clouds float by in the sky without following them.
• Seeing boats go by on a quiet river without boarding them.
• Observing vehicles pass by on a country road without chasing them.

The effect is to quiet the incessant chatter of the "monkey mind" and enter a state of deep calm and peacefulness. Attention shifts from thinking about past or future to awareness in the present moment. Typical advice is to practice for about 20 minutes twice a day. Although there may be a structured introduction with a certain number of sessions, the intent is to establish a lifelong practice and foster trait mindfulness (Shapiro, Brown, Thoresen, & Plante, 2011; Shevlov, Suchday, & Friedberg, 2009).

Beyond these basics, there are variations in conceptualization and practice (Keng, Smoski, & Robins, 2011). Some seek to empty consciousness of all content, toward a thoughtless awareness. Others seek to open themselves to noticing whatever comes without judging or following the content—the usual meaning of mindfulness. Consistent with Step 11, prayerful forms can be understood as opening oneself to the presence and influence of God or a Higher Power (Keating, 2009a). Mindfulness meditation can be practiced while walking, observing one's surroundings with nonjudgmental awareness (Nguyen Anh-Huong & Thich Nhat Hanh, 2006).

> The intent is to establish a lifelong practice and foster trait mindfulness.

Whereas clinical trials have found little benefit of relaxation training in addiction treatment (Miller & Wilbourne, 2002), recent research on meditation has been more encouraging. Randomized clinical trials of training in meditative practices have reported lowering of withdrawal symptoms and anxiety (Li, Chen, & Mo, 2002), reduced drug use, craving, and problems (Bowen et al., 2009, 2014; Brewer et al., 2011; Chiesa & Serretti, 2014; Garland et al., 2014; Witkiewitz, Warner, et al., 2014), and more rapid reinstatement of abstinence (Vidrine et al., 2016). This is part of a larger literature on the salutary effects of meditative practice on health, psychological wellness, and self-regulation (Brown, Ryan, & Creswell, 2007; Galante, Galante, Bekkers, & Gallacher, 2014; Keng et al., 2011). As with many interventions, the degree of adherence to meditation (e.g., regularity of practice) appears to be related to benefit (Gryczynski et al., 2018).

Although there has been substantial neuroimaging research on meditation (Cahn & Polich, 2006; Chiesa & Serretti, 2010; Tang, Holzel, & Posner, 2015), the mechanisms by which it may impact addiction treatment outcomes are only beginning to be understood (DiClemente, 2010). Candidate routes of influence include reduction in stress and rumination (Brewer, Bowen, Smith, Marlatt, & Potenza, 2010; Davis et al., 2018; Zgierska et al., 2008), delay discounting (Ashe, Newman, & Wilson, 2015), decoupling of craving from use (Elwafi et al., 2013; Spears et al., 2017), alteration of cognitive and affective processes (Bowen, Witkiewitz, Dillworth, & Marlatt, 2007; Elwafi et al., 2013; Garland, Froeliger, & Howard, 2013; Khanna & Greeson, 2013; Witkiewitz & Bowen, 2010), acceptance of present experience (Baer, 2003; Bien, 2010), and enhancement of positive emotion and reappraisal (McConnell & Froeliger, 2015). To the extent that addictive behaviors have been used to cope with aversive mental states, their mere suppression is likely to be temporary unless alternative coping behaviors are substituted (Toneatto, Vettese, & Nguyen, 2007). Mindful attention is sometimes focused on the physical, mental, and emotional experiences that trigger craving and use, without attaching to or identifying with the thoughts and sensations (Witkiewitz, Bowen, Douglas, & Hsu, 2013; Witkiewitz, Bowen, et al., 2014) as a way of diminishing cue reactivity (Carter & Tiffany, 1999).

> Mindful attention can focus on triggers for craving and use without attaching to them.

Meditation or mindfulness may be unfamiliar to many of your clients, and its relevance to addiction may be unclear to them. On the other hand, some may already have a meditative practice. Here is an example of how you might introduce this option to a client.

PRACTITIONER: I wonder if you have ever heard about or maybe even tried practicing something called "meditation" or "mindfulness."

CLIENT: It sounds like something they do in a monastery!

PRACTITIONER: That's one place it was practiced for many centuries, but now it's being taught in health care and used by ordinary people like us.

CLIENT: In health care?

PRACTITIONER: Yes. Would it be all right if I take a few minutes to tell you about it?

CLIENT: Sure.

PRACTITIONER: There has actually been a lot of scientific research on the health benefits of meditation. It's been shown to reduce stress, improve heart health, and decrease depression and anxiety. It can be very relaxing, and help you let go of stresses in your life. Can you see how that might be useful to people recovering from addiction?

CLIENT: Maybe. I do get stressed out, and sometimes that's why I drink.

PRACTITIONER: Right! So it might be an alternative to drinking for you when you're feeling distressed.

CLIENT: But does it really help with addiction?

PRACTITIONER: I don't know if it's for you, but I do think it's one good tool to have in recovery, and not just when you're feeling stressed. Ideally, it's something that you practice every day, and it seems to help reduce urges to drink. I think you've had some experience with the 12 steps, and meditation is mentioned in Step 11 as a regular practice. Does that sound familiar?

CLIENT: Yeah—prayer and meditation, I think.

PRACTITIONER: That's right. It's something you can make a regular part of your life.

CLIENT: But I'm not really the praying type.

PRACTITIONER: You don't want to have anything to do with prayer.

CLIENT: Well, it's just not something I do.

PRACTITIONER: I respect that. Meditation has been part of many different world religions, and it can also be practiced without any religious overtones. One book about meditation is just called *The Relaxation Response*.

CLIENT: How long does it take?

PRACTITIONER: You can practice it in as little as 15 minutes a day. Some people fit it in at the beginning or end of their day. I guess the real question, though, is whether it's something you'd like to experience, to try out and see if it seems possible for you.

CLIENT: Would I have to go somewhere else?

PRACTITIONER: Actually, I can help you get started here. I've been practicing mindfulness meditation myself for several years now, and I like how it has changed me. Are you curious?

CLIENT: I guess I'm willing to try it.

A final note here is that mindfulness meditation can also be useful for treatment providers. For professional integrity, if you are going to recommend meditation to your clients, you should be familiar with its practice.

BOX 12.1. Personal Reflection: Contemplative Practice

I was well into retirement before I began a regular practice of meditation. The prompt was a 2-year "living school" with the Franciscan friar and teacher Richard Rohr. I had certainly heard about meditation and knew friends who had been practitioners, but I wasn't sure that it was a good fit for me. Nevertheless, I gave it a try. At first I was waiting for something to happen, but soon I remembered Gahan Wilson's famous *New Yorker* cartoon of an old monk seated next to a young novice and saying: "Nothing happens next. This is it." Next I wanted to turn it into an achievement: I was going to get really *good* at meditating! Nope. Then I made it into a duty, something that I *had* to do every day, and of course I resisted it. Eventually I stopped trying or expecting to make anything happen and settled into a peaceful state of willingness and openness. I'm still a relative novice, but I like the gradual changes I'm experiencing in myself.

—W. R. M.

Like music instructors, those who teach mindfulness should be experienced practitioners themselves. The kind of deep empathic listening and client-centered approach described in Chapter 4 is itself a contemplative practice, focusing full attention without judgment (unconditional positive regard). The trait of mindfulness in clinicians has been found to predict better fidelity in the practice of motivational interviewing as well as improved treatment outcomes (Arlt, 2017). Mindfulness practice has also been found to reduce stress and burnout among health care professionals (Cohen-Katz et al., 2005; Shapiro, Astin, Bishop, & Cordova, 2005). Improving the ratio of cortical to limbic activation can be good for both counselors and clients!

KEY POINTS

🕯 Meditation is meant to become a regular life practice, as indicated by Step 11 of the 12-step program.

🕯 Various forms of meditation have certain common elements as well as differences in emphasis.

🕯 Mindfulness is a discipline of observing and accepting thoughts or feelings that arise without following, judging, or attaching to them.

🕯 People with a regular meditative practice are less likely to use, have problems with, or become dependent on psychoactive substances.

🔖 Clinical trials now support adding mindfulness meditation to the menu of evidence-based options for treating addiction.

🔖 Regular meditative practice can also benefit treatment providers.

Reflection Questions

Q How might you make meditation available to the people you treat as one option on a menu of evidence-based methods to support recovery?

Q What has been your own personal experience with meditative practices?

Q What do you think are potential benefits and obstacles to adding regular meditative practice in one's life—either your clients' or your own?

CHAPTER 13

Contingency Management

A quandary in escaping from SUDs is that the benefits of sobriety tend to be delayed, whereas the reinforcement that drugs offer is fairly immediate. Drug effects include positive reinforcement (such as a desired state like a high, stimulation of the brain's reward circuitry) as well as negative reinforcement (relief from an undesired state like drug withdrawal or unpleasant feelings or memories). Complicating this picture is the phenomenon of *delay discounting* (Vuchinich & Heather, 2003) which is exacerbated by substance use: potential future rewards lose their value with delay, whereas immediate rewards become more salient. Fortunately, delay discounting diminishes over time in recovery (Quisenberry, Eddy, Patterson, Franck, & Bickel, 2015; Quisenberry, Koffarnus, Franck, & Bickel, 2015). The challenge is how to accumulate enough sobriety to tip the balance.

One evidence-based way of accomplishing this is contingency management (COM), sometimes also called "motivational incentives." It is based on the principle of positive reinforcement: behaviors that are rewarded are more likely to continue or increase whereas those that are not rewarded tend to decrease or stop. In COM people are rewarded for adhering to a defined desirable (target) behavior such as submitting a drug-free urine or an alcohol-free breath test, completing a homework assignment, or finding and maintaining employment. When missing the target behavior (e.g., submitting a drug-positive urine screen or skipping medication doses or appointments), there is no punishment; reward is simply withheld.

Like parents, providers sometimes wonder whether it is proper to reward people for what they should be doing anyhow. In the case of addiction, however, what the person is already doing (typically substance use) is reinforcing in itself, otherwise it would have stopped naturally. Incentives to move toward sobriety are, in essence, competing with the sometimes substantial positive and negative reinforcement derived from substance use. The aim is to increase alternative health-promoting behaviors such as staying drug-free, attending treatment or mutual help meetings, spending time in events incompatible with substance use, and in general maintaining a lifestyle that promotes sobriety. Immediate reinforcement tends to be more effective than delayed incentives for increasing health-promoting behaviors more generally (Herrmann et al., 2017)

> Behaviors that are rewarded increase; behaviors not rewarded decrease.

Practicalities of Delivering COM

Vouchers: Every One a Winner

One common COM approach encourages positive behaviors by offering incentives in the form of vouchers that can be exchanged for goods, services, or other preferred items as determined by the client in consultation with the provider. Vouchers may also contain points that are redeemable at an office or shop located within the treatment facility. Higher point values can be assigned to more challenging goals like obtaining and maintaining a job.

Vouchers can have an *escalating* value, so that with each consecutive positive behavior (e.g., counseling sessions attended, medication doses taken, drug-free urine samples submitted) the value of the voucher increases. For example, the first target behavior might have a $1.00 value, the next $2.00, and so on. In this case, the value of vouchers is reset to the starting level when a target behavior is missed.

Drawing for Prizes

Cost is one drawback of a voucher system where every target behavior is rewarded. A less expensive but equally effective approach involves drawing slips or cards from a "fishbowl," sometimes called a *prize-based* approach (Petry et al., 2005). With each positive behavior (such as submitting a drug-free urine sample) the person gets to draw a slip from a box or bowl that contains incentives of various values (Petry, 2012). These might range from just a positive comment like "Good job!" to a monetary value between $1.00 and $100.00. This is essentially a variable reinforcement schedule, which tends to maintain behavior at least as well as receiving a small reward every time. To save costs, most prizes are small, with very few having a larger cash value. As with escalating vouchers, clients may be allowed an increasing number of draws based on the number of consecutive target behaviors achieved, resetting to just one draw if a positive behavior is missed. Drawn slips may also contain points that can be exchanged for nonmonetary incentives. Research has indicated that in head-to-head comparisons prize-based and voucher-based incentives can be equally effective (Rash, Stitzer, & Weinstock, 2017).

Specifying Target Goals

There may be value in breaking down target goals into smaller steps or intermediate components such as scheduling of job interviews, attending medical appointments, and participating in activities that are incompatible with drinking or drug use (Reback et al., 2010). Success with intermediate goals can enhance readiness and confidence to pursue further goals. Target behaviors can be scaled from low impact (such as scheduling an appointment with a health care provider) to high impact (e.g., maintaining abstinence and employment for 2 months). Achieving a higher-impact goal results in additional prize draws or higher voucher value, and as described above a reset procedure can be included to deter reversal of gains. Similarly, progress in successive approximations (such as gradually reducing use) can be recognized rather than reinforcing only perfection. This can afford clients greater opportunity for success and bolster motivational readiness and self-efficacy (McDonell et al., 2017; Reback et al., 2010).

> Success with intermediate goals can enhance readiness and confidence to pursue further goals.

How Effective Is COM?

A meta-analysis of 19 studies concluded that adding COM to treatment programs significantly improves clients' short-term outcomes (Benishek et al., 2014). COM has shown benefit in a wide variety of treatment settings including intensive outpatient programs, methadone clinics, sheltered housing, and group treatment programs for diverse clients experiencing problems with alcohol, cocaine, cannabis, nicotine, methamphetamine, and other drugs (Benishek et al., 2014). It has also been be used to decrease alcohol/drug use by contingency management of disability payments (Budney, Brown, & Stanger, 2014; Ries et al., 2004) that otherwise might facilitate drug use (Shaner et al., 1995). COM has been applied effectively with adolescents (M. D. Godley et al., 2014), in treating co-occurring medical, mental health, and SUDs, and at-risk HIV/AIDs behaviors (Rash et al., 2017), and to address related issues including job skills training, medical care, and housing that help to prevent recurrence of substance use problems (Herrmann et al., 2017). Beneficial effects have emerged from adding COM to treatment for cocaine use disorders (Garcia-Rodriguez et al., 2009; Secades-Villa et al., 2013). Based on encouraging efficacy data, the U.S. Department of Veterans Affairs initiated an expansion of COM in their treatment programs (Petry, DePhilippis, Rash, Drapkin, & McKay, 2014).

How Long-Lasting Are COM's Effects?

One reasonable concern regarding the use of COM is that the desired behavior will stop as soon as the contingency and reinforcement end (Tuten, DeFulio, Jones, & Stitzer, 2012). In fact, external rewards can even undermine internal motivation (Deci, Koestner, & Ryan, 1999). A meta-analysis in addiction treatment (Benishek et al., 2014) found that the effect size of COM decreased from 0.46 at the end of treatment to 0.33 at early follow-up, and by 6 months the outcomes of COM and control conditions were no longer different. The benefits of COM do not completely disappear as soon as contingencies are removed, and several studies have observed enduring effects 3–12 months after contingencies end (Dougherty et al., 2015; Halpern et al., 2015; Murphy, Rhodes, & Taxman, 2012; Secades-Villa, Garcia-Rodriguez, Lopez-Nunez, Alonso-Perez, & Fernandez-Hermida, 2014). Posttreatment benefits of COM have also been observed in reducing HIV risk behaviors (Hanson, Alessi, & Petry, 2008; Petry, Weinstock, Alessi, Lewis, & Dieckhaus, 2010), alleviating psychological symptoms (Petry, Alessi, & Rash, 2013), and improving quality of life (Petry, Alessi, & Hanson, 2007). Adding motivational interviewing to COM appears to prolong the impact on substance use (Sayegh et al., 2017).

Another possibility for extending the impact of COM is to gradually fade reinforcement rather than abruptly discontinuing it (Cooney et al., 2017). The frequency and value of vouchers can be slowly diminished, and supplemented with ample nonmaterial reinforcement and social recognition. In a prize-based approach, drawings can occur less frequently and the percentage of higher-value prizes can be decreased. Some have recommended extending COM for longer periods or reintroducing it at distal points over the course of treatment. In certain situations such as employment-based abstinence programs, it might be cost-effective to continue contingencies indefinitely (DeFulio & Silverman, 2011).

Nevertheless, COM primarily gives clients a head start, a boost in experiencing early success with change, and other treatment methods may be needed to help clients make the transition from substance use to sobriety. COM can help retain and encourage change while other treatment components and the natural rewards of sobriety take effect. In essence, it can help to "buy time" for other treatment to work.

Combining COM with Other Approaches

COM could be combined with virtually any other treatment method described in this book. What else does your client need besides a head start on sobriety? What would support long-term change in establishing and maintaining a drug-free lifestyle (M. D. Godley et al., 2014)? What challenges are not addressed by COM alone? One study found that adding motivational interviewing increased the efficacy of COM in promoting smoking cessation after residential addiction treatment (Rohsenow et al., 2015). In a 1-year follow-up of treatment for cannabis use disorders, a combination of COM with cognitive-behavioral therapy and motivational interviewing was more effective than either component alone (Budney, Roffman, Stephens, & Walker, 2007). Similarly, a combination of COM with sustained-release bupropion was more effective than either component alone in helping adolescents to stop smoking (Gray et al., 2011).

Combining COM and other effective psychosocial and pharmacological treatments may be particularly useful with special populations who may lack the social and economic resources needed to sustain abstinence once the contingencies are removed (Montgomery, Carroll, & Petry, 2015). During and after the period of COM, such populations may benefit from ongoing case management, which has been shown to be a valuable adjunct in both pharmacotherapy and behavioral treatment in studies with disadvantaged or underserved populations (Barry, Sullivan, & Petry, 2009; Bride & Humble, 2008; Montgomery et al., 2015).

We note, however, that combination treatments are not always more effective than their individual components (Anton et al., 2006). In one study (Carroll et al., 2012) adding COM to cognitive-behavioral therapy (CBT) was less effective than either component alone in treating cannabis use disorders. The authors concluded that adding CBT to COM "backfired," perhaps by overwhelming their court-referred clients.

For Whom Is COM Most Effective?

The intensive monitoring demands of COM may not be a good match for some types of clients—for example, those seen in nonspecialty settings (e.g., primary care) primarily for medical concerns and not seeking help for SUDs. When COM proved ineffective with a mandated population, the authors speculated that the intensive monitoring of COM may have been overwhelming in combination with the economic, legal, housing, and medical issues their clients were facing (Petry, Barry, Alessi, Rounsaville, & Carroll, 2012).

COM may be unhelpful for clients who already show little or no drug use during treatment. In essence, they don't need COM and it might even undermine autonomous motivation for change. In contrast, those having

---

BOX 13.1. Contingency Management for Persons
with Co-Occurring Disorders

A COM program was implemented with individuals having psychiatric and substance use disorders. The overall goal of the program was for clients to achieve and
maintain independent functioning. In this program, Social Security disability payments were arranged so that frequency (not the amount) of benefits was contingent
on demonstrating improvement in several areas of functioning such as managing
finances, attending treatment, adhering to the medication regime, and reducing
alcohol and drug use. Preliminary findings showed that individuals who participated in the program demonstrated improvement in managing their finances and
reducing alcohol and drug use as compared to individuals who received disability
payments via *the usual* method (i.e., without contingencies).

Based on Budney, Brown, and Stanger (2013).

---

greater difficulty abstaining early in treatment appear to benefit from
higher-incentive COM (Herrmann et al., 2017; Petry et al., 2012).

Interventions for SUDs among homeless people have sometimes made
housing contingent upon continued abstinence. This runs contrary to a
"Housing First" perspective, that getting homeless people into stable housing is a prerequisite for changes in their health and social problems. A study
with 2,154 people experiencing both homelessness and mental illness found
that Housing First (with housing not being contingent on abstinence) was
equally effective regardless of the presence or absence of concomitant SUDs
(Urbanoski, Veldhuizen, et al., 2018).

There is a need for innovative and effective methods to strengthen and
extend the benefits of COM to a broader range of people with SUDs,
including African American and Latino groups (Montgomery et al., 2015),
methamphetamine users (Reback et
al., 2010), and individuals with multiple drug use and co-occurring disorders (McDonell et al., 2017; Petry &
Martin, 2002).

> Those having greater difficulty abstaining
> early in treatment benefit from higher
> incentives.

Implementing COM

Even though COM has shown encouraging efficacy in numerous studies,
its use does vary dramatically between and within agency settings (Cunningham et al., 2017; Taxman, 2012). A recent survey indicated that even
among settings where staff have been trained in COM, only about half

were actually using it (Aletraris, Shelton, & Roman, 2015). In part the obstacles to using COM are attitudinal:

- "Rewarding people for abstinence is contrary to our treatment values and principles."
- "Relying on external rewards will keep clients from taking personal responsibility for their problem and their recovery."
- "It may work as long as you offer bribes, but as soon as the rewards end so does the client's sobriety."

Providers may accept the importance of positive recognition for progress but remain reluctant about offering tangible rewards (Hartzler, Jackson, Jones, Beadnell, & Calsyn, 2014). Some programs hold regular recognition events and offer certificates or pins to acknowledge achievements. Weight loss groups often recognize and celebrate steps of progress along the way toward a long-term goal. Many 12-step groups offer pins or coins celebrating various lengths of sobriety. It is not necessary, by the way, to "reset" such intangible recognition to zero when, as frequently happens, progress is not continuous. Recovery often occurs through progressively longer periods of sobriety interspersed with shorter, less frequent, and less severe episodes of use (see Chapter 21).

Another obstacle to implementing COM is the additional cost involved. The costs of training and implementing any new treatment procedure should be weighed against its effectiveness and the benefits to be gained by clients. The costs of COM can include more frequent monitoring of drug use, staff time and training, and acquiring the cash or other material rewards to be used. In a traditional voucher program clients could earn as much as $1,000 by providing negative drug specimens over 12 weeks of treatment (Petry, Alessi, Barry, & Carroll, 2015). As mentioned earlier, this cost can be substantially reduced by using the partial reinforcement schedule of a prize-based system, without compromising COM effectiveness. Another cost-saving method is to reserve COM only for clients who are most likely to benefit from it (Cunningham et al., 2017; DeFulio & Silverman, 2011; Petry et al., 2012; Rash et al., 2017).

The research described above suggests a variety of responses to potential barriers in implementing COM. These are summarized in Box 13.2.

COM Training

To facilitate the implementation of COM within treatment programs, it helps to have a cadre of providers well trained in COM skills. Broader exposure of staff to the scientific evidence for and practicalities of this method can increase acceptance of COM by providers with initially negative reactions (Aletraris et al., 2015).

BOX 13.2. Responding to Challenges in Implementing COM

Challenges	Possible Solutions
Offering tangible reinforcement incentives	Offer nontangible incentives (e.g., access to recreational activities) only; allow clients to choose between tangible or nontangible incentives
COM costs	Target the intervention to subgroups more likely to benefit from COM (e.g., individuals who test positive for drug use at intake)
Duration of benefits	Maintain contingencies for longer periods or at distal points; increase the magnitude of reinforcement incentives for individuals with high severity alcohol or drug use problem
COM for special populations	Combine COM with other effective pharmacological and psychosocial interventions (e.g., case management and COM for underserved populations); adapt COM to the special needs of particular groups such as mandated clients
Changing negative attitudes of providers toward COM	Involve providers in the design and implementation of COM studies; expose and train providers in COM.
Availability and feasibility of employing accurate measurement devices in COM	Test the reliability and validity of novel technological devices such as biosensors and biomarkers in COM.

As with other treatment methods, solid training can increase staff skillfulness with COM, which in turn predicts better treatment outcome (Hartzler, Beadnell, & Donovan, 2015). Research is proceeding to discover more effective methods for COM training (Henggeler, Chapman, Rowland, Sheidow, & Cunningham, 2013) and free research-based web-based training resources are available (Promoting Awareness of Motivational Incentives [PAMI]: *www.bettertxoutcomes.org/bettertxoutcomes/PAMI.html*).

Final Thoughts

There has already been much progress in the development and utilization of COM in addiction treatment. Having provider involvement in the design and implementation of COM treatment and research can facilitate more positive attitudes toward COM (Walker et al., 2010). Toward this end, the federally supported Patient Centered Outcomes Research Institute (PCORI; *www.pcori.org*) was formed to expand the role of providers in treatment outcome research. Their mission is to encourage collaborative involvement in comparative outcome clinical trials. Researchers are required to partner with providers in forming the research questions, developing the design, and implementing the interventions in comparative outcome studies.

Much can be learned from future research on how best to structure schedules of reinforcement, and beyond the technology (Hartzler et al., 2015), the therapeutic skills that facilitate or impede the efficacy of COM (Miller & Moyers, 2015). More will be discovered about how COM may benefit high-risk and high-cost populations such as people with co-occurring mental illness and substance use (Srebnik et al., 2013).

Advances in technology may also improve COM, particularly with regard to accurately and immediately measuring substance use. Urine toxicology assesses only a snapshot window of time. Already-available technological innovations show promise in providing accurate and immediate feedback via biosensors (e.g., Barnett, Tidey, Murphy, Swift, & Colby, 2011) and biomarkers (e.g., Hahn et al., 2012).

KEY POINTS

♣ COM competes with the immediate reinforcement offered by substance use.

♣ People are more likely to engage in health-promoting behavior when incentives are immediate and frequent than when relying on delay of gratification.

♣ Schedules and magnitude of reinforcement incentives can be adapted to particular populations and linked with appropriate goals to improve treatment outcomes.

♣ Breaking down target behaviors into small components or scaling them at different levels provides more opportunities to reinforce progress and experience success.

♣ Combining COM with effective psychosocial and pharmacological treatments can strengthen and extend the benefits of both.

♣ COM is more likely to benefit clients who have positive drug tests at entry and have greater difficulties in abstaining early in treatment.

♣ Exposure to and training in COM can increase providers' understanding, acceptance, and use of this method.

Reflection Questions

Q Having read this chapter, what is your own personal opinion now about using COM as a component of addiction treatment?

Q How might you respond to the following objections of colleagues regarding COM?

- "Rewarding people for abstinence is contrary to our treatment values and principles."
- "Relying on external rewards will keep clients from taking personal responsibility for their problem and their recovery."
- "It may work as long as you offer bribes, but as soon as the rewards end so does the client's sobriety."

Q Where do you think COM might be most helpful in specialty and nonspecialty settings that treat people with SUDs?

CHAPTER 14

A Community Reinforcement Approach

There are at least two striking facts about the community reinforcement approach (CRA). The first is that for decades it has been one of the most strongly supported addiction treatment methods in terms of evidence of efficacy in clinical trials. The second is that for a long time, relatively few addiction treatment professionals had ever heard of it.

CRA: The Big Picture

Central to CRA is the principle of positive reinforcement: that when a behavior leads to rewarding consequences, it is likely to be repeated. The underlying perspective of CRA is relatively simple: in order for a person to give up a significant reinforcer like drug use, the alternative needs to be more appealing. That is, a life without drugs needs to be more rewarding than a life of drug use.

There is good reason for CRA's focus on positive reinforcement rather than negative consequences. Indeed, if suffering and punishment cured addiction, there would be far less of it. Most of the people we see for treatment have experienced substantial, sometimes astonishing, levels of adverse effects of drug use: family, health, financial, social, legal, and/ or psychological problems. It is a central puzzle of addictions why these behaviors persist despite such high levels of negative consequences. In his history of Australia, Hughes (1987) described the defiant willingness of convicts there to incur beatings, torture, and even the threat of execution in order to obtain tobacco and alcohol. Attempts to punish away substance use are notoriously ineffective and can even backfire.

There is no mystery, though, as to why psychoactive drugs are reinforcing. Caged laboratory animals will self-administer nicotine, cocaine,
opiates, and amphetamine without further encouragement. Certain animal
strains also show strong preference for alcohol, whereas others avoid it. All
of these drugs in some way access the brain's central reinforcement systems
that signal, "Do that again!" (Koob, 2005; Volkow, Koob, et al., 2016).
Beyond this direct reinforcement, which often occurs within minutes or
even seconds of drug administration, there can also be powerful psychosocial reinforcers for drug use. Other
real or imagined desirable effects of
drugs can include relaxation, suppression of memories, sexual facilitation,
and feelings of well-being or power. Family and friends may encourage
substance use and help to insulate the user from its negative consequences.
Drugs are problematic precisely *because* using them involves positive reinforcement. One need not look beyond animal models and basic principles
of learning for an explanation of how and why people can become addicted
to such drugs (Logan, 1993).

> Life without drugs needs to be more rewarding than a life of drug use.

Yet if drugs are so powerfully reinforcing in their own right, why
doesn't everyone become addicted? Most people who are exposed to potentially addictive drugs don't use them habitually or become dependent on
them. Most American soldiers who used heroin while deployed in Vietnam
abruptly discontinued use on return home (Robins et al., 2000; Robins,
Helzer, & Davis, 1975). Though the tens of millions of annual prescriptions
for opioid analgesics have generated a U.S. epidemic of misuse and mortality (Dart et al., 2015), short-term prescription use does not normally lead
to continued use or dependence, and some individuals use addictive substances in a moderate or "controlled" manner (Zinberg, 1984). Laboratory
rats do self-administer psychoactive drugs when isolated in small cages,
but the "rat park" experiments found that they shunned available morphine when living in a large reinforcement-rich open space with other rats
(Alexander, Beyerstein, Hadaway, & Coambs, 1981; Alexander, Coambs,
& Hadaway, 1978). Deprivation of natural freedom and reinforcement is
one way of understanding the strikingly similar and devastating patterns
and effects of alcohol use among diverse displaced indigenous populations
(including the homeless) around the world (Alexander, 2008; Daugherty,
Love, James, & Miller, 2002).

CRA fundamentally seeks to increase drug-free positive reinforcement
and to undermine rewards associated with drug use. Family members are
taught how to avoid inadvertently reinforcing substance use (see Chapter
15). CRA can incorporate certain medications that interfere with the usual
positive consequences of drug use (see Chapters 3 and 18), such as those
that block receptor systems (e.g., naltrexone) or impose adverse effects
(e.g., disulfiram; Azrin, 1976). Reducing sources of positive reinforcement
for drug use is one avenue toward change. CRA has also been combined

with COM (Chapter 13) to provide direct positive reinforcement for early abstinence (Higgins & Abbott, 2001). The primary focus in CRA, however, is connecting clients with natural alternative sources of positive reinforcement that do not involve substance use, and ideally are incompatible with it. In short, the goal is to help people construct a life that is joyful, rewarding, and meaningful without using drugs.

As we will review later in this chapter, CRA has been used effectively in both residential and outpatient settings, with adolescents and adults, with homeless individuals, and in treating dependence on alcohol, heroin, cocaine, and multiple drugs. In outpatient contexts, the special procedures of CRA typically require between six and 18 sessions. Often CRA begins with motivational counseling to enhance the person's readiness for change (see Chapter 10). In Chapter 15 we will also describe how CRA has been used effectively to work through significant others (SOs) even when their loved one refuses to get treatment.

> Prescriptions for opioid analgesics have generated an epidemic of misuse and mortality.

CRA Procedures

CRA draws on a menu of procedures that are used flexibly, as appropriate to the individual's situation. Therefore, the length and content of CRA treatment are not prescribed. For some people, a few of the procedures may suffice to establish and maintain sobriety. For others, more extensive life changes are needed.

Functional Analysis

One defining characteristic is that CRA begins with a careful *functional analysis* of drinking or drug use, examining both the antecedents and the consequences of substance use. With regard to antecedents, when is the person most likely to use (or use to excess)? Are particular times of day, days of the week, feelings, places, or companions especially associated with use? Sometimes the use of one drug triggers the use of another. Smoking and drinking are often closely linked, for example, and resumption of cocaine use frequently occurs in the context of drinking alcohol. One way to assess antecedents is to ask about the person's "triggers" for drinking or drug use. In group counseling, we have generated a list of such triggers, writing them on the left side of a board or paper.

With regard to consequences, the interest here is particularly in the positive and rewarding consequences of use. "What do you *like* about alcohol?" or "What do you hope will happen when you use marijuana?" Here again one can generate a list, either in individual or in group counseling. We do this on the right side of the board or paper.

Next it can be helpful to make connections between these two columns: the point is that drugs are often used to get the person from one state (the trigger situations) to another (the consequences). This can be illustrated by drawing lines from each element in the left-hand list to a corresponding goal in the right-hand list. Each item may have more than one partner in the other list. It also happens that there are items in one list that do not seem to have a partner in the other, in which case it is usually possible to fill in a missing component. Box 14.1 provides one example of a list that could be generated by a group.

After creating and discussing the list of triggers and consequences, brainstorm alternative ways of getting from one point to another, or to cope in a manner that does not require the use of drugs. These are, in essence, "new roads" (Miller & Pechacek, 1987). As long as a person has only one way (a drug) to get from point *A* to point *B,* he or she is by definition psychologically dependent on the drug. An important goal of functional analysis is to identify how the person has been using drugs and the functions that the drugs have served, and then to find new ways to serve those needs.

As you consider alternative behaviors, it can also be useful to do a functional analysis of these as well. When, where, and with whom is the person most likely to engage in these alternative behaviors? What are the possible positive consequences? This process recognizes that the person is already engaging in some positive activities that do not involve substance use.

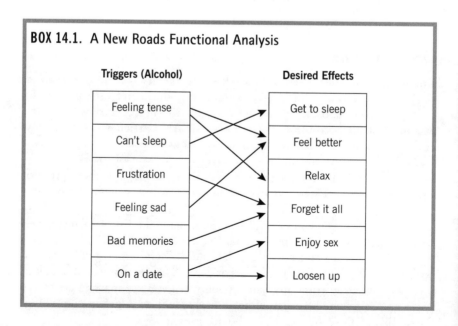

BOX 14.1. A New Roads Functional Analysis

Happiness Survey

In considering alternative sources of positive reinforcement, one useful tool is a happiness or life satisfaction survey, which is another characteristic procedure in CRA. This is a simple list of life areas that the person rates from 1 (completely unhappy or dissatisfied) to 10 (completely happy or satisfied). The scale might look like the one shown in Box 14.2, although the specific items can be adjusted to your own setting and population.

Areas of dissatisfaction that are identified on this form can become goals on a treatment or case management plan, as areas to strengthen positive reinforcement. "My drinking" or "my drug use" can also be included on this survey, to gain a sense of the person's current satisfaction or dissatisfaction with substance use.

Sobriety Sampling

One sound motivational principle in counseling is not to ask clients to do what they are unwilling to do. This does not mean that you should approve of the status quo, but before you ask clients to do something, assess and work on their motivation to do so (Chapter 10). If a client is unwilling to consider long-term abstinence, the method of successive approximation is one way to proceed. What step in this direction might the client be willing

---

BOX 14.2. Current Happiness Scale

My work or education	1	2	3	4	5	6	7	8	9	10
My financial situation	1	2	3	4	5	6	7	8	9	10
My social life	1	2	3	4	5	6	7	8	9	10
My family life	1	2	3	4	5	6	7	8	9	10
My love life	1	2	3	4	5	6	7	8	9	10
My spiritual life	1	2	3	4	5	6	7	8	9	10
My friends	1	2	3	4	5	6	7	8	9	10
My spouse/partner	1	2	3	4	5	6	7	8	9	10
My personal freedom	1	2	3	4	5	6	7	8	9	10
My emotional life	1	2	3	4	5	6	7	8	9	10
My overall happiness	1	2	3	4	5	6	7	8	9	10

to take? That is the basic idea behind the CRA method of sobriety sampling (Meyers & Smith, 1995). In essence, the counselor and the client negotiate a period of abstinence that the client is willing to try.

Start by asking clients what might be some advantages of being drug-free for a period of time. You could describe this activity as taking a vacation from drugs. Perhaps it has been some time since the client has experienced sobriety, and this is a chance to experience what it is like. It can demonstrate to others the person's desire to change, and decrease immediate levels of interpersonal conflict. Following principles of MI (Chapter 10), it is better to elicit the positive benefits of sobriety from the client rather than presenting them yourself. A period of sobriety also quickly clarifies the ways in which the client has become dependent on substance use for coping, for a sense of well-being, and for managing symptoms. If the trial period of sobriety proves challenging, the specific difficulties that are encountered can be quite instructive. Box 14.3 offers a questionnaire that you could use to help clients consider possible advantages.

The point is to negotiate an initial trial period of abstinence that seems manageable and to which the client will agree. It might be a specific number of weeks, or even days. Remain in close contact with your client during this period, particularly during the first few days. If there is indication of physical addiction and the possibility of serious withdrawal (e.g., from alcohol or sedatives), the client will need close monitoring during early abstinence (see Chapter 6). Even if the client's long-term intention is to cut down rather than abstain (see Chapter 11), there are good reasons for a trial period of abstinence at the outset (Miller & Muñoz, 2013; Sanchez-Craig, 1996).

> It is better to elicit the positive benefits of sobriety from the client rather than presenting them yourself.

Monitored Medication

For certain drugs there are medications available to help in maintaining abstinence (see Chapter 18). Disulfiram (trade name Antabuse), for example, when taken daily induces discomfort and illness only if the person drinks alcohol. It thus serves as a significant deterrent to alcohol use, which may also help the person to refrain from other drug use (e.g., cocaine or other stimulants) for which drinking is a trigger (Carroll et al., 2004; Carroll, Nich, Ball, McCance, & Rounsaville, 1998). Another drug, naltrexone (trade name Revia), effectively binds opioid receptors, blocking the desired effects of heroin, and also apparently reduces the reinforcing effects of alcohol.

One limitation on the effectiveness of these medications, of course, is that clients discontinue them, or are reluctant to take them in the first place. MI (Chapter 10) can be used to strengthen motivation for a trial

BOX 14.3. Possible Advantages of a Drug-Free Trial Period

Here are some advantages that people sometimes experience by trying a period of being drug-free. How important *to you* might each of these be?

	Not at all important	A little important	Somewhat important	Fairly important	Very important
1. I could save some money	1	2	3	4	5
2. I could find out how it feels to be drug-free	1	2	3	4	5
3. People who care about me would be happy I'm doing it	1	2	3	4	5
4. I might find out how drugs have been harming me	1	2	3	4	5
5. It would demonstrate to myself and others my sincere desire to change	1	2	3	4	5
6. I could feel better about myself	1	2	3	4	5
7. I could discover what the longer-term challenges are going to be for me in recovery	1	2	3	4	5
8. I could learn more about what drugs have been doing *for* me—why I have needed them	1	2	3	4	5
9. I could give my body a break, a rest from drugs	1	2	3	4	5
10. I'm tired of living the way I have been	1	2	3	4	5
11. I could get through the early symptoms of withdrawal	1	2	3	4	5
12. My head would be clearer to do some things I need to do	1	2	3	4	5
13. I'd have fewer conflicts and arguments with people	1	2	3	4	5
14. I would be more in control of myself	1	2	3	4	5
Other reasons of your own:	1	2	3	4	5
15.	1	2	3	4	5
16.	1	2	3	4	5

period of such medication, similar to the strategy of sobriety sampling. Many clients find, for example, that they experience little or no desire to drink when they know they have taken disulfiram. Taking such medications can also demonstrate commitment to one's probation officer, family members, and loved ones.

CRA includes another procedure that can be quite effective in maintaining adherence: supportive monitoring by a loved one of the client's medication taking. The loved one is given brief training on how to administer the medication in a way that ensures it is taken (Azrin, 1976; Meyers & Smith, 1995). The client and loved one agree to a specific time when they will be together to complete the daily routine. The loved one's role is not that of an enforcer but rather a reinforcer, providing appreciation, support, and encouragement for the client's continued commitment to change as demonstrated by taking the medication. There is a further agreement that if either party declines to participate in the daily routine, the other will contact the counselor promptly. (Given the half-life of most medications used in this way, this immediate contact gives you a chance to intervene before substance use resumes.) Although medication is not an essential part of CRA (Meyers & Miller, 2001), this procedure can be quite helpful in getting clients through the more difficult early weeks of abstinence.

Use of Time

A diagnostic aspect of behavioral dependence is that it consumes large proportions of a person's time. Substance-dependent people spend a lot of time obtaining, using, recovering from, and coping with the consequences of using drugs. Consequently, when drug use stops, they find that they suddenly have a lot of time on their hands. It is important to anticipate this situation and help your clients plan for positive alternative ways to use their time.

A prime goal, of course, is to have the person spend time in activities that bring positive reinforcement without substance use. What brings this person joy? A general guideline is: Do things that you enjoy, and do them with or around other people who are not drinking or using drugs. To be sure, enjoyable solitary activities are also fine, but there is added value in having fun with others that is not associated with substance use.

Clients may at first be at a loss to think of ways for spending time and having fun that don't involve biochemistry. Here it can be useful to have a menu at hand. There are various long lists of possible reinforcers available (e.g., Lewinsohn, Muñoz, Youngren, & Zeiss, 1992; Miller, 2004) such as shown in Box 14.4, or you can construct your own. In cities, the newspapers often print a weekly list of local groups, activities, meetings, clubs, and entertainment. The key is to help your clients identify activities that they do enjoy, have enjoyed, or might enjoy, and then to start sampling them. Help clients as well with the follow-through process, perhaps

BOX 14.4. A Menu of Possibly Pleasurable Activities

Here are many different ways in which people sometimes enjoy themselves. Underline some options that you have enjoyed in the past or might enjoy in the future.

Take a drive to see something new
Relax and read the newspaper
Help your child with homework
Plant something to watch it grow
Go for a walk
Take a nap
Build something from wood
Feed the birds or ducks
Hang a hummingbird feeder
Enjoy a special dessert
Go for a run
Get up early to watch the sun rise
Walk a dog
Play frisbee
Sew something
Have a relaxed breakfast
Spend an hour in a favorite store
Have a makeup demonstration
Visit a shopping mall
Add one new item to your wardrobe
Pamper your feet in a basin of warm water
Massage your feet with a cooling lotion
Write a letter to someone who helped you
Work on a quilt
Pray
Visit an old friend
Cook a favorite meal
Lie on the grass
Go out for a special meal
Rent a funny movie
Play tennis
Try a new recipe
Go to a yard sale or garage sale
Have your own yard sale
Go skateboarding or rollerblading
Go roller skating or ice skating
Have coffee with a friend
Visit a museum
Walk along the water

Visit someone who is homebound
Walk or ride a bicycle path
Buy a small gift for a friend or child
Find a place for a moment of solitude
Make a pizza
Visit the library
Play a card or board game
Buy thick fluffy new bath towels
Put fresh sheets on the bed
Hunt for bargains at a thrift store
Trade backrubs for 20 minutes
Take a relaxing hot bath
Indulge in your favorite childhood treat
Enjoy one perfect flower in a vase
Compliment someone
Babysit for someone who needs relief
Send a care package to a student
Call someone special in your family
Write to an old friend
Go to a movie, perhaps with a child
Make a big bowl of popcorn
Have or give an oil massage
Listen to your favorite music
Read a book you've heard about
Bake a batch of cookies
Make some food for a friend
Add an item to your collection
Hum or sing
Listen to a favorite CD
Write in a diary or journal
Ride a motorcycle
Play golf or miniature golf
Clean out your purse
Read old letters you have kept
Read poetry
Write poetry
Start a memory box
Read your favorite children's book
Rearrange the furniture

(continued)

Thank you to Shelby Steen for compiling this list.

BOX 14.4. *(continued)*

Call a friend who makes you laugh
Make biscuits or tortillas
Daydream a little
Enjoy the quiet of an early morning
Have lunch with a friend
Roll down a hill
Polish your nails a new color
Grow (or shave off) a beard or mustache
Try a new hairstyle
Enter a contest
Search your family history
Volunteer to be a coach
Paint a room
Wash and wax your car
Lie under a tree and watch the sky
Do some gardening
Take a class
Play a musical instrument (or learn to)
Visit a wildlife refuge
Visit (or volunteer at) the zoo
Go horseback riding
Look at maps for places to visit
Cover a bulletin board with family pictures
Meditate
Go camping
Search the Web
Take a creek walk—the stream is your
    path
Pick fresh fruit or berries
Make homemade ice cream
Read a favorite magazine
Go to a demonstration in a store
Play tennis
Go to a gym and work out
Go to a sporting event with someone
Spend an hour alone with your child

Be creative—try out a new kind of art
Make a family scrapbook
Build a swing in a tree
Refinish old furniture
Call someone you'd like to talk to
Send a card to a someone you care about
Wash your windows
Have a picnic in the park
Find a good spot and watch the night sky
Go fly a kite
Go dancing
Sing in a chorus
Go downtown
Go to an open house
Have dinner at a romantic restaurant
Give and receive a foot massage
Visit an aquarium
Ski or play in the snow
Build a fire
Work on a car or truck
Plan a holiday or trip
Smile
Find shapes in the clouds
Draw a cartoon
Roast hotdogs and marshmallows
Cut, chop, or carve wood
Go for a swim
Listen to a favorite radio station or
    program
Frame a picture
Put your feet up
Skip stones across water
Go to the mountains
Ride a train
Go to a talk or concert

by connecting them with contact people who can help them get acquainted and be comfortable with initial experiences.

Interpersonal Relationships

Close relationships can be a primary source of positive reinforcement (and also, of course, of stress and conflict). Because interpersonal relationships so importantly influence both substance use and recovery, CRA includes helping clients to develop and strengthen relationships that will support sobriety. This involves two common components of cognitive-behavioral relationship counseling: strengthening positive communication and problem-solving skills, and participating together in enjoyable activities that do not involve substance use (see Chapter 15). Having both the client and the SO complete the same happiness survey (see Box 14.2) allows you to compare their areas of satisfaction and dissatisfaction, providing areas for focus in communication training and problem solving. There is a particular focus on increasing positive communications such as compliments, appreciation, affection, and pleasant surprises, and decreasing negative communication patterns such as nagging, criticizing, threatening, and blaming.

Job Finding

Nathan Azrin, who introduced CRA, also developed effective methods for helping clients to become employed or find a more rewarding job (Azrin & Besalel, 1982). This has become a key component of CRA, and with good reason. Stable employment is a strong predictor of sobriety. Counseling methods for helping clients find rewarding employment are described in Chapter 11.

Sobriety Skills

Abstinence is the absence of a behavior. It is, in a way, doing nothing. Displacing a previously preferred behavior sometimes requires behavioral coping skills that your clients may need assistance in developing. For example, a newly abstinent person may experience invitations or social pressure to use alcohol or other drugs, and refusal skills are important in responding to such occasions. As discussed above in the "new roads" analysis, it is common for people to use psychoactive drugs as a coping strategy. When abstaining they will continue to encounter situations that require coping, and may not have effective alternative responses. This often becomes apparent during the early weeks and months of sobriety. In essence, the general strategy is to strengthen the client's skills for responding effectively in expected and unexpected situations that could trigger resumed use. This is the principal focus of Chapter 11.

Practicalities

As is apparent by now, CRA involves a menu of procedures that are used flexibly to address the needs of each individual. It makes no sense to construct a one-size-fits-all CRA program in which all clients are given the same skill training, job club, relationship counseling, monitored medication, and so forth. The question is, "What will it take *for this client* to tip the balance of reinforcement away from drug use and toward sobriety?" A few components are offered for all clients in CRA: motivational counseling, a sound functional analysis, and clear goal setting (e.g., sobriety sampling). Beyond that, CRA relies on the creativity of the counselor and client to choose, from a menu of procedures, those most likely to solve problems and address needs of the individual client (Meyers & Smith, 1995; Miller, 2004).

There is, in CRA, a strong emphasis on encouragement and positive reinforcement during the process of counseling itself. The counselor is characteristically upbeat and affirming, acknowledging any and all efforts that the client makes to move in a positive direction. Timeliness of response is also important. When a window of opportunity opens and a client is ready to move, the counselor should be ready to go. Motivation does not wait for waiting lists. Similarly, if a spouse or client calls to say that they have

---

BOX 14.5. Personal Reflection: Learning the CRA

In searching during the 1970s for addiction treatment methods with a strong track record of efficacy, I came across outcome studies of CRA with strikingly positive findings. I didn't need statistics to see that these were large improvements over standard practice at the time. CRA was only one of many innovative clinical contributions of Nathan Azrin, a widely respected behavioral scientist and a student of B. F. Skinner. Reading the research articles, however, gave me very little understanding of how this treatment was actually done. There were only brief descriptions of the procedures, with no real sense of how the method looks in practice.

It was my good fortune, then, when one of Azrin's own students, Bob Meyers, came to work at the addiction treatment center where I was doing research. He had been a therapist in the most recent clinical trial of CRA (Azrin, Sisson, Meyers & Godley, 1982). In watching him demonstrate and work with clients I was struck by aspects of the practice of CRA that were not emphasized in the research articles. He was a consistently empathic, friendly, positive, and *reinforcing* presence. He listened well to clients, recognizing and encouraging any small step toward recovery. Clients *enjoyed* working with him. "So *that's* how you do it," I thought. Both the menu of practical procedures and the therapeutic relationship matter. Either one without the other is missing something (Miller & Moyers, 2015; Moyers, Houck, Rice, Longabaugh, & Miller, 2016).

—W. R. M.

missed the daily medication monitoring routine, the counselor tries to see them that day or the next. A little attention right away can avert the need for much more treatment later.

The Efficacy of CRA

Across five decades there has been strong evidence that CRA not only works, but adds significantly to the effectiveness of approaches with which it has been compared. Every clinical trial of CRA to date has been positive, showing significant benefit. A series of early studies found CRA to be more effective than treatment as usual for alcoholism in both inpatient (Azrin, 1976; Hunt & Azrin, 1973) and outpatient settings (Azrin, Sisson, Meyers, & Godley, 1982; Miller, Meyers, Tonigan, & Grant, 2001). Other studies have found large effects for CRA with people experiencing homelessness (Slesnick, Prestopnik, Meyers, & Glassman, 2007; Smith, Meyers, & Delaney, 1998), as well as efficacy with Native Americans and Alaskans (Campbell et al., 2015; Venner et al., 2016) and Aboriginal Australians (Calabria et al., 2013). Four trials have shown CRA and contingent incentives for abstinence to be significantly more effective than traditional approaches in treating cocaine dependence (Higgins et al., 1994; Higgins et al., 1995, 1993, 1991; Higgins, Wong, Badger, Haug Ogden, & Dantona, 2000), and the addition of contingent vouchers increased the efficacy of CRA (Secades-Villa et al., 2013). Relative to treatment as usual, opioid-dependent people treated by CRA have been more likely to complete withdrawal management and remain heroin-free (Abbott, Moore, & Delaney, 2003; Abbott, Weller, Delaney, & Moore, 1998; Bickel, Amass, Higgins, Badger, & Esch, 1997). Procedures have been developed for monitoring the fidelity of CRA (Smith, Gianini, Garner, Malek, & Godley, 2014), and treatment outcomes have been specifically linked to the delivery of CRA procedures: the more CRA treatment procedures used, the greater the change in substance use (Garner, 2009). A multisite trial also showed an independent contribution of CRA modules beyond the impact of therapist empathy (Moyers et al., 2016).

The application of CRA with adolescents (A-CRA) has expanded since the publication of our first edition (Godley, Smith, Passetti, & Subramaniam, 2014). A-CRA significantly reduced substance-related problems (relative to usual treatment) with youthful offenders involved in justice systems (Henderson et al., 2016). Benefits of A-CRA have also been reported in reducing cannabis use among youth (McGarvey et al., 2014). Adolescents with concomitant psychological problems showed significantly *greater* benefit from A-CRA, compared with those with only SUDs (Godley et al., 2014). Engaging and training peers of A-CRA clients significantly reduced alcohol use for both the emerging adults themselves and for their peers

(Smith, Davis, Ureche, & Dumas, 2016). This builds on the pioneering research of Natasha Slesnick and colleagues applying A-CRA with homeless youth (Slesnick, Kang, Bonomi, & Prestopnik, 2008; Slesnick, Meyers, Mead, & Segelken, 2000; Slesnick et al., 2007).

Another important product of CRA is the community reinforcement and family training (CRAFT) method for helping and working through family members and significant others even when the identified substance user refuses to seek treatment (Meyers, Miller, Hill, & Tonigan, 1999; Smith & Meyers, 2004). The CRAFT method is described in more detail in Chapter 15.

KEY POINTS

🔖 CRA helps people rearrange their lives so that sobriety is too good to give up.

🔖 CRA focuses on reinforcement for positive alternatives to substance use.

🔖 COM (Chapter 13) is also an effective tool for reinforcing sobriety, which can be combined with CRA.

🔖 CRA has been supported in every clinical trial in which it has been tested to date.

🔖 CRA has worked with particularly difficult-to-treat populations: those refusing to seek treatment; the homeless; adolescents; people with cocaine, heroin, and polydrug dependence; and those with concomitant disorders.

🔖 Training of significant others through CRAFT (Chapter 15) can engage initially unmotivated substance users in treatment and improve outcome.

Reflection Questions

❓ In your own community, what enjoyable activities are available that are not associated with substance use?

❓ Why is positive reinforcement more effective than punishment in changing addictive behaviors?

❓ How comfortable are you with sobriety sampling when clients are not ready to commit to long-term abstinence?

CHAPTER 15

Working with Significant Others

A person's addiction adversely affects more people than the one who is diagnosable, and sometimes many more. The stress of living with and caring about someone snared in addiction has long been recognized (Jackson, 1954) and can take its toll on physical and mental health (Orford, Velleman, Natera, Templeton, & Copello, 2013). Collateral harm to family members and significant others [SOs] can include psychological, physical, social, and relationship harm (Enser, Appleton, & Foxcroft, 2017; Orford, 2017). In this regard, affected family members may seek and benefit from health services whether or not their loved one accepts treatment for addiction. This chapter is about starting with concerned family members and other SOs.

As will be discussed in Chapter 16, including an SO in addiction treatment can improve outcome, even with brief intervention (Jiménez-Murcia et al., 2017; Monti et al., 2014; Shepard et al., 2016). But what can you do if the person who is experiencing addiction refuses to get help? Every addiction treatment program receives desperate phone calls from people concerned about someone's substance use. They have tried everything to get their loved one to seek help, but to no avail. The problems continue to mount, and they want to know what to do. How should you respond? Three approaches that have been fairly common in North America are:

1. Tell them that the drinker/drug user has to be the one to take the initiative, and to have the person call when he or she is ready.
2. Refer the caller to Al-Anon for support.
3. Arrange for an "intervention" in the original style of the Johnson Institute in which the person is confronted by family and others

with the consequences of his or her substance use and urged to seek treatment.

Here is what is known about each of these three approaches.

1. *Wait for the substance user to get ready.* Predictably, when the caller is told that the loved one has to be the one to make the call him- or herself, it's unlikely to happen. Sometimes the family will increase their pleas or pressure, but few call back.

2. *Refer to Al-Anon.* It is clear that participating in Al-Anon can be helpful and supportive to the concerned SO, who may show improvement in physical symptoms, depression, stress, and general well-being. That is good in itself, but it does not directly address the original reason for the SO's call. Participants in Al-Anon are usually advised that they are powerless to influence the drinker, to detach, and to desist from efforts to change their loved one. It is unsurprising, therefore, that while the SOs themselves improve, only about one in eight of their loved ones may get into treatment within a year (Miller, Meyers, & Tonigan, 1999).

3. *Conduct an "intervention."* What happens when the family is counseled to prepare for a confrontational meeting with the drinker/drug user? Early reports indicated that when the family went through with the full intervention, a high percentage of their loved ones were persuaded to enter treatment. It is also the case, however, that even with highly skilled counselors, the vast majority of families decide not to go through with the confrontational family meeting. This was the principal reason why, in the only randomized trial, only 30% of families counseled in this way succeeded in getting their loved one into treatment (Miller, Meyers, & Tonigan, 1999).

Working *through* SOs

A different approach is to work with the concerned SOs (usually one or more family members), not only to provide them with help themselves, but also to use their own influence to help their loved one. We have found that these SOs are some of the most rewarding and collaborative clients we have treated. They are motivated not only by their own suffering, but by their loving concern for the person affected by SUDs.

Is it possible to influence someone's substance use by working through his or her SOs? The answer clearly is "yes." José Szapocznik and colleagues found that they were equally able to influence family dynamics and substance use outcomes via a "one-person family therapy approach" versus conjoint therapy including the whole family (Szapocznik, Kurtines, Foote,

Perez-Vidal, & Hervis, 1986; Szapocznik, Kurtines, Foote, Perez-Vidal, & Hervis, 1983). Edward Thomas and colleagues took this a step further, developing and testing a "unilateral family therapy" to work through spouses when their partners with alcohol use disorders were unwilling to seek treatment (Thomas, Adams, Yoshioka, & Ager, 1990; Thomas & Santa, 1982; Thomas, Santa, Bronson, & Oyserman, 1987). In the SO group receiving unilateral family therapy, eight of 13 drinkers (62%) entered treatment or cut their drinking at least by half (or both) within 4 to 6 months, whereas none did so in a delayed treatment control condition.

> Significant others can use their own influence to help their loved ones.

In Chapter 10 we discussed the predictable result when you tell people that they have a problems and what they should do about it. The normal human response is defensive, to argue against a need for change. The phenomenon of psychological reactance is the "well-established inherent tendency to act contrary to recommendations from others . . . even where they agree" (de Almeida Neto, 2017). Yet concerned SOs (like counselors) can easily fall into this "righting reflex" of arguing for change, with the usual result that the person with addiction digs in deeper to defend the status quo. This pattern, once attributed to the inherent pathology of alcoholism (Steiner, 1984), is an avoidable interpersonal tussle as family members try to cope with the chaos of addiction.

The key is to help SOs find a middle ground between control and detachment, which can be a very tricky balance. In a Dutch randomized trial (Smeerdijk et al., 2012), parents of young adults with recent onset schizophrenia were trained in motivational interviewing skills to help their children reduce cannabis use, which exacerbates psychotic symptoms. Through 15 months of follow-up (Smeerdijk et al., 2015), young adults showed significantly greater reduction in quantity and frequency of use and in craving for cannabis when parents were trained in MI (Chapter 10). Parental distress was also significantly reduced in the MI-trained group. Helping SOs find a middle ground to influence loved ones' substance use is also the purpose for which community reinforcement and family training (CRAFT) was developed, as described in the next section.

> Help SOs find a middle ground between control and detachment.

Community Reinforcement and Family Training

Taking a behavioral approach, Sisson and Azrin (1986) taught seven concerned SOs to modify reinforcement contingencies at home in order to influence alcohol use, and prepared them for rapid initiation of treatment at an opportune moment. In six of the seven cases (86%), the drinker entered treatment, whereas none did so in a randomly assigned comparison group.

Furthermore, those entering treatment had already reduced their drinking by more than half, closely paralleling the unilateral family therapy findings described above.

This inspired Bob Meyers to further develop the CRAFT method building on the work described in Chapter 14. The crux of CRAFT is encouraging family members that they *can* make a difference, and teaching them specific ways in which to use the considerable social influence that they do have (Meyers & Wolfe, 2004; Smith & Meyers, 2004). In particular, SOs are taught how to provide positive reinforcement for sobriety and to avoid inadvertently reinforcing the loved one's substance use. SOs are also prepared to watch for windows of motivational opportunity and how to encourage their loved one to seek help at those times. When the person finally does agree to seek help, it is important that treatment be readily accessible. When a new window of readiness opens, it is no time to put someone on a waiting list!

Some of the basic principles of CRAFT are common sense when viewed from the perspective of reinforcing the right stuff:

- Do not buy or otherwise provide the person with alcohol/drugs, or provide money that can be used to buy them.
- Do not protect the person from the natural negative consequences of substance use.
- Be sure to give positive feedback and reinforcement when the person is not using.
- Schedule time and activities together that compete with ordinary periods of drinking or drug use.
- Withdraw from the person's presence and be careful not to provide reinforcement when he or she is using.

Positive reinforcement of abstinence is often sorely missing (see Chapter 13). Cigarette smokers may get negative attention when smoking in public, but when they quit smoking nobody may notice that they are *not* doing something. Even more important, perhaps, is to help the person develop new and rewarding activities to fill the time previously occupied by addiction.

In the first randomized trial (Miller, Meyers, & Tonigan, 1999), CRAFT was compared with two other methods for helping SOs when their loved one refuses to seek help for an alcohol use disorder. It was not difficult to recruit 130 concerned SOs through referrals and announcement of the service through public media. The three approaches tested were:

- Al-Anon facilitation therapy to help SOs get involved in the fellowship and program of Al-Anon (Nowinski & Baker, 1998; Nowinski et al., 1992; see Chapter 17).

- The family intervention described by the Johnson Institute (Johnson, 1986).
- CRAFT (Meyers et al., 1999)

Each of three treatments was delivered and supervised by separate therapists trained in the approach that "reflected their own orientation and experience" (p. 692). By 6-month follow-up, 64% of drinkers whose SOs were in the CRAFT condition had entered treatment for their alcohol problems, as compared with 13% in Al-Anon facilitation and 30% with the Johnson intervention. The lowest engagement rate for any CRAFT therapist (50%) exceeded the highest engagement rate for any therapist in the Al-Anon (17%) or Johnson intervention condition (36%). As found by Sisson and Azrin (1986), initially unmotivated drinkers upon entering treatment had (by SO report) already cut their alcohol use by half on average. In a parallel randomized trial with SOs of treatment-refusing drug users (Meyers, Miller, Smith, & Tonigan, 2002), treatment entry within 6 months was 68% in the CRAFT condition, and 29% with Nar-Anon facilitation therapy.

It is important to note that in these clinical trials, the SOs benefitted equally from the treatment methods being compared. For example, in all three conditions (Miller et al., 1999), SOs showed significant reductions in depression, anger, and family conflict, with significant reported improvement in family cohesion and relationship happiness. The SOs themselves benefitted from any one of these forms of support. The substantial difference is in whether their loved one received treatment.

From trials in four nations it is now well replicated that CRAFT successfully engages initially unmotivated substance users by working unilaterally through their loved ones (Bischof, Iwen, Freyer-Adam, & Rumpf, 2016; Dutcher et al., 2009; K. C. Kirby, Marlowe, Festinger, Garvey, & McMonaca, 1999; Meyers et al., 2002; Miller et al., 1999; Roozen, 2010; Sisson & Azrin, 1993; Waldron, Kern-Jones, Turner, Peterson, & Ozechowski, 2007). Successful engagement rates vary across studies and by individual therapists, but in all cases CRAFT has yielded a substantially higher rate of engagement than is achieved through either Al-Anon facilitation or a family "intervention." It is not necessary to wait for people to "hit bottom"!

Offering CRAFT to supportive SOs can also be beneficial once the substance user is engaged in treatment. Providing CRAFT to the parents of adult opiate users during withdrawal management, for example, improved treatment retention (Brigham et al., 2014). In essence, SOs are learning specific skills to support their loved one's sobriety.

As with other complex treatments, CRAFT is not readily learned just by reading about it. Guidelines in implementing CRAFT are available for counselors (Smith & Meyers, 2004), and we recommend obtaining specific training if possible to gain competence in using these methods. In many geographical areas there may not yet be providers who have been adequately trained in CRAFT procedures. A self-help CRAFT guide is available for family members to use on their own (Meyers & Wolfe, 2004). In a randomized comparison of delivery methods, the treatment engagement rates were 60% for SOs offered CRAFT in group therapy format (71% for SOs who received at least one session of CRAFT), as compared with 40% with self-directed CRAFT, and both groups reported improvement in family functioning (Manuel et al., 2012). Progress is also being made on computer-assisted delivery formats (Brooks, Ryder, Carise, & Kirby, 2010; Campbell et al., 2012).

> CRAFT engages substance users by working through their loved ones.

Treating SOs

When someone is being treated for addiction problems, including an SO can benefit both clients and improve treatment engagement, retention, and outcome. We address this aspect of treatment in the next chapter (16). We have focused here on the situation where SOs are concerned about a person with addiction problems who is not yet receiving professional care. In this situation, engaging and motivating the SO is not usually a problem. It is the SO who initiates contact seeking advice. It is often welcome news to SOs that there *is* something they can do, and they may be more than willing to do what they can. Seeing the SO alone is likely, if nothing else, to benefit her own health and well-being. If a diagnosis is needed to warrant treatment or reimbursement beyond primary care, there are likely to be health issues, often stress-related, that can be addressed in their own right. In fact, SOs may first present with such psychological or other health concerns.

> Seeing the SO alone is likely to benefit her or his own health and well-being.

We acknowledge that it is unusual for a person to be "treated" for someone else's health problem, and this situation may not fall within current guidelines of health care systems. In the larger picture, however, there are circumstances in which it makes sense to do so. Like many chronic conditions, addiction is more easily treated at earlier stages of development, and it is not unusual for SOs to recognize and be concerned about a loved one's health issues. There has been longstanding education, for example, about early recognition of cancer signs, and encouragement to come for care early. It is common that people with some chronic conditions, such as combat-related PTSD, are reluctant to seek treatment even though their condition inflicts suffering on family members. It is often family members who first become aware of hearing impairment and encourage evaluation.

With addiction, we have an evidence-based method for engaging the affected individual in treatment earlier than would otherwise occur, and even for changing addictive behavior through the training of concerned SOs. The outcome is likely to be decreased long-term suffering and impairment for the person with addiction and for family members as well.

KEY POINTS

🖈 It is unnecessary to wait for someone with addiction to "hit bottom" or become "motivated" for treatment.

🖈 Family members and SOs are often the first to become aware of and concerned about addiction problems.

🖈 There are evidence-based methods to intervene through SOs to change addictive behavior and initiate treatment sooner than would otherwise occur. Compared to Al-Anon facilitation or an "intervention," CRAFT is consistently more effective in doing so.

🖈 Engaging SOs in treatment is likely to benefit both them and their loved one.

Reflection Questions

Q Within your own work context, how often does someone come to your attention who is being adversely affected by a family member's addiction?

Q What concerns would you have about working directly with SOs to help their loved one become engaged in treatment?

Q What is your own perspective on the assertion that family members are powerless to influence a loved one's alcohol/drug use?

CHAPTER 16

Strengthening Relationships

There is a long history of focusing solely on the individual "identified patient" in addiction treatment. The person with an SUD attends individual treatment sessions or participates in group sessions alongside others struggling with similar issues. Sometimes programs have offered a "family night" to educate concerned significant others (SOs), but treatment usually focuses on the individual with "the problem."

This is understandable from the clinician's perspective. Including an SO in treatment sessions adds a layer of complexity. You have to manage not only the individual client, but also the family member and the dynamics of their relationship. Furthermore, many providers of addiction treatment have had little or no training in couple or family counseling. Some systems even preclude reimbursement for conjoint sessions.

Yet there are good reasons to formally include a client's SO in addiction treatment, and it is actually quite feasible to do so (Magill et al., 2010; O'Farrell, Schumm, Murphy, & Muchowski, 2017; Schumm, O'Farrell, Kahler, Murphy, & Muchowski, 2014). One reason is that when an evidence-based approach is used, involving a loved one/partner can significantly increase the individual's prospects for recovery (McCrady, Epstein, Hallgren, Cook, & Jensen, 2016). SOs can be supportive in the process of recovery. Addiction issues may not be isolated to one person in the family; sometimes an SO has a substance use problem of his or her own. Furthermore, struggles with addiction are just hard on family members and relationships, and timely attention to these issues can prevent a host of problems later.

Recovery and Relationships

In 12-step meetings it is common to hear about relationships breaking up during the first year of recovery. This is a disturbing message and, for those sitting in a meeting and contemplating a change in their substance use, it might even be a deterrent. Imagine if part of the informed consent process for individual treatment were a caution against the "side effects" of recovery: *Warning: Sobriety may be harmful to your relationships.*

Yet it's true, and maybe that warning should be part of the consent process for those who engage in treatment that does not include the SO in a meaningful way. In addition to the anecdotal accounts circulating among recovery groups, research has shown that a disproportionate number of relationships do end *after* addiction treatment (O'Farrell & Fals-Stewart, 2006).[1] Why is this so? Substance use and related consequences can be tremendous stressors in a relationship (Cranford, 2014). If the substance use is a primary source of conflict between a couple, shouldn't the relationship become stronger once stable recovery is achieved?

Chances are that substance use is not the only source of stress in a relationship. Even when the substance use itself is removed, other problems may linger, surface, or even intensify. Perhaps the couple grew apart while one was actively using or in treatment. Even if the relationship preceded the development of addiction, it can be hard to remember what it was like before. Perhaps one or both decided that the relationship was no longer worth the investment of working through difficulties. It is also possible that the SO may not be ready to set aside past hurts and move forward. Conflicts that had been dammed up for years may be released once substance use is out of the way. A recovering person coming home to an SO loaded with built-up resentment could yield a cascade of conflict and relationship distress (Gottman, 1994, 2014). Newfound sobriety also can require a redistribution of power and roles within a relationship, with the recovering person ready and expecting to resume functions that had been taken on by the partner.

It is worth noting that most relationships do stabilize or improve rather than deteriorate once addiction is treated. Nevertheless, relationship problems persist or get worse often enough that it is definitely worthwhile to focus on improving relationship quality when treating addiction.

There is yet another good reason to focus on the relationship during substance use treatment: in research examining the main reasons why

---

[1]Tragically, claims of falsification of data arose against Dr. Fals-Stewart before his untimely death. Aware of this concern, we checked the veracity of research in which he collaborated and have been assured that the studies we cite in this book were properly conducted, supervised, and verified by senior colleagues and the research team.

people *resume* substance use, interpersonal conflicts with an SO are a frequent precipitant (Barber & Crisp, 1995; Hunter-Reel et al., 2009; Maisto, O'Farrell, Connors, & McKay, 1988). It is a destructive cycle. Relationships seem to be at risk for breaking up during the recovery process and, at the same time, conflicts within relationships can endanger someone's recovery. A modified warning might read: *Caution: Recovery may be harmful to your relationships, and your relationships may be harmful to your recovery.* To be most effective, then, it seems important to address not only the individual's substance use, but also the primary relationship in ways that are more conducive to stable recovery.

This is also consistent with the broader approach to conceptualizing addiction presented in Chapter 2 and throughout this book. Rather than viewing addiction just as individual pathology, many factors influence whether a person will develop and maintain addiction, and changes in these factors can positively or negatively influence the process of recovery. Relationship conflict appears to be one of these significant factors. By concurrently addressing both addiction and relationship functioning, outcomes for both can be significantly improved.

> Most relationships improve once addiction is treated.

A History of Ideas about Families and Addiction

It has long been recognized that addiction and family disturbance co-occur, but *why* is this so, and what are the implications for treatment? Theories abound, leading to dramatically different implications for intervention (McCrady, 2006). Early writings on this subject typically focused on men with alcohol problems and their wives, and the implicit underlying question was "What is going on with these women?" Various ideas have been proposed over the years.

Spouse and Family Pathology

The *disturbed spouse hypothesis* posited that wives had deep-rooted personality problems themselves as a result of developmental disturbances in their childhood. Based on clinical impressions, this psychodynamic hypothesis arose around the 1940s and speculated that these women sought out alcoholic husbands in order to fulfill their own unconscious needs. One account, for example, described them as aggressive, domineering women who married in order to mother or control a man, and who therefore had an investment in the continuation of his drinking (Futterman, 1953). It would be expected, therefore, that a man's attempt to quit drinking would be undermined and sabotaged by his wife. Anecdotes (e.g., of a wife buying alcohol for her sober husband) were used to exemplify and support this view, and the term "enabling" came to be associated with family behaviors that promote the continuation of addiction. Related to the pathological spouse hypothesis was the belief that if the husband sobered up, then the wife would decompensate (Edwards, Harvey, & Whitehead, 1973). The logical intervention, given this view, would be individual psychotherapy for the spouse, focused on alleviating her personality disturbance and her need for her partner to remain addicted.

A similar idea was the *disturbed family hypothesis,* often linked to family systems theory (Bowen, 1991; Shorkey & Rosen, 1993). Here the pathology was not attributed to an individual partner, but rather to dysfunctional patterns of family interaction. The problem was seen as residing within the family system itself, with each member of the family having a particular pathological role that maintains the equilibrium of the system. As a unit, the family system works to preserve these roles because of the familiarity and comfort of knowing what to expect from each family member. The person with an addiction occupies an important role within the system, crucial to the family's identity and self-regulation. In this view, the family would be expected to sabotage recovery in an effort to restore the status quo and prevent deterioration of the family (Rotunda, West, & O'Farrell, 2004). The book *Games Alcoholics Play* (Steiner, 1984) described in detail such self-maintaining family dynamics, with supporting anecdotes. The logical intervention within this view would be therapy for the entire family in order to change its pathological interaction dynamics.

This view of family members as having unique pathology of their own reemerged in a new but closely related form in the 1980s: the *codependence hypothesis* (Wegscheider-Cruse, 1990; Woititz, 1984). In this view, addiction was conceptualized as a "family disease" wherein both the addicted person and his or her family members are afflicted with complementary and interlocking illnesses. The term "codependence" was coined to describe the personality pathology of family members, which was alleged to be a separate disease that predates and exists apart from the loved one's SUD. As with earlier psychodynamic views, codependence was attributed to early childhood factors such as poor parenting, related perhaps to addiction in the prior generation, and was said to share certain features of an addictive personality (Cermak, 1991). A wide variety of described symptoms of codependence included continual emotional pain, inability to recognize one's needs and illness and ask for help, a high tolerance for inappropriate behavior, and compulsive dishonesty and pretending (Carruth & Mendenhall, 1989). Codependence was also alleged to have a definable course of deterioration mentally, physically, psychologically, and spiritually. Physical consequences of codependence were thought to include gastrointestinal problems, ulcers, high blood pressure, and even cancer, so that left untreated, the disease of codependence would be fatal. Schaef (1992) claimed that the codependent person often dies before the addicted person. (We know of no scientific evidence for this claim.) It would follow from this view that family members such as "adult children of alcoholics" would require separate treatment to overcome their disease of codependence. In essence, the codependence/family disease perspective represented a blending of disturbed spouse and disturbed family hypotheses.

All of these hypotheses predict observable abnormal behavior in families of people with addiction, and thus are scientifically testable. Within these views, the normal outcome of a person sobering up through individual treatment should be *increased* pathology in either the spouse or the family as a whole. The disturbed spouse and codependence hypotheses also predict the presence of stable and measurable personality disturbance in the spouse or other family member, independent of the loved one's drinking or drug use. Supported mostly by anecdotes, none of these hypotheses have been confirmed by the weight of scientific evidence (Hurcom, Copello, & Orford, 2000; Paolino, McCrady, & Kogan, 1978). As we stated earlier, if you have to guess what will happen in a family when an addicted member sobers up, bet that things will get better rather than deteriorate. The typical outcome is that even if only individual addiction is treated, other life

---

BOX 16.1. Personal Reflection: Am I Crazy?

She came into my university office visibly upset. "The department secretary told me that you know something about addictions," she said, and I invited her to sit down. She explained that her father had recently been admitted to a local residential treatment program. "After I left home about 12 years ago, he started drinking more, and when he retired it really got bad." Two weeks into treatment, a counselor from the program called her to ask if she could come to family night in order to support her father's recovery. "I said of course I would, and I went last night. Some of the counselors took me aside, surrounded me, and told me that I have a fatal disease called codependence, and that people who grow up with an alcoholic are just as sick as he is." They described the symptoms to her, a few of which seemed to fit, but she protested that in general she felt normal and was quite happy with her life. "Then they told me that people who are codependent don't know what normal is, and this proved that I have it. I explained that Dad wasn't drinking much when I was still living at home, but they told me it didn't matter, and I definitely need treatment or I'll mess up my own kids. Am I crazy?" After talking with her a while longer, I explained that there had been an attempt to insert a diagnosis of "codependence" into the DSM, but the American Psychiatric Association had rejected it for lack of scientific evidence. I thanked her for being willing to help her father, and reassured her that I saw no reason for concern about her own mental health. She was clearly comforted to learn that she was not "crazy" or "terminally ill" herself.

—W. R. M.

problems will tend to improve (Miller, Hedrick, & Taylor, 1983). There are exceptions, of course. Some problems and families really do get worse, and it happens often enough to deserve clinical attention, but this is the exception rather than the rule. Furthermore, there is no scientific evidence that there is generally "something wrong" with the spouses or family members of people with addiction.

The Family Adjustment Model

Where did the field go so wrong in stigmatizing already-suffering family members? There is usually at least a kernel of truth from which mistaken ideas are grown. That kernel here seems to be the observation that spouses and other family members often *do* show high levels of emotional distress. But *why* is this so? Long ago Joan Jackson (1954) proposed that the psychological disturbance and behavior of spouses represent understandable reactions and adaptive attempts to cope with the progressive deterioration of their partners' substance use. This *stress-coping hypothesis* posits that what appears from the outside to be aberrant behaviors of a spouse or other family members actually represents a normal adjustive reaction to the addictive behavior of their loved one. Within Jackson's perspective, behaviors stigmatized as "enabling," such as providing substances, or protecting the loved one from negative consequences, are understandable attempts to adjust to and cope with the chaos of addiction.

How would one help within this perspective? Certainly, emotional support is in order for the family during the process of treatment, but family members can also play an important role in supporting recovery. One evidence-based approach here is to help SOs distinguish between actions that favor recovery and those that favor continued use and addiction (Meyers & Wolfe, 2004). In essence, you teach the family to reinforce sobriety. It is common to advise family members to refrain from doing things that make substance use easier or reinforce it (still sometimes pejoratively called "enabling" behavior). But just as important, if not more so, is for the

> There is no scientific evidence that there is generally "something wrong" with the spouses or family members of people with addiction.

family to provide positive reinforcement for sobriety, for nonuse, and alternatives to use. This is part of the CRAFT method, described in Chapter 15, that has also been used effectively to engage reluctant loved ones in addiction treatment.

Al-Anon: Loving Detachment

Like other 12-step programs, Al-Anon (and Alateen for younger family members) does not endorse any particular theory of the etiology of addiction or related family problems. Although SUDs are described as a "family disease" because they adversely affect those close to the person, family members are clearly not blamed or held responsible for their loved one's addiction. Meetings are free of charge, anonymous, and widely available. Separate "Nar-Anon" meetings are available in many areas for those whose loved one is involved with illicit drugs, although many such family members also attend Al-Anon or Alateen.

The response that is usually advocated in these 12-step meetings is one of "loving detachment" (Al-Anon Family Group Headquarters, 1976). The spouse or family member is encouraged to give up attempts to influence a loved one's drinking or drug use, accepting his or her own powerlessness to control the addiction, and looking to other members for strength and support.

Within the framework of teaching family members that they are powerless to influence addiction, the Al-Anon program does not usually focus on encouraging or facilitating the loved one's abstinence, or even on improving family relationships. Individuals are encouraged to focus on what they need to do to improve their own lives. Because of this focus, it is not surprising that family involvement in Al-Anon has not been found to facilitate the loved one's seeking of treatment. Studies have found, however, that family members themselves who are receiving "Al-Anon facilitation therapy" to support their involvement in Al-Anon do significantly reduce their emotional and physical distress and improve their coping (Miller et al., 1999).

Chicken and Egg: The Cycle of Substance Use and Relationship Distress

The causal connections between substance use and relationship distress are complex. The negative effects of substance use can produce relationship problems. Stress from relationship problems in turn can trigger or exacerbate substance use. Each affects the other in a destructive cycle. Consider these three scenarios and the interlocking chain resulting from each person's actions:

> A couple gets into a disagreement at a restaurant about whether the man has been working longer hours to spend more time with a female coworker. The fight escalates and the woman accuses the man of cheating. Though they had already had several drinks at dinner, once home the woman retreats to her bedroom where she takes painkillers and drinks another bottle of wine as a way to soothe herself and distract herself from the upsetting thoughts.

> Couple problems → increased use

> A man tells his wife that he is too hung over to go into the office and too sick to even call in to his employer. He rolls over in bed and tells

his wife to leave him alone. Realizing that he will be fired if he doesn't show up without calling in for the second time in 2 weeks, and that they won't be able to pay their monthly bills without his income, the wife calls his employer to say that he has a virus and won't be coming to work that day. She then fixes him breakfast in bed, gets the children ready for school, and before leaving for work herself leaves a note on the counter telling him that she hopes he feels better soon and that she loves him very much. He spends the day in bed watching television and has several beers to help with the hangover. By the time his wife returns home in the evening, he is intoxicated again.

Increased use → caretaking, affection → more use

A woman returns home from a 28-day inpatient treatment program. Barely through the door with her suitcase, her spouse begins lecturing her about all of the things he has been angry about for years and that she was never sober enough to hear in the past. It seems to her that each day he spends hours telling her the various ways she let him down. After weeks of what seems like endless shaming, she begins using again. With her resumed use, the man stops airing his complaints.

Recovery begins→ increased conflicts → drug use →
decreased conflict

In other words, relationship conflict and substance use can be a self-sustaining cycle, and it is not crucial to decide which is causing the other. Identifying who is to blame is not fruitful, although distressed couples sometimes want you to do so. The point is to interrupt the cycle and start it turning in a positive direction.

The Evidence for Family–Involved Treatment of Adults

Studies indicate that including a person's SO in treatment results in higher rates of retention, adherence, and abstinence than does individual treatment (McCrady & Epstein, 1996; McCrady et al., 2016; McPherson, Boyne, & Willis, 2017). Family visits (Smith et al., 2003) and medical visit companions (Wolff & Roter, 2008) are already being used in health care to facilitate care management. Although addiction treatment has often focused on the diagnosed individual alone, there are good reasons to routinely engage an SO in treatment when feasible.

Behavioral couple therapy (BCT) is the treatment method with the strongest research support for its efficacy in treating addiction in adults. A meta-analysis concluded that overall, BCT produces better outcomes than individual-based treatment (Powers, Vedel, & Emmelkamp, 2008). In addition to increased rates of abstinence, BCT yields better relationship functioning, defined as lower risk of separation and divorce, compared to typical individual-based treatment, and reduces social costs, partner violence, child abuse, and the emotional problems of couples' children (Fals-Stewart, O'Farrell, & Birchler, 1997; Karakurt, Whiting, VanEsch, Bolen, & Calabrese, 2016; Kelley, Bravo, Braitman, Lawless, & Lawrence, 2016; McCrady, Epstein, Cook, Jensen, & Hildebrandt, 2009; O'Farrell, Murphy, Stephan, Fals-Stewart, & Murphy, 2004; Sayers, Kohn, & Heavey, 1998; Schumm, O'Farrell, Murphy, & Fals-Stewart, 2009). BCT can also improve adherence to medications such as disulfiram (Azrin et al., 1982) and naltrexone (Fals-Stewart & O'Farrell, 2003).

There is surprisingly little evidence for involving the entire family unit in treatment. Rather, the treatments that work seem to focus on involving the spouse (O'Farrell & Fals-Stewart, 2006) or another concerned family member (Donohue et al., 2009; Smith & Meyers, 2004). With adolescents, there is strong evidence for involving the parents or caregivers, as we will discuss later in this chapter. We will now discuss BCT in more detail as a specific evidence-based method for SO-involved treatment for adults.

What Is BCT?

BCT is designed for married or cohabitating couples in which one person is seeking help for addiction. The primary purpose of BCT is to include the SO in treatment as a way to increase and reinforce behaviors that support abstinence and long-term recovery and also improve the couple's overall relationship quality.

Participants in studies that support BCT's efficacy have typically been couples who have been married or cohabiting for at least a year and are willing to work together to see if their relationship can be improved. Although BCT was designed for couples experiencing significant relationship distress, there is also evidence that it can be useful even when a couple is getting along well (McCrady & Epstein, 1996). Results from a pilot study indicated that behavioral family counseling, an adaptation of BCT involving family members other than the spouse, was effective in reducing substance use and improving treatment retention (O'Farrell, Murphy, Alter, & Fals-Stewart, 2010), but the preponderance of evidence is for involving the spouse or partner.

The primary reasons why BCT may not be appropriate for a couple relate to legal and safety issues. Domestic violence is more common in addiction treatment populations, and for this reason you need to be aware and take steps to protect each person's safety. Some concerns are more clear-cut; for instance, if there is a restraining order stating a couple may not have contact with each other, then these individuals should not be seen together in therapy unless an exception is granted and both are willing. Less clear-cut are situations in which there is a history of intimate partner violence. On the one hand, there is strong evidence supporting the efficacy of BCT with couples who have a history of partner violence (O'Farrell et al., 2004; Schumm et al., 2009). However, if there is an acute risk for domestic violence that could cause serious injury or be life-threatening, then couple treatment may be unwise. It's a professional judgment call. Fals-Stewart and Kennedy (2005) offered five exclusion criteria that indicate an acute risk of severe violence:

1. One or both partners report a fear of injury or death.
2. A history of violence has resulted in an injury requiring medical attention in the past 2 years.
3. Violence has been threatened or inflicted using a weapon such as a knife or gun.
4. One member of the couple expresses fear in participating in couple treatment because of concern that violence may occur.
5. One member of the couple expresses desire to leave the relationship due to the degree and severity of partner aggression.

BCT is a comprehensive treatment package that includes behaviorally oriented couple sessions in addition to other psychosocial and pharmacological clinical services. As part of a treatment package, it is not intended to replace individual treatment; it can be an adjunct to other services offered in your treatment setting. Relationship quality is promoted primarily by increasing shared positive activities while improving the couple's communication skills and decreasing hurtful interaction patterns. Each partner commits to do what he or she can to improve the relationship.

In its full traditional form, BCT consists of 12–20 weekly couple sessions, each of which lasts 50–60 minutes. Sessions tend to be moderately to highly structured, with the counselor setting the agenda at the outset of each meeting and giving the couple assignments to complete between sessions. Though effective, this intensity of treatment can be prohibitive for some settings and populations. Consequently, a brief BCT was developed and tested in comparison to standard BCT or individual-based therapy. This briefer six-session BCT had posttreatment and 12-month outcomes that were equivalent to those for standard BCT, and still superior to those for individual treatment (Fals-Stewart & Lam, 2008). Thus, it appears possible to reduce the intensity and cost of implementing BCT without undermining efficacy.

Initial BCT sessions typically focus on establishing a recovery contract to support sobriety and to decrease couple conflicts about past or possible future substance use. Once sobriety and attendance at BCT sessions have stabilized, the counselor adds relationship-focused interventions to increase positive activities and improve communication. Finally, when sobriety has been sustained for 3–6 months, the counselor plans for continuing recovery to prevent or minimize a return to use (see Chapter 21) and decreases the frequency of BCT sessions.

Learning BCT

Compared to individual therapy, couple therapy is challenging because there is now a third person in the room requiring your attention. It can be challenging to empathize equally with both partners and form a strong therapeutic relationship with both people, yet this is important in order to avoid one person feeling like you are "ganging up" or taking sides. BCT requires clear structure and control over the sessions to maintain the focus of therapy, which is to address the substance use first and foremost, and prevent interactions in session that are further hurtful. As discussed earlier, the use of substances can lead to a great deal of anger and resentment in a relationship. The couple should be aware of what the BCT sessions entail; sessions are not an opportunity to vent and ruminate, something they might expect from stereotypes of "couple therapy." Rather, the purpose of this treatment approach is to change the ways that they communicate and act toward each other from this point forward.

This takes time and practice. BCT is not readily learned by reading about it, and plenty can go wrong in couple sessions. As with other evidence-based treatments discussed in this book, we recommend both initial training and some ongoing feedback and coaching based on observed practice. That's what it takes to really learn most any complex skill (Miller et al., 2006). Is it worth it to take the time and expense of obtaining such training for treatment staff? We believe that the increased benefit of involving an SO in treatment more than justifies learning BCT.

The Four Tasks of BCT

Whether using the full BCT or the shorter six-session version, there are four main tasks to accomplish (O'Farrell & Fals-Stewart, 2006). The first is to build motivation for engaging in BCT and to discuss the BCT approach with the couple. Following engagement, the next treatment task is to have the addicted client achieve and maintain sobriety by implementing the recovery contract, teaching refusal skills, deciding together how to deal with stressful life situations without substance use, and addressing how the SO can support recovery. The third task is to have the couple improve the quality of their relationship by working with them to increase positive and rewarding activities and behaviors, decrease negative interaction patterns, and learn skills for positive communication and resolving conflicts within their relationship. The final task is to work with the couple to tailor a plan for continuing recovery following initial treatment. The continuing recovery plan may involve check-in visits and/or plans to continue activities practiced during treatment. Within these four tasks, there is a great deal of flexibility in which methods are used and in the type of skills training that would be most useful to the couple.

BCT techniques all follow a typical behavioral skill training format (see Chapter 11). When teaching each skill, you first describe the skill to the couple, giving a rationale for why this is important. Second, you show how to effectively use the skill through modeling. For example, in practicing drink refusal skills you would role-play as the client; making eye contact and saying "no" in a clear, firm, unhesitating voice, escalating refusal responses as needed. The third step is to have the couple practice the skill in-session while you offer positive reinforcement and coaching to give feedback on areas needing improvement. The couple is then instructed to practice this skill at home. When the couple returns, you review their real-world practice and offer further coaching and practice for areas that were difficult.

Engaging the Couple

None of this couple work is possible, however, unless you first engage the couple in treatment (see Chapter 4). To work with a couple, you must receive permission to contact the spouse (see Chapter 24 on confidentiality ethics) by talking with the client who is seeking or already in treatment. In this initial conversation, explore the person's thoughts about including his or her SO in the treatment process. Though many are happy to do so, it is also common for people to express fears and concerns about including their loved one in treatment. It's normal to have mixed feelings about long-term decisions such as changes in substance use or commitment to the relationship. All that is needed in these early sessions is the willingness to explore things further in joint sessions.

After this initial conversation and permission, talk directly to the SO to invite him or her for a joint interview to discuss treatment planning and explore the possibility of couple counseling. To build trust you may want to call the SO while the client is with you, so the client can hear exactly what you say. This also facilitates scheduling of the joint interview since everyone can give their availability and find a mutually agreeable time. If the client has already expressed interest, the SO can be invited to learn more about treatment and find out if it is a good fit for both partners. We do not, of course, recommend imposing any particular approach on a person; if someone is adamant that a specific approach is unacceptable, there are many other options; developing a treatment plan that the person is enthusiastic about is a much better strategy.

The next step is to meet with the couple and gain their commitment to working together to promote recovery and work on the relationship. Remember that the couple does not need to be experiencing serious relationship problems to be appropriate candidates; rather, the SO's involvement can be framed as a way to work together to promote recovery. If the couple decides to try BCT, determine some key areas for focus in order to individualize the intervention. Even though BCT is often highly structured in the order of sessions and home assignments, deciding which aspects to emphasize more than others is a matter for your clinical judgment. Also, individually tailored are recommendations for adjunctive support such as mutual help meetings (Chapter 17), urine drug screens or breath tests, and use of medications (Chapter 18). Typically, engagement includes the couple making promises to each other regarding the course of treatment, such as not threatening separation, refraining from violence and threats of violence, focusing on the present and future, and actively participating in all sessions and completing home assignments.

Four Broad Goals in BCT

What are the primary components of BCT? Four broad goals are to (1) support sobriety, (2) improve positivity of the relationship, (3) strengthen communication skills, and (4) manage changes, conflicts, and problems. The order in which these goals are pursued can be flexible. For example, managing conflict might be an early priority when a couple has a high initial rate of aversive interactions.

Supporting Sobriety

When they begin treatment, some couples may be having little contact with each other or frequent arguments. A recovery contract is one way to encourage a couple to talk together in a positive way every day about sobriety and recovery. One component that is often included is a discussion around trust. Each day, at a specific agreed-upon time, the client initiates this brief discussion. In the trust discussion, the client states his or her intent not to drink or use drugs that day, in the same tradition of the 12-step "one day at a time" (Alcoholics Anonymous World Services, 2001). The SO then expresses encouragement and support for the client's efforts to stay abstinent, and the client thanks the SO for supporting his or her efforts. To prevent substance-related conflicts that can trigger a return to use, both partners agree not to discuss past or possible future substance use, instead reserving these discussions for the therapy sessions. The daily recovery contract time can also be the occasion when medications to aid in recovery (e.g., disulfiram or naltrexone) are taken in the SO's presence. This represents an opportunity for the SO to thank the client for his or her commitment. The contract might also include any other daily or weekly behaviors such as attending AA meetings, completing urine drug screens, attending group or individual counseling, exercising, or spiritual counseling. The contract will likely evolve as certain components are added and removed. New weekly activities to support recovery can be added or substituted.

In addition to a recovery contract, specific behavioral skills can be introduced at the outset (e.g., Meyers & Smith, 1995; Miller, 2004). For example, you may decide to spend time teaching priority skills for alcohol/ drug refusal or coping with urges. If the person does resume substance use, intervene promptly before it persists (see Chapter 19). One approach is to have a plan in place so that either the client or the SO calls you if substance use recurs or seems imminent. Another area you might focus on would be a discussion of triggers for use and ways to avoid or cope with these cues. A functional analysis might be useful to figure out ways to get desired effects without using (Chapter 14). For example, if a couple is distressed about ongoing conflicts, how might they cope with that stress without substance use?

Substance use can be particularly difficult to avoid when exposure to substances is pervasive and frequent. Especially early in recovery, avoidance of high-risk situations is helpful. The safest plan, of course, is to avoid all contact with people and situations where alcohol and drugs are readily available, but this may not be feasible. Will there be alcohol in the home? Will it be served to guests? Will the SO also abstain in solidarity with the client? (It's very hard, for example, for one partner to quit smoking while the other continues.) Will the couple attend functions that include alcohol or other drugs? Some couples are able to use partial avoidance, while others may need major life readjustments to avoid people and places that might trigger a return to use, at least early in the recovery process.

It is also useful to help couples find alternative ways of coping with significant life stressors and identify supportive community resources (see Chapter 8). Some issues you may be able to address directly, whereas others may require referral to another resource. Start with problems that may show quick progress, and defer more complex problems until initial encouraging gains in abstinence and relationship skills have been made.

You may discover and need to address partner behaviors that encourage substance use. Avoid placing blame and shame. Partners often do such things inadvertently or with the best of intentions, perhaps to avoid conflict or protect the family from negative consequences. Help the couple to identify any such responses that have occurred in the past or may still be occurring. Then brainstorm alternatives with the couple so that they have a different way of responding (Meyers & Wolfe, 2004; Smith & Meyers, 2004).

Offer lots of encouragement and reinforcement for positive changes, even small ones. Acknowledge periods of abstinence, notice and comment on positive coping responses, praise small steps in learning. Also encourage the couple to share in mutually enjoyable activities when the client has not been using (Meyers & Smith, 1995; Noel & McCrady, 1993).

Increasing Relationship Positivity

A second common goal is to improve the positivity of the couple's relationship. These interventions are directed toward increasing enjoyable couple and family activities as a way to enhance positive feelings, goodwill, and commitment to the relationship. Notice and affirm statements that reflect communal coping (Rentscher, Soriano, Rohrbaugh, Shoham, & Mehl, 2017)—more first-person plural pronouns ("we") and fewer "I" and "you" statements. "We" language during sessions is correlated with improved substance use outcomes (Hallgren & McCrady, 2016).

John Gottman, who has spent decades studying happy and unhappy couples, has described methods for strengthening relationships. One simple but important method is to increase positive communications and actions. Over time, relationships can drift toward negativity, focusing on partners' shortcomings and pet peeves. Early in a relationship the partners tend to exchange many positive comments and actions. As these positives decline over time, the partners can come to feel taken for granted and unappreciated. Increasing positive activities is a way to reverse this common negative drift in relationships. The ratio of positive to negative comments made by partners is a fairly good indicator of relationship happiness. Increasing positives involves consciously and conscientiously practicing caring behaviors on a daily basis. The reciprocal role for each partner is to notice and appreciate the partner's caring actions. Together, these changes can greatly improve relationship satisfaction (Gottman, 1994; Gottman & Silver, 2015).

A common recommended step is for each partner to make a list of personal "P's and D's" (pleasing and displeasing actions). Each person generates a list of pleasing things that the partner could do or say, as well as displeasing things. (It can also be interesting for each to guess what would be on the partner's lists.) These are usually shared with each other first during a session, and then both partners begin keeping records of P's and D's they give and receive. The goal is to have the P's substantially outnumber the D's. Sometimes each person is asked to secretly choose one "caring day" in the week in which to particularly increase P's for the partner.

Each partner is also asked to notice and appreciate the other's P's. A helpful instruction here is to "catch your partner doing something nice" each day. When the couple returns for a session, you can ask each one to take turns describing pleasing things that the partner did in the preceding week, perhaps using an appreciative "I" message ("I appreciated when you . . ."; "I felt good when you . . ."; "I liked it when you . . .").

This method sounds fairly straightforward, but there's a lot of clinical know-how to making it work well. A variety of books provide more detailed practice guidelines for counselors (McCrady & Epstein, 2008; O'Farrell & Fals-Stewart, 2006) and for couples themselves (Gottman, Gottman, & Declaire, 2007; Gottman & Silver, 2015).

Another way to strengthen positivity of relationship is to share pleasurable activities. It is common for distressed couples to stop doing enjoyable things together. As one partner spends more time acquiring, using, and recovering from drugs, the couple spends less time together and becomes more distant from each other. The nonusing person may understandably begin avoiding social events with the partner for fear of embarrassing consequences. This can lead to parallel lives, a sign that the partners are withdrawing from their relationship. Reversing this negative drift requires increasing positive couple or family activities that do not involve alcohol/drug use. Couples who share more positive activities have better recovery rates after treatment (Moos, Finney, & Cronkite, 1990).

So how can you help to reunite a couple? Help them plan and share in activities that they enjoy together each week. This begins by having them identify activities they would like to do. If the couple is having trouble thinking of some activities they may enjoy, it may be helpful to provide them with a menu of local recreational activities. Remember that offering your own solutions for clients will often be met with "Yes, but . . ." reasons why that activity won't work. Instead, start with an open question of "What things might you enjoy doing together?" or have them brainstorm activities at home and bring the list to the next session to discuss. A goal is for the couple to have some enjoyable time alone together, while also having some quality time with their family and friends.

Strengthening Communication Skills

A third common goal in working with couples, beyond supporting sobriety and increasing relationship positivity, is to strengthen communication skills (McCrady & Epstein, 2008, 2009). Couples with a painful history of addiction often become angry and defensive with each other, with communications dominated by hostility and withdrawal. Strengthening communication skills involves both improving positivity and clarity of expression as well as fostering good listening skills. The speaker and the listener have important complementary roles. The speaker should clearly state what he or she wants, thinks, and feels. The listener should seek to understand the message without jumping to conclusions.

Effective listening helps each person feel understood, and prevents quick escalation of negative exchanges by slowing down the conversation and making sure that the message received by the listener is what the speaker intended (Miller, 2018; O'Farrell & Fals-Stewart, 2006). Good listening includes restating in one's own words the message that was heard, and seeking clarification by asking open questions (see Chapters 4 and 10). The first step is to *understand* what the partner is saying before responding. Also helpful are small acknowledging responses (e.g., "I know that bothers you") without jumping immediately to disagreement or refutation. This enhances the partner's feelings of being understood and valued (Gottman, 1994).

On the expressive side, the use of "I" messages is a common tool. Starting a statement with "I" focuses on one's own feelings, without blaming the other person (as is more likely to happen when the statement begins with "You"). One helpful formula originally suggested by Thomas Gordon (1970) is "I feel _____ (emotion) when you _____ (behavior) because _____ (specific reason)." The speaker takes responsibility for his or her own feelings and reactions (rather than saying, "You make me feel . . . "), and the specifics leave more room for problem solving instead of blaming.

During sessions it is important to practice, not just discuss, communication skills such as active listening and "I" messages. A good place to start when practicing listening and expressing skills is to discuss a neutral or positive topic. Don't start with the most contentious issues! The usual cycle is to first demonstrate the skill to be learned, then have the couple practice in session, and then assign a similar activity for home practice. Plan home assignments in such a way that they minimize the risk of negative escalation.

Managing Changes, Conflicts, and Problems

A fourth common goal in BCT is to manage and reduce negative interactions. Although increasing communication skills and shared positive activities usually will reduce negativity, it can also be useful to develop specific skills for requesting changes, resolving conflicts, and solving problems in the relationship.

REQUESTING CHANGES

Generalized, global, personal "You" messages (such as "You're lazy," or "You never care") tend only to create negative feelings, whereas being specific is more likely to result in a concrete change. Specific complaints and requests for change can be very healthy in a relationship (Gottman, 1994; Gottman & Silver, 2015). Such requests are most constructive (and likely to result in change) when they ask for specific behavior, and are stated positively. A positive request is to do *more* of something. If the request could be accomplished by general anesthesia—by doing nothing (e.g., "Stop being so messy")—try reframing it in the positive (e.g., "Please hang up your towel instead of leaving it on the floor"). Such messages are also *requests* and open for negotiation and compromise (e.g., "Would you be willing to . . . ?).

Once a couple has tried out monitoring and changing their P's and D's and more positive communication skills are in place, each partner can practice making a specific positive request for change. The usual approach here is not a *quid pro quo* where they agree to make certain changes if and only if the partner also makes specific changes. The problem with *quid pro quo* is that the whole thing can break down quickly into disagreements about whether each person is keeping up his or her part of the deal. Rather, each partner unilaterally focuses on making a requested change that is acceptable. Again, the more specific and positive these requests are, the more likely they are to be successful.

CONFLICT RESOLUTION

Conflict happens naturally in every relationship. It emerges when people have different thoughts, beliefs, or preferences. What matters in a relationship is how such conflicts are resolved. The skills here involve active negotiation, rather than trying to end conflict through avoidance or dominance. Again, effective communication skills provide a good foundation. It can be helpful for a couple to set a specific appointment and an amount of time (perhaps 20 minutes) to discuss a particular conflict. Have the couple practice the conflict first in your presence, with your feedback and coaching. The skills discussed above—such as making specific requests, using "I" messages, and active listening—are applicable here. Setting a specific amount of time averts the concern that the discussion will go on endlessly or escalate. It can also be useful to allow time-outs if certain signs of escalation emerge. Let them succeed with such a negotiation in your presence before you make it a home assignment.

PROBLEM SOLVING

Some problems may not involve heated conflicts or desires for change, but can still cause a lot of stress when they remain unresolved (e.g., financial problems, extended family problems, legal problems). If partners disagree on desirable solutions or don't know what to do, they may avoid dealing with a problem, and so it drags on. Such unresolved problems can build up in a relationship. Here it can be useful to teach some generic problem-solving skills. The usual steps are:

1. To describe specifically the problem and desired outcome(s).
2. To brainstorm—generate as many different possible solutions as possible, without rejecting or criticizing any of them.

3. To discuss and compare the various options. What would be the likely outcomes of each possible solution?
4. To agree on a solution or at least one next step.
5. To try out the chosen solution.
6. To evaluate how the chosen solution is going and make adjustments as needed.

A Continuing Recovery Plan

Of course, your sessions don't go on forever. Plan in advance when and how to begin stepping back to let the couple proceed on their own using their skills. You might begin scheduling sessions farther apart. Discuss termination in advance and invite the couple to discuss remaining concerns and their plans to continue strengthening their relationship. What will each partner do specifically to support sobriety and a strong relationship? You can discuss possible high-risk situations for returning to use, and an action plan to prevent that from happening (see Chapter 21). Leave the door open for them to call back or return, and consider scheduling a follow-up appointment to check on progress.

Family–Involved Treatment for Adolescents

Involving family members in treatment is perhaps even more important for adolescents than for adult clients. Involving the parents or caregivers yields substantially better outcomes than treating an adolescent individually (Kaminer, 2001; Rowe, 2012). The family of the adolescent can either significantly help or hinder the adolescent's engagement in treatment, and family factors such as home environment, family substance use, housing issues, and co-occurring disorders can have a profound impact on an adolescent's recovery from addiction (Henggeler, Melton, Brondino, & Scherer, 1997; Lawrence & Sovik-Johnston, 2010; Stormshak et al., 2011). Family-involved approaches also tend to have more enduring treatment effects with adolescents (Liddle, Dakof, Turner, Henderson, & Greenbaum, 2008).

Several effective family-based therapies have been developed, and represent the most thoroughly researched treatment methods for adolescent substance use (Baldwin, Christian, Berkeljon, & Shadish, 2012; Rowe, 2012). These include multisystemic therapy (MST; Van der Stouwe & Asscher, 2014), the adolescent community reinforcement approach (A-CRA; Godley, Hunter, et al., 2014; Godley, Smith, et al., 2014), brief strategic family therapy (BSFT; Robbins, Szapocznik, & Horigian, 2009; Szapocznik, Schwartz, Muir, & Brown, 2012; Szapocznik & Williams, 2000); multidimensional family therapy (MDFT; Liddle, 2016), and functional family therapy (FFT; Alexander, Waldron, Robbins, & Neeb, 2013; Slesnick &

Prestopnik, 2009; Waldron & Turner, 2008), all of which show encouraging efficacy with adolescents.

Though they have different names, these approaches have many similarities, and one common thread is a cognitive-behavioral family therapy approach (Kaminer, 2001). Another commonality is the integration of other services and addressing the multiple risk factors in the adolescent's life. In addition to reducing substance use, these approaches have also reduced long-term rates of rearrest and out-of-home placement for violent and chronic juvenile offenders (Henggeler, Schoenwald, Letourneau, & Edwards, 2002), reduced behavioral problems, increased involvement of more difficult families (Santisteban et al., 2003; Szapocznik, Hervis, & Schwartz, 2003), engaged runaway youth (Slesnick & Prestopnik, 2009; Slesnick et al., 2007), and increased positive peer relations and improved relationship and communication between parent and adolescent (Liddle, Rowe, Dakof, Henderson, & Greenbaum, 2009). The impact of these interventions can last well into adulthood, with effects on adult criminal conduct (Datchi & Sexton, 2013; Sawyer & Borduin, 2011). These approaches also seem to work well across cultures, particularly in those that emphasize family relationships (Santisteban et al., 2003). We highlight here three integrated family-based treatment models with good support for efficacy. A fourth, CRA, was described in Chapter 14, and has also been successful with adolescents.

> Family-involved approaches have more enduring treatment effects with adolescents.

Multisystemic Therapy

MST is a family- and community-based treatment approach originally developed to address the full spectrum of mental health needs of adolescents involved in the juvenile justice system, with the goal of reducing out-of-home placements and incarcerations. MST is a time-limited (typically 4–6 months), very intensive therapeutic program. It is unique in that MST therapists are full-time providers with small caseloads of approximately three families and are available to those families 24 hours a day, 7 days per week. To increase the family's access to treatment, services are provided in the family's home, in a treatment agency, or wherever the family feels most comfortable. This flexible arrangement allows the provider to have multiple contacts with the family during the week, sometimes even meeting daily.

A key feature of MST is its capacity to address multiple challenges facing children with mental health problems and their families. MST interventions are focused on the present and are behaviorally oriented, targeting specific and well-defined problems such as reducing criminal activity, delinquency, risky sexual behavior, and drug use. Although substance use has always been one of the behaviors addressed, MST has more recently been adapted to include A-CRA with COM so that providers are better able to treat adolescent substance use (M. D. Godley et al., 2014; S. H. Godley, Smith, et al., 2014). Urine screens, functional analyses to identify triggers and consequences of drug use, and skills training in drug refusal skills are integrated in this approach as a way to better target substance use.

In addition to addressing risk factors including substance use, MST focuses on developing protective factors to maintain therapeutic change, such as enhancing the adolescent's educational and vocational skills and developing pro-social peer relationships. By decreasing risk factors and increasing protective factors, interventions provide safety for the family, prevent violence, offer the family easier access to needed services, and increase the likelihood that the family will stay in treatment. The parental skills training also offers parents or caregivers the capacity to manage future difficulties and maintain change. MST has particularly received attention for its success in reducing long-term rates of rearrest and out-of-home placement for violent and chronic juvenile offenders (Henggeler, Schoenwald, Rowland, & Cunningham, 2002). Training and practice of MST are carefully regulated for quality control.

Brief Strategic Family Therapy

BSFT (Horigan, Anderson, & Szapocznik, 2016; Szapocznik, Muir, Duff, Schwartz, & Brown, 2015; Szapocznik et al., 2012) is a manualized brief intervention (8–24 sessions) to treat co-occurring adolescent behavioral problems such as aggressive and oppositional behavior, associating with antisocial peers, and drug use. It has been found to promote better engagement and retention in treatment, improve parent reports of family functioning, and reduce substance use in both parents and adolescents (Horigan et al., 2015; Robbins et al., 2011). BSFT is problem-focused and emphasizes modifying maladaptive patterns of family interactions and ineffective communication patterns that are presumed to be related to the adolescent's symptoms. For instance, if an adolescent's parents are fighting, the adolescent may act out so that the parents turn their attention toward the adolescent rather than continuing to fight with each other. In addition to these maladaptive interactions within the family, the communication between family members may also become ineffective and full of anger and animosity.

The BSFT counselor attempts to develop alliances with each family member and with the family as a whole, to understand family strengths and problem relationships that affect the adolescent's behavior or the ability of parental figures to correct the behavior, implement effective communication strategies to reduce negative family communication, and develop behavioral strategies to correct problematic family relations. Specific change strategies (such as building conflict resolution skills and providing parenting guidance and coaching) are implemented, and effective family behaviors and communication are reinforced through the use of home assignments to practice new behaviors.

Multidimensional Family Therapy

MDFT (Liddle, 2016) is an outpatient family-based treatment for adolescents with SUDs. The underlying assumption of MDFT is that adolescent drug use results from a network of developmental and environmental influences within the individual, the family, the community, and peers. The multidimensional approach therefore targets multiple pathways as a way to reduce substance use and increase pro-social behaviors. MDFT includes both individual and family sessions. Sessions can be held in the clinic, home, school, or by phone with the format and components modified to suit the individual needs of the adolescent.

Similar to the other family approaches that we have discussed, targeted outcomes of MDFT include reducing the impact of negative risk factors as well as promoting protective processes in as many areas of the adolescent's life as possible. During individual sessions, the therapist and the adolescent work on important developmental tasks such as decision-making skills, ways to more effectively communicate thoughts or feelings, and problem-solving skills to better deal with life stressors. Objectives for the adolescent include shifting from a drug-using to a drug-free lifestyle, improved functioning in developmental domains such as positive peer relations, healthy identity formation, bonding with school, and autonomy within the parent–adolescent relationship. Parallel to the adolescent's individual therapy, the MDFT therapist also works with the parents, who are taught how to be more effective in their parenting and to differentiate between controlling and influencing their child. Objectives for parental change include improved relationship and communication between parent and adolescent and increased knowledge about parenting practices such as limit setting.

KEY POINTS

🔖 Outcomes can be significantly improved by including an SO in treatment.

🔖 There is no scientific evidence that family members of people with addiction have unique or greater personal pathology relative to the general population, though of course they do often suffer distress and adverse consequences.

🔖 BCT focuses on skills for supporting sobriety, communication, resolving conflicts, and building a more positive relationship.

🔖 Parental or caregiver involvement is particularly important in treating substance use problems of adolescents.

🔖 Effective family-involved methods include MST, BSFT, MDFT, as well as the CRA.

Reflection Questions

Q Various views are discussed in this chapter regarding how families are involved in addiction. Which one(s) of these best reflect(s) your own current understanding?

Q How comfortable are you with including SOs when treating addiction? What are the biggest obstacles to your doing so?

Q What experience, if any, have you had with addiction in your own family, and how do you think this may influence your own work with individuals and families?

CHAPTER 17

Mutual Help Groups

Few areas of health are so richly supplied with peer support networks as the world of recovery from addiction. For three centuries—beginning with American Indian recovery circles in the mid-1700s—individuals recovering from SUDs have provided peer-based recovery to support one another and help those who are still suffering. Alcoholics Anonymous (AA) alone is arguably the world's largest mutual help network for any health topic, with over two million members and 115,000 regular meetings worldwide, half of them within the United States (Alcoholics Anonymous World Services, 2015). In North America, AA is the most commonly sought source of help for alcohol use disorders (Hedden et al., 2015). These networks, with which anyone treating addictions should be familiar, offer important resources to support recovery.

The term "mutual help" describes these networks because they consist exclusively or primarily of people who are themselves in or seeking recovery, and they exist for the sole purpose of helping those with addictions. "Mutual help" is more accurate than "self-help" because of the importance of reciprocal support in these networks, rather than trying to go it alone. Furthermore, within the 12-step fellowships, strong emphasis is placed on seeking help from outside oneself, as discussed below and in Chapter 23.

Mutual help groups are not "treatment" or "therapy" per se. They fall outside the context of people seeking help from expert professionals. Rather they represent either an *alternative* or an *adjunct* to formal addiction treatment. Many people do seek support from mutual help networks without ever entering formal treatment. It is furthermore the case that within the United States, a majority of those in treatment are likely to have been at least exposed to one or more mutual help groups. In many areas, mutual help groups are available every day free of charge, with growing presence on the Internet. This alone warrants knowing about mutual help resources for those you serve.

Recognizing that addiction can be a chronic condition with a lengthy course of recovery (see Chapter 2), mutual help groups offer an important source of continuing care for lasting change. Unlike most professional treatment, people can attend mutual help groups as long as they would like, during evenings and weekends or other high-risk times without the constraints of insurance coverage approval or sharing identifying information. Such services help people develop internal and social resources to maintain recovery, building what has been termed "recovery capital" (Kelly & Hoeppner, 2015).

Strong preconceptions about mutual help groups are common. Some have described AA in superlative terms, for example, as "medicine's crowning glory" (Martin, 1980) and "the only continuing and successful group dealing with alcoholism. . . . In comparison with other therapies, its success rate is nearly miraculous" (Madsen, 1974, pp. 156, 195). Others have viewed mutual help groups skeptically if not cynically, believing them to be ineffective or even harmful. In our view, neither extreme view is warranted. The large scientific literature on mutual help groups, particularly AA, described later in this chapter provides ample reason for professionals to be interested in and knowledgeable about these groups as an important resource for promoting and supporting recovery.

> Mutual help groups represent either an alternative or an adjunct to formal addiction treatment.

The Spectrum of Mutual Help Organizations

There is a wide array of mutual help groups covering a range of addictive behaviors including alcohol and other drug use, gambling, overeating, and compulsive sexual behavior. They also vary widely in conceptions of the causes of and remedies for addiction. What all of these varied groups share is the central idea of afflicted people helping each other to recover.

One way to conceptualize these groups is according to certain dimensions along which they differ (Humphreys, 1993; Nowinski, 1999). Here are a few:

• One obvious distinction is the addictive behavior on which they focus. Some are designed primarily or exclusively for people with a particular form of addiction such as gambling, alcohol problems, or cocaine use disorders. Others span a range of addictions.

• Mutual help groups differ in the extent to which they use trained or certified leaders to convey program content. Self-Management and

Recovery Training (SMART), for example, uses trained unpaid facilitators, and Women for Sobriety (WFS) relies on certified volunteer moderators. Twelve-step program groups elect a chairperson for a specified period of time and strictly prohibit the use of professional or paid leaders.

• Most groups are for people with addiction themselves. Others, such as Al-Anon, Alateen, and SMART Recovery Family and Friends, are for family members and significant others affected by a loved one's addiction.

• Mutual help groups vary in the extent to which they rely on spiritual beliefs and practices as useful in overcoming addictions. Twelve-step programs are explicitly spiritual in nature, whereas other programs, such as Secular Organizations for Sobriety (SOS), were developed specifically for people who are uncomfortable with or skeptical about spiritual approaches.

• Groups also differ in the extent to which they promote long-term connection among members. SMART meetings, for instance, are not intended to be long-term support groups and are more like classes. Participants are not expected to continue in them once the core curriculum has been covered. In contrast, 12-step programs encourage lifelong membership, sometimes with the belief that members who are not attending regularly are placing their recovery at risk.

• Mutual help groups vary in their emphasis on ego deflation versus self-enhancement. The 12-step programs value humility, surrendering self-control, accepting one's powerlessness, and admitting and addressing character flaws. Other groups, such as WFS, emphasize empowerment, self-confidence, and personal competence. There is an interesting theological parallel here. Traditional Protestant religions in which the 12-step programs were rooted often emphasize sin, confession, repentance, humility, and salvation through grace rather than through one's own merit. Feminist theology has explored whether this emphasis on ego deflation is more appropriate for males, whereas women, who have historically been more powerless and self-denying, may be more in need of empowerment (Donovan, Ingalsbe, Benbow, & Daley, 2013; Ruether, 1998).

• Finally, mutual help groups differ in their emphasis on abstinence. Most such groups, including all 12-step groups, regard total and lifelong abstinence as the only acceptable goal for change. Drinkwatchers and Moderation Management (MM) were developed for people wanting to reduce their alcohol use, with abstinence as one valid choice.

12-Step Groups

By far, the largest and most popular mutual help groups for addictions are those based on the 12 steps of AA (*www.aa.org*). Within the United States, nearly one in every 10 people attends an AA meeting during the course of their lifetime (Room & Greenfield, 1993). By the time Americans with alcohol problems enter professional treatment, a majority have already attended AA meetings (Tonigan et al., 1996). Beyond AA itself, there are dozens of other mutual help groups patterned after AA and based on the 12 steps, such as Narcotics Anonymous, Cocaine Anonymous, Gamblers Anonymous, and Sex Addicts Anonymous.

In understanding 12-step groups, a distinction must be made between the 12-step *program* and *fellowship*. The program encompasses the written beliefs and practices of the organization, usually referred to as the 12 steps and the 12 traditions. The 12 steps (see Chapter 23) are meant to be worked on sequentially and involve spiritual processes such as asking God for help, practicing prayer and meditation, making amends, and performing service to others. The 12-step program explicitly involves inviting and relying on a spiritual higher power to provide the strength and wisdom needed to sustain sobriety. Although the understanding of God or a higher power is left to the individual and is intentionally flexible so as to avoid unnecessarily alienating potential members, it is clear that the founders of AA intended a personal relationship with a transcendent presence (Kurtz, 1991). The 12-step program is meant to be practiced not only in regard to addiction, but "in all our affairs" as a more general approach for living.

In addition to the formal program just described, 12-step organizations also offer a more informal fellowship, which can be described as the pattern of interactions among members that includes sharing joys and hardships, helping out when others are in need, and enjoying social events together. Members are encouraged to have a sponsor, a mentor who has longer experience with sobriety and the program, to help them in progressing through the steps and to provide encouragement and support, particularly at times of risk for return to substance use. People at meetings often exchange phone numbers and other contact information to extend mutual support beyond the meetings themselves. Some have described the guidelines for recovery as a 12-step "six pack": (1) don't drink or use drugs, (2) go to meetings, (3) get a sponsor, (4) ask for help, (5) join a group, and (6) get active.

In addition to meetings, AA and other 12-step programs operate 24-hour telephone coverage through local service centers in many areas. In larger cities, meetings are typically available 7 days a week, morning, afternoon, and evening, and are always free of charge. Members traveling to other cities, states, or nations can usually find a 12-step meeting nearby where they are warmly welcomed. Increasingly, meetings are offered in virtual environments: via phone, text, discussion forum, or web-based audio and video to enhance accessibility. A list of these online meetings can be found at *www.aa-intergroup.org.*

Twelve-step meetings typically last about 60 to 90 minutes and may be either open or closed. Open meetings can be attended by anyone, but closed meetings are restricted to members—that is, anyone with a desire to stop their own addictive behavior. The format of the meeting may be one in which the formal program is reviewed (step meeting), might be devoted to hearing the experiences of one person's struggle with an addiction (speaker meeting), or could involve discussion of particular problems likely to be encountered in recovering from addictions (discussion meeting). Finally, some 12-step groups are geared toward particular demographic groups such as women, adolescents, gays and lesbians, medical professionals, atheists and agnostics.

Some Common Myths about 12-Step Groups

There are some common misconceptions about AA and other 12-step groups that warrant consideration here. The ways in which the 12-step program is practiced certainly vary across groups and individual members. This sometimes gives rise to anecdotes that can be incorrectly generalized to stereotypes about the 12-step program or fellowship. Here are some such myths.

1. *AA believes only in a traditional disease model and discourages people from receiving any other kind of treatment. This position will contradict what I am doing in treatment and confuse my clients.* In fact, AA has no official position with regard to the etiology of alcohol problems, and by policy it does not get involved in controversies. Twelve-step literature describes a broad range of possible factors contributing to addiction including biological, psychological, social, and spiritual factors. Occasional points of philosophical disagreement in AA meetings can be addressed by urging clients to learn all they can with an open mind and choose what helps them, consistent with the AA advice to "take what you need and leave the rest." In a 10-year follow-up of Project MATCH, clients who were most likely to be attending 12-step meetings were not those who had received 12-step facilitation, but rather those in cognitive-behavioral and motivational enhancement conditions (Pagano, White, Kelly, Stout, & Tonigan, 2013). Whatever advice we or others may give to people, they actively pursue what seems useful to them.

2. *People are pressured to discontinue their medications if they attend 12-step meetings.* Although injunctions against psychoactive medications are sometimes expressed by individual members in 12-step meetings (Rychtarik, Connors, Dermen, & Stasiewicz, 2000), such a prohibition is not supported by the core 12-step literature. Tonigan et al. (2003) found that despite what they might hear in meetings, 12-step attendees as a whole were *less* likely to reject medications for emotional problems than were clients in other forms of treatment. Thus, attending 12-step meetings is not incompatible with taking prescribed medications, nor is there evidence that

attendance has any detrimental effect on clients' attitudes toward doing so (Tonigan & Kelly, 2004).

3. *The 12-step program only works for religious clients. It won't help nonreligious people, even if they can be persuaded to attend.* Actually, people's religious beliefs do not predict whether they will benefit from 12-step programs (Connors, Tonigan, & Miller, 2001). In a study with long-time members in Narcotics Anonymous, only 29.6% of participants described themselves as religious (Galanter, Dermatis, Post, & Santucci, 2013). The "Big Book" of AA directly addresses atheists (Alcoholics Anonymous World Services, 2001), and although agnostics and atheists are less inclined to attend AA, they are no less likely to benefit when they do (Tonigan, Miller, & Schermer, 2002). Clients who benefit from 12-step programs do tend to show changes in their spiritual beliefs and practices over time (Robinson, Cranford, Webb, & Brower, 2007; Robinson, Krentzman, Webb, & Brower, 2011).

4. *Clients who participate in 12-step programs are told that only someone who is in recovery can be an effective therapist for them.* Again, individual members may offer this opinion, but official AA literature does not support this view. The perspectives of other recovering people are among the benefits of attending 12-step meetings, but many studies confirm that personal recovery status makes one neither more nor less effective as a therapist, even when delivering 12-step facilitation therapy (Project MATCH Research Group, 1998d).

5. *Pressuring my clients to go to 12-step meetings can't hurt, even if they don't want to go.* Pressuring people into 12-step programs is unwise, particularly if clients express strong resistance or philosophical objection (Humphreys, 1993; Peteet, 1993; Tonigan et al., 2002). Coercing clients to attend 12-step meetings despite objections to religious content may even violate codes of professional ethics. AA has always been meant to be a voluntary association, and the few clinical trials studying coerced AA attendance have shown no differential benefit (Brandsma, Maultsby, & Welsh, 1980; Ditman, Crawford, Forgy, Moskowitz, & MacAndrew, 1967; Walsh et al., 1991). We concur with Glaser's (1993) admonition to clinicians treating alcohol use disorders that clients should be encouraged to try AA but no one should be required to do so. As discussed later in this chapter, various other organizations are available, and it is also the case that mutual help groups are not for everyone.

6. *There is no scientific evidence that AA helps people.* To the contrary, there is an abundant research literature on AA that generally shows a positive association between attendance and better outcomes (Donovan et al., 2013). Less is known scientifically about other 12-step programs besides AA. We turn now to a brief consideration of this research.

BOX 17.1. Personal Reflection: Learning about AA

In the 1970s when I entered the field of addiction treatment, there was a polemical battle raging. In one corner were the "traditionalists" who generally endorsed a disease model of the etiology of alcoholism, regarded lifelong abstinence as the only acceptable treatment goal, and lauded AA as the golden road to recovery. In the opposite corner were the "revisionists" who typically regarded drinking as behavior subject to the same rules of learning as any other response, touted "controlled drinking" as a treatment goal option, and demeaned AA as outdated, unscientific mumbo-jumbo (Maltzman, 2008). We seldom met in the same venue. Each camp had its own professional meetings at which to despise and denounce the other. I was professionally born and raised in the behavioral camp and dismissed AA without investigation. One traditionalist averred in print that concerned colleagues ought to do "an intervention" to shake people like me out of our denial.

It didn't happen, but over time I did have the good fortune to meet and work with bright and compassionate colleagues who introduced me to the world of Bill W. I am grateful to my friend Ernie Kurtz for his patient conversations with me. When we collaborated to publish an article about AA (Miller & Kurtz, 1994), *both* of us had colleagues asking us incredulously, "What on earth are you doing working with *him*?" I went to AA meetings, felt the heart in them, and began reading in earnest not only the AA literature but also the voluminous research about AA. With Barbara McCrady I organized a scientific conference on AA research (McCrady & Miller, 1993), and we visited the home office of AA in New York together. For two decades I also had the privilege of collaborating with my friend and colleague Dr. Scott Tonigan to do and foster AA research.

Bill W. (W. W., 1949) welcomed collaboration with clinical professionals and encouraged AA members to participate in research (Alcoholics Anonymous General Service Office, 2002). The more I read his gentle writings about how to work with others, the more it sounds to me like motivational interviewing, and so different from the in-your-face confrontational methods that have sometimes been practiced and promulgated in the name of "12-step" treatment. I will never have an insider's understanding of alcoholism or AA, but I have come to a heartfelt appreciation of the breadth and depth of AA, and its untiring ministry to those who continue to suffer. In this sense, I became a friend of Bill W.

—W. R. M.

Research on 12-Step Groups

Many studies have examined the relationship between sobriety and 12-step group attendance. These studies are necessarily correlational, evaluating the extent to which these two factors—attendance and outcome—covary, without establishing whether one causes the other. The usual finding across this body of research is a modest inverse relationship: attending more 12-step meetings is associated with lower levels of addictive behavior in the same or subsequent periods of time. The largest number of studies pertains to AA and drinking outcomes. Across several decades of research, in both older (Emrick, Tonigan, Montgomery, & Little, 1993) and more recent studies, very frequent AA attendance predicts higher rates of abstinence in the first year (Fortney, Booth, Zhang, Humphrey, & Wiseman, 1998; Johnson & Herringer, 1993; Tonigan, 2001), 3 years after treatment (Chi, Kaskutas, Sterling, Campbell, & Weisner, 2009; Kelly, Stout, Zywiak, & Schneider, 2006), and 5 years or longer after treatment (Gossop, Stewart, & Marsden, 2007; Moos & Moos, 2006; Pagano et al., 2013).

Over the past 30 years, 12-step research has advanced a step farther from correlational studies to analyses within prospective controlled trials. These longitudinal studies have found that AA attendance predicts subsequent abstinence, whereas abstinence does not predict subsequent AA attendance (Magura, Cleland, & Tonigan, 2013; McCrady, Epstein, & Kahler, 2004; McKellar, Stewart, & Humphreys, 2003). This sequence is consistent with a positive prospective influence of AA participation on treatment outcome. AA attendance also predicts long-term sobriety apart from treatment (Moos & Moos, 2005; Timko, Moos, Finney, & Lesar, 2000). There is converging evidence that this is not simply self-selection biases, but rather that AA has a direct impact on subsequent abstinence (Humphreys, Blodgett, & Wagner, 2014).

From AA's perspective, people recover from alcohol use disorders through a spiritual awakening resulting from a combination of working the steps, having a sponsor, and believing in a higher power. Participation in AA does produce changes in spirituality, which in turn accounts for some of the impact of AA on outcome (Kelly, Stout, Magill, Tonigan, & Pagano, 2011). Yet there are other theories that also explain how AA works, and research efforts are examining the mechanisms through with AA helps people recover. Recent findings indicate that much of AA benefit is explained by factors that are similar to the mechanisms operating in formal treatment, including enhancing coping skills to better tolerate sources of distress and tension, building and maintaining motivation, and increasing self-efficacy (Blonigen, Timko, Finney, Moos, & Moos, 2011; Kelly, 2017; Kelly, Hoeppner, Stout, & Pagano, 2012; Kelly, Stout, Magill, Tonigan, & Pagano, 2010). Further, AA promotes changes in social networks by helping people gain ties with nondrinking individuals and enhancing social networks that are supportive of abstinence (Kelly et al., 2012; Longabaugh et al., 1998).

Clients who do receive formal treatment tend to have better outcomes when they also attend AA (Dawson et al., 2006; McCrady et al., 2004; Timko et al., 2000). Taken together, there is ample reason to encourage people in treatment for alcohol use disorders to also try AA. Studies are fewer regarding 12-step attendance and subsequent illicit drug use or gambling, but findings are generally similar to those for alcohol (Christo &

Franey, 1995; Gossop et al., 2007; McKay, Alterman, McLellan, & Snider, 1994; Toumbourou, Hamilton, U'Ren, Stevens-Jones, & Storey, 2002; Wells et al., 2014).

It is not simply the number of meetings attended that predicts benefit from 12-step programs. Attendance is modestly correlated with other 12-step practices such as prayer and reading core literature (Morgenstern, Kahler, Frey, & Lavouvie, 1996; Toumbourou et al., 2002). A broader concept is *involvement* in the 12-step program and fellowship. An analysis of multiple studies of AA found that reaching out to others for help, having a sponsor, and working through the first four steps of AA were significant positive predictors of benefit (Tonigan & Rice, 2010; Witbrodt, Kaskutas, Bond, & Delucchi, 2012). Studies have found that AA attendance per se did not predict posttreatment abstinence, whereas AA involvement did (Majer, Jason, Ferrari, & Miller, 2011; Montgomery, Miller, & Tonigan, 1995).

Are there particular kinds of clients who are more likely to benefit from a 12-step group? One clear finding is that AA is especially beneficial for people whose social networks do not support abstinence (Longabaugh et al., 1998; Toumbourou et al., 2002). In essence, it provides clients with an instant social support network that is rooting for their sobriety.

In sum, there is good reason to encourage clients with SUDs, whether religious or not, to sample 12-step meetings. As stated earlier, we believe that no one should be required or coerced to attend, but there is good reason to expect that such mutual help groups may improve clients' chances for stable sobriety.

> Reaching out to others for help, having a sponsor, and working through the first four steps of AA are predictors of benefit.

Facilitating Mutual Help Group Attendance

It makes a difference whether and how you encourage clients to sample mutual help groups. Here are a few things to keep in mind in this regard.

1. If not already involved in one, people are most likely to try out mutual help groups while they are still in treatment. Said another way, if you don't encourage clients to sample mutual help groups while they are in treatment, they are unlikely to do so afterward (Tonigan et al., 2003). The period of active treatment is a window of opportunity to encourage mutual help involvement.

2. Mutual help groups vary widely, so that it makes sense to sample several rather than just one. Even within AA, there are large differences in the social environment from one group to another (Montgomery et al., 1993; Moos, Finney, & Maude-Griffin, 1993; Tonigan, Ashcroft, &

Miller, 1995). You can't know what AA is like just by going to one meeting, any more than you know what churches are like by attending one service, or colleges by attending one class. There is a natural process over time of finding a "home group," the place where one feels most welcome, supported, and at home.

3. Similarly, don't just try once to encourage mutual help involvement and then give up. One practical guideline is a "three strikes" approach, in which clients who initially decline a referral to a mutual help group are asked if they would be willing to revisit the issue further along in treatment (Miller, 2004). As the name implies, the counselor is advised to try three times to refer to a mutual help group. This should be done, of course, in a way that does not engender discord (see Chapter 4).

4. If you want people to try out a mutual help group, do more than just provide information. One of the largest treatment effects ever reported in the alcohol literature involved procedures for encouraging clients to attend AA (Sisson & Mallams, 1981). Half of the male clients in this study (randomly assigned) were advised to attend AA and given a list of the local meeting places and times. The other half were given the following systematic encouragement procedure. The counselor had prearranged help from volunteers who were themselves AA members. While the client was still in

> If you don't encourage clients to sample mutual help groups while they are in treatment, they are unlikely to do so afterward.

the office, the counselor (with the client's permission) telephoned one of these volunteers and then gave the phone to the client. The volunteer introduced himself, offered to accompany the client to a first meeting and provide transportation, and arranged a meeting time. In the advice group, no one attended an AA meeting; in the systematic encouragement group, everyone got to a first meeting—no statistical analysis needed!

What should you tell people to expect when attending 12-step meetings? First and foremost, explain that people often do benefit from attending, even if they don't agree with every aspect of the program. For example, as mentioned earlier, atheists and agnostics who go to AA show just as much benefit as theists do. Explain the strong emphasis in AA on personal choice, to "take what works and leave the rest," and that the only requirement for membership is a sincere desire to abstain. The program does not encourage hostile confrontation or "cross-talk" (uninvited advice or arguments), and participants are not required to speak or to disclose personal information.

Even for those who try AA, many do not stay with it in the long run. In the Project MATCH study, for example, 95% of those in 12-step facilitation did attend AA during treatment, but 41% of these were no longer doing so at 9 months (Tonigan et al., 2003). Very similar findings were reported in another study with 2,778 men treated in 12-step-oriented programs (Kelly & Moos, 2003), of whom 91% attended at least one meeting. Of these attenders, 40% were no longer attending after 1 year. Longitudinal research, however, shows that dropping out of AA (not regularly attending) is not the same as disaffiliation. Some prior AA attenders still describe themselves as AA members and report that they continue to live the 12-step program (Tonigan, 2003). This suggests that some people internalize the 12-step program and continue to practice it, even though not regularly attending meetings.

Clients with concomitant addiction and major mental disorders offer a special challenge (see Chapter 20). For some clients with psychological problems, groups may feel intimidating or rejecting. In many areas there are mutual help or professionally facilitated support groups especially for people with dual diagnoses (e.g., "double-trouble" 12-step groups). Refer to such groups with cautious optimism, and of course use your clinical judgment.

> People often benefit from attending AA meetings, even if they don't agree with every aspect of the program.

12-Step Treatments

What you do during treatment makes a difference in whether people will attend and affiliate with a mutual help group. Some professionals and programs describe themselves as 12-step-oriented, which can have a variety of meanings. Many encourage clients to become involved in the fellowship and practice the 12-step program. The design for Project MATCH included developing and formally testing a 12-session outpatient 12-step facilitation (TSF) therapy to parallel what was then the most commonly reported American program philosophy. TSF is delivered by a professional counselor and is designed to help clients find, attend, and become comfortable and involved in AA meetings. It reviews core 12-step beliefs and literature, discusses etiquette for meetings, helps clients know what to expect in AA, and encourages them to sample a variety of meetings. The therapist's primary goal is to help the client become engaged and involved in AA as a long-term recovery program (Nowinski & Baker, 1998; Nowinski et al., 1992).

It is fair to say that none of the nine principal investigators in Project MATCH was an ardent promoter of TSF. All had previously worked with behavior therapies. The study was very carefully executed, and all three treatments were delivered by therapists who were trained and believed in the approach that they were delivering. TSF was designed and supervised by professionals who were highly knowledgeable and enthusiastic about a 12-step approach. A total of 1,726 clients were randomly assigned to receive TSF, cognitive-behavioral, or motivational enhancement therapy.

As discussed in Chapter 7, all three treatments yielded excellent and similar results, with no significant differences between them on the two primary outcome measures (Babor & Del Boca, 2003; Project MATCH Research Group, 1997a, 1998a). On an outcome measure of most interest to AA, however—the percentage of clients who remained totally abstinent—the 12-step treatment maintained a significant advantage of about 10 percentage points throughout the course of follow-up. Thus, this methodologically strong clinical trial indicates that TSF was at least as effective as two state-of-the-art treatments with which it was compared. A national collaborative trial of treatments for cocaine dependence similarly found that a combination of individual and group drug counseling based on a 12-step approach was significantly more effective than either cognitive or psychodynamic psychotherapy in combination with the same group counseling (Crits-Christoph et al., 1999).

Further evidence emerged from a large naturalistic study examining outcomes for 3,698 men treated for alcohol problems at 15 U.S. Department of Veterans Affairs hospitals (Ouimette, Finney, & Moos, 1997). The programs in which they had been treated were classified as 12-step, cognitive-behavioral, or mixed (both) in orientation (five of each type). As in Project MATCH, overall outcomes were very good, with significant improvement on all 11 measures. At 1-year follow-up, 25% of those treated in 12-step programs were abstinent, compared with 18% in cognitive-behavioral programs and 20% in mixed programs, a statistically significant difference. Those receiving 12-step treatment also showed significantly lower health care utilization in the year after discharge (Humphreys & Moos, 2001).

Similar findings were reported in a clinical trial comparing group therapies for cocaine use based on a cognitive-behavioral or a 12-step approach (Wells, Peterson, Gainey, Hawkins, & Catalano, 1994). Clients were assigned in order of admission to one group until it was filled, then the next clients were assigned to the other condition. Both groups showed substantial improvement, with no between-group differences in outcome at 6 or 12 months on cocaine, marijuana, or alcohol use. In a Ukrainian randomized trial, adding 12-step-oriented outpatient treatment to withdrawal management (vs. no additional treatment) substantially reduced posttreatment drinking (Vlasova et al., 2011).

In a trial assessing the effects of adding a 12-session TSF to treatment as usual in an outpatient dual diagnosis program, greater participation in TSF was associated with greater reduction in substance use, and greater 12-step group participation also predicted decreased frequency and intensity of drinking (Bogenschutz et al., 2014).

Treatments delivered in these TSF studies involved far more than simple referral to attend AA. Such referral without systematic encouragement in some form is unlikely to help clients attend and benefit from mutual-help groups (Sisson & Mallams, 1981).

Religious Mutual Help Groups

Because 12-step programs are described as "spiritual but not religious" and are nondenominational, avoiding dogmatic faith statements, members of religious faith communities sometimes prefer recovery programs that are specifically consistent with their own religious beliefs. Both Overcomers Outreach (OO; *www.overcomersoutreach.org*) and Alcoholics Victorious (AV; *www.alcoholicsvictorious.org*) are mutual support groups that bridge 12-step philosophy and biblical teachings. OO meetings are held in churches and may focus on many problems including use of pornography, gambling, depression, and substance use. Meetings are open, and current religious faith is not a requirement to attend, although meetings are explicitly focused on encouraging devotion to Jesus Christ as the higher power and biblical teachings as a means of overcoming addiction. AV meetings are more specifically focused on alcohol/drug problems. Similarly, the Calix Society (*www.calixsociety.org*) was founded in 1947 to provide Catholics with a faith-consistent mutual support group to augment the 12-step program. Meetings are typically facilitated by priests who assist members in using the 12 steps in a manner consonant with Catholic teachings (Nowinski, 1999). Searching the Web readily yields resources adapting the 12 steps to many other faiths including Buddhism, Judaism, Mormonism, and Islam. We are aware of no scientific studies of the effectiveness of such religiously based mutual help groups.

Secular Mutual Help Groups

In contrast, some people find 12-step programs to be *too* "religious" (e.g., Copeland, 1997). All of the organizations described next were developed in part as secular alternatives for people who for whatever reason find that a 12-step approach doesn't fit or work for them. In pooled data from the 2000, 2005, and 2010 National Alcohol Surveys (Zemore et al., 2014) 34% of those who reported resolving an alcohol problem indicated attending a mutual help group alternative to 12-step groups. In a survey comparing 12-step group members to members of mutual help alternatives, those participating in alternative groups tended to be less religious and generally higher in education and income (Zemore, Kaskutas, Mericle, & Hemberg, 2017). These groups vary widely in availability, but all maintain a website, some of which include online chat rooms. What all of them have in common, as of this writing, is extremely limited scientific evidence. In a longitudinal study comparing 12-step groups with alternatives of WFS, LifeRing, and SMART, findings indicated that these programs were as effective as 12-step groups for those with alcohol use disorders (Zemore, Lui, Mericle,

Hemberg, & Kaskutas, 2018). We describe alternative secular groups in alphabetical order.

LifeRing Secular Recovery

LifeRing Secular Recovery (*www.lifering.org*) has its roots in the SOS (described below) and is an abstinence-based network of individuals seeking to recover from alcohol or other drug use (Nicolaus, 2012). Founded in 2001, its model emphasizes social-cognitive change strategies informed by cognitive-behavioral therapy and dialectical behavior therapy. Meetings are held across the United States, Canada, the United Kingdom, Ireland, and Sweden. There is also an active Internet community with e-mail lists and online meetings.

The LifeRing approach focuses on empowering the "sober self," living in sobriety and facing the challenges of recovery, and developing a personal recovery program across nine different domains. Meetings are peer-led with participants sharing details from their week and peers offering questions, comments, and feedback. In one study, those affiliating with LifeRing (as compared to 12-step members) had lower odds of total abstinence, a difference that became nonsignificant when controlling for baseline recovery goal (Zemore et al., 2018).

Moderation Management

MM is currently[1] the only mutual help organization that targets nondependent problem drinkers with moderation as a potential goal (Kishline, 1994; Lembke & Humphreys, 2012). It was developed specifically for people who do not have lifelong abstinence as a personal goal, but who want to reduce their drinking to a problem-free level. The program begins with 30 days of abstinence, a procedure originally tested in Canada by Martha Sanchez-Craig (1980, 1996; Sanchez-Craig et al., 1996) to break habitual drinking patterns in preparation for moderation. The guidelines essentially follow behavioral methods for self-management of drinking (Hester, 2003; Hester & Delaney, 1997; Miller & Muñoz, 2013). MM provides services both in face-to-face and online formats.

The introduction of MM triggered impassioned controversy in the 1990s (Humphreys, 2003), renewing longstanding debates regarding abstinence and moderation goals (Fingarette, 1988; Heather & Robertson, 1984; Marlatt, 1983) and more recently harm reduction (Klaw, Horst, & Humphreys, 2006; Miller, 2008; Tatarsky & Marlatt, 2010). Media attention was fueled when in 2000 the founder of MM, Audrey Kishline, opted

---

[1] A prior Drinkwatchers International organization (Barrison, Ruzek, & Murray-Lyons, 1987; Winters, 1978) is apparently inactive.

for abstinence, resigned from MM, joined AA, and 2 months later drove while intoxicated, causing a tragic car crash in Washington that killed two people and resulted in her imprisonment. Pundits variously blamed either AA or MM for what Ms. Kishline acknowledged to be her personal responsibility (Kishline & Maloy, 2007).

Research to date indicates that MM does indeed tend to engage those with milder alcohol use disorders, particularly women and youth, who are disinclined to seek treatment or accept a lifelong abstinence goal (Humphreys, 2003; Humphreys & Klaw, 2001), although this pattern may be shifting over time (Kosok, 2006). This low-severity group is precisely the subpopulation who are more likely to sustain moderation than abstinence (Miller & Muñoz, 2013). In this sense, MM appears to attract a relatively underserved population most of whom have never been treated for alcohol problems, though most had previously attended AA (Humphreys & Klaw, 2001).

Very little is known about the outcomes of people who participate in MM. In one trial testing the online resources of MM alone versus in combination with a web-based protocol (*www.ModerateDrinking.com*), there was a significant overall reduction in alcohol-related problems and consumption in both groups and better outcomes on percent days abstinent in the group utilizing both resources (Hester et al., 2011). Most professionals might discourage more severely dependent drinkers from trying MM. The MM website (*www.moderation.org*) is more permissive in this regard, leaving the choice up to the individual (where, of course, it does reside), but does indicate that moderation is more feasible for people with less severe problems. Indeed, a series of studies of moderation-oriented treatment identified a level of dependence above which no one had succeeded in maintaining problem-free moderation[2] (Miller, Leckman, Delaney, & Tinkcom, 1992; Miller & Muñoz, 2013).

Those with less severe problems and dependence were most likely to establish stable moderation. Many who tried moderation and found it difficult tended ultimately to abstain and said that the experience of trying moderation had helped convince them of the wisdom of abstention (Miller et al., 1992). Alcoholics Anonymous (Alcoholics Anonymous World Services, 2001) describes failure at moderation as one way in which people realize their alcoholism, and clearly recognizes the difference from problem drinkers who are able to moderate their drinking (Humphreys, 2003; Miller & Kurtz, 1994). Interestingly, in studies of treatment with a moderation goal, abstinence outcomes were not limited to those who tried moderation and

---

[2]In these studies, moderation was defined as averaging less than three standard drinks per day, with blood alcohol peaks below .08%, with no evidence of problems or dependence symptoms related to current drinking, by consensus of two interviewers (a psychologist and a psychiatrist) who evaluated each person independently.

failed. More-dependent people who ultimately abstained often had simply found moderation not worth the white-knuckle effort that it required of them.

Secular Organizations for Sobriety

As of 2004, SOS was estimated to be the largest non-12-step mutual help group in the United States, albeit with still less than 1% of the membership of AA (Humphreys et al., 2004). SOS was founded in 1986 by James Christopher to provide a secular-humanist alternative to the spiritual focus of the 12-step program. The practice of SOS groups is similar to 12-step groups in the focus on mutual support and healthy interpersonal interactions, but the SOS program separates the concept of sobriety from spirituality. Distinctly secular-humanist, SOS encourages mutual support for members as well as the use of science-based methods for achieving abstinence. Avoiding religious terminology and practices, the objectives of SOS (Connors & Dermen, 1996) focus on peer support for abstinence and providing a safe atmosphere for individuals to share experiences related to sobriety. Information about SOS meetings and philosophy can be found at *www.sossobriety.org*

Self-Management and Recovery Training

SMART is a more recent secular nonprofit organization offering both face-to-face and online meetings to teach rational-emotive (Ellis & Velten, 1992; Trimpey, Velten, & Dain, 1993) and cognitive-behavioral coping skills, as well as a web chatroom format (*www.smartrecovery.org*). SMART-trained volunteer facilitators lead the meetings, focusing on practical coping skills for achieving and maintaining abstinence such as problem solving, refuting irrational beliefs, and responding to urges. Meetings are free of charge, although as in 12-step meetings a free-will collection may be taken. Meetings are open to the public unless specifically announced as closed meetings, and walk-ins are welcome.

SMART incorporates a range of evidence-based behavioral treatment and self-management strategies (Horvath, 2000; Horvath & Yeterian, 2012). A comparison of participants in SMART groups with AA participants found, not surprisingly, that the former were less spiritually oriented and perceived greater personal control over their alcohol use.

The historic roots of SMART lie in an organization known as Rational Recovery (RR), founded in 1986 by a social worker named Jack Trimpey. During its first decade, RR groups met with both educational and mutual help purposes. In 1999, however, Trimpey ordered the disbanding of all RR group meetings, summarily denouncing mutual help groups, spiritual approaches to recovery, and professional treatment. A court battle led to a parting of ways, with SMART breaking off from RR (which remains a for-profit organization offering books, classes, and online services) (Trimpey et al., 1993). A caution regarding RR is that, given its program philosophy (*www.rational.org*), RR participants are likely to be encouraged to shun both professional treatment and mutual help groups. This is not true of SMART, which publicly supports evidence-based treatment methods.

Evidence is sparse for the effectiveness of RR, with no controlled studies to date. A national sample of 433 people attending RR groups were surveyed before the mutual help format was disbanded, thus representing a reasonable proxy for subsequent SMART Recovery groups (Galanter, Egelko, & Edwards, 1993). A majority of those who had been in RR groups for at least 6 months reported continuous abstinence for the prior 1 month (77%) and 6 months (58%). A small pilot study assessed 20 participants in an RR group before and after the class. Significant reduction in substance use was reported, along with increased openness to acknowledging substance use problems (Schmidt, Carns, & Chandler, 2001).

In the only longitudinal study to date comparing outcomes for participants in various mutual help groups, 647 people with lifetime alcohol use disorders were surveyed online across 1 year of follow-up (Zemore et al., 2018). Relative to 12-step participants, those in SMART Recovery were generally less likely to be maintaining continuous abstinence, a statistical difference that appears to be driven by baseline outcome goals. Endorsement of a total abstinence goal, which predicted subsequent abstinence, was less common among SMART participants. Regardless of mutual help group choice, longer and more consistent group attendance was associated with longer self-reported abstinence from alcohol. In a clinical trial, 189 problem drinkers participating in SMART showed large reductions in drinking at both 3-month (Hester, et al., 2013) and 6-month follow-up (Campbell, Hester, Lenberg, & Delaney, 2016), with no additional benefit for those randomized to receive a web-based application based on SMART Recovery.

Women for Sobriety

Much has been written about the special needs of women in recovery from addictions (Beckman & Amarno, 1986; Finkelstein & Mora, 2009; Kaskutas, 1994; Lisansky, 1999). In mixed-gender treatment groups women may feel more stigma and guilt about their drinking than men do (Wilsnack, 1973). Women with SUDs also have a very high incidence of experiencing sexual abuse (Beckman, 1993; Simpson & Miller, 2002), which can render mixed-gender groups stressful. WFS is an alternative recovery program for women only, addressing addiction as a coping mechanism that women may turn to in response to life and relationship problems. WFS seeks to build self-esteem, reduce negative thinking and guilt, and encourage competence, self-acceptance, and personal responsibility for recovery. Founded by Jean

Kirkpatrick (1999), WFS is a secular abstinence-based program with meetings facilitated by trained volunteer moderators.

In a survey with 600 women in WFS groups, Kaskustas (1994, 1996) found that women who affiliate with WFS do so for various reasons other than simply achieving or sustaining sobriety, and 60% stated they would be able to remain abstinent without attending WFS (Kaskutas, 1994). Among other reasons for attending WFS, women in this survey identified receiving support from other women, the positive and self-enhancing focus of the program philosophy, the unique benefits of an all-woman milieu (including cross-generational sharing and strong female role models), and the felt safety of the environment. Stated reasons for not attending AA included that they found 12-step programs too negative and male-oriented, felt as though they didn't fit in, and did not like discussion of God or spiritual themes. Nevertheless, nearly a third of the women in this survey reported attending *both* AA and WFS meetings, consistent with the WFS philosophy that these programs can be complementary. Despite the apparent contradiction in program philosophies along the ego deflation versus self-enhancement continuum, women attending both groups appreciated the wide availability of AA groups, the opportunity to enjoy friends and fellowship, and additional support for sobriety. Of those attending both, only about one in five mentioned coercion as a reason for attending AA.

In summary, if it is available in your area, consider WFS as a mutual help resource for your female clients, especially those who might be uncomfortable in mixed-gender groups or who are uncomfortable with spiritual themes. Locations of groups and more information about WFS can be found at *www.womenforsobriety.org.*

Practical Considerations

As indicated earlier, the best window of opportunity for getting clients engaged in a mutual help group is *during* treatment. This is the time to encourage people who are unfamiliar with or disengaged from mutual help groups to try or retry them, perhaps sampling a variety of groups.

You can be more clear and credible if you are yourself familiar and comfortable with the resources available. A first step is to find out what mutual help groups are available in your service area or online. Most such groups welcome professional visitors who want to learn and make referrals, unless they are explicitly closed (some 12-step) or specialized meetings (e.g., women only in WFS). Have a cancellation? Sample chat rooms on mutual help websites to which you might refer clients. Find out where and when face-to-face groups meet in your area and keep a schedule or website links handy. Some groups also have literature or fliers that you can keep in your office to distribute. If you are in a larger city, the local AA service office can often informally advise you by phone about meetings that might be a good match for a particular kind of client. For example:

CLINICIAN: I have a client I'd like to get to an AA group. She's a middle-aged professional, divorced, kind of shy, no prior AA, and pretty skittish about religion, so a church might not be the best meeting place for her to start. Have any suggestions?

AA PHONE VOLUNTEER: Why don't you suggest the noon brown-bag discussion meeting tomorrow over at the university? They're really friendly, there are some professional women who've got years of solid sobriety, and they're great with newcomers. There's also a step meeting that's good for newcomers, every Tuesday and Thursday night at 7:00 at the Serenity Club downtown. Do you know where that is?

In accord with the systematic encouragement procedures described earlier in this chapter, it's great if you can find some longer term participants who would be willing to talk with newcomers and accompany them to a meeting. A same-gender match is generally advised.

Also prepare your client in advance to not generalize from first impressions. It is common for people to shop around among meetings, which can be very different from each other, before finding a group that suits them. Groups differ not only in content and format, but also in their interpersonal atmosphere on dimensions such as warmth, cohesiveness, expressiveness, and aggression (Montgomery et al., 1993; Tonigan et al., 1995).

If you are in recovery yourself, should you share this information with clients? In the addiction treatment field it is quite common to do so, but professionals do vary in their preferences on whether, when, and how to do this. Conventional wisdom is that it's unwise to refer your client(s) to your own home group, although of course you can't prohibit them from attending if they happen in. If that should occur, it is best to offer a friendly greeting but not call the person by name or reveal that you have a professional relationship. Then discuss the situation at your next session—privately if it is a group session.

KEY POINTS

🔖 Involvement in the 12-step program of AA is consistently correlated with subsequent abstinence from alcohol. Less is known about other mutual help groups.

🔖 People are most likely to try mutual help groups when encouraged to do so during treatment.

- Twelve-step facilitation therapy (a special form of treatment that involves far more than encouraging people to attend) has been found to be at least as effective as other evidence-based treatment methods.

- A variety of both religious and secular mutual help groups have been developed.

- Groups vary widely in structure, content, and social climate, so that clients are well advised to investigate several before deciding whether and which to attend or participate in online.

Reflection Questions

- What do you know about mutual help groups that are available in your community or on the Internet? Which have you visited and what was your experience?

- Of the common myths about 12-step groups discussed in this chapter, which (if any) have you found to be most prevalent among your professional colleagues?

- What (if anything) surprised you about the research findings discussed in this chapter?

CHAPTER 18

Medications in Treatment

As effective medications have been developed, pharmacotherapy has played an increasingly important role in the treatment of addictions. A report by the President's Commission on Combating Drug Addiction and the Opioid Crisis (2017) recommends that the use of medications should be expanded based on the evidence that it can help to improve treatment retention, reduce heroin use and related mortality, decrease criminal activity, and prevent the spread of infectious disease. Yet only a minority of privately funded addiction programs offer medications as a treatment option.

Medications can be used to manage the negative effects of withdrawal, reduce cravings and urges to drink or use drugs, and/or impede the reinforcing effects of alcohol or other drugs. They can help clients become less preoccupied with substance use and decrease impulsive drinking and drug use, which in turn increases the likelihood of maintaining a longer period of abstinence.

This chapter examines the current state and recent advances in pharmacotherapies for addiction problems. We emphasize in particular how medications can be used as part of addiction treatment to address various symptoms and problems, enhance self-efficacy, and heighten a commitment to change. We examine the evidence for the efficacy of various kinds of medications and how they can be combined in productive ways with behavioral interventions.[1]

---

[1]While the term "medication-assisted treatment" is in current usage, to us it suggests a second-class status for pharmacotherapies in addiction treatment. No one describes "psychotherapy-assisted treatment."

Medications for Withdrawal and Maintenance

People with severe physical dependence may need medications to reduce the aversive effects of stopping or reducing their use of alcohol and other drugs. As is true more generally in addiction treatment, medication to manage withdrawal is only a first step or one part of the stabilization process (see Chapter 6), and should be accompanied by psychosocial interventions in order to clarify the benefits and risks of the medication (such as side effects), to facilitate medication and treatment adherence, to enhance motivation and skills to reduce substance use, and to maintain recovery (Agosti, Nunes, & O'Shea, 2012; Barber & O'Brien, 1999; Carroll & Kiluk, 2012; Carroll & Weiss, 2017; Heffner et al., 2010; Weiss et al., 2014; Wilcox & Bogenschutz, 2014).

Medications that attenuate withdrawal tend to be longer acting *agonists,* those that have similar effects to the problem drug. For this reason, they can be used not only for withdrawal management, but also as an aid in the reduction, cessation, and prevention of substance use. Thus, these medications can be used for immediate withdrawal (see Chapter 6), for gradual tapering of use over time, and/or for longer-term maintenance (see Chapter 21).

Alcohol Withdrawal Medications

Pharmacologically managed withdrawal is unnecessary for most people with alcohol use disorders. A minority of clients in a typical treatment population will have sufficiently severe alcohol dependence to require pharmacological management for safe withdrawal, and even this can in most cases be done in a medically supervised outpatient setting (see Chapter 6). Although a majority of clients can complete alcohol withdrawal with mainly supportive (i.e., nonpharmacological) care, severe alcohol withdrawal is a serious medical condition, with potential consequences including seizures, delirium, and death (Kosten & O'Connor, 2003).

Effective medications are available to suppress seizures and delirium as well as the discomfort of alcohol withdrawal, and their use may also improve ultimate treatment outcome (O'Malley & Kosten, 2006). There is no evidence that allowing people to suffer during withdrawal benefits their recovery, and of course there is a medical risk in doing so. Medications such as benzodiazepine, chlordizaepoxide, and lorazepam are effective in treating alcohol withdrawal. Other medications such as beta-adrenergic blocking drugs, anticonvulsants, and antipsychotics can also be used to alleviate withdrawal symptoms and complications.

Instruments for predicting the likely severity of alcohol and other drug withdrawal are discussed in Chapter 6. Such scales are useful both in predicting severity of withdrawal and in titrating medications, adjusting treatment to the individual client (Swift, 2003).

Remember that withdrawal management is only a preparation for recovery, an opportunity and responsibility to engage the person in treatment beyond stabilization. Used alone, it rarely changes substance use problems, leading to the familiar and expensive *revolving door* of people returning for dozens, even hundreds of episodes of supervised withdrawal.

> There is no evidence that allowing people to suffer during withdrawal benefits their recovery.

Medications to Attenuate Alcohol Use

Medications can be used to reduce cravings for and reward from substance use, thus helping clients to initiate and sustain recovery. Establishing an initial period of abstinence is an important part of stabilization, interrupting prior use patterns and enabling clients to benefit from psychosocial treatment. The medications described here have been tested with various clinical populations and have demonstrated efficacy in suppressing the use of alcohol or other drugs.

Disulfiram

Disulfiram (trade name Antabuse) has long been used in treating serious alcohol use disorders. The World Health Organization has recognized disulfiram as an important component of a treatment approach for help-seeking individuals with a serious alcohol use disorder (Brewer & Steel, 2018). It can be readily adapted and used with behavioral treatments to reduce heavy drinking and to achieve and sustain abstinence (Azrin et al., 1982). Disulfiram has been used effectively with various special populations such as heavy drinking methadone-maintained clients, opioid users, and clients in sensitive professions such as physicians and pilots (Brewer & Steel, in press).

Disulfiram works by selectively blocking the metabolism of acetaldehyde, a by-product produced as the body breaks down ethyl alcohol. The resulting buildup of acetaldehyde produces highly unpleasant and potentially dangerous symptoms such as nausea, vomiting, racing heart, lowering of blood pressure, and shortness of breath (Ait-Daoud & Johnson, 2003; Burnett & Reading, 1970). The strategy assumes that clients, knowing that they will have such an aversive reaction if they drink, will refrain from using alcohol. Disulfiram is *not* intended to be used as an "aversion therapy," because ideally the person would never experience the disulfiram–ethanol interaction. (During the 20th century, clients were sometimes given disulfiram and then alcohol while hospitalized as a "challenge" to let them experience the unpleasant interaction, but this is no longer done.) The person must be abstinent for at least 12 hours before taking the initial dose without significant medical or psychological contraindications. The intended use of disulfiram is to help the person achieve an initial period of abstinence by taking the medication daily (Barber & O'Brien, 1999; Strain, 2009), which in turn can facilitate psychosocial treatment during Phase 3 rehabilitation (see Chapter 7).

Clinical trials of disulfiram for alcohol dependence have produced mixed results (Brewer, 1992; Miller & Wilbourne, 2002). What seems clear is that clients who faithfully *take* disulfiram fare better than those who do not (Fuller & Gordis, 2004; Garbutt, West, Carey, Lohr, & Crews, 1999). Medication adherence is the principal problem. Studies suggest that men who are older, more socially stable, have more severe alcohol problems, and attend Alcoholics Anonymous may be more likely to adhere to and do well on disulfiram (Swift, 2003).

Additional measures can be taken to increase disulfiram adherence. Pharmacist-supervised daily administration can be used, with the obvious inconvenience that the person must come to the pharmacy daily. An effective alternative is to engage a supportive significant other (SSO) monitor in a daily disulfiram ritual with the client. The SSO's role is not to nag or enforce, but rather to witness and lovingly encourage daily dosage (Azrin, 1976; Azrin & Besalel, 1982; Meyers & Miller, 2001; Meyers & Smith, 1995). SSO-monitored disulfiram has been found to significantly increase abstinence when added to psychosocial treatment (Brewer, 1992; Meyers & Miller, 2001). People who do not have such an SSO or who have had several unsuccessful treatment experiences may benefit from daily disulfiram supervised by clinical staff to establish an initial period of abstinence (Fuller & Gordis, 2004; Swift, 2003).

Another potential use of alcohol sensitizing medications is as a protective measure taken as needed. This has been done both with disulfiram and also with citrated calcium carbimide, which is available in Canada (trade name Temposil). In this situation, the client does not take the medication every day but carries a supply and pops a tablet if feeling in danger of drinking. Clients report that this strategy helps them to "make the decision once rather than a hundred times" in a day.

Disulfiram has also been used successfully as an aid in treating cocaine dependence, and acceptance of the medication may be better when cocaine rather than alcohol is the primary drug of choice (Carroll et al., 1998). One obvious mechanism is that drinking is a common antecedent to resumed cocaine use, so that suppressing alcohol use may improve cocaine abstinence. Disulfiram may also have a direct pharmacological effect on cocaine use and craving. In a randomized trial, clients receiving behavioral or interpersonal psychotherapy showed significantly greater reduction in cocaine use when they were also given disulfiram than when receiving placebo

(Carroll et al., 2004). Interestingly, the impact of disulfiram on cocaine use in this study was not attributable to changes in alcohol use. Another clinical trial found that it was necessary for disulfiram dosage to be no less than 250 mg for the drug to suppress cocaine use in methadone-maintained clients (Oliveto et al., 2011).

Disulfiram is a generic medication that is, in our view, underutilized in helping clients to achieve stable abstinence. Its cost varies by country, and is far less than typical expenditures on alcohol.

Naltrexone

Naltrexone appears to be a useful aid in treating alcohol use disorders presumably by blocking the rewarding aspects of drinking that are mediated through opiate receptors. Clinical trials have shown significant albeit modest benefits, and side effects are typically mild (the most frequent being temporary nausea). Naltrexone appears to reduce the frequency and intensity of drinking, as would be expected if it reduces the rewarding effects of alcohol, and to help people return to achieve abstinence more quickly after drinking (Garbutt, 2009; Garbutt et al., 1999; Kranzler & Kirk, 2001). In a large rigorously designed multisite clinical trial known as the COMBINE study (Anton et al., 2006), naltrexone was significantly more effective than placebo when given within the context of medical management, a low-intensity primary care approach (Pettinati et al., 2005, 2004); benefits were still present a year after medication had been discontinued. It is worth noting that people who were admitted to these studies generally did not have other severe behavioral health disorders beyond alcohol dependence and were required to complete a brief period of abstinence prior to treatment. Retention rates have been low in some naltrexone trials (Garbutt et al., 1999; Oslin et al., 2008). In short, individuals benefitting from naltrexone in these studies may represent a more stable, manageable population than typically seen in alcohol treatment settings (Anton et al., 2006). In a Department of Veterans Affairs study with clients having more severe and chronic alcohol dependence, no benefits from naltrexone were found (Krystal, Cramer, Krol, Kirk, & Rosenheck, 2001).

Naltrexone seems to offer little or no benefit while clients are abstinent; it does not, for example, delay time to resumption of drinking. Rather, the mechanism may involve reducing the intensity of drinking by blocking the euphoric effects of alcohol when drinking. A controversial "Sinclair method" exposes clients to naltrexone while still drinking, and then advocates preventive daily or targeted dosing with naltrexone before drinking in order to reduce the intensity of alcohol use (Sinclair, 2001).

The Sinclair method per se has not thus far been tested in clinical trials for alcohol use disorders, but naltrexone has been tested on a "targeted" or "as needed" basis. In one study (Heinälä et al., 2001) medication conditions were crossed with cognitive coping skill training or supportive counseling. They found naltrexone significantly decreased a return to heavy drinking for clients receiving cognitive coping training (73% vs. 97% with placebo) but no medication effect was found for clients in the supportive counseling condition. In another study (O'Malley et al., 2015), young adult heavy drinkers received placebo or "targeted" naltrexone along with a brief screening and intervention for college students. These heavy drinkers took naltrexone (as needed before drinking) for a week, then daily dose plus an additional predrinking dose for 7 weeks. Naltrexone did not affect the percentage of drinking days, but did decrease drinks per drinking day (five vs. six with placebo) and estimated peak blood alcohol concentration (0.077 vs. 0.095g%)—statistically significant but obviously modest effects. A randomized trial of as-needed naltrexone found no effect (vs. placebo) on pathological gambling (Kovanen et al., 2016).

Extended-Release Naltrexone for Alcohol Use Disorders

An injectable form of naltrexone (trade name Vivitrol) has been offered for clients with serious alcohol use disorders. Administered once monthly, the injectable form offers an obvious advantage in increasing medication adherence. Research on this medication has been promising. In a multisite efficacy trial of injectable naltrexone, individuals who received the active medication had significantly fewer days of heavy drinking at follow-up than their counterparts in the placebo group (3.1 vs. 6 days, respectively; Garbutt et al., 2005).

Prescription and monitoring of this medication seems to be feasible and effective in primary care settings (Lee et al., 2010). Within the context of psychosocial treatment, it has also been used to reduce drinking during high-risk periods such as holidays (Lapham, Forman, Alexander, Illeperuma, & Bohn, 2009).

Acamprosate

Acamprosate (trade name Campral), which affects various neurotransmitters, particularly glutamate and GABA, is also approved for the treatment of alcohol dependence in the United States and in other nations. The results of clinical trials, however, have been quite mixed. Early studies conducted in Europe found that acamprosate (vs. placebo) significantly increased the proportion of already-abstinent clients who remained continuously abstinent (Lhuintre et al., 1990; Mason & Ownby, 2000; Sass, Soyka, Mann, & Zieglgänsberger, 1996; Whitworth et al., 1996). The findings of these Europe-based studies were not replicated in three large randomized trials. In an industry-sponsored multisite U.S. study, no advantage was found for acamprosate relative to placebo (Mason, Goodman, Chabac, & Lehert,

2006). Similarly, acamprosate showed no greater benefit than placebo for alcohol-dependent clients in the largest study, the federally supported multisite COMBINE trial (Anton et al., 2006) and in a 20-site randomized trial in the United Kingdom (Chick, Howlett, Morgan, & Ritson, 2000). A preliminary trial of acamprosate for cocaine dependence found no benefit (Kampman et al., 2011). A meta-analysis of effect sizes (Maisel, Blodgett, Wilbourne, Humphreys, & Finney, 2013) suggested that acamprosate may be more effective than naltrexone when the goal is total abstention from alcohol, although this was not based on studies directly comparing the two medications. The multisite COMBINE study, which did directly compare the two, found no such advantage for acamprosate. A meta-analysis of pharmacotherapies for reducing alcohol consumption found no efficacy of acamprosate (Palpacuer et al., 2018).

Topiramate

Advances in neuroscience research have suggested that neurotransmitters (such as GABA and serotonin) and receptor subtypes linked with the development of alcohol and drug problems may parallel those for other common psychological disorders such as depression and obsessive–compulsive behaviors (Schuckit et al., 1999). Consequently, medications found to be effective in treating other disorders have also been tested in addiction treatment. One such medication is the anticonvulsant topiramate (trade name Topamax) that is already approved for treating epileptic seizures. Topiramate's mechanisms of action were hypothesized to be relevant for treating alcohol and cocaine misuse. In a head-to-head comparison, topiramate was found to be superior to naltrexone across a number of outcomes such as craving (as measured by the Obsessive Compulsive Drinking Scale), drinks per drinking day, the Addiction Severity Index (ASI), number of heavy drinking days (Flórez et al., 2011), time to first drink, cumulative abstinence, and duration and weeks of heavy drinking (Baltieri, Daró, Ribeiro, & De Andrade, 2008). Topiramate (unlike naltrexone and disulfiram) also has the clinical advantage of starting medication without an initial period of abstinence.

Following on promising initial studies (Johnson et al., 2003), a 17-site clinical trial for alcohol dependence (Johnson et al., 2007) found that topiramate was more effective than placebo across a number of consumption measures including drinks per drinking day, percent of heavy drinking days, and percent of abstinent days.

> Medications can be used to reduce cravings for and reward from substance use.

The medication was also found to reduce craving on various obsessive–compulsive drinking scales that are highly correlated with self-reports of drinking. Although topiramate was clearly efficacious, the absolute proportion of clients with good clinical outcomes was low (as is common with other pharmacotherapies); the percentage of heavy drinking days over a 14-week study period was 43.8%. Although improved from baseline, clients continued to drink heavily about 3 days per week while receiving the active medication. In a single-site randomized trial, topiramate was more effective than placebo in producing clinically meaningful improvement with cocaine-dependent clients (Kampman et al., 2004).

Medications to Treat Opioid Use Disorders

Opiate Withdrawal and Maintenance Medications

Methadone Maintenance

Oral methadone is a well-known and effective medication that has been used to prevent opiate withdrawal symptoms and to promote long-term maintenance for individuals with opioid use disorders (Hser, Evans, Grella, Ling, & Anglin, 2015; McKeganey, Russell, & Cockayne, 2013; Pinto et al., 2010; Samet & Fiellin, 2015). Methadone relieves the aversive effects of opiate withdrawal (e.g., anxiety, agitation, insomnia, abdominal cramping, and diarrhea) and reduces motivation for opiate use. In addition to preventing opiate withdrawal, methadone also substantially reduces the euphoria or highs associated with opiate use (Batki, Kauffman, Marion, Parrino, & Woody, 2005). The best outcomes for methadone have been found when methadone has been given in conjunction with a behavioral intervention of demonstrated efficacy such as case management and related services (Carroll & Kiluk, 2012; McLellan et al., 1999; as discussed in Chapter 8 and later in this chapter).

When beginning this medication, clients are typically required to attend a methadone clinic daily to receive their dosage. This provides daily contact and the opportunity for additional evaluation, case management, and treatment services. Urine screening for illicit drug use is commonly required. When clients attend clinic reliably, are stabilized on methadone, and remain free from other drug use, they may be offered take-home methadone for up to 30 days, provided they continue to refrain from other drug use or criminal activity. The convenience of take-home doses serves as an incentive for continued adherence to program requirements and can alleviate potential problems with transportation, employment, and child care.

Buprenorphine

The development of buprenorphine (trade name Subutex) and the combination of buprenorphine plus naloxone (trade name Suboxone) provided an effective alternative to methadone for alleviating opiate withdrawal and weaning clients from opiate use. Buprenorphine offers several practical advantages over methadone. Its action is longer lasting, which means that the dosing schedule is less frequent—three times a week instead of every day (O'Malley & Kosten, 2006). Self-administration of the medication can be easily observed because buprenorphine is absorbed sublingually (under the tongue). Buprenorphine is generally considered to have a less euphoric effect as compared to methadone and therefore is less likely to be sold on the open market. In short, buprenorphine is fast becoming a treatment of choice in withdrawing clients from opiate use, whereas methadone continues to be used for longer-term maintenance therapy (Pinto et al., 2010).

Buprenorphine is administered in three phases: (1) induction, (2) stabilization, and (3) maintenance (Batki et al., 2005). The induction phase focuses on stopping opiate use by reducing the aversive effects of withdrawal. The stabilization phase focuses on eliminating withdrawal symptoms and managing any side effects. In this phase, clients are tested regularly for illicit drugs. In the maintenance phase, other treatment can be provided to address psychosocial aspects and prevent a return to illicit drug use (see Chapter 21). Buprenorphine dosage can then either be maintained or tapered down. Because withdrawal from buprenorphine is typically easier than from methadone, buprenorphine is preferable when the client's goal is to be drug-free rather than being maintained on a replacement medication. Unlike methadone maintenance, buprenorphine treatment can be conducted in physicians' offices and therefore may be preferable for clients not interested in participating in a structured methadone maintenance program (Hser et al., 2015).

Comparing Buprenorphine and Methadone

Studies have shown that individuals receiving methadone tend to fare better overall (less opioid use) than those in buprenorphine programs, due to higher dropout rates from buprenorphine treatment (Carroll & Weiss, 2017; Field & Rowe, 2017; Hser et al., 2015; Pinto et al., 2010). Summarizing comparison studies between methadone and buprenorphine, Field and Rowe (2017) found that retention rates were 50% lower in buprenorphine programs, with most dropouts occurring during the first month of treatment (Carroll & Weiss, 2017). This difference in retention may be attributable to the higher level of the structure (i.e., scheduled treatment sessions), social support, and close monitoring that typically accompany methadone maintenance. Among those who *remain* in treatment, however, individuals maintained on buprenorphine show lower opiate use and more sustained abstinence from illicit drugs, relative to those maintained on methadone (Pinto et al., 2010). It may be beneficial to provide a higher level of structure during the early months of buprenorphine maintenance in order to promote retention.

Naltrexone for Opioid Disorders

Naltrexone (U.S. trade name Revia) selectively blocks opiate receptors. If given to a person using heroin, it immediately triggers withdrawal and thus is used to reverse opiate overdose. Naltrexone blocks the effects of heroin, but does not provide comparable benefits of an agonist substitution therapy like methadone or buprenorphine–naloxone. While maintained on naltrexone, a person experiences no high from injecting heroin. It might seem, therefore, an ideal drug to treat opioid disorders, except for the problem that the vast majority of heroin users do not continue taking the oral medication (O'Malley & Kosten, 2006). This problem led to the introduction and development of an injectable, extended-release naltrexone (U.S. trade name Vivitrol) for treating opioid disorders.

Extended-Release Naltrexone for Opioid Use Disorders

Recent studies have shown extended-release naltrexone to be effective in suppressing opioid use, although retention in treatment is a significant problem (Jarvis et al., 2018). A multisite randomized controlled trial (Lee et al., 2018) examined the efficacy of extended-release naltrexone with a study population comprised of male outpatients, many of whom had criminal justice involvement (e.g., on probation or parole or released from prison in the last 12 months). To minimize potential coercion, clients were not recruited directly from criminal justice settings but from other recruitment or outreach channels including outpatient clinics, and through mass and social media resources. These clients were randomly assigned to extended-release naltrexone or usual treatment, which included supportive counseling and/or referral to buprenorphine and methadone treatment if preferred. Individuals given extended-release naltrexone showed less opioid use compared to those receiving treatment-as-usual over the 24-week treatment period. Another study with criminal offenders found that those who received extended-release naltrexone missed fewer court sessions and had fewer new arrests relative to their counterparts given usual care (Robertson & Swartz, 2018).

Comparing Injectable Extended-Release Naltrexone and Buprenorphine–Naloxone

So how does extended-release naltrexone compare with buprenorphine–naloxone in treating opioid use disorders? A rigorously designed study (Lee et al., 2017) enrolled 570 clients over 2 years. In an intention-to-treat analysis, the failure rates (defined as 4 consecutive weeks of any nonstudy opioid use or 7 consecutive days of use) were higher for extended-release naltrexone than for buprenorphine–naloxone (65% vs. 57%, respectively).

As in aforementioned buprenorphine versus methadone research, these differences were primarily related to more dropouts in the extended-release naltrexone condition. Dropout rates in the induction phase were 28% with extended-release naltrexone versus 6% in the buprenorphine–naloxone condition. This difference appeared to be due to the withdrawal management procedures required for extended-release naltrexone, where individuals had to be opioid-free for 3 or more days, to provide opioid negative urines, and to demonstrate no or minimal opioid withdrawal symptoms following a naloxone challenge. For people who successfully completed the induction phase, the two medications were equally effective. Over the 24-week treatment period, clients who used nonstudy opioids were 52% with extended-release naltrexone as compared to 56% with buprenorphine–naloxone. Clinical implications of these findings are discussed later in this chapter.

In another rigorously designed study conducted in Norway (Tanum et al., 2017), extended-release naltrexone and buprenorphine–naloxone were found to be equally safe and effective in maintaining treatment engagement, and in reducing heroin use and other illicit opioids and craving for opioids. In this study, participants had fewer difficulties completing the induction phase because many had already been through opioid withdrawal while in inpatient treatment or prison.

Medications to Treat Tobacco Use

Nicotine Substitution

Tobacco use and nicotine dependence are disproportionately high among people with other SUDs. Historically, addiction treatment programs often tolerated cigarette smoking, but legislation requiring the establishment of smoke-free environments has increased pressure to incorporate smoking cessation services in addiction treatment programs. Early concerns that smoke-free facilities (or efforts to treat nicotine dependence more generally) might compromise the efficacy of addiction treatment have proved to be unwarranted. To the contrary, smoking cessation can facilitate abstinence or help reduce drinking and other drug use (Bobo, Mcilvain, Lando, Walker, & Leed-Kelly, 1998). The reverse is not so: abstinence from alcohol or other drugs does not necessarily lead to reduction in smoking. Tobacco use may need to be addressed specifically and is obviously relevant to clients' long-term health and survival. Among smokers who are in recovery from other SUDs, tobacco is the most common cause of premature death and disability (Whitfield et al., 2018).

Most effective approaches for smoking cessation involve some form of nicotine substitution such as nicotine patches or chewing gum (Lancaster, Stead, Silagy, & Sowden, 2000). Here the drug that is being "substituted" is the same one that is the primary addictive substance in cigarettes:

nicotine. Substitution strategies are used because of the low success rate of total cold-turkey withdrawal from nicotine. Typically, clients are switched to an alternate source of nicotine and dosage is then gradually tapered over time to minimize withdrawal symptoms. Some clients, however, continue to use a nicotine substitution source at least periodically, to deal with ongoing experienced nicotine cravings. More effective programs combine behavioral interventions with nicotine substitution and tapering. The website *www.treatobacco.net* provides information for health professionals about evidence-based methods to help clients quit smoking.

> Smoking cessation can facilitate abstinence or help reduce drinking and other drug use.

Partial Agonists

An alternative strategy to nicotine substitution is a partial nicotinic agonist intended to provide some of the dopamine release that is afforded by nicotine, while also blocking nicotinic receptors so that nicotine itself has less positive impact. This partial agonist strategy parallels the use of buprenorphine for opioid dependence. The partial nicotinic agonist varenicline (trade name Chantix), along with counseling, appears promising as an aid in attaining smoking abstinence (Evins et al., 2014; Gray et al., 2015; Tonstad, 2006). More recent research has suggested that varenicline could be also be used as an aid in recovering from a serious alcohol use disorder (Litten et al., 2013; O'Malley et al., 2018). Dopamine agonists are also being tested as aids in abstaining from other stimulants such as methamphetamine and cocaine (Pérez-Mañá, Castells, Vidal, Casas, & Capellà, 2011).

Adapting Medications to Clients' Treatment Needs

The development and testing of new medications for addiction treatment is currently a very active area of research. While it seems unlikely that any medication will be found to cure drug problems by itself, new discoveries will continue to emerge from research, providing promising adjuncts for treatment.

It is also worth saying that many medications have been tested and found ineffective. An astonishing array of pharmacotherapies have been evaluated in clinical trials for substance use problems including antidepressants, anxiolytics, lithium, hallucinogens, and even antibiotics, with little success (Carroll & Kiluk, 2012; Miller & Wilbourne, 2002; Miller, Wilbourne, et al., 2003; Palpacuer et al., 2017; Wilcox & Bogenschutz, 2014).

Combining Medications for Addiction Treatment

There may be advantages in combining medications that have different purposes and mechanisms of action. Some are designed to suppress use, some to alleviate craving, and still others to diminish adverse consequences associated with substance use. Nevertheless, it should not be assumed that two medications are better than one. In treating people with concomitant alcohol use and other behavioral health problems, the combination of disulfiram and naltrexone was no more effective than either medication alone (Carroll & Kiluk, 2012). Similarly, adding acamprosate did not improve alcohol use outcomes, relative to naltrexone alone (Anton et al., 2006). Some medications may impact more than one kind of substance use. Varenicline, for example, may suppress both alcohol and tobacco use (O'Malley et al., 2017). Polydrug use might also be impacted by combined medications; heavy-drinking opioid users had lower severity of withdrawal symptoms (anxiety, perspiration, shakiness, nausea, stomach cramps and craving) and better retention in treatment when given low-dose naltrexone along with methadone, relative to those receiving methadone alone (Mannelli et al., 2011). Different medications can be combined, of course, to target specific concomitant disorders. Pharmacotherapies described in this chapter might be used to attenuate substance use along with those discussed in Chapter 20 to treat a concomitant psychological disorder.

Selecting a Medication for Substance Use

There are a number of issues to consider in selecting a medication. A major consideration is the duration of abstinence required before starting a medication regime. Such was the case in the extended-release naltrexone versus buprenorphine–naloxone study discussed above. The sizeable proportion of clients dropping out of the extended-release naltrexone condition during the induction phase accounted for outcome differences between the two conditions. The major implication here is that without sufficient support and monitoring, clients may not maintain a sufficient period of abstinence to start or be stabilized on a medication. In fact, it has been suggested that buprenorphine–naloxone be used with people who have difficulty meeting the abstinence requirement for extended-release naltrexone. Once withdrawal is complete, they could be started on extended-release naltrexone (Volkow, 2017).

Another consideration is how treatment programs regard a decrease in drinking or drug use. When only total abstinence is acceptable, people may stop taking their medication if any drug use occurs, believing that treatment is not working or viewing themselves as treatment failures. An alternative model is to view the medication as a mechanism to improve decision-making capacities by reducing urges and craving, negative mood, impulsivity and related stress, and to enhance self-efficacy and coping capacities to maximize self-regulation (Carroll & Kiluk, 2012; Kenney, Bailey, Anderson, &

BOX 18.1. Clashing Perspectives on Treatment Research: Lessons Learned

We have both been involved in clinical trials testing combinations of medication and behavioral treatment, studies that brought together pharmacotherapy and psychotherapy researchers. In the process we learned a lot about divergent perspectives and contrasting values on how treatment studies should be conducted.

Pharmacotherapy researchers were naturally focused on outcomes during treatment while clients were still taking the medication. Once the medication ends, treatment is over. Psychotherapy researchers were interested in changes during treatment, but were much more concerned with how well the effects of treatment were maintained long after treatment sessions had ended. In pharmacotherapy research, if a client shows significant improvement during treatment and then the benefit disappears once treatment ends, it is proof that the medication *works*. The very same pattern is often considered to be a failure of psychotherapy—proof that treatment *didn't* work!

What about the content of treatment? In psychotherapy studies the medication has already been developed and is usually administered double-blind. The clinician does not know what's in the capsule. However, in psychotherapy research, treatment cannot be delivered double-blind. The therapists know what they are delivering. Furthermore, it is necessary to specify carefully what treatment will be provided, often by developing a therapist manual. Then therapists must be trained to a competence criterion, and the delivery of therapy needs ongoing quality assurance such as recording and monitoring of sessions to demonstrate what was actually provided.

How intensive should a behavioral treatment be? Psychotherapy researchers are naturally concerned that clients should have sufficient exposure to the behavioral treatment to maximize benefits and show an effect above and beyond the medication. Our pharmacotherapy colleagues, on the other hand, were concerned that too much exposure to behavioral treatment could mask the effects of the medication.

Who should be treated? Pharmacotherapy researchers need clients who are willing to take medication and likely to adhere to a complex dosing regime. This can screen out less stable individuals, many of whom may be reluctant about medication or unable to adhere to the requirements of a pharmacotherapy trial. Psychotherapy researchers may be more concerned to have a study population that is representative of clients commonly seen in "real-world" settings.

Finally, regarding outcome measures, our pharmacotherapy colleagues were understandably focused on the symptoms directly targeted by the medication under study (such as substance use and craving). Psychotherapy researchers were concerned with these as well as a broader array of psychological, social, spiritual, and quality of life measures.

What different treatment outcome studies will be designed depending on the values of the researchers! We learned much from each other.

—A. Z. and W. R. M.

Stein, 2017). In other words, the medication is just one component (albeit an important one) of treatment to facilitate decreased substance use and adverse consequences (Wilcox & Bogenschutz, 2014). Thus, we turn our attention to combinations of medications and behavioral treatments.

Combining Medications and Behavioral Treatments

As mentioned earlier, medications are seldom prescribed alone in addiction treatment, but are typically used in combination with some form of behavioral treatment. There are several good reasons for doing so. One of the main limitations of pharmacotherapies is that high adherence rates are important, but often difficult to achieve. Behavioral treatment can have as one of its goals to increase medication adherence (Heffner et al., 2010; Miller, 2004; Pettinati et al., 2004). Clients ordinarily need reliable exposure to a medication regime in order to experience benefit, and supportive counseling can help with adherence. A stable period of abstinence in turn allows clients a greater opportunity to benefit from the motivational and behavioral treatments to achieve lasting change. Medications and behavioral treatments may also focus simultaneously on different aspects of addiction (e.g., cravings and lifestyle changes), thereby complementing each other. In both pharmacological and behavioral treatment, retention and adherence are associated with better treatment outcome, and thus these treatments may interact in a synergistic way.

Pharmacotherapy may be helpful in establishing abstinence and diminishing urges or cravings, but the sudden absence of substance use raises other issues that medication may not address (see Chapters 11 and 14). How will the person spend the substantial time that was previously devoted to getting, using, and recovering from the effects of alcohol or other drugs? With whom will he or she share time and activities, particularly when a change of friends is needed? How will

> Medications are seldom prescribed alone in addiction treatment, but are used in combination with behavioral treatment.

the person cope with feelings and situations that previously triggered use? How can relationships be repaired that have been damaged by addictive behavior? What will be the new sources of fun, pleasure, and meaning in life? Medications are not designed to solve these problems, and ignoring them is a recipe for failure. The methods described in Chapters 8–17 can be combined with pharmacotherapy for an integrated approach.

Research on Combined Treatments

There is accumulating evidence that combining behavioral and pharmacotherapies for addiction can be beneficial (Carroll & Kiluk, 2012; Carroll &

Weiss, 2017; Chick et al., 2000; Pettinati, Volpicelli, Pierce Jr., & O'Brien, 2000; Volpicelli, Pettinati, McLellan, & O'Brien, 2001; Weiss et al., 2014; Zweben & Zuckoff, 2002). Pharmacotherapy trials have successfully incorporated behavioral components to facilitate medication adherence and improve treatment outcomes (Carroll, 1997; Pettinati et al., 2005). Forms of behavioral treatment that have been combined with pharmacotherapies include (1) COM with disulfiram for cocaine-dependent clients (Carroll et al., 1998); (2) CRA (see Chapter 14) with disulfiram for alcohol-dependent clients (Azrin, 1976; Azrin, Sisson, Meyers, & Godley, 1982; Meyers & Miller, 2001); (3) motivational and behavioral therapy with naltrexone for alcohol-dependent clients (Anton et al., 2006); (4) MI and compliance enhancement therapy with a selective serotonin reuptake inhibitor (Heffner et al., 2010); and (5) motivational (Saunders, Wilkinson, & Phillips, 1995) behavioral family therapy (Dattilio, 2009), or individual counseling with case management and social services for methadone maintenance clients (McLellan et al., 1998, 1999; Morgenstern et al., 2009). Indeed, it is rare to find a pharmacotherapy study for substance use problems that does not also provide a behavioral intervention.

One series of trials, for example, provided open-label naltrexone to clients who also received either supportive therapy (analogous to primary care) or cognitive-behavioral therapy over a 10-week period (O'Malley et al., 2003). Clients who responded positively to either of the behavioral treatments (i.e., no more than 2 days of heavy drinking and adhered to the medication regime 60% of the time) were followed for an additional 24 weeks and given either naltrexone or placebo under double-blind conditions. Results showed that responders who had received CBT maintained their treatment gains throughout the 6-month period with or without naltrexone. In contrast, responders who had received supportive therapy maintained their initial gains only if they were continued on naltrexone during the follow-up period. Apparently, CBT provided benefits beyond those from medication or supportive therapy alone.

Recent studies have shown that when combined with medication, the level of intensity of a behavioral intervention can be an important factor in improving treatment outcomes. In particular, individuals with more severe addiction problems and/or residing in an unstable environment may require a more intensive behavioral intervention along with an effective medication in order to produce clinically meaningful change (Carroll & Weiss, 2017). Such clients often miss treatment appointments, do not provide negative urine tests, have poor adherence with a medication regime, and encounter interpersonal and intrapersonal problems over the course of treatment. They may lack the requisite social stability and support to sustain gains derived from medication alone. Having adequate exposure to a more intensive behavioral approach can help them improve individual and social coping resources, which are important mediators of behavioral change (Nielsen, Hillhouse, Mooney, Ang, & Ling, 2015)

To illustrate, in a study conducted by Roger Weiss et al. (2014), individuals categorized as having a more severe opioid use disorder (dependence on prescription opioids plus heroin) who received buprenorphine–naloxone were more likely to have a sustained period of opioid abstinence if they were adequately exposed to coping skills counseling, relative to their counterparts who received medical management alone (66.7% vs. 35%, respectively). No such difference was found for clients with a less severe opioid disorder (prescription opioids only without history of heroin), who fared well with brief medical management with a medical practitioner who reviewed medication side effects and withdrawal symptoms, addressed medication nonadherence, and provided ongoing support for change. Adding a motivational interviewing component might provide additional benefits in medication management (Heffner et al., 2010; Zweben, Piepmeier, Fucito, & O'Malley, 2017).

In the COMBINE study mentioned above, no additional benefits were found in adding a more intensive, comprehensive behavioral treatment termed the "combined behavioral intervention" (CBI; Miller, 2004), to the naltrexone plus medical management intervention. Similarly, clients receiving CBI showed no additional benefit from naltrexone (vs. placebo). It is noteworthy that clients seen in the COMBINE study did not have other SUDs or behavioral health disorders and generally appeared to be a more stable or manageable population than might typically be encountered in community practice.

Integrating a behavioral treatment and pharmacotherapy can optimize benefits from addiction treatment (Anton et al., 2001; Azrin et al., 1982; Chick, Howlett, et al., 2000; Meyers & Miller, 2001; O'Malley et al., 2003; Pettinati et al., 2000, 2004; Witkiewitz, Maisto, & Donovan, 2010). Studies also indicate that severity of addiction is an important consideration in the combination of behavioral therapies and pharmacotherapies. At least for clients with less severe addiction problems, the unavailability of intensive behavioral treatment need not be a barrier to providing an effective medication (Anton et al., 2006; Carroll & Kiluk, 2012; Schwartz, Kelly, O'Grady, Gandhi, & Jaffe, 2011).

Implementing Pharmacological Interventions in Treatment Settings

Pharmacotherapies obviously require the involvement of a licensed medical provider who can prescribe and monitor medication—something that many addiction treatment agencies have lacked historically. If you already work in a setting with both behavioral and medical expertise available, collaborate as a team. If not, it is worth considering how such collaboration might be arranged with colleagues in your area. Programs currently without medical staffing can make a broader range of therapies available to clients by establishing collaborative consultation. Conversely, if you work in a medical setting (e.g., primary care) without staff who have expertise in health behavior, consider how you might integrate behavioral health consultation into your practice (Blount, 1998; Dunn & Ries, 1997; Ernst et al., 2007; Willenbring & Olson, 1999).

Issues in Integrated Treatment

What issues need to be considered in offering effective medications along with behavioral interventions? How does one administer a medication, ensure the safety of clients, and facilitate medication adherence? This section offers some guidelines for including medications in treatment for SUDs.

Medical Evaluation

Obviously a medical examination and evaluation are important in choosing appropriate medication and ensuring its safety. This includes consideration of any preexisting health conditions such as liver or kidney disease, hypertension, or heart disease. It is also important to review all other medications (both prescription and nonprescription) to consider potential drug interactions. Prior experience with specific medications (e.g., their effectiveness, and any adverse reactions) can be important. Behavioral factors such as psychological symptoms, past experience with taking medications (e.g., adherence to the medication regime), and overall motivation for change are also relevant considerations.

The Therapeutic Relationship

Medications are prescribed and monitored within the context of a therapeutic relationship. A strong working alliance can help in explaining important information about the medication, clarifying misunderstandings, preventing misuse of medication, and improving retention and adherence to the prescribed regime.

Formulating a Plan for Medication Use

When medication is only part of treatment, it is important to consider how it fits within the larger treatment plan. It can be important for nonmedical members of the treatment team to understand the purpose and plan regarding medications, and to help encourage adherence. When two or more medications are used concomitantly or sequentially, develop a specific plan for when and how each one is to be taken. It is wise to check in early and periodically to monitor adherence and discuss any adverse reactions or other problems.

As discussed earlier, some medications are used intermittently as needed. In this case, the plan should specify the circumstances under which it should be used (e.g., to forestall drinking or drug use), as well as the appropriate dose and method for taking it (Boyer, 2012).

Developing a Medication Adherence Plan

A variety of factors can affect whether medications are taken as prescribed and intended. These include the person's:

- Overall motivation for change.
- Knowing the purpose and importance of the medication.
- Understanding how it is to be taken.
- Unpleasant side effects.
- Ability to afford and obtain the medication.
- Lifestyle factors that interfere with reliable adherence.

Before prescribing and starting a pharmacotherapy, review and address potential obstacles to adherence. When and how will the person take the medication? What reminders might be used? How will the person respond to side effects? Can a family member help with adherence? If the person is ambivalent about the goals of treatment (and therefore about taking the medication), strategies from Chapter 10 may be helpful.

It can also be useful to administer the four-item Medication Adherence Questionnaire (MAQ) in conjunction with a behavioral intervention. The MAQ (Morisky, Green, & Levine, 1986) is a widely used device to identify distinct previous patterns of nonadherence and to predict future medication adherence problems (Culig & Leppée, 2014). Responses to the items of the MAQ have been linked with particular intervention strategies to address adherence challenges and strengthen commitment to the medication regime (Zweben et al., 2017). The MAQ questions are as follows:

1. "Do you ever forget to take your medication?"
2. "Are you careless at times about taking your medicine?"
3. "When you feel better, do you sometimes stop taking your medication?"
4. "Sometimes if you feel worse when you take the medicine, do you stop taking it?"

The MAQ yields two factors: unintentional nonadherence (items 1 and 2) and purposeful nonadherence (items 3 and 4).

To illustrate, if an individual answers "No" to all items, affirm and reinforce the response by reviewing the benefits of the medication (e.g., improved health) and offer supportive statements (e.g., "It sounds like you are ready to stick with the treatment plan."). If a person answers "Yes" to either forgetfulness or carelessness (item 1 or item 2), discuss specific issues related to unplanned nonadherence such as going on a trip, changing hours of employment, and having a very busy work schedule; then develop an action plan to attend to these matters. Motivational interviewing methods such as open-ended questioning, reflective listening, and affirming may be helpful here.

With someone who tends to discontinue the medication when feeling better (item 3), explain that this feeling is not unusual and discuss the value of adherence, evoking the person's own ideas as to why it would be good to see the medication regimen through. For example, you might ask, "How has the medication helped you?" and "How might you sustain such improvement?" In short, different motivational responses can be linked with particular items (Zweben et al., 2017).

Treatment in Nonspecialist Settings

We have previously emphasized the potential and advantages of treating addictions within the context of regular health care and social services. Specialist addiction treatment programs simply cannot meet the needs of the full spectrum of alcohol/drug problems that pervade society. SUDs should be screened for and addressed wherever people receive general health and social services (Hilton et al., 2001; Miller & Weisner, 2002; Weisner, Mertens, Parthasarathy, Moore, & Lu, 2001b), where people with addictions are typically seen first, and earlier in the development of problems. Many people with SUDs are reluctant or refuse to seek specialist care, but are willing to talk to a primary provider about their substance use.

The development of effective pharmacotherapies has made it more feasible to address addictions within primary health care. Most health professionals involved in primary care have neither the time nor the training to provide comprehensive treatment for addictions, but they *can* screen, evaluate, prescribe, and monitor (Saitz, 2005; Saitz, Horton, Larson, Winter, & Samet, 2005; Samet, Friedmann, & Saitz, 2001). This is the *normal* role of a primary care practitioner in treating a chronic illness. Chronic conditions are often first diagnosed in primary care. If a patient is diagnosed with asthma, diabetes, cancer, or heart disease and is then treated by a specialist, ongoing care and monitoring are still provided as part of primary care. For this reason, it is important to foster closer relationships and collaboration of behavioral health professionals within mainstream health care systems.

Clearly, people with addictions can benefit from pharmacotherapy delivered within primary health care (Saitz, 2005). In the studies described earlier in this chapter, clients who benefited from topiramate and naltrexone received only supportive therapy, such as could be provided within primary care, while receiving the medication. Those taking topiramate were not required to be abstinent prior to receiving the drug and all clients had been drinking at enrollment (Johnson et al., 2007). These findings indicate that addiction treatment can be delivered, or at least begun, in nonspecialist medical settings. Most people with addiction problems never receive specialist treatment, and only 12% of addiction treatment programs offer alcohol pharmacotherapies, for reasons including lack of medical staff, cost, and ideology (Abraham, Rothrauff, & Roman, 2010). Combining medications and primary care supportive therapy can improve access to effective treatment for many individuals with addiction problems seen in medical settings.

Integrating on-site behavioral health providers in medical settings can further facilitate access to effective care. Although pharmacotherapy is often better than no treatment, many people with SUDs can benefit from additional treatment that behavioral health professionals are trained and able to provide. Such care can be offered on-site at primary care clinics when behavioral health specialists work in those settings. Close collaboration makes it feasible for a person to be diagnosed and receive initial treatment in primary care, then be referred with a "warm handoff" for specialist treatment, and return for ongoing monitoring and case management (Samet et al., 2001). Integrating care can be accomplished in a cost-effective manner through cooperation between a medical professional and a case manager. The former provides medical management, and the latter facilitates medication adherence while keeping medical staff informed of any change in symptoms or side effects that may warrant a dosage change or further medical evaluation. The case manager also coordinates care with other professionals who are providing services during active treatment. With appropriate training, the case manager can help to educate clients and their families as well as offer referral sources about the importance of medications in addiction treatment.

Much remains to be known about how best to integrate these services for people with addictions. It will be helpful to learn more about how to (1) determine what behavioral treatment modalities are more effective with what pharmacological agents; (2) sequence medications and behavioral interventions to address different symptoms and problems that may stem from substance use; and (3) adapt or modify the combined approach to help nonresponders who are not benefiting from initial treatment. Important questions also remain regarding the long-term cost-effectiveness of a combined approach particularly in generalist practice settings. More treatment is not necessarily better treatment, and sometimes combinations of treatments are not more effective than an evidence-based pharmacotherapy or behavioral treatment alone (Anton et al., 2006). Further experience with stepped care will help clarify what treatment is enough for whom, and how best to help those who do not respond to initial treatment (Sobell & Sobell, 2000).

KEY POINTS

🗲 Effective medications are available to reduce or prevent withdrawal symptoms and help clients safely through withdrawal.

🗲 Substitution drugs can also be used for longer-term maintenance.

🗲 Pharmacotherapies are available to help reduce urges to drink or use drugs, facilitate initial abstinence and treatment participation, enhance motivation, and maintain change.

🗲 Pharmacotherapies can be seen as complementary to rather than a replacement for psychosocial interventions.

🗲 Pharmacotherapy also can improve access to effective treatment for many untreated individuals with addiction problems who are currently seen in health care settings.

Reflection Questions

Q What attitudes have you encountered with regard to the use of pharmacotherapies in addiction treatment? What is your own current attitude?

Q If you are not a prescribing professional yourself, what are the various ways in which the clients you serve can access pharmacotherapies?

Q What could you do to help clients who are on pharmacotherapy take their medication reliably as prescribed?

PART IV

PROFESSIONAL ISSUES

B eyond the treatment tools described in Part III, there are particular issues that often arise when treating addictions. In this final section we alert you to particular professional aspects of practice in this field. First, in Chapter 19 we describe 11 specific practical issues that can arise, and how to respond to them: resumed use, coming to sessions under the influence, missed appointments, responding to "resistance," detecting early warning signs, gradualism, raising your own concerns, interacting with correctional systems, interprofessional communication, supporting treatment adherence, and crisis intervention. Chapter 20 explores the complexities of treating addiction plus other disorders with which it co-occurs. In Chapter 21 we consider one of the major challenges in addiction treatment: helping clients maintain the initial changes they make during treatment. Because addiction treatment is often delivered in group as well as individual sessions, Chapter 22 is devoted to the unique challenges of working with groups. More than in many health fields, the spiritual side of recovery has been a prominent subject in addiction treatment, and we address that topic in Chapter 23. Then we close this text with two final chapters: one on ethical issues in addiction treatment (Chapter 24), and the other (Chapter 25) on the challenges of implementing evidence-based treatment methods in ongoing practice.

CHAPTER 19

Stuff That Comes Up

It happens. In fact, it's the norm. You're cruising along well with treatment when suddenly you hit some unexpected turbulence. It doesn't necessarily require a course correction, but you do have to decide how to respond. This chapter suggests some practical strategies that can be useful when "stuff" happens.

Resumed Use

A familiar situation in addiction treatment happens when clients have set a goal for change and then deviate from their intention. Usually there has been a period of abstinence and then the person starts drinking or using again. This is very common and not in itself reason for discouragement (yours or the client's). People with some periods of low-risk drinking have outcomes just as good as for those who continuously abstain during treatment (Witkiewitz et al., 2017). Even occasions of heavy drinking are no reason for despair. Outcomes are worst when clients keep drinking or using heavily throughout treatment, an indication that it's time to try a different approach and perhaps explore sobriety sampling (see Chapter 14). A recurrence of substance use is very common, and not a reason to withdraw or withhold treatment. People are not "discharged" from AA for drinking; the message is "keep coming back."

It seems odd, then, that treatment professionals and programs have sometimes responded to resumed use in such a punitive manner. Renewed use has sometimes been seen as reason to reduce maintenance medication doses, revoke privileges, or even terminate treatment. These would be strange professional responses to a recurrence of symptoms in someone with hypertension, diabetes, or asthma. If anything, a resumption of prior problems would suggest a need to *increase* dosage (Maremmani, Balestri, Sbrana, & Tagliamonte, 2003) or provide intensified or different treatment. Further, don't assume that resumed use means that treatment (let alone the person) is a failure (see Chapter 21). The course of recovery is seldom smooth, and a certain number of bumps are to be expected along the way. A message we like to give to clients is, "I will work with you until we find what works for you."

We recommend a restorative rather than a critical or a punitive approach when responding to resumed use. This involves reviewing the situation for lessons learned. It is also important to keep recurrent use in perspective. All that has happened is that the person violated a rule that he or she or you had (at least apparently) adopted as a goal. So how is it best to respond when people deviate from their goal of abstinence or moderation? We suggest three simple questions:

1. "What's up?"
2. "What's new?"
3. "What's needed?"

"What's Up?"

First, seek to understand what happened. Voice tone matters. The simple question "What happened?" can be asked in a manner that sounds curious and supportive, or judgmental and shaming. (Try asking it with different voice inflections.) The basic mindset is a problem-solving approach starting with a review of how the client understands what occurred. What seemed to trigger resumed use? What was the person thinking or feeling at the time? What has he or she thought about since?

An important point in responding to resumed use is to help the person (and significant others) not overinterpret or be demoralized by what has happened. What really matters is what happens next. Language can make a difference here. Framing resumed use as a "failure," "relapse," "falling off the wagon," and such may add negative emotion but not hope. A cognitive issue to watch for with resumed use is the "rule violation effect"—the classic downfall of New Year's Eve resolutions. The very term "relapse," which we no longer recommend using (see Chapter 21), incorrectly implies that there are only two possible outcomes: perfection and disaster (Miller, 1996b, 2015b). Having broken a resolution, people may overgeneralize, catastrophize, or just plain give up: "Now I've done it! I'm off my diet"; "I have nothing to lose now; I blew my sobriety"; "I guess I just can't do it." In fact, imperfection is the norm for human beings, and it's possible just to get back on track, to return to the original plan (Kurtz & Ketcham, 1992;

Witkiewitz et al., 2017). We are generally inclined to treat resumed use for what it is—behavior and choice—and move on to problem solving.

"What's New?"

It is also common for resumed use to reflect something new, some kind of change. Were the person's hopes and expectations for sobriety somehow disappointed? Did the person discover that there was something he or she missed about using? Sometimes new feelings or problems emerge with abstinence that had previously been masked by use. Often resumed use occurs when people encounter a new situation for which they were not quite prepared. Here are a few things to consider exploring:

1. What was happening just before the resumed use that might have triggered it? Where was the person, and with whom? What was the person feeling, thinking, and doing? Explore these questions in a nonjudgmental manner. They are not "excuses," but clues to what else may be needed to support the person's long-term recovery.
2. How conscious was the person of making the decision to use? What contributed to that decision? "What were you thinking?" is not for shaming and blaming, but for understanding "apparently irrelevant decisions" and thought processes that increase the risk of resumed use (Cummings et al., 1980).
3. What did the person hope or expect would happen with resumed use? Did it happen? What if anything did the person enjoy about using (smoking, drinking, etc.)?
4. What, if anything, did the person do at the time to try to avoid using? What else could he or she have done, but didn't do?
5. What are the client's other hunches about the resumed use? Is there anything else happening in the person's life that made substance use look more attractive?
6. How did the person react to the initial use? What did he or she think, feel, and do after violating the plan?
7. Perhaps most important question is "What's next?" What does the person want, hope for, and choose to do now?

Make sure that you understand the client's goals. If abstinence is your goal but not your client's, then continued use is unsurprising. Clarify what your client wants, using motivational methods described in Chapter 10. Does the resumed use reflect a shift in the person's motivation and goals for change? It is normal for motivations to fluctuate over time. Try to distinguish here between motivational shifts that *preceded* the event, and

> Imperfection is the norm for human beings.

responses (such as demoralization) to the event itself. Explore what the person wants, needs, and hopes for, and as appropriate renew commitment to change goals. Have the person's original motivations changed? If commitment to change seems shaky, it may be useful to explore the consequences of continued use versus resumed abstinence. In the style of MI, you would particularly seek to hear from the person the advantages of resumed abstinence (or moderation, if that was the goal), and the risks and disadvantages of returning to prior use patterns. Beware the scenario where you champion a particular goal while the client argues against it.

"What's Needed?"

Two nonjudgmental questions that are often asked in a restorative approach are:

1. "Who has been affected by what you did, and in what ways?"
2. "What do you think you need to do now in order to make things right or get back on track?"

A period of "sobriety sampling" may reveal feelings or situations that previously triggered substance use, and for which substance use was an attempt to cope, perhaps the only tool that the person knew for handling a particular feeling or situation (which is a working definition of psychological dependence). Here again it can be useful to conduct the "new roads" functional analysis of the person's use described in Chapter 14, an exercise that can also be done with groups. The point is to identify different ways for the person to respond to the "trigger" situation, and better ways to get from there to a desired outcome without engaging in addictive behaviors.

> With abstinence, new problems can emerge that had previously been masked by use.

What other responses are possible if this or a similar challenge arises again? Then develop a plan for resumed progress (see Chapter 21).

Coming to a Session Intoxicated

People in treatment for SUDs sometimes come to sessions under the influence. This is no more surprising than patients with diabetes coming to the doctor's office with a high blood sugar level, or patients with hypertension presenting with elevated blood pressure. It is the very problem for which they are being treated, and it makes little sense to discharge people for the same reason they were admitted.

Nevertheless, intoxicated clients can pose some practical and ethical concerns. In group treatment sessions, it can be disruptive or disturbing to other clients when a participant is obviously under the influence of alcohol or another drug (see Chapter 22). Your workplace may have specific policies for how to handle this situation. There is a reasonable concern as to whether clients will benefit from or remember what happens in treatment, although emergency department studies have shown significant effects of even brief interventions when patients are intoxicated (e.g., Bernstein et al., 2005; Chafetz et al., 1962; Kohler & Hofmann, 2015).

Disagreement can arise regarding the presence and extent of intoxication, and perhaps the simplest way to resolve this is through on-site breath or urine testing. Some programs do routine or periodic testing prior to treatment sessions; others use immediate-result testing only when there is a question about intoxication. It is wise to make this procedure clear at the outset of treatment so that it is not a surprise.

Suppose you have administered a breath test that shows a client's estimated blood alcohol concentration (BAC) is double the legal limit for driving, and you know that the client has driven to the appointment. Here there is at least a moral if not a legal obligation to take steps to prevent the client from driving away under the influence. One possible sequence of responses is:

1. Ask the client to wait on site until the BAC has decreased to below the legal limit. (Even here there is risk, because the only truly safe BAC when driving is zero.)
2. Offer to call a relative or a taxi to drive the client home.
3. Inform the client (if this is your policy) that you are obliged to notify the police if he or she drives away under the influence.

In any event, schedule the next appointment and give the client a written note of the appointment time. You can also contact the client the next day to affirm your caring and interest in continuing treatment, and to reconfirm the appointment.

Missed Appointment

Missed appointments are common in addiction treatment. When someone misses a scheduled appointment, respond right away to proactively re-engage him or her rather than waiting for clients to get back in touch (Miller, 2004). Depending on your own or agency policy, you can try immediately to reach the client by phone, text, e-mail, or social media. Here are some things you can do once you do make contact:

- Review (in a nonjudgmental fashion) the reason(s) for the missed appointment.
- Express your eagerness to see the person again.
- Affirm the client for prior attendance, progress, motivation, etc.
- Listen for client change talk and reflect it (see Chapter 10).
- Encourage optimism about positive change.
- Reschedule the appointment.

It can also be effective to send a personal handwritten message (not a form letter) with the appointment time and some of the above encouragement. This can significantly increase the chances that your client will return (Nirenberg et al., 1980; Panepinto & Higgins, 1969).

> Re-engage clients proactively rather than waiting for them to get back in touch.

Responding to "Resistance"

As mentioned in Chapter 2, we encourage letting go of the concept of client "resistance." To label clients as "resisting" has at least the overtone of blaming them for it: either they are being intentionally oppositional, or it's a function of personality defenses. Either way it sounds like the client's fault. In fact, it takes two for resistance to occur; no one stands alone in a room and resists.

Nevertheless, the situation that gets labeled as "resistance" is a common one; there is some point of disagreement. Perhaps there is a goal, idea, or treatment approach that you wish your clients would share, but they do not concur, at least not yet. (Warren Farrell once quipped that when clients disagree with their therapist it is called "resistance." When they subsequently come to agree with the therapist it is called "insight.") In MI (Chapter 10), resistance is deconstructed into *sustain talk* (a normal part of ambivalence: motivations not to change) or *discord* (tension in the therapeutic relationship).

Our first suggestion is not to push when you experience some reluctance from your client. Disagreeing, challenging, confronting, even just teaching or directing are likely to increase rather than decrease defensiveness (Glynn & Moyers, 2010; White & Miller, 2007). Our advice here runs counter to the popular idea of "confronting resistance and denial." Pushing back is just likely to evoke reactance and strengthen resistance (Brehm & Brehm, 1981; Karno & Longabaugh, 2005).

Reflecting

The simplest and often effective response to discord or persistent sustain talk is to reply with reflective listening (Chapter 4). Without any tone of sarcasm, offer a simple or complex reflection of what you think the client may mean. Here are four examples:

1. "I don't see why I have to be here."
   "This doesn't make much sense to you."
2. "I really don't have any problem with drugs."
   "Using drugs has never caused any problems for you."
3. "I don't listen to anybody who isn't in recovery."
   "You're really not sure if I can help you."
4. "I've tried to quit and I just can't do it."
   "It's been really difficult for you."

One artful type of reflective response is a *double-sided reflection* that puts together both sustain talk and change talk that the client has expressed. Two hints here: (1) It's usually better to put an "and" in the middle instead of a "but" (the word "but" is a bit like an eraser, discounting what went before); (2) usually put the client's reluctance at the front end followed by change talk that you have heard.

- "So you don't see any real problems with your drinking, and at the same time you do see some of your wife's concerns as legitimate."
- "You're happy with the way you've been living your life, and you also would like to get your probation officer off your back."
- "It's hard to imagine how you'd get through the day without more medicine, and it sounds like you also understand why I'm worried about prescribing more."

Emphasizing Self-Determination

Another good response to resistance is to acknowledge and honor the person's autonomy, the choice and control that he or she actually has (Ryan & Deci, 2008). This is simply truth telling: People do get to decide how they will behave. Three examples:

1. "Look, I'm not going to quit smoking, OK?"
   "And that's your choice. No one else could ever decide that for you."
2. "I really don't want to be here."
   "In fact, you don't have to be. You could go somewhere else and I can help you find services that suit you better if you wish."
3. "I don't listen to anybody who isn't in recovery."
   "Then, I can listen to you."

Taking Partial Responsibility

Sometimes discord is the issue—there is some tension in your working alliance. Discord statements often have the word "you" in them. Here a reasonable response is to take partial responsibility for the experience, recognizing that it takes two notes to create dissonance. Taking partial responsibility costs you nothing and can go a long way to alleviate discord.

1. "You just don't understand how hard this is for me."
   "OK, I'll do my best to listen more carefully. Tell me what I've been missing so that I can understand better."
2. "Are you telling me that I'm an addict?"
   "No, sorry if I gave you that impression. I don't really care about labels. What I care about is you—what's going on in your life and what, if anything, you might want to do about it."

What's common to these different ways of responding to experienced resistance is that you don't let it become a power struggle. Ultimately it is the client who decides what to do, and you are a companion along on the journey.

Detecting Early Warning Signs

A sizeable proportion of clients do not stick with their original plan. Willingness to take certain steps (e.g., taking medication, attending mutual help meetings, avoiding high-risk situations) may shift over time. Significant life changes can disrupt original plans, and detecting and addressing these adherence challenges can avert a return to substance use or withdrawal from treatment.

Missed or cancelled visits or arriving late for session can be an early signal of emerging problems. Another warning sign can be increased defensiveness or evasiveness, which might be manifested in persistently talking about irrelevant issues ("chatting"). Attending to such signs may prevent premature dropout. Case monitoring (see Chapter 8) can be helpful here. Explore whether these possible warning signs may be connected to other problems or concerns the client is having. Discussing these matters openly and directly may reduce future nonadherence by facilitating trust and change (Stout, Rubin, Zwick, Zywiak, & Bellino, 1999). Case management can also help stabilize clients' living situations so that they can attend treatment. In some cases it may be helpful to involve family members or supportive others to facilitate the client's treatment (see Chapter 16).

A particularly good approach for detecting early warning signs is to ask clients to provide ongoing feedback after each visit. The Outcome Questionnaire and the briefer Outcome Rating Scale are simple client feedback tools with well-established reliability and predictive validity (Bringhurst, Watson, Miller, & Duncan, 2006; Lambert et al., 1996; S. D. Miller, Duncan, Brown, Sparks, & Claud, 2003). Comparing clients' ratings from session to session can alert you to a perceived lack of progress, and obtaining such regular feedback has been shown to improve both retention and outcome (Lambert et al., 2001; S. D. Miller et al., 2006; S. D. Miller, Duncan, Sorrell, & Brown, 2005). Feedback-informed treatment (FIT) scales can be obtained free of charge from *www.scottdmiller.com*.

Gradualism

It is common in addiction treatment for clients and their therapists to entertain different goals (or at least hopes) for change. A harsh approach has been to refuse treatment to (or even discharge) anyone who does not agree to accept stated program goals such as total abstinence from all psychoactive drugs. An alternative palliative approach is to work with people "wherever they are," seeking at least to prevent or diminish harm to themselves or others.

A helpful perspective here is *gradualism*—successive approximations toward better health (Kellogg & Kreek, 2005). This is a common perspective in managing chronic illnesses like diabetes or hypertension, where sudden error-free perfection is rarely expected. Instead, good progress is reflected in gradual changes in health behavior, with corresponding improvement in physical measures such as blood glucose level and reduction in risk for adverse outcomes of uncontrolled diabetes. Gradual and progressive improvement is also normal in psychotherapy, with "two steps forward and one step back." Although sudden transformational changes do occur (Forcehimes, 2004; Miller & C'de Baca, 2001), the step-by-step "educational variety" of change described by William James (1902) and honored in A. A. is far more common.

So what efforts to promote gradual, progressive changes are comfortable for you? Box 19.1 offers some examples that have been implemented in clinical practice. How acceptable to you is each of the described services? Ethical considerations with "harm reduction" are discussed in Chapter 24.

> Good progress is reflected in gradual changes.

BOX 19.1. Would You?

How acceptable to you would each of the following services be?

This is unacceptable or unethical to me.				It's OK with me if I don't have to do it myself.				I would be willing to do this myself.		
0	1	2	3	4	5	6	7	8	9	10

_____ Operate a free needle exchange program to provide clean syringes to injection drug users and safely dispose of their used needles.

_____ Provide heroin users with naloxone rescue kits, similar to those used in emergency rooms, to use if witnessing a heroin overdose. (Many heroin overdose deaths happen in the presence of at least one other drug user, who is often reluctant to call for help.)

_____ Offer free testing of drugs with unknown content, to identify for users or parents what's in them.

_____ Provide a substitution drug like buprenorphine if the person is willing to taper off toward abstinence.

_____ Provide a safer maintenance drug like suboxone or methadone for longer-term use instead of heroin.

_____ Help a client gradually taper down his or her use of a drug toward an ultimate goal of abstinence. (Does it make a difference to you if the drug is nicotine, alcohol, marijuana, or cocaine?)

_____ Provide free condoms for people in addiction treatment. (Does it make a difference to you if the client is an adult or an adolescent?)

_____ Encourage heroin-dependent adults to register with a medical service that dispenses heroin to be injected on-site, if you know that doing so would reduce (1) overdose deaths, (2) property crime, (3) the need to recruit other users in order to support one's own habit, (4) medical consequences of using drugs of unknown strength and purity, (5) violence associated with buying from drug dealers, and (6) the market for illegal sale of heroin.

_____ Work with a marijuana user who is currently unwilling to quit, to try cutting down and see how it goes.

If an injection polydrug user is willing to come to treatment sessions but is not willing to accept a goal of total abstinence, would you be willing to work with this person to:

_____ Get HIV testing?

_____ Use only clean needles from a needle exchange and never share needles?

_____ Switch to a less risky route of administration (e.g., from injection to snorting)?

_____ Quit using some drugs (e.g., methamphetamine, heroin) but not others (e.g., alcohol, marijuana, tobacco)?

_____ Focus on quitting one drug at a time (e.g., methamphetamine, alcohol, nicotine)?

Raising Concerns

Even within a person-centered approach there come times when you experience a concern that you want to express to your client. Perhaps you foresee a potential problem or obstacle, you sense an unspoken issue, or you have reservations about how your client plans to proceed. How can you raise such concerns in a respectful therapeutic manner?

Jumping right in with a directive or confronting style can evoke defensiveness and set back your working alliance:

- "Look, that plan of yours just isn't going to work!"
- "It sounds to me like you're in denial."
- "What is it that you're hiding from me?"

Nevertheless, you want to express your concern. You may even feel a professional obligation to do so and note it in the records. A good first step is to ask permission:

- "You know, there's something that worries me here, and I wonder if it's OK to tell you what I'm concerned about."
- "I have a couple of thoughts about your plan. Is it all right if I share them with you?"

It can also be helpful to give the person permission to ignore or disagree with you. Again this is just truth telling—they already can ignore or disagree, but giving permission can increase the likelihood that they will hear what you have to say.

- "I don't know if this will make any sense to you, but there's something I've noticed in working with other people that might be helpful."
- "This may or may not concern you, and that's fine, but there's something that is bothering me about our conversation today."

You can follow this preface with asking for permission, and 99% of the time clients will say OK. But in the rare event that you feel urgently obliged to give your information or advice even if the client says "No," you can just preface your comments with such an acknowledgment of the person's autonomy and then proceed. State your concern clearly and briefly. Then if the client doesn't reply, ask what he or she thinks about what you said.

An example of such an urgent concern is potential suicide risk, a familiar issue for professional helpers. If you find yourself wondering whether a client may be suicidal, by all means ask. Another helpful preface in raising a sensitive topic like this is to normalize it.

"I find that often when people are feeling as down as you are, they begin thinking about ending their own life. It might just be thoughts about death as a relief, or people even think about exactly how they would do it. I wonder if you've had this experience?"

Interacting with Correctional Systems

It is common in specialist addiction treatment programs for clients to enter under some duress, whether from family, an employer, or the courts. In the United States about half of people entering formal addiction treatment are referred by a judge, attorney, or probation officer. This is not in itself a reason for concern. Relative to voluntary self-referred clients, those mandated by the courts tend to have somewhat less severe addiction problems at intake, which makes sense because they are coming sooner than they might otherwise. Clients who perceive that they have been coerced into treatment may have lower initial levels of intrinsic motivation (Jones, Hayhurst, & Millar, 2017). Nevertheless, on average, treatment outcomes for mandated people are at least as good as those for voluntary clients (Kelly, Finney, & Moos, 2005).

Legal coercion, however, can impose some reporting requirements. Most often the treating agent or program must periodically confirm that the person has been attending and participating as recommended. Sometimes the referring agent may also require more detailed progress reports. It is important to understand clearly what the referring agent requires, and to file reports in a timely manner.

Interprofessional Communication

People suffering from addictions frequently have other significant problems as well: family, financial, legal, economic, medical, and psychological. There is a need to make and receive referrals, exchange information, and coordinate care (see Chapter 8). This involves communicating with a broad range of professional colleagues.

A first issue in any such communication is client consent. Regulations for the protection of confidentiality in addiction treatment can be even more stringent than those generally required in health care (see Chapter 24). Clients must consent in writing to particular types of communication with specified individuals or agencies, and signed consent forms are retained with client records. Without such consent it is improper even to acknowledge whether a person is under your care. Early in consultation, anticipate the people or agencies with whom you may need to exchange information and obtain clients' consent to do so, clearly defining the purpose of such communication. People for whom clients may consent to confidential communication can include family members, health care providers, case workers, attorneys, clergy, and social service agencies. When receiving a referral it is appropriate, as a professional courtesy, to acknowledge the referral. Further communication with the referring agent would be with client consent only. See Chapter 24 for emergency and other conditions in which reporting information without client consent may be permitted or required.

Courtesy and promptness are appropriate when replying to requests for communication once you have obtained proper consent. Usually information is provided in written form with copies retained in hard copy or electronic client files. To obtain information from professional colleagues, provide a written request specifying the information needed and providing a copy of the client's signed consent. Clients are often required to obtain, complete, and sign the agency's own consent form before information will be released.

Supporting Adherence

Clients cannot benefit from a treatment they have not received. Greater adherence to treatment is associated with better outcomes, whether it is attending sessions, taking prescribed medication, or completing take-home assignments. Doing something, taking steps toward one's own recovery, predicts greater change (Bohart & Tallman, 1999). In clinical research when people are prescribed (unbeknownst to them) a placebo medication, the extent to which they faithfully take their "doses" predicts successful outcome (Zweben et al., 2008).

Rather than the term "compliance," we prefer the term "adherence" (sticking to it) to describe how fully and well people participate in a particular treatment or change effort. Adherence is a common challenge in treating SUDs. On average, 44–60% of those beginning addiction treatment leave within the first month (Carroll, 1997; Greenfield et al., 2007). In some settings, the modal (most common) number of treatment sessions completed is one. This is good reason to provide something that is likely to help in the very first contact, but obviously if people do not return, they cannot benefit from the intended treatment. Adherence can be particularly difficult for people with serious concomitant medical and psychological problems (Weiss, 2004). Individuals with co-occurring addiction and psychological problems tend to fare better in settings that address both areas, rather than in addiction-specific programs (Mueser, Drake, Turner, & McGovern, 2006; see Chapter 20).

It is tempting just to blame clients for being unmotivated and not doing what they are supposed to, but in fact there is much that you can do to support better adherence and thereby improve outcomes. A person-centered approach and motivational interviewing can strengthen your working alliance with clients and enhance readiness to change, which in turn predict better adherence and outcomes (see Chapters 4 and 10). Provide a client-friendly environment from the very first contact: a welcoming and courteous reception staff, an attractive and safe waiting area, a cup of coffee (AA has known this for a long time), and prompt appointment times. Instead of making clients fit into a single fixed program, offer a menu of options from which clients can choose. People who have a choice among options are more likely to stay and adhere to what they have chosen. Consider whether what you (or your program) have to offer is consistent with the person's own needs, hopes, and expectations. A clash of expectations often leads to adherence problems. Some individuals initially want to cut down on their drinking and do not fit with a program that accepts only lifelong abstinence. Some may be willing to take medication but don't want behavioral therapy, whereas for others the reverse is true. Some folks are uncomfortable with groups, and others prefer them. It matters what's on the treatment menu and how much flexibility you have in individualizing treatment plans.

Crisis Intervention

As treatment proceeds, life continues to happen. Crises can emerge that may or may not be related to clients' presenting concerns, but can disrupt the course of care. Dealing with an acute crisis is often a higher priority for clients than whatever was already happening in treatment. If you already have an established working alliance, it is natural to join with the client's concern and focus attention on how to respond.

A first consideration is the immediate safety of clients and their significant others. If in your opinion there is imminent danger (like suicidality or violence), take appropriate professional steps to protect those involved (see Chapter 24). Is there other action that should be taken immediately? Is assistance needed from other professionals experienced with particular kinds of crises (such as rape, bereavement, or victim advocacy)?

Unexpected crises can also be highly stressful and disorienting. Suddenly all the pieces of life seem to have been thrown up in the air. There can be a shaking of the foundations that have given the person's life structure and meaning. In this case the pressing focus of counseling may not be on making particular choices or change, so much as on confusion reduction (Gilmore, 1973).

Meanwhile, your own calm, structured presence can be a real support. Here are some commonly recommended steps in responding to a crisis (Miller, 2004, p. 118).

1. *Listen.* Rely on reflective listening to gain an understanding of what has happened and how the people involved are reacting.
2. *Assess.* What is needed? Are there immediate safety issues to address? Is there danger of suicide or other violence? What additional information is needed?
3. *Help with understanding.* Help clients and significant others understand what is happening to them. Make the situation comprehensible. As appropriate, normalize events and reactions.
4. *Focus on problem solving.* After listening, assessing, and helping with understanding, focus on practical problem solving. What needs to be done first? How can the immediate crisis be abated? Develop a specific plan to address short-term and longer-term problems.
5. *Mobilize social support.* Who besides yourself can offer practical and emotional support for the client? What family or community resources are available to provide additional support? Link the client up with these sources of support.

Crises are sometimes accompanied (and exacerbated) by the client resuming substance use. In this case, recommendations at the beginning of this chapter can be useful.

KEY POINTS

🔖 Much as we may think of treatment as a smooth linear process, things come up along the way that require therapeutic response.

🔖 Just as symptom recurrence is common in chronic disease management, resumed use is normal in addiction treatment. The key is to help clients get back on track quickly with a nonjudgmental restorative approach.

🔖 It often happens that a client comes to treatment under the influence. Have a clear compassionate response plan that clients understand in advance.

🔖 When clients miss an appointment, responding promptly in a supportive manner can substantially improve retention.

🔖 What therapists experience as "resistance" is not a client trait but an interpersonal phenomenon. Pushing against or confronting it only tends to strengthen it. Some "rolling with" responses from MI include reflecting, emphasizing self-determination, and taking partial responsibility.

🖈 There is a gentle way to raise concerns with your clients that recognizes and honors their autonomy.

🖈 Information exchange is often needed with other professionals and with correctional colleagues and systems. Have a clear understanding with clients about what will and won't be communicated and obtain proper consent.

🖈 Faithful adherence to change plans is a common challenge in addiction treatment (and in human nature). There are various ways counselors can help people follow their best intentions.

🖈 Life crises can arise during treatment and temporarily require a clinical response in order to keep longer-term goals from being derailed. A common flow in crisis response is:

1. Listen.
2. Assess.
3. Help with understanding.
4. Focus on problem solving.
5. Mobilize social support.

Reflection Questions

🖎 In your own experience, what situations most often arise that tend to interrupt or jeopardize the smooth flow of treatment?

🖎 When you want to raise a concern or disagree with a client, how do you usually do it?

🖎 What are three things that you do (or could do) to help clients more closely adhere to agreed-upon steps toward recovery?

🖎 To what extent do you agree or disagree with (or find yourself ambivalent about) the authors' view that the term "relapse" should be retired from addiction treatment? Why is that?

CHAPTER 20

Treating Co-Occurring Conditions

People struggling with SUDs often have more than one diagnosable condition. Various terms have been used for this common situation. Some terms like "mentally ill chemical abuser" are highly stigmatizing. "Dually diagnosed" can have multiple meanings in health care; for example, for concurrent developmental and mental disorders. In the context of addiction treatment, we prefer the broader term "co-occurring," which simply acknowledges that people can have different conditions at the same time, without referring to any particular combination. One person might be struggling with posttraumatic stress disorder (PTSD) and an opioid use disorder, another with borderline personality disorder and an alcohol use disorder, and yet another with attention-deficit/hyperactivity disorder (ADHD) and a nicotine use disorder. All of these combinations would be co-occurring conditions. We note that some have restricted *dual diagnosis* to addiction plus a *serious* mental illness, a category that includes bipolar disorder, schizophrenia, and severe depression. SUDs also co-occur with a host of medical problems, but for purposes of this chapter we focus on concomitant mental health issues.

Addictive disorders are associated with higher prevalence of many other mental health problems. In the United States about 41% of people with SUDs have another diagnosable mental disorder (Bose et al., 2016). Thus, when treating addictions, you are likely to encounter a broad range

> Almost half of people with SUDs have another mental disorder.

of co-occurring conditions. Relative to the general population, people with an SUD are twice as likely to suffer from a mood or anxiety disorder, antisocial personality disorder, or conduct disorder (Grant et al., 2015, 2016). Co-occurring disorders also increase with the number of drugs used

(Burdzovic, Lauritzen, & Nordfjaern, 2015) and with severity of the addictive disorder (Bakken, Landheim, & Vaglum, 2007; Grant et al., 2015; Whiteford et al., 2015). It's fair to say that co-occurring conditions are the norm rather than an exception.

The same applies in mental health services. SUDs are the most common diagnosis in the general population, and the most frequent co-occurring disorder among people with a serious mental illness (Hasin & Grant, 2015). For example, about half of people diagnosed with schizophrenia also develop an SUD at some point in their lifetime (Grant et al., 2015, 2016; Hartz et al., 2014), and this concurrence rate may be increasing (Hasin & Grant, 2015; Nesvåg et al., 2015). The good news is that effective treatment for addiction can improve the course of the co-occurring behavioral health problem (Bergman, Greene, Slaymaker, Hoeppner, & Kelly, 2014; McGovern et al., 2015).

Which Came First?

Is the substance use a cause or a result of the mental disorder, or do both result from some third factor? All of these are possibilities. The two conditions may be independent of each other, or one may be secondary to another and subside when the primary is treated. Some clinicians try to determine which emerged first in time, although this can be challenging and still does not resolve the question of independence. It is often unclear whether substance use influences development of these other conditions or vice versa. People who use multiple drugs simultaneously tend to have more behavioral health problems. In a 10-year longitudinal study in Norway, for instance, researchers examined changes in psychological symptoms over time and their association with poly-substance use. Over time, mental distress increased in a dose-response fashion with the number of substances being used (Andreas, Lauritzen, & Nordfjaern, 2015).

The combination of two disorders is generally more serious than either condition alone. When substance use and mental disorders co-occur, the course of each problem is worsened (Swann, 2010). Co-occurring conditions also tend to be more severe and have a greater effect on clients' quality of life than does a single diagnosis (Brown, O'Grady, Battjes, & Farrell, 2004; Burns & Teesson, 2002; Kessler, 1995) Those with co-occurring conditions tend to be worse off than those with substance use or psychological problems alone on a variety of dimensions including health, employment, housing, and suicide attempts (Mericle, Ta Park, Holck, & Arria, 2012; E. R. Walker & Druss, 2017) and struggling with concurrent conditions is a leading cause of disability (Erskine et al., 2015; Whiteford et al., 2015). As a barrier to treatment, stigma for people with mental disorders can be compounded by still more negative public attitudes toward SUDs (Barry, McGinty, Pescosolido, & Goldman, 2014). Despite the need for effective treatments to address both issues concurrently, people with SUDs are often excluded from clinical trials evaluating the effectiveness of treatments for one condition or the other (Baingana, al'Absi, Becker, & Pringle, 2015). Treating those with co-occurring conditions is certainly more challenging than treating people with a single disorder.

Why Are Co-Occurring Conditions So Common?

The Self-Medication Hypothesis

A popular explanation for co-occurring conditions is the self-medication hypothesis described in Chapter 11: that people are using alcohol, tobacco, or other drugs in an attempt to manage their other symptoms. This explanation has a certain intuitive appeal in that these drugs are psychoactive, and indeed many people report that substance use offers them some symptom relief (e.g., "It helps my anxiety"; "I feel less depressed"). It would seem to follow logically that people with depressive symptoms would prefer stimulants, and those with anxiety symptoms would choose more anxiolytic substances. Research findings, however, do not support such clear associations between the person's symptoms and the particular substances used (Conway, Swendsen, Husky, He, & Merikangas, 2016; Lembke, 2012). Drugs of choice tend to be influenced more by peers, and use persists despite fluctuations in symptoms over time (Mueser et al., 2006). In addition, many people report continuing use despite their clear awareness that the drug actually makes their other symptoms worse. This is just a specific example of the more general puzzle of addictions: that people continue using in the face of clear adverse consequences.

Although the self-medication hypothesis doesn't seem to be a satisfactory general explanation for co-occurring conditions, it still may be correct in specific cases and is worth considering. Perhaps the more general question is what is motivating someone with a co-occurring disorder to use particular substances. Even if drug use does not directly alleviate psychological symptoms, people may *believe*, for example, that nicotine improves cognitive function or that alcohol alleviates depression. It is not necessary that the drug *actually* yields the desired effect, but only that the person believes it does so. Alcohol, for example, tends to produce both stimulant and depressant effects depending on dose and time since consumption (Holdstock & de Wit, 1998). Within this *biphasic* effect, drinkers may remember (and drink for) the initial stimulant effects, with selective forgetting of the depressive rebound that occurs later and with higher doses (an ironic meaning of "happy hour"). A list of perceived motivations for drinking is provided in Box 20.1. In any event, attempting to self-medicate psychological symptoms does not in itself explain the high rates of co-occurring conditions.

> It is not necessary that the drug actually yields the desired effect, but only that the person believes it does.

BOX 20.1. Desired Effects of Drinking

Tracy L. Simpson, PhD, Judith A. Arroyo, PhD, William R. Miller, PhD, and Laura M. Little, PhD

Drinking alcohol can have many different effects. What results or effects have you wanted from drinking alcohol *during the past 3 months?* Read each effect/result of drinking on the left and indicate how much this was an effect of drinking you *wanted* during the past 3 months.

During the past 3 months, how often did you want this effect from drinking alcohol?	Never 0	Sometimes 1	Frequently 2	Always 3
1. to enjoy the taste	0	1	2	3
2. to feel more creative	0	1	2	3
3. to change my mood	0	1	2	3
4. to relieve pressure or tension	0	1	2	3
5. to be sociable	0	1	2	3
6. to get drunk or intoxicated	0	1	2	3
7. to feel more powerful	0	1	2	3
8. to feel more romantic	0	1	2	3
9. to feel less depressed	0	1	2	3
10. to feel less disappointed in myself	0	1	2	3
11. to be more mentally alert	0	1	2	3
12. to feel good	0	1	2	3
13. to be able to avoid thoughts or feelings associated with a bad experience	0	1	2	3
14. to feel more comfortable in social situations	0	1	2	3
15. to get over a hangover	0	1	2	3
16. to feel brave and capable of fighting	0	1	2	3
17. to be a better lover	0	1	2	3
18. to control my anger	0	1	2	3
19. to feel less angry with myself	0	1	2	3
20. to be able to think better	0	1	2	3
21. to celebrate	0	1	2	3
22. to control painful memories of a bad experience	0	1	2	3

(continued)

From Miller (2004). This instrument is in the public domain and may be reproduced without further permission. For psychometrics, consult Doyle et al. (2011).

BOX 20.1. (continued)

During the past 3 months, how often did you want this effect from drinking alcohol?	Never 0	Sometimes 1	Frequently 2	Always 3
23. to be able to meet people	0	1	2	3
24. to sleep	0	1	2	3
25. to be able to express anger	0	1	2	3
26. to feel more sexually excited	0	1	2	3
27. to feel less shame	0	1	2	3
28. to feel more satisfied with myself	0	1	2	3
29. to be able to work or concentrate better	0	1	2	3
30. to relax	0	1	2	3
31. to forget about problems	0	1	2	3
32. to have a good time	0	1	2	3
33. to stop the shakes or tremors	0	1	2	3
34. to be able to find the courage to do things that are risky	0	1	2	3
35. to enjoy sex more	0	1	2	3
36. to reduce fears	0	1	2	3
37. to feel less guilty	0	1	2	3

SCORING INFORMATION

Sum the scores for these four items in each scale:

	Scale	Items				Totals
A	Assertion	7	16	25	34	
D	Drug Effects	6	15	24	33	
M	Mental	2	11	20	29	
N	Negative Feelings	9	18	27	36	
P	Positive Feelings	3	12	21	30	
R	Relief	4	13	22	31	
S	Self-Esteem	10	19	28	37	
SE	Sexual Enhancement	8	17	26	35	
SF	Social Facilitation	5	14	23	32	
	Total Score					

Genetic Vulnerability

Another hypothesis suggests that people with co-occurring conditions may have genetic vulnerabilities that increase the likelihood of developing both disorders. The use of particular substances may act as an epigenetic factor to activate specific genes associated with certain disorders (Brown et al., 2015). Gene expression can also interact with a person's environment so that when certain stressors (including drug use) are present, the person will develop the disorder.

If vulnerability to a disorder is sensitive to the effects of certain drugs, even use at a level that might be considered low to moderate could trigger mental disorders (Mueser et al., 2006). An anecdotal example is a person who experiences a first psychotic episode during or after taking a hallucinogenic drug. The vulnerability was there, but symptoms were triggered by the drug experience. This in turn may have a *kindling* effect such that experiencing a first episode places the person at increased risk for further or more severe episodes—something that appears to be true of major depression (Muñoz et al., 2009) and alcohol withdrawal-induced seizures (Becker, 1998; Becker & Hale, 1993). Seizures are also associated with increased risk for psychosis (Smith & Darlington, 1996). Given these factors, people with serious mental illness may reach a threshold for serious negative consequences of substance use at a much lower level than others do (Mueser et al., 2006).

Neurocognitive Factors

Research has also examined developmental factors that may affect brain development, increasing risk for mental illness and co-occurring substance use. One proposed factor is the neurocognitive impairment of self-regulation. Generalized self-regulatory deficits that are observable in the first decade of life predict a host of later problems and diagnoses including SUDs (Brown, 1998; Diaz & Fruhauf, 1991; W. R. Miller & Brown, 1991; Moffitt et al., 2011; Tarter et al., 2003). Impulsivity, inhibitory control deficits, and other neurocognitive problems are commonly observed in many mental disorders including personality disorders, schizophrenia, and bipolar disorder. Therefore, a common neurocognitive vulnerability may underlie risk for co-occurring conditions.

Developmental Factors

Yet another possibility is that there are timing-specific exposure effects in development. The brain experiences dramatic developmental change during adolescence and early adulthood, and the use of substances while the brain is still undergoing maturation may increase risks of the later development of an SUD and concurrent mental health disorder (Volkow et al.,

2016). Early (including *in utero*) exposure to a drug may affect brain development and increase risk of developing a mental disorder; similarly, early emergence of mental health problems may affect brain development and increase the risk of developing an SUD. In this bidirectional model, the mental illness and substance use worsen or sustain each other in a reciprocal fashion (Smith & Randall, 2012).

Environmental Factors

A fourth hypothesis regarding co-occurring conditions is that an underlying vulnerability from adverse experience independently increases the risk for both the addiction and the concomitant disorder. A variety of common vulnerability factors have been proposed including environmental stressors such as child abuse and trauma (Simpson & Miller, 2002), peer aggression (Moore et al., 2014), poverty or deprivation, and other adverse childhood experiences. The impact of such events obviously varies across individuals. Those very low in harm avoidance, a characteristic of antisocial personality disorder, may not experience negative consequences as intensely as others do, and so the threat of punishment or other adversity may not be so great a deterrent (Miranda, Meyerson, Myers, & Lovallo, 2003).

In sum, various hypotheses have been proposed to explain co-occurring conditions, and the evidence thus far does not support any one of these as the whole story. Chances are that each contains some element of truth, and science may yield new insights to further inform treatment. In the meantime, much is already known about how to help people with co-occurring conditions.

What Disorders Are Overrepresented?

Certain disorders are particularly overrepresented among people with SUDs (Hasin & Grant, 2015). Some of the most common are mood disorders (major depression, bipolar disorder), anxiety disorders (PTSD, generalized anxiety disorder, panic disorder), thought disorders (schizophrenia and schizoaffective disorder), and personality disorders (borderline personality and antisocial personality). We briefly consider each of these diagnostic groups and key issues and concerns that they can raise in addiction treatment.

Mood Disorders

The most common concomitance is with mood disorders, particularly among women (Hasin & Grant, 2015; Lai, Cleary, Sitharthan, & Hunt, 2015). Major depression is more common than other mood disorders, affecting 9% of men and 17% of women (lifetime prevalence in the general population) (Hasin & Grant, 2015). A diagnostic complication is that the effects of intoxication and drug withdrawal include mood disturbance. Dysphoria, for example, can result from alcohol or other depressant drug use, or from cessation of stimulants. Stimulant-induced episodes of mania can include paranoid symptoms that last from hours to days. Since nearly all psychoactive drugs have some effect on mood, it is unsurprising to find mood disturbances associated with alcohol/drug use and withdrawal.

It is a mistake, however, to assume that mood disturbances are merely secondary to substance use. Independent mood disorders are common in addiction treatment populations and may appear, persist, or even worsen with abstinence. Drug use in turn can exacerbate the swings of affective disorders, specifically the highs of mania and the lows of depression. In almost all studies of completed or attempted suicide, alcohol or drug use and major depression are among the top associated conditions. Having both conditions simultaneously leads to one of the highest statistical risks for suicide. When you are working with someone who suffers from a mood disorder and addiction, it is important to assess and reassess danger to self or others because the use of psychoactive substances can lower inhibitions and result in impulsive action.

Anxiety Disorders

Like mood disorders, anxiety disorders are common co-occurring conditions affecting people with SUDs. The lifetime prevalence of anxiety disorders ranges from 0.2% for agoraphobia to over 9% for specific phobia and PTSD (Hasin & Grant, 2015). Psychoactive drugs can increase psychomotor stimulation and manifestations of anxiety including generalized anxiety and panic attacks. Anxiety symptoms that are merely alcohol- or drug-induced and withdrawal-related anxiety usually resolve within a few days or weeks.

Again, it is unwise to assume that anxiety symptoms are merely side effects of substance use. Independent anxiety disorders co-occur with addictions at a much elevated rate, as does a history of child abuse, trauma, and PTSD (Simpson & Miller, 2002). In individuals with both drug and alcohol use disorders, nearly half have diagnosable PTSD (Grant et al., 2015, 2016). The co-occurrence of PTSD and substance use may be due, in part, to lifestyle factors associated with substance use, including exposure to criminal behavior and traumatic experiences. Substance use can also be motivated by a desire to manage, avoid, or escape from the suffering related to PTSD and other anxiety disorders. Furthermore, physical withdrawal from drugs can mimic anxiety (see Chapter 6), which in turn can reinforce continued use. Rebound from benzodiazepine or alcohol use, for example, can increase anxious arousal, convincing users that they need more frequent and higher doses. If medicating is the only means clients have for managing anxiety symptoms, they are vulnerable to resumed use when encountering even normal life stressors.

Schizophrenia Spectrum and Other Psychotic Disorders

Among people with a lifetime diagnosis of schizophrenia or schizophreniform disorder, almost half have also met criteria for an SUD (Grant et al., 2015). Again, there can be confusion as to whether psychotic symptoms represent a primary disorder or are secondary to substance use or withdrawal. Symptoms of substance intoxication and withdrawal can strongly mimic symptoms of thought disorders, including hallucinations, paranoia, agitation, or delirium. These tend to resolve relatively quickly. Yet it is important to be alert for independent thought disorders that preceded substance use or persist well into abstinence. As discussed above, it is also possible for drug use to trigger the first episode of what becomes an independent disorder.

People with acute psychotic symptoms are most likely to be taken to mental health facilities, but may also present in addiction treatment systems. The first priority is typically to stabilize the crisis and determine whether the person needs emergency medical care, hospitalization, or withdrawal management (see Chapter 6). Often, people with psychoses are also experiencing social problems such as homelessness or housing instability, victimization, poor nutrition, and poverty, and these immediate crises may need to be addressed. Also assess the risk of danger to self or others, considering any current hallucinations or thought disorders.

A thorough assessment should follow as soon as feasible. Collateral information from family or significant others is especially helpful when clients' speech and thought patterns are disorganized and their ability to give a history is impaired. Inquire for a history of significant medical disorders, loss of consciousness or head trauma, and behavioral health problems.

Personality Disorders

People with Cluster B personality disorders (American Psychiatric Association, 2013) have very high incidence of concomitant SUDs. Personality disorders are diagnosable in about a quarter of those with an alcohol use disorder and in over half of those with both drug and alcohol use disorders (Grant et al., 2015, 2016). The most common co-occurring personality disorder among substance using clients is antisocial personality disorder followed by borderline personality disorder (Hasin & Grant, 2015).

Individuals with antisocial or borderline personality display impulsivity and high-risk behaviors which, when combined with substance use, can be quite dangerous. Chaotic patterns of substance use are typical in this population and increase a variety of risks including violence, injury, and infection from unprotected sex or contaminated needles.

Avoiding Misdiagnosis

Across these conditions there is a common issue of distinguishing the effects of drug use and withdrawal from those of co-occurring disorders (McKetin, Hickey, Devlin, & Lawrence, 2010). This involves some skill in differential diagnosis, and provisional diagnoses are appropriate early in the evaluation process, given the number of diagnoses that can be mimicked by drug effects (see Box 20.2). A diagnosis of a separate (not substance-induced) disorder is clearest when there is evidence of symptoms prior to the onset of substance use, if symptoms persist for a month or more after acute withdrawal, or the symptoms are in excess of what would be expected given the type and amount of substance used.

Waiting until the withdrawal process has fully subsided is one approach to differential diagnosis and gives perhaps the clearest indication of what additional conditions may require clinical attention. It is possible, of course, that persisting problems are severe enough during the first month to require a more rapid clinical decision and treatment, particularly if symptoms are worsening. After initial stabilization, it is usually easier to construct a time line of when substance use and psychological symptoms began. What was the person's quality of life during substance-free periods? Meeting diagnostic criteria for a disorder prior to the onset of substance use is strong evidence for an independent disorder. Remember, however, that onset during substance use does not rule out an independent disorder (e.g., the first episode of which may have been triggered by substance use).

Approaches to Treating Co-Occurring Conditions

The Quadrant Model

The quadrant model offers a useful framework for conceptualizing subgroups of people with co-occurring conditions by understanding the severity of each disorder (McDonell et al., 2012; McGovern, Clark, & Samnaliev, 2007). Four different subgroups (see Box 20.3) correspond to combinations of high and low severity of mental and SUDs. The idea behind the quadrant model is that those who differ in the severity of their addiction and psychiatric disorders have different treatment needs and may require different treatment settings.

- *Quadrant I.* These individuals display low severity of both substance use and mental illness. They may not seek treatment at all, and if they do they are usually treated in nonspecialist settings, with specialist consultation as needed.

- *Quadrant II.* These individuals display low substance use severity and high mental illness severity, and are usually seen in mental health

BOX 20.2. Drug Effects That Can Mimic Mental Disorders

	Some Possible Psychiatric Symptoms during:		
	Intoxication	**Acute Withdrawal**	**Protracted Withdrawal**
Alcohol	• Euphoria • Mood lability • Disinhibition • Slurred speech	• Agitation • Anxiety • Tremors • Insomnia • Hallucinations • Delirium	• Mood instability • Hostility • Fatigue • Low sexual interest • Sleep disturbance
Stimulants	• Euphoria • Impulsivity • Grandiosity • Paranoia • Rapid pressured speech	• Depression • Fatigue • Agitation • Sleep disturbances	• Anhedonia • Lethargy • Dysphoria • Anxiety
Hallucinogens	• Sensory dissociation • Visual hallucinations • Panic • Paranoia • Delusions	• Anxiety • Delirium	• Depression • Flashbacks
Cannabis	• Euphoria • Agitation • Lethargy • Grandiosity (high doses) • Perceptual distortions	• Irritability • Depression • Anxiety	• Irritability • Depression • Anxiety
Inhalants	• Euphoria • Slurred speech • Psychomotor retardation	• Insomnia • Agitation • Anxiety • Hallucinations	• Anxiety • Depression • Irritability
Sedatives	• Euphoria • Disinhibition • Mood lability • Slurred speech	• Mood instability • Depression • Anxiety • Insomnia • Hyperactivity	• Anxiety • Depression • Perceptual distortions • Depersonalization
Opioids	• Euphoria • Indifference • Apathy	• Agitation • Irritability • Anxiety • Depression • Anhedonia • Insomnia • Delirium	• Anxiety • Depression • Sleep disturbance

From Sacks and Ries (2005).

BOX 20.3. The Quadrant Model

		Psychiatric severity	
		Low	High
Substance use severity	Low	I	II
	High	III	IV

settings. A collaborative or integrated model is preferred, in which substance use and mental health service providers collaborate, or where services are blended with a single team of providers.

• *Quadrant III.* These individuals have high substance use and low psychological severity, and are most often seen in addiction service settings. Similar to Quadrant II, a collaborative model is preferable, offering integrated treatment of disorders.

• *Quadrant IV.* People in this quadrant have severe substance use and severe mental illness. They may be seen in mental health clinics or hospitals, correctional facilities, and emergency departments. They may also be bounced back and forth between mental health and addiction treatment facilities. It is for people in this quadrant that an integrated service model is most vital.

Integrated Treatment Models

The problem of deciding where to send people from each quadrant is a byproduct of the historic isolation of addiction treatment from other health care systems. It has been relatively rare for specialist addiction treatment services even to be co-located with mental health or primary care systems. Thus, referring agents, clients, and their families have had to choose which system to access. This has resulted in referrals back and forth, sequential treatment of one and then the other problem, or at best parallel treatment within two different systems. Some enter treatment through mental health services, where it is discovered that substance use is also part of the clinical picture. In this case, they might be referred to an addiction treatment program to resolve that problem first. Many such referrals are not completed because of client reluctance, stigma, or practical barriers like waiting lists. This is changing as chronic care management perspectives emerge similar to those for diabetes and hypertension, a possibility enhanced in the United States through the Patient Protection and Affordable Care Act mandating substance use treatment as a normal part of health care (Croft & Parish, 2013).

Another barrier to integrated treatment has been a function of professional specialization. For decades, SUDs in the United States were treated primarily by specialist counselors whose training and expertise were focused on addictions. Educational requirements (as well as salaries and status) were lower for addiction counselors than for professionals working in other health care settings, including mental health. Even in the early 21st century, it was controversial in state laws whether a bachelor's degree should be required for addiction counselors—a contention that would be unthinkable for the treatment of virtually any other life-threatening illness. Conversely, those trained in mainstream mental health professions such as psychology, psychiatry, and social work rarely received adequate preparation, training, or even encouragement to treat addictions, the most common disorders they would encounter throughout their careers (Miller & Brown, 1997). In other developed nations, SUDs have been addressed by mainstream health care professionals. The professionalization of addiction treatment has been occurring in the United States as well, both with gradually increasing educational and training standards for addiction counselors and with greater inclusion of addiction training in medicine and mental health professions. "Behavioral health" has come to describe expertise and services in both addiction and mental health, and addiction specializations and journals have emerged within health professions including psychology, psychiatry, medicine, social work, and nursing.

Since the 1980s, integrated outpatient or day treatment programs have emerged for people with co-occurring severe disorders (Quadrants III or IV), which combine services within a single system of care. Integrated residential facilities have also been developed (Drake, Mueser, Brunette, & McHugo, 2004). In 2016, about 47% of addiction treatment facilities in the United States reported providing programs specifically tailored toward co-occurring conditions (Substance Abuse and Mental Health Services Administration, 2017).

Integrated treatment models combining mental health and addiction services are optimal in addressing co-occurring disorders (Eack et al., 2015; Farren, Snee, & McElroy, 2011; Horsfall, Cleary, Hunt, & Walter, 2009; Weiss & Connery, 2011). Unlike parallel treatment, integrated treatment uses the same team of providers combining mental health and addiction treatments in the same setting to offer coordinated care. The uncertainty surrounding etiology and clinical presentation hints at the complexity of co-occurring conditions: they are so intertwined that it makes sense to deal with them simultaneously rather than trying to isolate which symptoms should be treated first and by whom. By having the same treatment providers in one centralized location, treatment-related stress is minimized, and engagement and retention can increase.

Integrated cognitive-behavioral therapy (ICBT) is a manual-guided therapy for addiction and PTSD that includes education, mindfulness practices, and cognitive restructuring over 8–12 sessions. A randomized trial compared standard care alone (intensive outpatient treatment) to standard care plus ICBT or standard care plus individual addiction counseling. PTSD symptoms were reduced equally in all three groups, yet ICBT resulted in better SUD outcomes (McGovern, et al., 2015).

Similarly, integrated dual disorder treatment (IDDT) is designed for people with co-occurring conditions as a way to address both disorders simultaneously, in the same clinic, and by the same team of treatment providers. The multidisciplinary team meets regularly to discuss the person's progress and coordinate all aspects of recovery. Different services are offered at different stages of treatment. For example, for someone ambivalent about engaging in treatment, the focus is on providing practical help, outreach, and crisis intervention. As a way to build an alliance with clients, clinicians engage in assertive outreach in the community where a client lives. As clients progress through stages of IDDT they are given access to comprehensive services including case management, behavioral health counseling, medical services, supported employment, and family services. Continuous access to services is one feature that sets IDDT apart from other interventions. People are able to receive services throughout their lifespan, even when symptoms are mild or infrequent (essentially a primary care model). Staying connected with the care system is an important aim in itself; people are not discharged if they stop taking their medications or continue using substances. IDDT essentially mirrors a chronic disease management approach.

An integrated approach seems to work well across the board for concomitant substance use and mental disorders with one possible exception: people with antisocial personality disorder. One study (Frisman et al., 2009) suggested that people with antisocial personality disorder benefit when assertive community treatment (ACT) is added to IDDT, showing greater reduction in alcohol use and incarceration than with IDDT alone. For people without antisocial personality disorder, IDDT worked equally well with or without the addition of ACT.

So what is ACT (Horsfall et al., 2010)? It is a more intensive treatment approach developed particularly for helping people with more severe disorders function in the community. A significant difference between ACT and other treatment models is that ACT takes treatment to the person rather than always asking the person to come in for treatment. The goal of ACT is to help people avoid crisis situations in the first place or, if that proves impossible, to intervene quickly at any time of the day or night to keep crises from turning into unnecessary hospitalizations. Another way ACT differs from IDDT is the inclusion of peer support specialists as part of the multidisciplinary team. These individuals have had personal successful experience with the recovery process and can offer a variety of recovery approaches from their own lived experience of receiving services.

Some Helpful Perspectives

Here are some points to consider in treating people with co-occurring conditions. They are useful considerations in addiction treatment more generally, but can be especially helpful with concomitant disorders in all four quadrants.

1. Think of recovery as something positive beyond the disorders, just as peace is more than the absence of war and health more than the absence of illness. What are the person's broader goals and values (see Chapter 23)? What would "recovery" or a "good life" mean to this person? Some continuing symptoms are likely, and are not incompatible with a path to recovery.

2. While men and women tend to show similar retention in treatment, there are gender differences that warrant attention. For example, women may enter treatment with greater severity on psychological measures (Choi, Adams, Morse, & MacMaster, 2015).

3. When cognitive difficulties are present, give smaller bits of information and use some repetition, particularly by presenting the same thing in different ways or by giving specific examples. It can be helpful to use a behavioral approach in which you first demonstrate the behavior to be learned, then have the client practice during the session. This way you can offer suggestions and troubleshoot any difficulties the person is having with the new skill. Another suggestion is to break down goals into smaller concrete steps in the right direction. Asking questions to ensure that the person is actively processing the information and frequently reviewing the material are other ways to help clients who may have cognitive difficulties.

4. Empower clients within a broad perspective of helping them to self-manage their symptoms. Educating and involving the family, caregivers, and significant others is also important as a way to promote understanding of the symptoms and effects of mental illness, substance use, and the medications used in treatment. Such involvement and support for the family can also reduce their stress. Organizations like the National Alliance on Mental Illness (NAMI) offer support and outreach to family members affected by mental illness.

5. Mutual help groups can be an important adjunct to treatment. Particularly explore groups that are specifically designed for people with co-occurring conditions. Groups such as Double Trouble in Recovery (DTR) can provide greater acceptance, understanding, and support than may be encountered in addiction-focused groups (Bogenschutz et al., 2014). A

> What would "recovery" or a "good life" mean to this person?

significant benefit of DTR (as compared to traditional 12-step programs) is the increased understanding of the importance of managing psychological conditions through the use of pharmacotherapy. DTR groups tend to encourage clients to practice adherence to their medications. Participation in DTR groups can have both direct and indirect beneficial effects on several important components of recovery, including medication adherence, abstinence, and quality of life (Magura, 2008; Magura et al., 2008).

Medications in Treating Co-Occurring Conditions

Historically, some counselors or mutual help groups have been skeptical about or even opposed to the use of psychoactive medications in addiction recovery. This remains a controversial issue in addiction treatment, although views are changing. Opposition to the use of medications in addiction treatment arose in part from a confusion of therapeutic medications with "drugs of abuse." Indeed, there is some overlap in that some therapeutic medications can be and are misused, whereas others are not. In part there has also been a perception that people ought to be able to recover "on their own" without using chemicals. The same argument was not made regarding insulin for people with diabetes, or for medications to reduce blood pressure and cholesterol, but ambivalence has been greater about psychoactive medications, even among clients themselves.

There is a large difference between an unprescribed drug used to get high and a medication taken as directed to manage a diagnosed disorder, many of which have little potential for physical dependence or street value. Effective medications are available and are an important component of treatment for severe mental disorders including psychoses (such as schizophrenia), mood disorders (like major depression and bipolar disorder), and anxiety disorders (such as PTSD, panic disorder, and generalized anxiety disorder). It is, we believe, unethical to deny effective treatment options to people suffering from mental disorders because they also have a concomitant (or history of) SUD. Even if you are not the prescriber of such medication, it is important to have a working knowledge of the main classes of psychotropic medications, their uses, side effects, and possible interactions with illicit substances. An understanding of these medications will also help you know how to respond when a client expresses ambivalence about taking medication. You might, for instance, encounter a client who is upset after being criticized in a 12-step meeting for continuing to take medication such as an antidepressant. This is a situation where it is good to have a working knowledge of the main classes of psychotropic medications and understanding of the difference between drugs used to get high and those used to manage a mental disorder.

Antidepressants

Medications used to treat depression are known (sensibly) as antidepressants. Some examples are fluoxetine (trade name Prozac), sertraline (trade name Zoloft), mirtazapine (trade name Remeron), and amitriptyline (trade name Elavil). There are several major classes of antidepressant medications. For many years, tricyclics were the first-line agents used to treat depression and are still used in certain cases. Tricyclics (like amitriptyline, desipramine, and impramine), however, can produce anticholinergic side effects like dry mouth and abnormal heart rhythm, and can be extremely toxic with overdose. Selective serotonin reuptake inhibitors (SSRIs) are currently the preferred first choice to try in the treatment of depression with the notable exception that in individuals with opioid use disorders and depressive disorders, the evidence is stronger for the efficacy of tricyclics than for SSRIs (Brady & Verduin, 2005). SSRIs (like fluoxetine and sertraline) have fewer side effects, improving patient acceptance and compliance with treatment. Serotonin–norepinephrine reuptake inhibitors (SNRIs) like venlafaxine (trade name Effexor) and selective dopamine reuptake inhibitors (SDRIs) like bupropion (trade name Wellbutrin) are also commonly prescribed with concomitant mood disorders and addiction. Some possible side effects of SSRIs, SNRIs, and SDRIs are nausea, headaches, insomnia, and sexual dysfunction. Because monoamine oxidase inhibitors (MAOIs; like those with trade names Marplan, Nardil, and Parnate) can produce lethal reactions when combined with certain drugs or foods, they are usually used only for patients who do not respond to other antidepressant medications.

There is little professional controversy about the use of antidepressants for patients with co-occurring depression and addiction. Most antidepressants are relatively safe and there is no real potential for misuse of these medications. There have been some reports of antidepressants like SSRIs causing suicidal ideation. For patients who are using substances and prone to impulsive actions, this is something to monitor, especially with adolescents. Alcohol should be avoided by those taking antidepressants. The MAOIs uniquely can cause fatal interactions with certain foods (including cheese and chocolate), beer, and many prescription and illicit drugs. In all cases, patients taking antidepressants should be medically monitored.

Anxiolytics

Anxiolytics are medications used to treat disorders in which the prevailing symptom is anxiety. First-line pharmacological treatment of most anxiety disorders involves use of an SSRI, followed by an SNRI or a tricyclic.

For people with a history of SUDs, there have been good reasons for caution in the long-term use of benzodiazepines like chlordiazepoxide (trade name Librium) and diazepam (trade name Valium), particularly because of their similarity to alcohol (which is what makes them useful in managing alcohol withdrawal). Benzodiazepines can produce tolerance and dependence, particularly for people with a history of addiction. Alcohol and benzodiazepines show cross-tolerance and inhibit each other's metabolism so that their combined effects can be multiplied rather than additive.

Why, then, might benzodiazepines be prescribed for people with a history of addiction? The reason is their efficacy in managing concomitant anxiety disorders that persist or worsen in abstinence. They work well in alcohol withdrawal to prevent seizures, and have a low risk of inducing physical dependence when used over the short term. Benzodizepines are rarely a primary drug of choice; their misuse tends to be in combination with other drugs. There is a growing problem with the use of benzodiazepines and opioids in combination, increasing risk of death due to overdose. Best practice is to use benzodiazepines primarily for the short term, avoiding them for people with active use of other substances.

Stimulants

Stimulants, particularly methyphenidate (trade name Ritalin) are effective in treating attention-deficit/hyperactivity disorder (ADHD), which is a common co-occurring condition. Because stimulants have street value and are subject to misuse, there has been concern that using them to treat ADHD in youth and adults could increase the risk of developing SUDs. However, untreated ADHD is itself a risk factor for future SUDs. An alternative treatment is to start with a medication like buproprion (trade name Wellbutrin), guanfacine (trade name Tenex) and atomoxetine (trade name Straterra), which are efficacious treatments with decreased risk of inducing physical dependence. There are longer acting medications such as osmotic-release oral system (OROS)—methylphenidate and extended-release amphetamine salts if first-line approaches are not successful.

Antipsychotics

Antipsychotics are medications used to treat major mental and emotional disturbances such as psychoses. Typical antipsychotics like haloperidol have good efficacy, but do increase risk for enduring extrapyramidal side effects (EPS) and tardive dyskinesia, and may also intensify the rewarding properties of drugs (Samaha, 2014), which offers a reason to avoid these medications in people with schizophrenia and a concomitant SUD. More recent "atypical" antipsychotics (such as those with the trade names Geodon, Seroquel, and Abilify) also have good efficacy with lower risk of EPS and tardive dyskinesia, and are also being increasingly used to treat bipolar disorder and depression. There is no risk of addiction with these medications and no known significant interactions with alcohol or illicit drugs. Like all medications, however, the atypicals can have significant side effects including metabolic abnormalities like diabetes, weight gain, elevated cholesterol, and high blood pressure.

Mood Stabilizers

In general, the first-line pharmacotherapies for bipolar disorder are mood stabilizers, which include lithium (trade name Lithobid), valproate (trade name Depakote), and carbamazepine (trade name Tegretol). These medications are typically used to control symptoms of mania and hypomania. Lithium is the oldest, and must be monitored carefully because of its potential toxicity. Valproate and carbamazepine appear to be generally safer and at least as effective as lithium, but tend to have sedating effects, so patients taking these medications have to be careful with alcohol consumption. There is no risk of misuse of these medications and no known interactions with illicit drugs.

Medication Nonadherence

Low adherence to prescribed medication is a widespread challenge in medical practice that undermines treatment effectiveness (McDonald, Garg, & Haynes, 2002). Failure to take medications as prescribed is a frequent cause of recurrence of major mental disorders, and is also a problem in addiction treatment (as described in Chapter 18). Strict adherence is also vital in the treatment of infectious diseases that are more prevalent in addiction treatment populations, including TB, hepatitis, and HIV. People may dislike or fear side effects, believe that a medication is not working, or discontinue it when symptoms abate in the belief that it is no longer needed. As discussed earlier, some clients may believe (or be told) erroneously that any medication will endanger their recovery from addiction. Poor adherence can also arise from disorganization, inattention, or apathy related to the concomitant conditions.

There is much you can do to support medication adherence in your clients, even if you are not a medical professional yourself (see Chapters 8, 9, 18, and 21). Certainly, patients should be urged to stay in regular contact with their prescribing physician(s) to monitor progress and discuss any concerns. Involving supportive family members or SOs can improve medication adherence (see Chapters 15 and 16). Explore your clients' beliefs and concerns about medications they are taking, check in about and encourage adherence, and brainstorm ways to improve it. Direct communication and collaboration with the prescribing physician(s) are often appropriate.

A Closing Note of Optimism

Throughout this chapter we have been discussing the complexities of treating people with concomitant substance use and mental disorders. This is indeed a professionally challenging area, but we want to close with the note that the prognosis for successful treatment is *good*. In a 10-year prospective study of clients with severe and persistent mental illnesses and SUDs treated concomitantly (Xie, Drake, McHugo, Xie, & Mohandas, 2010), 86% had at least one 6-month remission period, and for those who achieved at least 6 months of abstinence, the average duration of continuous remission was 6 years. Remission from addiction was associated with better outcomes on employment, independent living, positive peer affiliations, and life satisfaction. As is the case with SUD treatment in general (Miller, Walters, et al., 2001), there were very large reductions in substance use and improvements in life functioning even among those who did not maintain perfect abstinence after treatment.

KEY POINTS

- Substance use and other psychological disorders commonly co-occur. Each one increases risk for the other.

- Simultaneous integrated treatment of addiction and a concomitant mental disorder is preferable. Treating one improves outcomes in treating the other.

- The effects of intoxication and drug withdrawal can mimic, trigger, or exacerbate other conditions.

- Prescribed medications can be both effective and appropriate in treating disorders that co-occur with addictions.

Reflection Questions

Q How comfortable and prepared are you to treat clients in each of the four quadrants (Box 20.3) described in this chapter?

Q Of the people you see in your daily work, what percentage would you estimate have an SUD as well as another psychological disorder?

Q How would you define "recovery" for people with co-occurring conditions?

CHAPTER 21

Facilitating Maintenance

He came to treatment reluctantly, under pressure from his wife who had threatened to leave him and take the children if he didn't seek help. He clearly met criteria for a moderate to severe alcohol use disorder. An initial assessment revealed some early neurocognitive and liver impairment, and he decided on abstinence as his goal, particularly to keep his family together. Because he was participating in a clinical trial, we obtained daily drinking data from 3 months before treatment through 15 months of follow-up. Prior to treatment he had been consuming 96 standard drinks per week on average. During week two of treatment he stopped drinking abruptly with no apparent withdrawal symptoms and remained abstinent until week 16 near the end of treatment, when he drank on two consecutive days (two and five standard drinks). He went back to abstaining again for 3 months, then had four drinking days in a row (total of 13 standard drinks), before returning to abstinence. During the remaining 7 months of follow-up he had a total of five more drinking days, with the heaviest being seven standard drinks, and at month 15 he had been abstinent for 4 months. In a clinical trial where outcomes are dichotomized as either abstinent or relapsed, his treatment was a failure. On the study's survival curve, he was classified as "relapsed" at week 16 even before treatment had ended, and remained so because a status change on a binary survival curve is irreversible. Yet even a cursory examination of his data shows that his drinking had changed dramatically (see Box 21.1). Compared to pretreatment levels, his alcohol use had decreased by 89% during treatment and by 96% during follow-up. By DSM criteria, he was in continuous remission from month 2 onward, with no remaining symptoms of alcohol use disorder. So was treatment a success or a failure?

331

BOX 21.1. Success or Failure?

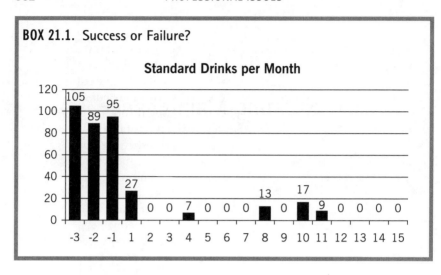

This mixed picture is a common scenario, even the norm in addiction treatment. In a summary of 12-month outcomes for 8,389 people treated for alcohol use disorders, only 24% had remained completely abstinent (Miller, Walters, et al., 2001). By binary standards that is a 76% failure rate. Yet for those who did not totally abstain, alcohol use had decreased by 87% on average, a dramatic and medically meaningful change. The 1-year death rate was 1.5%. Mortality can be higher with illicit drugs. In an opiate substitution treatment program, the comparable annual mortality figure was 3% (P. G. Barnett, Trafton, & Humphreys, 2010). For almost any chronic illness, 24% complete remission and an 87% reduction in symptoms for the rest would be regarded as remarkable success. This is not unique to alcohol use disorders. Per-year remission rates have been estimated at 22% for opioid dependence and 45% for amphetamine dependence (Calabria et al., 2010). If Box 21.1 were blood pressure levels of someone with hypertension, the patient would be congratulated for excellent adherence.

McLellan observed that addiction treatment has been held to a peculiar standard for success in comparison with other chronic behavior-related diseases (McLellan et al., 2000; McLellan, McKay, Forman, Cacciola, & Kemp, 2010). When the onset of a treatment (such as a medication) for a chronic illness results in a significant reduction in symptoms and clinical indicators (like blood pressure or glucose), and then discontinuation of treatment subsequently results in a return to pretreatment levels, that is classic evidence that the treatment *works*. The same pattern with addiction treatment is often regarded as a dismal failure.

Retiring "Relapse"

We believe that the term "relapse" has outlived its usefulness in addiction treatment. It implies, inaccurately, that there are only two possible outcomes: success or failure, perfection or disaster. This standard is not used in managing chronic illnesses. A hypoglycemic crisis may put someone with type 1 diabetes in the emergency room or hospital, but no one whispers that this person has "relapsed" or that treatment has failed, even if the crisis was a direct result of the person's own choices. In treating asthma, a remarkably successful outcome of diagnosis and treatment would be for the person to *never* have another asthma attack, but a more typical outcome of asthma management is fewer, less severe attacks spaced farther apart in time, so that the person lives a longer life with better quality, and ultimately dies of some other cause. In primary care, when someone being treated for hypertension has a high blood pressure reading, the term "relapse" is not likely to be found in case notes. Instead attention is focused on what adjustments need to be made in treatment and self-management.

> The term "relapse" has outlived its usefulness.

There is also a moralistic, pejorative connotation to the term "relapse." Relabeling substance use as a "relapse" adds nothing useful to the simple description of behavior (Maisto, Witkiewitz, Moskal, & Wilson, 2016), and it invokes potentially demoralizing overtones of shame, blame, and failure that are unlikely to inspire change. As discussed in Chapter 19, such dichotomous thinking can trigger the self-fulfilling prophecy that Marlatt termed the "rule violation effect" (Marlatt, Witkiewitz, & Donovan, 2005): Once a rule has been broken, all is lost. In a prospective treatment study, clients who endorsed a dichotomous disease model of alcoholism were significantly more likely to "relapse" even after other predictive factors (like severity) had been taken into account (Miller et al., 1996).

"Relapse" thinking can even be demoralizing for treatment staff. After any single episode of stabilization or rehabilitation, most people will use again, usually within the first few months after initial treatment. We create a needlessly (and inaccurately) gloomy public and professional impression of addiction treatment if any recurrence of prior symptoms constitutes failure. Imperfection is human nature (Kurtz & Ketcham, 1992). Who wants to work in a field with a 76% (or, in tobacco cessation, a 90%) failure rate? In contrast, when examining overall outcomes (not behavioral survival curves), the prognosis for recovery from SUDs is very good, comparing favorably with that for most chronic illnesses. One reason why we, the authors, have collectively spent more than a century in this field is that treatment outcomes are so good.

So our recommendation is to stop using the term "relapse" in relation to addiction treatment. Don't just search for euphemisms for the same thing.

Retrain your *thinking* about outcomes to correspond with the scientific data. Simply describe behavior: the person drank, the client used a drug, period. DSM-5 (American Psychiatric Association, 2013) included criteria for SUDs to be "in remission," defined as the absence of any symptoms (other than craving) for at least 3 months (early remission) or 12 months (sustained remission). The total absence of substance use is not required to classify a person as being in remission.

Rethinking Addiction Treatment

Although addiction is often described as a chronic condition, its treatment has not yet adjusted accordingly. Too often treatment has been thought of as a discrete event, a particular dose such as 21 days of residential care or 12 weeks of outpatient treatment that is sandwiched in between intake and discharge, as if one were treating an infection. Treatment for SUDs, like that for other chronic conditions, should begin with the very first contact (see Chapter 4) and continue with ongoing management to help people maintain their own changes and health. Within a good health care system, someone who presents with symptoms of a life-threatening condition like heart disease will receive immediate attention, but care does not end with that episode of treatment. To be effective, addiction treatment should follow a similar path. Needless to say, it doesn't make sense to terminate people from treatment for the same reason that you admitted them. Imagine if we "fired" patients from treatment for cancer, heart disease, diabetes, or asthma because their symptoms had returned! If addiction is a chronic condition, then we should treat it like one.

Understanding an illness as chronic does not absolve people of responsibility for their own health, of course. To the contrary, the successful management of chronic illness normally requires quite a lot from the patient. The course and outcomes of chronic disease are strongly related to the person's own health behavior: taking prescribed medications, managing diet and weight, keeping appointments. The same is true of health in general. Maintaining good health has much to do with lifestyle: diet, exercise, checkups, stress, and moderation.

Both addiction and recovery emerge over time within a person's ongoing life course. Typically, SUDs develop gradually, and it is common for their severity to wax and wane over a period of years. To be sure, there are fortunate individuals who have a sudden discrete, even mystical, experience that ends their substance use once and for all (Alcoholics Anonymous World Services, 2001; Forcehimes, 2004). For most people, however, recovery and sobriety involve successive changes over time, often with two

Addiction is a chronic condition; we should treat it like one.

steps forward and one step back (Hibbert & Best, 2011). Members of AA describe themselves as still recovering, not recovered, and sobriety as involving far more than abstinence (Dodge, Krantz, & Kenny, 2010). Although people tend not to seek treatment (if ever they do) until their problems are well developed, self-change efforts often begin much earlier and can extend over many years (Venner & Miller, 2001). It takes time to adjust one's life after having a heart attack or being diagnosed with diabetes. Recovery from addiction can similarly be a long and continuing journey. Smokers often have three or four serious quit attempts before they finally stop. Similarly, people with alcohol/drug problems often go through several episodes of treatment before stable remission. The dichotomous "success rate" of any particular treatment event is, therefore, much lower than the rate of eventual recovery from addiction, and specific treatment episodes are only a small part, timewise, of the recovery process. If addiction is truly like a chronic illness, then it is a mistake to quote success rates or wonder how many treatment episodes are required to "cure" it. Chronic illnesses are not cured by treatment episodes, but are managed over time to support the person's health and quality of life, and medical care is only a part of the picture. With such chronic conditions, long-term health has very much to do with motivation for and practice of self-care.

Phase 4 Treatment: Maintenance

In Chapter 7 we described four phases of addiction treatment: (1) palliative care, (2) stabilization, (3) rehabilitation, and (4) maintenance. Treatment is not over at the end of rehabilitation (Phase 3). The efficacy of residential rehabilitation, for example, is widely acknowledged to depend on whether people receive continuing outpatient care back home (once termed "aftercare"). In this sense, the initial phases of specialist treatment for stabilization and rehabilitation might be described as "forecare."

Helping people to experience an initial period of weeks or months of sobriety is an important first step toward maintenance. Within the transtheoretical model of change (Prochaska & Norcross, 2013), making the initial changes required to escape from SUDs is termed the *action stage*. That is not the whole story. Stopping smoking, drinking, or other drug use is not all that difficult to achieve in itself. Even for severely dependent people, withdrawal that was once an agonizing ordeal is now a reasonably straightforward process (see Chapter 6). The challenge in addiction, as with weight loss, is maintaining changes, and this may require significant changes in behavior and lifestyle.

Some preparation for maintenance can be done during the rehabilitation phase, paralleling a "pre-mortem" strategy in project management. A premortem analysis anticipates problems that could arise to disrupt recovery so that preventive steps can be taken. Sometimes alcohol or other drugs were being used as a way to cope with life problems that then persist into sobriety. In this case it can be important to help clients learn new coping strategies to replace substance use in these situations (Chapter 11). The "new roads" assessment presented in Chapter 14 is one way to anticipate and address these challenges. A variety of Phase 3 strategies have been tested to help clients avoid a return to problematic substance use during Phase 4 (Abbott et al., 2003; Marlatt & Donovan, 2005).

Follow Up

The maintenance phase itself is likely to be less intensive than stabilization or rehabilitation, and may resemble primary care: routine follow-up visits to review health status and adjust or intensify treatment as needed. Indeed, the maintenance phase of treatment might occur within primary health care. In a health maintenance system where patients return for various kinds of care on a regular basis, it's easy enough to ask, "How's it going with _____ ?"

Scheduling routine maintenance visits has been common practice in dentistry, eye care, chronic disease management, and automobile maintenance, but rarely in specialist addiction treatment systems except during clinical trials. Nevertheless, there are good reasons to consider building this into a continuum of care, to check back *routinely* and *proactively* on how people are doing. Because most people who resume drinking, smoking, or drug use do so within 3 months after initial treatment, one option is to check back routinely at 2 months and perhaps again at 4 months. These need not be long contacts, and they can even be done by telephone (McKay et al., 2010, 2011). We find that most people appreciate the continued concern and interest. We particularly noticed this in doing follow-up visits in our clinical trials. Even though people knew that we were seeing or calling them primarily to collect research follow-up data, they often perceived and appreciated it as continuing care. Scott and Dennis (2009) found in two randomized trials that adding quarterly "recovery management checkups" based on motivational interviewing was effective in reengaging clients in treatment when needed and significantly increased abstinent days across 2 years of follow-up. Emerging problems may be more easily remedied when they are detected and addressed early. This should be a reimbursable service just as it is in primary health care. Quarterly recovery management checkups have been found to be cost-effective in maintaining recovery with treated clients and released offenders over 2–4 years of follow-up (McCollister et al., 2013, 2014).

We also recommend taking a broader quality-of-life view in such follow-up visits. Don't just ask about substance use. People are more likely to maintain recovery if their new life of sobriety is just too good to give up. A brief happiness survey (Chapter 14) might be included in checkups.

Case management (Chapter 8) can be implemented to connect clients with needed community resources.

Staff morale is yet another good reason for routine follow-up visits. If you wait for clients to return or be brought to your attention, you are most likely to see only those who are in serious trouble. When you follow up everyone who has been treated, you get a clearer and encouraging picture of just how much better most clients are faring. On average they are healthier, happier, and enjoying better relationships. This is one of the joys we have experienced in addiction treatment research where we sought to interview everyone we had treated. You don't need subtle psychological instruments to detect the changes that people experience in recovery.

Many people do well during maintenance (Phase 4) with little or no additional help. There is no reason to require everyone to stay in active treatment for a certain period of time or to jump over a fixed number of hurdles. For some people, making the initial decision to quit and getting through the stabilization period (Phase 2) is sufficient. When asked how to have a successful addiction treatment program, the director of a prominent private rehabilitation center once quipped, "Be the place where people go once they have finally decided to quit." For some, Phase 3 treatment is sufficient, and for others it is not. Maintenance (Phase 4) should be a normal part of addiction treatment services.

Keep the Door Open

One general guideline for helping people in the maintenance phase after initial stabilization or rehabilitation is just to keep the door open. Don't communicate the message that treatment is over, the process finished, or that clients are now on their own. Neither do we recommend telling people that they may "relapse," or scaring them into additional treatment. A reasonable middle ground is to keep the door open and the light on, inviting them back whenever they want additional consultation. If you can schedule routine follow-up visits, all the better. A readily available visit or two may help clients stay in remission.

And is it really necessary to "discharge" clients and close cases? Some administrative structures may require it, but your dentist, eye doctor, and primary care provider don't normally close your file unless you die, move away, or change providers.

> Keep the door open and the light on, inviting them back whenever they want additional consultation.

Use the Client's Wisdom

Most people are reasonably good judges of their stability, a fact that is particularly evident in research on self-efficacy. If you ask clients how likely they are to still be a nonsmoker (or sober, or drug-free) 3 months from now, their probability estimate is a reasonably good predictor of that specific outcome. Estimates lower than 80% provide some reason for concern and further exploration. Short of routine follow-up visits, ask clients when they would like to check back.

Maintenance Strategies

What recovery support services make a difference (Humphreys & McLellan, 2011)? Sometimes the skills and strategies needed for successful maintenance are different from those that worked to get stabilized and sober in the first place. Fortunately, many of the tools needed in Phase 4 have already been discussed in prior chapters. Here are some general maintenance strategies.

Self-Help Materials

Something as simple as self-help materials can support continuing recovery. One review found that abstinent smokers were half again as likely to remain abstinent when provided with self-help resources, as compared with unaided quitters (Agboola, McNeill, Coleman, & Leonardi Bee, 2010). "Bibliotherapy" has also been evaluated in treating alcohol use disorders (Apodaca & Miller, 2003). Drinkers randomly assigned at the end of treatment to receive a self-help book (Miller & Muñoz, 2013) continued to reduce their alcohol use by half during 12 weeks of follow-up, whereas those receiving the same behavioral treatment but no self-help materials simply maintained their posttreatment level of drinking (Miller, 1978).

As a clinical tool, interactive journaling extends bibliotherapy by offering readers frequent structured opportunities to respond to and integrate material being presented (Miller, 2014). In one randomized trial, providing substance-dependent offenders with an interactive journal prior to release from jail significantly reduced recidivism rate by 15 percentage points (Proctor et al., 2012).

> Something as simple as self-help materials can support continuing recovery.

Mutual Help Groups

A good resource for maintenance is the mutual help groups that can be found in many communities (see Chapter 17). Encourage people to try out available groups as a source of ongoing support during the maintenance phase. How many meetings should a client attend? People who stick with AA after treatment tend to be those who attended at least two meetings a week during Phase 3 treatment (Tonigan, 2003). That is far fewer than the "90 meetings in 90 days" sometimes recommended or even mandated. Here again the client's own wisdom is a good resource, and ultimately people settle into their own patterns of involvement.

Maintenance Medications

Some medications are designed specifically to help people avoid their previously preferred drugs over the short or longer term (see Chapter 18). Disulfiram, methadone, buprenorphine, naltrexone, bupriprion, and nicotine replacement are all examples (Taylor, Leonardi-Bee, Agboola, McNeill, & Coleman, 2011). One general strategy is to transfer the patient from his or her previously preferred drug to the maintenance medication (a common approach in withdrawal management), then gradually taper the dose over time. A second strategy is long-term maintenance on the medication. Agonist (substitute) medications are also generally addictive, but offer important advantages in terms of their pharmacological properties. Some medications, for example, have a longer half-life and avoid the rapid high followed by an abrupt crash. Also, unlike street drugs, the content and dose are known, decreasing risk of overdose. Antidipsotropics like disulfiram can be maintained at a protective dosage over time, or taken in anticipation of high-risk situations.

Case Management and Continuing Care

Besides mutual help groups and medications, what kinds of services can be helpful in maintaining sobriety? We do not recommend any standardized set of services here. Instead we suggest a flexible menu of options from which clients can choose on the basis of their needs and preferences. In one public treatment system we literally presented such a menu to the people we served, empowering them to choose the options that met their needs. Helping clients to address the particular problems they face can aid maintenance of treatment gains (McLellan et al., 1997, 1998).

The perspective of case management (Chapter 8) continues to be of value in Phase 4 maintenance. People with SUDs often have a broader range of social, legal, financial, health, and spiritual issues to deal with and can benefit from services far beyond those that directly address addiction. It can be useful to survey the range of services that clients may need and to develop a plan for accessing these in order of priority.

Self-Monitoring

Another strategy is to use self-monitoring as an early warning system. Keeping a daily record, particularly for the first few months of sobriety, can alert the client to emerging concerns before they turn into renewed substance use problems. Within a community reinforcement approach (Chapter 14), for example, a general goal is for the person to be happy in sobriety, and simple daily mood monitoring on a 1–10 scale has been used to watch for slippage that could signal a drift toward renewed problems. You might instruct the client to call you if mood ratings fall below a certain point for 2 days in a row. Another obvious target for daily monitoring would be cravings or urges (see Chapters 6 and 11). For clients seeking to maintain moderate drinking, daily monitoring of alcohol use should be continued for a few months after Phase 3 treatment (see Chapter 11). This parallels the common method of keeping detailed food diaries as part of a weight loss program. The essential strategy here is to keep track of anything that could signal a drift toward prior patterns of substance use and to take steps early to head off problems.

Dealing with Old and New Problems

Some problems do abate with sobriety. Others such as chronic pain may continue or even worsen (Witkiewitz et al., 2015). Without alcohol or other drugs on board, the symptoms of PTSD may return with a vengeance, and mood disorders may become more apparent or severe. The financial, legal, family, social, employment, educational, and medical consequences of prior use can come home to roost during recovery. Conventional AA wisdom likens this to the inertia of a train wreck: after the locomotive has come to an abrupt stop, the boxcars continue to hit for some time thereafter.

Part of the challenge here is treating other disorders that have coexisted with addiction. As discussed in Chapter 20, this may be best done concomitantly with addiction treatment. However, some disorders are difficult to recognize or address while the person is still using. Addressing these in an effective and timely manner during Phase 4 can diminish the risk of resumed substance use. Here is yet another good reason for routine follow-up visits.

KEY POINTS

🔖 Resumed use is common following addiction treatment and need not be characterized pejoratively as a "relapse." Even among people who do not maintain perfect abstinence from alcohol, posttreatment drinking is normally reduced by 87% on average.

🔖 During maintenance (Phase 4 treatment), people can be offered strategies to retain the good changes they have made, which may be different from what helped them initially.

🔖 Recurrence of substance use and problems is a reason to resume or intensify treatment, not withdraw it.

🔖 Maintain follow-up contact with people who have been under your care and keep the door open for ongoing consultation.

Reflection Questions

Q Think about a change you have made and then maintained. What have you done to maintain it?

Q How could you arrange to make routine follow-up calls or checkup visits with people who have completed Phase 3 treatment?

Q What are your personal reactions when someone you have treated resumes substance use?

CHAPTER 22

Working with Groups

Could bringing people together to learn from each other also help them to change? A physician named Joseph Pratt asked this question in 1905, bringing together 15 tuberculosis patients to educate them about their disease and allow them to discuss their shared experience. Pratt reported positive results from this form of treatment, and soon thereafter group therapy began to grow in popularity (Rutan, Stone, & Shay, 2014). The addiction field was an early adopter of group therapy, which became one of the first formal treatments for alcohol use disorders (Voegtlin & Lemere, 1942). Its popularity has remained over the years, and group therapy continues to be the most common form of treatment for alcohol and other drug problems in both inpatient and outpatient treatment settings (Burlingame et al., 2016; Wendt & Gone, 2017, 2018).

In Chapter 17 we discussed mutual help groups such as AA. In this chapter we turn to group treatment led by a therapist. Group therapy is not itself a kind of treatment, but simply a context in which to deliver particular treatment methods with two or more unrelated individuals at the same time. Group therapy can also be done with couples or families, but in this chapter our primary focus is on groups of unrelated individuals.

The Rationale for Group Treatment

Cost-effectiveness is one obvious potential advantage of group treatment, allowing health care professionals to work with a group of people simultaneously rather than individually. This permits more efficient use of professional time and can decrease individual cost per session. Another practical advantage is the decreased impact of individual no-shows because the group continues and the professional's time is thus occupied. Given these advantages, if group and individual therapy have comparable outcomes, group delivery would be more cost-effective.

In addition to potential economic advantages, group therapy allows clients to benefit from each other's experiences, and certain types of treatment such as social skills training (Chapter 11) may be particularly appropriate for group formats. Furthermore, there are aspects of addiction that may render group therapy advantageous. It is common for people with alcohol/drug problems to feel and be disconnected from others. As addiction progresses there is a tendency to detach from important relationships and activities. In AA, a familiar term is "terminal uniqueness," describing someone's perception of extreme alienation and separateness from peers. If addiction involves isolation from others, it seems intuitive that a group therapeutic approach may offer a foundation for relatedness.

There are some potentially powerful healing forces that are unique to group therapy. A group can foster feelings of community, encouragement, mutual hope and optimism, and a sense of commonality and belonging. People who are averse to authority may find it easier to receive information and feedback from peers than from a therapist. One of the underpinnings of 12-step programs (Chapter 17) is that members benefit from interacting with others who have had similar experiences. The process of cooperating and being useful to others also facilitates the transition from being dependent to being dependable and helping others.

Research on the Effectiveness of Group Therapies

The fact that a treatment approach is practical, economical, and popular does not mean that it's effective. With such widespread use in addiction treatment—according to recent surveys, group therapy is offered at over 90% of SUD treatment facilities (SAMHSA Office of Applied Studies, 2010)—it is surprising that group therapy is far less studied than individual approaches (Wendt & Gone, 2017, 2018). This is due in part to some unique methodological challenges in evaluating group treatment. In clinical trials with closed groups, for example, researchers must recruit enough participants to fill groups before they begin, which can delay the start of treatment and thus endanger retention. If open groups are used, the constantly evolving membership imposes significant challenges in treatment and in interpretation of findings (as discussed later in this chapter). Another difficulty is that the interdependence of group members makes data analytic approaches more challenging. For instance, imagine how the presence of one highly disruptive group member might change the dynamics of a whole group, affecting others' participation, retention, and outcomes. Such factors make it more difficult to determine the efficacy of group therapies and the factors that influence outcomes.

Nevertheless, there is a growing body of clinical research to help guide evidence-based practice in group therapy. It is apparent that all group therapies are not equally effective, and as with individual treatment for addiction (Miller & Moyers, 2015), there is a growing literature on the importance of therapist factors in group treatment. The person who provides group treatment—specifically what they do during facilitation of the group—makes a difference (Crits-Christoph, Johnson, Connolly Gibbons, & Gallop, 2013).

Evidence on Specific Group Therapies

Over the years a wide variety of group psychotherapies have been tried in the treatment of addictions, including psychodynamic (Khantzian, Halliday, & McAuliffe, 1990), confrontational (Yablonsky, 1965, 1989), educational/didactic and client-centered (Ends & Page, 1957), gestalt (Browne-Miller, 1993; Brownell, 2012), group process (Yalom & Leszcz, 2008), interpersonal (Weissman, Markowitz, & Klerman, 2000), cognitive (Beck et al., 2001), motivational (D'Amico et al., 2015; Santa Ana, LaRowe, Armeson, Lamb, & Hartwell, 2016; Velasquez, Maurer, Crouch, & Diclemente, 2001; Wagner & Ingersoll, 2013), and behavioral (Epstein & McCrady, 2009; Kouimtsidis, Reynolds, Drummond, Davis, & Tarrier, 2007; Petry, Weinstock, & Alessi, 2011). There is also wide variability in the evidence base for these various approaches. Some have fairly solid evidence of efficacy. Others have been well supported when delivered as individual therapy, but have not yet been properly evaluated in group format. Still others have little evidence of efficacy in any delivery format (Miller & Wilbourne, 2002; Miller, Wilbourne, et al., 2003).

One long-standing approach is the didactic group using educational lectures and films to convey information such as the harmful short-term and long-term effects of substance use. In a review of 381 clinical trials of alcohol treatment efficacy (Miller, Wilbourne, et al., 2003), such educational approaches were found to be the *least* effective of the 48 treatment methods studied. Of 39 published trials, 34 showed no beneficial effects. Similarly, insight-oriented psychotherapy ranked 46th, and all published studies were negative for both confrontational counseling and process group therapy.

Why would so many studies find no benefit, or occasionally worse outcomes, with therapies that are intended to provide knowledge, insight, or confrontation? One possibility is that addiction is not attributable to a lack of knowledge, insight, or contact with reality. Another is that any benefit of relatively weak treatment methods may be overridden by the effects of exposure to others acting in a similarly unhealthy or destructive manner

(Roback, 2000). Particular concern has been raised about the potentially adverse effects of exposing adolescents to deviant peers in a group format (Dishion, McCord, & Poulin, 1999). Although meta-analytic reviews suggest that peer influences outside treatment are much more significant than within-group influences (Weiss et al., 2005), it is still important to understand that negative peer influences are a risk inherent in the group format, particularly if the treatment being offered is relatively weak.

So what does work? Thus far the most strongly supported group therapy for addiction focuses on teaching cognitive-behavioral coping skills to promote drug-free life quality (Carroll & Rounsaville, 2006). Studies of such behavioral skill training report outcomes from group formats to be at least as good as those from individual behavior therapy (Graham, Annis, Brett, & Venesoen, 1996; Marques & Formigoni, 2001; Miller & Taylor, 1980). Indeed, some studies report better outcomes from group formats when compared to individual behavioral therapy (Burlingame et al., 2016). McKay et al. (1997), for example, found that individuals treated in groups had higher rates of abstinence at 6 months than those treated individually. Individual and group therapies may exert different and additive effects. In a national collaborative trial, individual plus group drug counseling was superior to two forms of psychotherapy and to group counseling alone in reducing cocaine use over a year of follow-up (Crits-Christoph et al., 1999). Cognitive-behavioral groups seem to reduce the intensity of resumed drinking or drug use and appear to be most effective for those with more severe substance use, greater levels of negative affect, and greater perceived deficits in coping skills (Carroll, 1996). Given this level of empirical support, we offer some guidance about cognitive-behavioral group therapy later in this chapter.

There is now also good evidence that motivational interviewing (MI) can be delivered effectively in a group format for both adults (Shorey, Martino, Lamb, LaRowe, & Santa Ana, 2015; Velasquez, Stephens, & Ingersoll, 2006; Wagner & Ingersoll, 2013) and adolescents (D'Amico et al., 2015; D'Amico, Osilla, & Hunter, 2010; Feldstein Ewing, Walters, & Baer, 2013; Naar-King & Suarez, 2011) to reduce substance use and related consequences. Treatment process research supports the importance of change talk in MI outcomes (see Chapter 10), and a group setting may provide an opportunity for synergistic effects of change talk among participants (D'Amico et al., 2015; Shorey et al., 2015), an issue discussed later in this chapter.

In between well-supported cognitive-behavioral and MI groups and the less effective methods mentioned earlier is an intermediate set of group approaches. These are methods that have been reasonably well supported as individual therapies but less is known about their efficacy in a group format. In each case there has been some research on group treatment, but not enough evidence yet to be confident that they work reliably in group contexts. Nevertheless, it is encouraging that they are effective in individual format, and that research more generally suggests similar outcomes from group and individual therapies. These include interpersonal (Weissman et al., 2000), 12-step facilitation (Crits-Christoph et al., 1999; Nowinski, 2003), and behavioral couple therapy (McCrady & Epstein, 2008; O'Farrell & Fals-Stewart, 2006).

Practical Decisions

Having considered the evidence base for various group approaches, we turn now to a discussion of some decisions that must be made when treating groups regardless of the method bring used. There are quite a few such decisions to be made with any group, and the choices that you make do matter. How many people will be in the group? Can people join along the way? Is it acceptable for people in the same group to be working toward different goals? These are some of the questions we discuss in this section. Some group therapy approaches have specific guidelines for these decisions, whereas others may be determined by your own agency or personal preference. In any event, it is helpful to think these issues through before you begin a group.

Duration and Frequency of Treatment

Research indicates that most client improvement as a result of group therapy occurs within a relatively brief period of about 2–3 months (Garvin, Reid, & Epstein, 1976). There may also be managed care or treatment program guidelines that determine the length of treatment. In the United States, for example, most outpatient treatment programs provide 8–20 sessions and most inpatient programs are limited to 2–4 weeks. The number of sessions per week is also usually determined by program goals and constraints. It may, for instance, be feasible to have sessions multiple times per week for people in residential or intensive outpatient treatment, whereas a once-per-week format may be more feasible for employed people in outpatient treatment. Depending on the content covered in the group, sessions might last between 45 and 120 minutes. A shorter length is common for cognitive-behavioral groups, whereas longer sessions might be more appropriate for a process group.

Where Groups Are Held

Accessibility is an important element for outpatient groups. A place that is difficult to find and is logistically complicated (e.g., lack of easy parking or public transportation) creates challenges for clients and can decrease their eagerness to attend the sessions. Ensuring that the location is safe is another important consideration. What is the neighborhood like? Are group members safe walking to and from the group? A telephone should be available for emergencies.

Group Size

Groups can range from two people to a large audience attending a didactic group. Skill training groups should be sized so that members can practice the skills they are learning and group members can receive adequate attention and feedback from the facilitator. With the presence of a co-facilitator, the group size may be somewhat larger.

Leaders

A group can be led by one individual, co-led by two facilitators, or led by one primary facilitator with the presence of a secondary facilitator. Some research suggests that members of co-facilitated groups may experience greater benefits than those with individual leaders, perhaps because of the complexities of following multiple interactions (Kivlighan et al., 2015). Two leaders are able to provide different social role models and can share in problem solving during challenging sessions. An added benefit is that co-leadership allows for the group to meet even when one leader is unavailable. A co-facilitator can also provide immediate support for an individual in crisis while the other leader continues the group.

Treatment Goals

Another issue is whether individual treatment goals within the group must be homogeneous. Suppose, for example, that clients are at different levels of motivation for change. Should you form groups of people with similar readiness (e.g., contemplation vs. action stage groups) or is it better to have heterogeneity? Those who are at earlier stages of readiness or recovery may benefit from interacting with others who are farther along. Such a mixed membership also removes the need for clients to switch groups as they progress. On the other hand, the differing needs and interests of people at varying stages can be frustrating, particularly for clients who are farther along. There are similar issues in deciding whether a group focuses only on one particular problem (such as substance use) or addresses a broader range of life concerns.

Clients also vary with regard to their goals regarding substance use (e.g., Lozano, Stephens, & Roffman, 2006). Some choose total abstinence as their immediate and lifetime goal. Others are initially willing to reduce their use or to choose less risky drugs or routes of administration, but do not accept lifelong abstinence as their immediate goal (Logan & Marlatt, 2010; Tatarsky & Marlatt, 2010). Furthermore, clients may have different goals for different drugs; for example, abstinence from heroin, mainte-nance on methadone, and reduction in alcohol use (Abellanas & McLellan, 1993). Does a therapy group encompass people with such differing goals? Some programs, by virtue of their treatment philosophy or clientele (e.g., probation), accept only total abstinence from alcohol and all illicit drugs as a treatment objective. Other programs seek to serve a broader spectrum of clients and work with harm-reduction goals for those who choose not to abstain. In the latter case, you need to decide whether to construct groups that have homogeneous or heterogeneous individual goals. Homogeneous groups may increase focus and diminish discomfort or confusion related to differing goals. Heterogeneous groups allow people to learn from each other and remove the need to switch groups if treatment goals change.

Physical Contact

What are the standards about touch within the group? Some people find a hug or a hand on a shoulder to be comforting during a difficult discussion or at the end of the session. Personal histories and cultural backgrounds can also contribute to very different interpretations of what touch means. Though physical violence is explicitly prohibited, the group should discuss feelings related to physical contact and establish group rules related to appropriate and inappropriate touch within the group.

Contact Outside of the Group

Development of intimate relationships between members of ongoing ther-apy groups is generally discouraged if not prohibited. In some models of group therapy, any personal contact outside of the group is discouraged. This is another decision for you as a group leader: whether to encourage supportive networks among group members, discourage them, or take a neutral stance. Whatever you decide, of course, group members may still choose to communicate outside the group.

Open versus Closed Groups

With open or revolving group membership, people enter whenever they are ready for the clinical interventions provided in the group. Revolving mem-bership groups are frequently found in short-term residential treatment pro-grams because as people are admitted and discharged, the membership of the group changes. In closed-enrollment groups, by contrast, all members are enrolled before the group begins and membership remains constant.

　　There are pros and cons to both closed and open groups. In open-enrollment groups, members are permitted to begin treatment at differ-ent times. An open-group format removes the need for a waiting list and also decreases problems due to attrition. A practical problem with open groups is that new people may enter at each meeting so that membership is constantly changing, which can affect group dynamics and trust. If the group has a structured cycle of content, people are also entering that cycle at different points, and it is thus difficult to build on content from one meeting to the next. Closed enrollment minimizes the disruptive effects of changing group membership, capitalizes on group cohesion, and permits a developmental sequence within the group. Attrition is common in addiction treatment, however, so membership in a closed group can wane over time. A closed format also requires new clients to wait until a new group is formed. Both of these problems can be alleviated by periodically admitting new members to an otherwise closed group.

Time-Limited versus Ongoing Groups

A further decision regards time-limited versus ongoing groups. Time-limited groups meet for a predetermined number of sessions, whereas ongoing groups typically continue within the structure of a treatment program and offer people access for an indefinite period. Time-limited groups are particularly appropriate when there is a certain amount of content to be covered. (Remember, though, that educational/didactic lectures generally have very little impact on outcome.)

Therapist Self-Disclosure

How much should therapists reveal about themselves within group therapy? Individual styles vary, ranging from little or no self-disclosure (as is common within a psychodynamic framework) to a high level of spontaneous participation (as in a humanistic or encounter group). Our rule of thumb is to use a level of personal disclosure that will facilitate the work of the group at that moment in time. Rachman (1990) distinguished between judicious self-disclosures (appropriate level of detail, focus remains on the client) and excessive self-disclosures (those that shift the focus to the therapist). There is also a distinction between revealing things about your own *past history* (such as telling a story from your own life or recovery) and sharing your immediate reactions to clients or observations about group process *in the present moment*. In general, have a clear, conscious, strategic reason for whatever self-disclosure you offer.

Talking Rules

Each group has formal or informal rules about who may talk when. In a didactic group, for example, participants might raise a hand to indicate when they want to ask a question or make a comment. Some groups have a formal turn-taking process, such as going around so that each participant has a chance to talk (or pass). Others use a "talking stick" that is passed from person to person (not necessarily in a fixed order) that designates the holder as the only person who has the floor. The most open format allows anyone to talk at any time. While participation might intuitively seem important as a way to engage and benefit from the group, self-disclosure and degree of participation in the group are actually unrelated to the degree of one's benefit from group treatment, so people should not feel pressured (Crits-Christoph et al., 2013).

Groups also have formal or informal rules about what members are to say, and how to say it. One such issue is "cross-talk"—whether members may comment on (criticize, agree or disagree, correct, suggest, confront, etc.) what another member has said. Cross-talk is discouraged in most 12-step groups, where members are expected to focus on their own experience. In some types of groups, however, cross-talk can be an important part of therapy. Group members may have suggestions for how a person might make a change, or see a connection between someone's current comment or dilemma and another area in which the person has been successful. A potential downside of cross-talk is the tendency for people to get off the subject or interrupt other group members to insert their own feelings/thoughts about an issue. Group members should be generally encouraged to talk in ways that are not critical, demeaning, or confronting.

In certain types of group therapy, particularly in ongoing or closed groups, members may be taught certain ways of responding to one another. In an MI or other person-centered group, for example, the therapist may respond primarily with "OARS" (Chapter 4): Open questions, Affirmations, Reflections, and Summaries. Clients can also learn to respond to each other in these same basic ways, and of course these skills can carry over into everyday relationships.

Diversity

A further important consideration is the extent to which a group should be homogeneous or heterogeneous on certain characteristics, such as gender. Women may fare better and be more likely to stay in same-sex groups than in mixed-gender groups, whereas men appear to do equally well in mixed or all-male groups (Stevens, Arbiter, & Glider, 1989). This may be related to common barriers that women may face in engaging and remaining in treatment, such as child care, safety issues, and greater stigma. Another possible reason why women may have better outcomes in same-gender groups is the high co-occurrence of substance use and traumatic events among women (Greenfield, Cummings, Kuper, Wigderson, & Koro-Ljungberg, 2013; Simpson & Miller, 2002). Because most perpetrators are male, women are often more willing to disclose and discuss their victimization (and its relation to substance use) in same-gender groups. Women may also generally defer and talk less in mixed-gender groups where men tend to dominate the conversation. In a randomized trial, women with alcohol use disorders showed equally good outcomes in individual or all-female group cognitive-behavioral therapy (Epstein et al., 2018).

Another diversity issue has to do with race, ethnicity, and culture. Some professionals believe that it's better for all members of a group including the facilitator(s) to be from the same or similar ethnic–cultural background. Certainly, language is important in clear communication, but beyond this there is little evidence that therapists have better outcome with clients of the same cultural background, or that racial–ethnic uniformity improves group outcomes (Salvendy, 1999). People with the same skin tone or socioeconomic background are still quite diverse in other ways. For this reason, a client-centered approach (see Chapter 4) is useful, regarding each person as unique and the expert on his or her own life. In determining the outcomes of the group and its members, the overall spirit of the interaction (openness, respect, autonomy) is far more important than a priori matching on client characteristics (Brooks, 1998).

Nevertheless, it is important to be sensitive to people who differ from the majority of group participants in some way. One example of cultural differences may be the concept of time. In Native American culture, for example, there is a tendency to have a relaxed attitude about time. How will you work with people who are late to groups? How might you find ways to accommodate traditions such as socializing or rituals involving food, music, or prayer? Think and ask about ways in which others' backgrounds or experiences may influence their participation in the group and affect the group dynamic. For example, people approach issues like anger and assertiveness in very different ways depending on their cultural background and individual experiences.

As discussed earlier, one more issue for group uniformity or diversity is readiness for change. Some groups have been designed specifically for clients at an early stage of change (e.g., precontemplation or contemplation; Velasquez et al., 2013). Should stage of change be a factor determining group placement? There are some advantages and disadvantages in trying to structure a group in this way. Having group members who are all at a similar stage of change (e.g., precontemplation or contemplation) allows you to focus on the issues appropriate to that stage (e.g., ambivalence). On the other hand, homogeneity at the precontemplation level could foster group alliances to resist change. It is also important to keep in mind that people may move back and forth among the stages of readiness, even within a single therapy session (Rollnick, 1998).

Intoxication

Most providers and programs do not permit clients to participate in a group session if they are visibly under the influence of alcohol or another drug. Certainly, coming to treatment intoxicated can interfere with the individual's and group's ability to benefit. A possible policy here is that the person may not attend group when intoxicated, but can come back or make up the session when sober. If someone comes to the group under the influence of alcohol or drugs, the person should be asked in a nonjudgmental manner to leave and to return for the next session in a condition appropriate for participation.

It is important to have clear standards for how intoxication is determined to avoid arguments about whether or not the person is under the influence. For alcohol, an on-the-spot breath test is feasible, and instant urine test cups for multiple drug classes are also available. The final criterion, however, is your own judgment as the group leader. You can announce this procedure in advance, with apologies for any "false positive" errors you may make.

It is also important to ensure an intoxicated individual's safety by helping the group member to find a safe way home (see Chapter 19). Coordinate backup assistance with other providers, a co-facilitator, or support staff in your agency should this occur, to minimize disruption within the group. Having a brief discussion regarding feelings and thoughts that this situation triggered for group participants is an appropriate focus for a small portion of the session.

Discord

Responding effectively to discord is an important skill in doing group therapy. The discussion in Chapter 19 regarding responding to "resistance" is pertinent here, paralleling processes that occur in individual therapy.

> Discord may appear as anger, interrupting, defensiveness, arguing, ignoring, shutting down, or even leaving the room.

Because discord is interpersonal, the opportunities for it to arise are multiplied in group therapy. Remember that discord occurs in response to communications from you or other group participants. It may appear as anger, interrupting, defensiveness, arguing, ignoring, shutting down, or even leaving the room. Such client behaviors do predict poorer treatment outcome if not handled appropriately, and so it is important to respond effectively without strengthening or further increasing disharmony.

It is normal for alliances to develop among clients within groups, and they can be beneficial as mutual support. A group leader does need skill, however, for managing alliances that work against change, as when some group members join in opposition to you or each other. Beyond the methods described in Chapter 4, one group dynamic strategy is to comment in a nonconfrontational way on this alliance, validate the concerns, and shift to a problem-solving focus (Rosenberg, 2015)—for example:

> "John commented that he isn't feeling understood and then Sam and Bill said they were feeling the same way. The three of you seem pretty

discouraged, and I want to be sure that you feel heard here. How could we be communicating and listening better? What ideas do you have?"

A different problem is presented when group members respond to each other in unhelpful ways and thus elicit defensiveness. It can feel like a tug-of-war if you are using an empathic style that seems to be overshadowed by confrontational comments made by other group participants. Prohibiting cross-talk is one way to prevent this behavior. Another strategy is to teach group members specific nonviolent ways of communicating with other group members (see Chapter 4; Rosenberg, 2015). We will offer other ideas from an MI-based approach to group therapy later on in this chapter.

Let clients know the decisions you have made about the above issues. On some issues you may prefer to have the group make a decision. Some additional practical considerations are shown in the checklist in Box 22.1.

Getting the Group Started

Once you have thought about these practical details and you have a plan for the size, length, membership, and nature of the group, it remains to decide how people will be screened, admitted, and oriented to the group. If you work within an agency, there are probably procedures already in place for connecting individuals with treatment options, and we offer here some general considerations for integrating clients into a group.

Pregroup Interview

We recommend that you, as group leader, meet individually at least once with each prospective group member prior to his or her entry to the group. This allows you to introduce yourself, get to know a bit about the person, and provide information about the purpose and rules of the group. A general question to consider together is whether this group is a good fit for this person's needs and goals. The individual pregroup interview is also an opportunity to strengthen motivation for change (Chapter 10). It is useful to ask about any prior experiences with group therapy and the person's hopes and concerns about participation in the group. There are some practical issues to troubleshoot at this point as well. Does the meeting time and place of the group conflict with other responsibilities? Are there transportation problems or other obstacles to participation? You are also evaluating how this person is likely to function in and benefit from a group format in general. Some characteristics of people who may be a less-good fit with group therapy include:

- Refusal or lack of interest in the group.
- Strong personal discomfort in groups.

BOX 22.1. Group Structure Checklist

How often will the group meet?

How long will group meetings last?

Will membership be open or closed?

How will clients be screened, admitted, and oriented to the group?

If an open group, how will new members be introduced and integrated?

Will the group be of predetermined length (number of sessions) or ongoing?

Will there be a fixed sequence of topics to be covered?

Will meetings be held in a safe and accessible location?

How large will the group be (number of participants)?

Who will be the group leader(s)?

Will membership be homogeneous or heterogeneous with regard to:

Gender?

Stage of readiness?

Treatment goals?

Other client characteristics?

What is not allowed (weapons, drugs, violence, etc.) in the group?

What will be the norms and rules with regard to:

Arriving on time (or late)?

Privacy and confidentiality?

Use of cell phones?

Missed sessions?

Physical touch?

Contact outside of group sessions?

Talking (e.g., raise hand, turn taking, no restrictions)?

Reasons for termination from the group?

How will you handle:

Self-disclosure?

Discord?

Cross-talk?

A member coming to group intoxicated?

What will the leader(s) be required to report (to courts, threats, child abuse, etc.)?

- Severe impulse or anger control problems.
- Unwillingness to respect group rules, including confidentiality.
- Suicidal or in acute crisis.
- Language or hearing issues that would make it difficult to follow the conversation.
- Youth who may be adversely influenced by group contact with deviant peers.

If the group format isn't a good fit, what other options are available to the person? If the person is unsure about his or her willingness or desire to be in a group format, ask open questions followed by reflective listening statements (Chapter 4) to understand this person's situation and consider whether this is a good fit for both the individual and the group.

Admission to the Group

If this is a closed group and all participants are starting at the same time, you can introduce and orient everyone in the first meeting. When new members join an ongoing group, consider how they will be introduced to the group. Will you simply introduce them by first name and ask the group to welcome them? Do new participants tell a bit about their story? Do all members of the group introduce themselves to a new person in some way? Perhaps each person would say how long they have been in the group and what they have gained from it thus far. In your individual pregroup interview, you can explain these group entry procedures and expectations.

Orientation

Each participant needs to be oriented to the group. When all members are beginning a closed group together, this is done in the first session. With open groups, however, each new member needs an orientation before entry. Typically, you won't want to take up much group time to do this for every new member, so most of it is accomplished in the individual pregroup interview.

One element of orientation is to explain the practical aspects of the group, in essence the decisions that you have made about the issues discussed in the preceding section of this chapter. You may prepare a written group agreement that states the group rules and conditions, for each member to sign prior to or at the beginning (essentially an informed consent to treatment). The rules contained in such an agreement should be clearly stated, particularly with regard to any specific consequences of violations. The content of this agreement is informed by agency policy, applicable laws, and appropriate legal counsel. Some leaders develop the group agreement through a collaborative approach, allowing group members to contribute to its creation, which may increase adherence as members work toward consensus (Yalom & Leszcz, 2008).

The ethical standards that apply to individual therapy also apply to group therapy (see Chapter 24). Though these legal and professional requirements are familiar to you, group members may be unaware of these standards and would benefit from a discussion of what information about them might be shared, under what circumstances, and why. One ethical issue particularly important to the group setting is confidentiality. Members should be admonished not to discuss anything outside of the group that might reveal the identity of other members. Group members will hear private information shared by others, and in order to facilitate an atmosphere of trust, group members need to feel safe enough to disclose their feelings and problems. Other legal requirements that are important to explain include the necessity of reporting instances of child or domestic abuse and taking action when people threaten to harm themselves or others. There may also be specific requirements related to reporting missed sessions or premature termination for people who are mandated to treatment.

Termination

There are generally three ways in which clients terminate their participation in group therapy. The first and happiest is successful completion of the group. The second is premature termination, when a client unilaterally decides to drop out of treatment or simply stops coming. The third is a decision to terminate for cause, either unilaterally by the facilitator or jointly with the client.

Coming to the End of Group Therapy

Termination of individual or group therapy, even when known in advance and expected, can raise strong feelings, and an important part of the closure process in a closed group is to address these issues within therapy as the group's work is coming to an end. Within an open-enrollment group, termination is an ongoing issue as individual members complete the group and leave at different times. Here it may be helpful to have an individual closure session as well as a ritual for the group to say good-bye to completing members.

Premature Termination

As in individual counseling, a member in group therapy may fail to show up without notice. It is important to have clear procedures for responding promptly when this happens, particularly if attendance has been mandated by a court or external agent. In general, we recommend taking the initiative after a missed appointment to contact the person as soon as possible by telephone, e-mail, or handwritten letter to ascertain the reason and welcome the person back to the group (see Chapter 19).

The first month is an especially critical time for retention in addiction treatment (Margolis & Zweben, 1998), and a preparation/role induction session may be particularly helpful (Zweben et al., 1988) to build readiness and motivation for group work. Another factor that increases retention is the availability of wrap-around services such as child care and transportation, barriers that often impede successful treatment engagement. Most of the case management issues and strategies discussed in Chapter 8 apply in group work as well.

Termination for Cause

Finally, a client may be terminated early from group treatment for specific reasons. Termination may occur by mutual agreement between client and facilitator; for example, the client's life circumstances may have changed (obtained or lost a job, moving to another city). A facilitator or program may also decide unilaterally to remove a client from a group for a serious violation of the group agreement (e.g., violence during a group session). Such rules apply equally to all group members, and are made clear in advance.

As stated earlier (Chapter 19), we do not recommend terminating clients from treatment because of substance use, which in essence would be discharging people for the same reason that they were admitted. We instead suggest following the example of the 12-step fellowships and welcome people on the basis of their desire for sobriety, not their current pattern of use. How to handle a client who comes to group intoxicated is a decision to be made and announced at the outset. If a person comes to group under the influence more than once, consider whether a different or additional form of treatment may be needed.

> We do not recommend terminating clients from treatment because of substance use, which is in essence discharging them for the same reason they were admitted.

With any termination, it is also good practice to help people find whatever additional services they need. Even completion of a particular treatment is no guarantee that gains will be maintained. Discharge planning considers what continuing support clients may want and need, and includes proactive efforts to link them with services (see Chapters 6–8). When clients decide unilaterally to drop out of treatment, you can still communicate an open-door policy to welcome them

> Welcome people on the basis of their desire for sobriety, not their current pattern of use.

back should they choose, or to help them find other services. When it is necessary to remove a person from a group for cause, it is often possible to continue that person in some other form of treatment. In the situation where a unilateral decision is made to terminate clients from treatment altogether, there is a beneficent responsibility to help them get care elsewhere.

The Successful Group Facilitator

What makes an effective group facilitator? Mostly the therapeutic skills are the same ones that characterize a more effective individual facilitator. An empathic, client-centered communication style is beneficial in group therapy. An empathic style within a group context means being interested in, listening respectfully to, and skillfully reflecting content that is offered by group members. Conversely, early research from encounter groups indicated that one type of facilitator stood out from all the rest in having more harmful effects and poorer outcomes: an adversarial, confrontational group leader (Lieberman, Yalom, & Miles, 1973). Blaming, criticizing, labeling, and shaming are to be avoided in group as well as in individual therapy (Chapter 4).

Group therapy, however, is more complex than individual counseling. In a group setting, the therapeutic alliance involves multiple relationships— member to member, member to group, and member to leader—and the responsibility to maintain rapport within the group is challenging (Burlingame, Fuhriman, & Johnson, 2002). In group therapy this rapport is often termed *cohesion,* describing the benefits of a healthy environment where the emotional experience is that of acceptance, empathy, support, predictability, and honesty (Moos et al., 1993). As is true in individual therapy, therapists are often inaccurate in predicting clients' views of the group relationship (Chapman et al., 2012).

Beyond the skills that you use in individual therapy, group treatment requires some additional know-how. One significant change is that the group environment is more fast-paced than individual therapy, and interactions between group members require creativity and spontaneity. The increased number of people also requires more redirection to ensure that certain group members do not dominate the interactions or get the group off-track. Self-awareness and self-monitoring are other important aspects of successful facilitation of group therapy, and a co-facilitator can also help in perceiving bias. For example, one common finding is that male group leaders are more likely to call on male rather than female members.

Yalom derived a factor analysis with a large number of leader variables for group therapy and categorized them into four basic leadership functions that were related to successful treatment outcome (Yalom & Leszcz, 2008):

1. Acceptance—encouraging members to reflect in safety on their own experience, including maladaptive aspects, and express themselves openly and honestly. Yalom called this "emotional stimulation," and it obviously overlaps with the clinical skill of accurate empathy.
2. Caring—warmth, compassion, and genuineness.
3. Meaning attribution—helping clients develop their ability to understand themselves, each other, and people outside the group, as well as what they might do to change things in their lives.
4. Executive function—setting limits, rules, norms, goals, and managing time.

Beyond training in a particular type of psychotherapy (e.g., cognitive-behavioral), Yalom suggested observing experienced group therapists and having intense clinical supervision for the first few groups you conduct.

As group facilitator, you are also a model for clients in how to respond to others. The first few sessions are a particularly important period in this regard, as you model the behavior that is expected and establish group norms. Depending on the type of group, you may or may not directly teach participants positive skills for responding to each other, but you are always modeling a way of being with others. It is also important to intervene promptly to prevent negative communication patterns from emerging and being normalized in the group.

It is human nature to respond to people in different ways and to fluctuate in one's response depending on current mood and recent experience. Within a therapeutic group, however, it is important to respond as consistently and reliably as possible. Respond empathically and respectfully to what clients offer. Avoid favoritism, maintain clear and consistent boundaries, and enforce ground rules for speaking. It can be helpful to record some group sessions and review the recording afterward to listen for consistency in how you respond and for adherence to group rules. This makes it possible to hear things that you may have missed while you were so busy leading the group.

Cognitive–Behavioral Skills Training

Beyond these general factors that are relevant to all types of group therapy, we now turn to a more specific consideration of cognitive-behavioral treatment (CBT), the most empirically supported form of group psychotherapy for addiction. CBT groups are intended to develop and strengthen behavioral and cognitive coping skills so that the person is better equipped to have a rewarding life without relying on psychoactive drugs. There is typically emphasis on identifying environmental and intrapersonal risk situations and practicing skills to cope with them successfully (as discussed in Chapters 11 and 14).

A potential disadvantage of group treatment is that there is less individual attention given to each person, and it can be easy for clients to be passive and tune out. Group treatment is necessarily less individualized, and the skills that you are addressing may already be solidly in place for some but not other participants. Plan for activities that engage as many people as possible. Prevent long periods of passivity by having people take turns and work on individual worksheets. Some group CBT approaches have client workbooks (e.g., Daley & Marlatt, 1999; Miller & Mee-Lee, 2010; Safren, Sprich, Perlman, & Otto, 2005) as well as facilitator guides. Other therapist resources include worksheets and handouts for clients (Miller, 2004; Monti, Kadden, Rohsenow, & Cooney, 2002). A key is to find ways to engage the group in such self-exploration processes rather than simply conducting individual therapy in a group setting.

Many CBT groups progress through a cycle of content, covering and practicing a variety of coping skills. This is possible even in open-format groups, where clients enter at different points in the cycle. You can prepare people for this structure in a pregroup individual session, and let them know where in the cycle they are entering. In open groups, people enter anywhere in the cycle and complete the group when it comes back around to the point where they entered.

A typical sequence in introducing a new skill is "tell–show–try." First explain what the skill is and how it works. Next demonstrate it. You go first, and show how the skill looks in practice. It can be fun here to invite participants to do their worst—to give you challenging situations to which you respond with the skill to be learned. It's also OK to struggle a bit here—to make mistakes, stop, and discuss how to do it better. A general social learning principle is that a "coping model" who responds well but imperfectly is generally more effective than a "mastery model" who exudes total competence (Schunk, 1991). Finally, let participants try out the skill. Usually skills are broken down into specific steps that build on each other. When clients are trying out a new skill, don't let other participants be too challenging. It is tempting for clients to pose impossibly difficult scenarios, in part because they are trying to imagine how they themselves might cope. Set it up so that people succeed as they learn a new skill. Take it in small steps, and give lots of positive reinforcement. Comment on what the client did well, perhaps make a small suggestion to try, and then again emphasize positive aspects of what the person did. Group CBT can be integrated with motivational approaches (L. C. Sobell & Sobell, 2011).

Motivational Interviewing Groups

There are many ways in which group MI is similar to individual MI. First and foremost, it involves a different way of thinking about people and approaching their ambivalence about change (see Chapter 10). Beyond a foundation of empathy and a spirit of partnership and collaboration, there are specific skills to help people move in the direction of change. MI-consistent practice increases the ratio of client change talk to sustain talk, which in turn predicts substance use outcomes (D'Amico et al., 2015; Miller & Rollnick, 2013). Change-supportive responses of others in the room can also increase this ratio (Apodaca et al., 2013). When a facilitator skillfully evokes and reflects change talk from one client, group members may follow suit and offer more change talk. This change talk cascade within the group affects individual-level outcomes (D'Amico et al., 2015)

There are learnable skills to support change talk and manage sustain talk within a group (Wagner & Ingersoll, 2013). When counselors learn to differentially attend to and reflect change talk, their clients express more change talk (Glynn & Moyers, 2010; Moyers, Houck, Glynn, & Manuel, 2011) and less sustain talk (Moyers et al., 2017). Key skills here are first recognizing change talk when you hear it, then learning how to evoke and respond to it (Miller & Rollnick, 2013; Rosengren, 2018). If you hear "When I drink I do stuff that I wouldn't normally do, but I also really like how it makes me more outgoing," the skill is in tuning your ear to hear the change talk within the statement and reflect that pro-change piece (i.e., "You do things you regret."). Asking open questions is another key skill, particularly when the questions are ones that evoke change talk. For instance, "How are you able to keep from using when you are somewhere alcohol is available?"

> When counselors attend to and reflect change talk, clients express more change talk.

Clearly, it is possible for counselors to influence this balance of client change talk and sustain talk levels within individual sessions (Glynn & Moyers, 2010; Moyers et al., 2009, 2011, 2017). If this is an important aspect of MI, how can this be accomplished in a group context where individual talk time is more limited? There are learnable skills to support change talk and manage sustain talk within a group (Rosengren, 2018; Wagner & Ingersoll, 2013). Whether in group or individual sessions a skillful MI practitioner responds in ways that differentially encourage change talk, which requires skills of recognizing, selectively evoking, and responding to it. It is also important to manage counterchange statements (sustain talk) so as not to strengthen them when they occur. Groups of heavy drinkers, for example, can devolve into swapping drinking stories and minimizing risk, essentially encouraging each others' sustain talk, which can result in outcomes worse than no treatment at all. A natural temptation is to offer counterargument, which only tends to accelerate this dynamic. Skillful MI group facilitation instead guides clients' own discussion back toward change, within the collaborative, affirming, and empathic spirit of MI.

KEY POINTS

🎗 On average, outcomes from group or individual counseling are similar.

🎗 Didactic (lecture and film) and confrontational groups appear to have little or no beneficial impact on outcome.

🎗 Many practical issues in group treatment warrant advance consideration and decisions (e.g., size, open vs. closed, duration and frequency, goals, talking rules).

🎗 As in individual treatment, the counseling style of the group leader can have a substantial impact (for better or worse) on client outcomes.

🎗 Cognitive-behavioral skill training is a well-supported form of group treatment.

🎗 Reflecting change talk and asking open questions are key skills when conducting MI groups.

Reflection Questions

🝆 How is leading a therapy group different from doing individual counseling?

🝆 On the list of practical decisions that one must make before beginning a group (Box 22.1), what are your own personal preferences? Why?

🝆 What do you think are the main potential advantages and disadvantages of group versus individual treatment?

CHAPTER 23

Addressing the Spiritual Side

Addiction and spirituality are mysteriously intertwined. There is a widely shared view, particularly within the United States, that spirituality is central to understanding and overcoming addiction, and individuals in addiction treatment frequently cite spirituality as a helpful influence during recovery (Heinz et al., 2010). Certainly, this view lies at the heart of the 12-step program, which is discussed later in this chapter. In a letter to Bill W., cofounder of AA, Carl Jung (1961/1975) quoted the ancient aphorism *spiritus contra spiritum* to mean that there is something mutually exclusive about alcohol (spirits) and healthy spirituality—each tends to drive out the other. Correlational data from a wide variety of studies support this inverse relationship. Religious involvement has been one of the strongest protective factors against the development of SUDs, accounting for as much shared variance as family history of addiction (Borders, Curran, Mattox, & Booth, 2010; Gorsuch, 1995; Gorsuch & Butler, 1976; Miller, 1998; Salas-Wright, Vaughn, Maynard, Clark, & Snyder, 2017). People with an SUD have reported relatively low levels of current religious and spiritual involvement, compared to the general U.S. population (Hilton, 1991; Larson & Wilson, 1980; Walters, 1957). Indeed, it is the very definition of behavioral dependence that a drug occupies an increasingly central place in the person's life, gradually displacing prior involvements, relationships, and priorities, including spiritual or religious ones. Involvement in AA after treatment is modestly but rather consistently associated with sustained abstinence (Emrick et al., 1993; Tonigan et al., 2003; Witbrodt et al., 2014).

Less clear from a scientific perspective is a causal role of spiritual factors in the etiology of and recovery from addiction (Connors et al., 2001;

Miller & Thoresen, 2003; Tonigan, Miller, & Connors, 2001). In one recent study, the more incoming college students were contending with spiritual struggles such as doubting their faith or feeling punished by God, the greater risk they had for a variety of addictive behaviors, from gambling to substance use (Faigin, Pargament, & Hisham, 2014).

> Religious involvement has been one of the strongest protective factors against the development of SUDs.

Spirituality does tend to change and grow over the course of recovery (Bonelli & Koenig, 2013; Brown, Jr., 1990; Robinson et al., 2011; Robinson et al., 2007; Schoenthaler et al., 2015; Tonigan, Rynes, Toscova, & Hagler, 2013), as do physical, psychological, and interpersonal health. Levels of spirituality may also be greater in individuals who are successfully abstaining from substances compared to those who continue with substance use (Jarusiewicz, 2000; Schoenthaler et al., 2015). Whether these spiritual changes are causes, effects, or merely concomitants of abstinence is unclear. Perhaps all of these relationships are true in part.

Yet, while many professionals and programs acknowledge the importance of spirituality, in practice relatively little time is usually spent addressing this side of addiction. Typically, the discussion of spirituality begins and ends with a recommendation to attend a 12-step meeting. Of the many special issues that arise during addiction treatment, attending to the spiritual aspects of recovery in addiction treatment is a topic that deserves some attention.

> Spirituality changes over the course of recovery.

What Is Spirituality?

For most of human history, spirituality and religion were equated, a perspective that was evident in William James's (1994/1902) classic volume *The Varieties of Religious Experience*. Within the latter half of the 20th century, however, spirituality came to be differentiated from religion in common usage (Hill et al., 2000). *Spirituality* began to refer to the individual's subjective experience of that which transcends human existence, be it of God, a Higher Power, a realm of spirit, meaning in life, or an ultimate reality. *Religiousness*, in turn, came to refer to involvement in traditional institutional religion. It thus became meaningful to characterize oneself as *spiritual but not religious*, which is also a common description of the 12-step program.

From a scientific perspective, one way to conceptualize spirituality is as a latent construct like personality or health, which has multiple measurable dimensions of belief, behavior, and experience (Miller & Thoresen, 1999, 2003). Within this view, individuals are not characterized as being *spiritual* versus *not spiritual,* or as possessing a certain degree of spirituality. Instead, every person is located somewhere along the various dimensions of spirituality. As with health and personality, there is a large scientific literature on reliable measures of spirituality and religiousness (Hill & Hood, 1999; Hill & Pargament, 2003; Hood, Hill, & Spilka, 2009). Involvement in traditional institutional religion is but one aspect of a person's spirituality.

Of U.S. residents, 89% profess belief in "God or a universal spirit"; over half report membership in a church, synagogue, or mosque; and three-quarters describe religion as "very important"(53%) or "fairly important" (22%) in their lives (Gallup, 2017). In contrast, the percentage of mental health professionals involved in religion tends to be much lower than that of the people they serve (Delaney, Miller, & Bisono, 2007). Through the 20th century, health professions increasingly distanced themselves from religion, and interest in spirituality became out of vogue, regarded at times as unprofessional or unscientific. Behavioral health professionals comfortably explored clients' drug use, sexuality, finances, family relationships, feelings, and fantasies, but rarely their religion or spirituality (Miller, 1999). This was less true in addiction treatment, however, owing in part to the broad influence of the 12-step program, which openly refers to God and emphasizes a spiritual path to recovery (Kurtz, 1991; Miller, 2003).

Exploring Spirituality

Often health professionals are unsure of how to ask people about their spiritual/religious side, but it's not difficult. A simple question such as "What role, if any, has religion or spirituality played in your life?" can open the door to exploring both prior and current religious involvement. The "if any" gives implicit permission for the answer "None." It is also useful to find what exposure a client may have had to AA or another 12-step program, because many have at least sampled one. "Have you ever been to an AA meeting?" and if so, "What was that like for you?" (see Chapter 17). Asking, "Do you believe in God?" or "Do you pray?" (the majority of Americans say they do) may give you some indication of the person's potential receptiveness to a 12-step program.

It is also possible to explore spirituality more broadly. In considering what open questions to ask, it can be helpful to have an organizing framework to guide your exploration. One good option proposed by psychologist Paul Pruyser (1976) centers around seven key themes that can be explored in understanding a person's spirituality. Don't misappropriate a diagnostic model here, thinking that you must explore all seven themes or prescribe remedies. Pruyser's themes just represent possible content in exploring spirituality, and it is likely that some will be more productive than others.

Following are the seven themes, recast somewhat, that highlight core human experiences corresponding to each. It is common for people to use "God language" in talking about these themes, but if religious-sounding language is off-putting for a particular client, you can ask just as easily about the related core human experiences.

Theme 1: Awareness of the Sacred

Spirituality involves a search for the sacred, the transcendent, and one's relationship to it. What, then, does this person regard with reverence, as sacred or holy? For what does he or she make significant sacrifice, or would be willing to do so? To what, if anything, does this individual acknowledge dependence or ascribe ultimate worth? This can be a significant theme in recovery precisely because behavioral dependence on a drug represents progressively giving the drug central and ultimate value in one's life. What will fill the vacuum when substance use is no longer central? A core spiritual experience to explore here is that of awe, reverence, or unspeakable joy. This is a common component of mystical experience and spiritual transformation (James, 1902/1994; Maslow, 1971; Miller & C'de Baca, 2001). When and how has this person felt awe or wonder apart from the use of drugs?

Theme 2: Providence

Whatever the person's conception of the holy, how does he or she understand its disposition or intentions? Is God (or the universe, the world, a higher power) a good and friendly reality, or dark and punishing, or removed and indifferent? What or whom do they trust? What is expected of them, and what is owed to them? In what do they hope? Where (if at all) do they see light and promise? What happens after death? The corresponding core experience here is benevolence. When have they deeply felt benevolent intentions—toward them, or their own toward others? When and whom have they deeply trusted?

Theme 3: Faith

The focus here is not necessarily on "a faith," a particular religion or creed, although certainly this can be important. Rather, what does this person have faith in, believe in? To what is he or she committed? To what extent does the person feel secure and anchored versus adrift? How inclined is the person to encounter and explore new ideas and perspectives, or does the person seem closed down, with little freedom to move? What is the person's "ultimate concern"? A core human experience here is deep security.

This is not to be confused with certainty, the absence of doubt. Rather, in the midst of life's storms, when has the person still felt in some sense safe, grounded? A related experience is the courage of commitment, of devotion to something larger than oneself.

Theme 4: Gratitude

What is the person's experience of feeling blessed (or cursed)? For what is he or she grateful? Is there a sense of sufficiency, of having "enough" (in material goods, recognition, relationships, love) or a tone of deprivation, entitlement, and hunger for more? Has the person "earned" and deserved that which he or she has? There is, of course, the opposite stance of inability to accept grace, of ultimate undeservingness. A core human experience here is unmerited grace. When has the person needed and experienced forgiveness? When has the person extended forgiveness, and why? When has he or she been blessed? Related is the experience of contentment, of *day-enu*—enough—to be satisfied with what one has.

Theme 5: Repentance

To what extent does this person take responsibility for his or her own actions and circumstances? Again, there are two extremes. At one extreme, the person experiences excessive remorse and responsibility. At the other end, the person perceives little or no responsibility for adversity and assumes a victim role. At issue is conscience, or the self-monitoring and self-dissatisfaction that lead to recognition of a need for change. Related core experiences in this domain include remorse, regret, and contrition—normal human displeasure with self in reaction to actual or perceived guilt or wrongdoing.

Theme 6: Connection

In what ways, if at all, does the person feel connected to fellow human beings, to humanity in general, or to all of creation? Our need to bond with others and feel understood is increasingly starved in an environment and a culture that tends to cut us off from connection or offer only the parody of it through social media. At the low end is a "dog-eat-dog" individualism, a sense of being isolated, estranged, disconnected from, or in competition with others. At the higher end is the experience of interconnectedness and interdependence, a sense of community or a mystical experience of oneness with all of humanity or the universe. Core human experiences in this domain include caring for others and being cared for, reverence for life, and union.

Theme 7: Vocation

Finally, what is the person's sense of purpose in life? Is there something that God wants from him or her, or from all human beings? What is it that the person hopes for or is called to do with his or her life? Core experiences in this domain include a calling or a sense of belonging with particular tasks or talents, satisfaction (or dissatisfaction/restlessness) with how one's time is spent, and a sense of meaning and purpose (or lack thereof) in one's life.

Some possible questions for exploring each of these themes are suggested in Box 23.1.

12–Step Spirituality

AA, the original 12-step program, grew out of the mutual support of its two cofounders, Bill W. and Dr. Bob Smith, and had its origins in a spiritual movement known as the Oxford Group (Kurtz, 1991; Lean, 1985). The structure of 12-step groups is discussed in Chapter 17; our focus here is on the broad spirituality that serves as their foundation.

AA is an unapologetically spiritual program. It is, in fact, not a treatment but a way of living. Substance use is mentioned only in the first of the 12 steps (see Box 23.2). The rest describe spiritual processes: awareness of and relationship with God, self-examination, confessing shortcomings, openness to being transformed, making amends, prayer and meditation, and conveying the program to others who are still suffering. AA states that abstinence is only a beginning of this lifelong process of spiritual growth toward serenity. There are also 12-step programs that are focused more on illicit drugs (such as Narcotics Anonymous and Cocaine Anonymous) and other addictive behaviors (like Gamblers Anonymous, Sex and Love Addicts Anonymous).

From a 12-step perspective, the core of addiction lies in *character*. "Selfishness—self-centeredness! That, we think, is the root of our troubles" (Alcoholics Anonymous, 1976, p. 62). Much discussed in 12-step circles are "defects of character" as being at the heart of the pathology of addiction, faults such as obsession with power and control, resentment, dishonesty, defiance, and grandiosity. The long-term remedy, then, is a change of heart, the development of positive virtues such as forgiveness, humility, honesty, patience, responsibility, and wisdom (Peterson & Seligman, 2004; Tonigan et al., 2013; Webb & Trautman, 2010), through ongoing living of the 12-step program.

AA is not affiliated with any religion. The 12-step program, however, has deep roots in Judeo-Christian spirituality and its historic practices of contemplative prayer, confession, and meditative study (Keating, 2009a;

BOX 23.1. Some Spiritual Themes, Core Experiences, and Avenues for Exploration

Pruyser's Themes	Core Spiritual Experiences	Possible Open Questions for Exploration
Awareness of the Holy	Awe Reverence Bliss Joy	"What do you regard as sacred or holy?" "What gives you a sense of awe or wonder?" "For what/whom are you willing to make significant sacrifices?" "When in your life have you felt a deep sense of joy?"
Providence	Benevolence Trust Hope	"What do you imagine God is like?" "What image do you have about what happens after death?" "What or whom do you trust?" "What gives you hope?"
Faith	Deep security Safety Courage Commitment	"To what/whom are you most committed in life?" "How safe do you feel in your life?" "What or whom do you believe in, have faith in?" "What things are you anxious about?"
Gratitude	Grace Blessing Forgiveness Contentment	"For what are you most grateful?" "When in your life have you felt truly blessed?" "When has it been hard for you to forgive someone?" "When have you experienced forgiveness from someone?"
Repentance	Remorse Regret Contrition	"In what ways could you be a better person?" "What things in your life have you regretted?" "When have you felt guilty or ashamed?" "When have you seen a need for change in yourself and done it?"
Connection	Belonging Caring Being loved Union	"In what ways do you feel connected to other people?" "Where do you feel most at home, like you belong?" "Whom do you care for?" "Who cares for you?"
Vocation	Meaning Purpose Calling	"How do you understand your purpose in life?" "How do you spend your time? Why?" "What do you want to do with the years of your life?"

BOX 23.2. The 12 Steps of Alcoholics Anonymous

1. We admitted we were powerless over alcohol—that our lives had become unmanageable.
2. Came to believe that a Power greater than ourselves could restore us to sanity.
3. Made a decision to turn our will and our lives over to the care of God *as we understood Him*.
4. Made a searching and fearless moral inventory of ourselves.
5. Admitted to God, to ourselves, and to another human being the exact nature of our wrongs.
6. Were entirely ready to have God remove all these defects of character.
7. Humbly asked Him to remove our shortcomings.
8. Made a list of all persons we had harmed, and became willing to make amends to them all.
9. Made direct amends to such people wherever possible, except when to do so would injure them or others.
10. Continued to take personal inventory and when we were wrong promptly admitted it.
11. Sought through prayer and meditation to improve our conscious contact with God *as we understood Him*, praying only for knowledge of His will for us and the power to carry that out.
12. Having had a spiritual awakening as the result of these steps, we tried to carry this message to others, and to practice these principles in all our affairs.

The 12 steps of AA and a brief excerpt from *Alcoholics Anonymous Comes of Age* (page 341) are reprinted with permission of Alcoholics Anonymous World Services, Inc. ("AAWS"). Permission to reprint these excerpts does not mean that AAWS has reviewed or approved the contents of this publication, or that AAWS necessarily agrees with the views expressed herein. AA is a program of recovery from alcoholism *only*—use of these excerpts in connection with programs and activities which are patterned after AA, but which address other problems, or in any other non-AA context, does not imply otherwise.

Rohr, 2011) to maintain "conscious contact with God" and conformity to God's will. AA is very permissive regarding how the individual understands God or a Higher Power, and the fellowship welcomes atheists and agnostics, who appear to benefit just as much as others when they do participate (Tonigan et al., 2002).

As a spiritual program for living, the AA program is meant to be internalized and practiced throughout all of one's life. As discussed in Chapters 7 and 17, a manual-guided form of 12-step facilitation (TSF) therapy was developed to encourage clients' entry and engagement in the fellowship of AA (Nowinski, 2003; Nowinski & Baker, 1998). TSF was designed to introduce clients to AA, help them work through the first three to five steps of the program, and get established with a sponsor in a home group. Clients assigned at random to TSF on average fared at least as well as those in cognitive-behavioral or motivational enhancement therapies (Babor & Del Boca, 2003).

Transformational Change

The reference in Step 12 to a "spiritual awakening" bespeaks another phenomenon that is observed in recovery, that of sudden transformation. William James (1902) described two kinds of change that occur in human life. The first, more common and familiar, is a step-by-step process of successive approximations that he called the "educational" or "volitional" variety of change. Most people most of the time change in this way: gradually, in small steps, like the learning of a new language or skill.

Sudden and seemingly permanent transformations do occur, however. James and his contemporary George Coe documented dozens of these sudden and striking transformations. The occurrence of epiphanies and sudden transformation is familiar in most world religions, and is also found with some frequency in autobiographies (Bidney, 2004; White, 2004). This was certainly the experience of Bill W., who found his own sobriety in this way when from a hospital bed he prayed for help:

> Suddenly the room lit up with a great white light. I was caught up into an ecstasy which there are no words to describe. It seemed to me, in the mind's eye, that I was on a mountain and that a wind not of air but of spirit was blowing. And then it burst upon me that I was a free man. Slowly the ecstasy subsided. I lay on the bed, but now for a time I was in another world, a new world of consciousness. All about me and through me there was a wonderful feeling of Presence, and I thought to myself, "So this is the God of the preachers!" A great peace stole over me and I thought, "No matter how wrong things seem to be, they are all right." (in Alcoholics Anonymous World Services, 1957, p. 63; reprinted by permission)

Miller and C'de Baca (2001) interviewed 55 people who had experienced such "quantum change," on average 11 years earlier, with a further 10-year follow-up for a two-decade retrospective (C'de Baca & Wilbourne, 2004), concluding that such transformations appear to be permanent, a kind of one-way door through which people pass. Their experience is quite different from that of the white-knuckle struggle to avoid a return to substance use that is so common in early recovery. Such stories of sudden spiritual transformation are frequently encountered within AA (Forcehimes, 2004), although AA clearly recognizes and honors the gradual "educational" variety of spiritual awakening and recovery as being the more common path.

Reconnecting with Religious Roots

Recovery from addiction involves reversing the process of isolation through which the person's life became centered on substance use or other addictive behavior, gradually pushing out other activities, involvements, and relationships. Abstinence creates a vacuum, removing what had been the person's primary use of time, energy, and devotion. It is important therefore for the recovering person to connect or reconnect with other sources of pleasure, meaning, and engagement (see Chapter 14).

It is common for people to have become particularly detached from whatever religious roots they may have had as their behavioral dependence progressed. Substance use generally competes for the time, talent, energy, and resources that might otherwise be invested in social relationships. Beyond this general trend, people may distance themselves from religion because their substance use and related behavior clash with religious values. Some have experienced outright judgment and rejection from religious quarters, and carry emotional scars. For such people, AA's characterization as being "spiritual but not religious" may make it safer to re-explore spiritual terrain.

For people who have simply drifted away from their religious roots, however, reconnection with their spirituality and a religious community may be a helpful part of recovery (Schoenthaler et al., 2015). Religious communities and activities typically do not involve drinking or other drug use, and thus they offer an alternative to a prior addictive lifestyle. Like AA, they can also provide a positive social network supportive of sobriety. Also like AA meetings, congregations vary widely in warmth, structure, dogmatism, and acceptance, and it can be useful for a person to sample a number of different ones to find a spiritual home.

Clergy can also be helpful and supportive in the recovery process, particularly those with a loving understanding of addiction. Individual clients may carry heavy baggage from negative religious experiences. In combination with the low self-esteem common in addictions, such experiences may convince a person that he or she is unforgivable, unworthy, unlovable, or is being rejected and punished by God. A loving and knowledgeable pastor, rabbi, imam, or chaplain may be able to help people work through such spiritual obstacles. If the client has no home congregation, you could offer referral to clergy whom you trust. In this regard, it is useful to meet members of the clergy from various religious backgrounds and discuss addiction with them, in order to develop a list of religious professionals to whom you can refer with confidence.

Spiritual Disciplines

In most Western treatment settings, people come from a wide variety of religious backgrounds. For some, religion is central to their cultural identity. In Hispanic and African American communities, for example, religion tends to play a major role in cultural life. The spiritual disciplines of world religions, which have been in practice for centuries if not millennia, offer paths to spiritual growth. Several of these have a prominent role in 12-step programs: prayer, meditation (discussed in Chapter 12), surrender, confession, and reconciliation.

Is it effective to promote the practice of spiritual disciplines during the stabilization and rehabilitation phases of addiction treatment? The sizeable correlational literature showing an inverse relationship of addiction and spiritual practice is encouraging in this regard. To find out, we offered individual direction in the use of spiritual disciplines to people during and following residential treatment for SUDs. Clients who were interested and willing to participate were assigned to receive or not receive up to 12 sessions of spiritual direction in addition to treatment as usual. In two randomized trials, contrary to our expectations, we found absolutely no benefit, whether the additional sessions were offered by professional spiritual directors or by treatment program staff (Miller, Forcehimes, O'Leary, & LaNoue, 2008). Even on spiritual health measures, we saw no change. In retrospect, our expectations were rather naïve. These people had just completed withdrawal and had a plethora of pressing life concerns to deal with: finding jobs, a place to live, safety, and child care, in addition to maintaining their newfound sobriety. On Maslow's (1943, 1970) hierarchy of human needs, they were down at the bottom of the pyramid addressing basic needs, and we were up at the top talking about spirituality and meaning in life. Furthermore, we acted as if an acute intervention could be enough (the same error often made in treating addiction). Spiritual development is a lifelong process, and not one to be addressed well in a few sessions. Although the whole 12-step program is spiritual, the disciplined practice of prayer and meditation appears later, at Step 11. Perhaps a better time to work on spiritual disciplines is in the maintenance phase, rather than early in stabilization or rehabilitation (see Chapter 7).

> Spiritual development is a lifelong process.

Spiritual Questing through Psychedelics

Although certain psychoactive drugs have been prohibited in some religions, various substances have also been used across diverse cultures as vehicles in the search for the sacred. Volunteers receiving psychedelics in controlled, supportive settings have reported profound and meaningful spiritual experiences during these medication sessions as well as robust and positive long-term changes (Doblin, 1991; Griffiths et al., 2008; Richards, 2008). Bill Wilson openly experimented with LSD for several years as part of his receptivity to anything that might help alcoholics recover (Kurtz, 1991, 1999). Eight clinical trials in the 1960s and 1970s tested psychedelics in treating alcohol use disorders, with mixed results (Miller & Wilbourne, 2002).

In addiction research there has been a recent resurgence of interest in the potential therapeutic value psychedelics (Bogenschutz, 2013, 2017; Bogenschutz et al., 2015; Johnson, Garcia-Romeu, Cosimano, & Griffiths, 2014; Krupitsky et al., 2007). In one trial examining the use of two or three doses of psilocybin in helping people overcome nicotine use, 80% of participants were abstinent at 6 months, results unheard of in smoking cessation treatment (Johnson et al., 2014). These results are consistent with a proof-of-concept study of psilocybin treatment for alcohol use disorders (Bogenschutz et al., 2015). Much remains to be learned about the efficacy, safety, and therapeutic mechanisms involved in controlled psychedelic experiences.

Exploring Values

Another aspect of the spiritual side of human nature is what people most value, that which is of "ultimate concern" to them (Emmons, 2003; Tillich, 1973). What is most important or sacred to this person sitting across from you? What do your clients most want in life for themselves and those they love? What are the values that guide them? In behavioral dependence, the drug itself gradually becomes the person's ultimate concern, the center of life, displacing all that was dear and sacred before. The process of recovery and a life of sobriety involve discovering or rediscovering the sacred—that which is of ultimate importance.

It can be useful, therefore, to help your clients clarify what matters most to them. Various tools have been developed for this purpose (Kirschenbaum, 2013; Rokeach, 1973). A simple but effective tool is a values card sort, which consists of a set of cards each describing something that may be important to people. Various lists have been developed for different populations, or you can develop your own. The list in Box 23.3 consists of a hundred values from which to choose. You may wish to use fewer cards and modify the language for the populations you serve. Typically, the client sorts the cards into three to five piles based on their personal importance. If the highest importance pile is large, you can ask the person to choose from it the five to 10 values that are most important, most central to his or her identity. These can then be rank-ordered from most important (1) on down.

BOX 23.3. A Values Card Sort

William R. Miller, Janet C'de Baca, Daniel B. Matthews, and Paula L. Wilbourne

These values are usually printed onto individual cards that people can sort into three to five piles such as "Most Important," "Very Important," "Important," "Somewhat Important," and "Not Important." It is wise also to provide a few empty cards so that people can add values of their own. These items are in the public domain and may be copied, adapted, or used without further permission.

1. ACCEPTANCE	to be accepted as I am
2. ACCURACY	to be correct in my opinions and beliefs
3. ACHIEVEMENT	to have important accomplishments
4. ADVENTURE	to have new and exciting experiences
5. ART	to appreciate or express myself in art
6. ATTRACTIVENESS	to be physically attractive
7. AUTHORITY	to be in charge of others
8. AUTONOMY	to be self-determined and independent
9. BEAUTY	to appreciate beauty around me
10. BELONGING	to have a sense of belonging, being part of
11. CARING	to take care of others
12. CHALLENGE	to take on difficult tasks and problems
13. COMFORT	to have a pleasant and comfortable life
14. COMMITMENT	to make enduring, meaningful commitments
15. COMPASSION	to feel and act on concern for others
16. COMPLEXITY	to embrace the intricacies of life
17. COMPROMISE	to be willing to give and take in reaching agreements
18. CONTRIBUTION	to make a lasting contribution in the world
19. COOPERATION	to work collaboratively with others
20. COURAGE	to be brave and strong in the face of adversity
21. COURTESY	to be considerate and polite toward others
22. CREATIVITY	to create new things or ideas
23. CURIOSITY	to seek out, experience, and learn new things
24. DEPENDABILITY	to be reliable and trustworthy
25. DILIGENCE	to be thorough and conscientious in whatever I do
26. DUTY	to carry out my duties and obligations
27. ECOLOGY	to live in harmony with the environment
28. EXCITEMENT	to have a life full of thrills and stimulation

(continued)

This material is in the public domain and may be reproduced without further permission.

BOX 23.3. *(continued)*

29. FAITHFULNESS	to be loyal and true in relationships
30. FAME	to be known and recognized
31. FAMILY	to have a happy, loving family
32. FITNESS	to be physically fit and strong
33. FLEXIBILITY	to adjust to new circumstances easily
34. FORGIVENESS	to be forgiving of others
35. FREEDOM	to be free from undue restrictions and limitations
36. FRIENDSHIP	to have close, supportive friends
37. FUN	to play and have fun
38. GENEROSITY	to give what I have to others
39. GENUINENESS	to act in a manner that is true to who I am
40. GOD'S WILL	to seek and obey the will of God
41. GRATITUDE	to be thankful and appreciative
42. GROWTH	to keep changing and growing
43. HEALTH	to be physically well and healthy
44. HONESTY	to be honest and truthful
45. HOPE	to maintain a positive and optimistic outlook
46. HUMILITY	to be modest and unassuming
47. HUMOR	to see the humorous side of myself and the world
48. IMAGINATION	to have dreams and see possibilities
49. INDEPENDENCE	to be free from depending on others
50. INDUSTRY	to work hard and well at my life tasks
51. INNER PEACE	to experience personal peace
52. INTEGRITY	to live my daily life in a way that is consistent with my values
53. INTELLIGENCE	to keep my mind sharp and active
54. INTIMACY	to share my innermost experiences with others
55. JUSTICE	to promote fair and equal treatment for all
56. KNOWLEDGE	to learn and contribute valuable knowledge
57. LEADERSHIP	to inspire and guide others
58. LEISURE	to take time to relax and enjoy
59. LOVED	to be loved by those close to me
60. LOVING	to give love to others
61. MASTERY	to be competent in my everyday activities
62. MINDFULNESS	to live conscious and mindful of the present moment
63. MODERATION	to avoid excesses and find a middle ground
64. MONOGAMY	to have one close, loving relationship

(continued)

BOX 23.3. *(continued)*

65. MUSIC	to enjoy or express myself in music
66. NONCONFORMITY	to question and challenge authority and norms
67. NOVELTY	to have a life full of change and variety
68. NURTURANCE	to encourage and support others
69. OPENNESS	to be open to new experiences, ideas, and options
70. ORDER	to have a life that is well ordered and organized
71. PASSION	to have deep feelings about ideas, activities, or people
72. PATRIOTISM	to love, serve, and protect my country
73. PLEASURE	to feel good
74. POPULARITY	to be well liked by many people
75. POWER	to have control over others
76. PRACTICALITY	to focus on what is practical, prudent, and sensible
77. PROTECT	to protect and keep safe those I love
78. PROVIDE	to provide for and take care of my family
79. PURPOSE	to have meaning and direction in my life
80. RATIONALITY	to be guided by reason, logic, and evidence
81. REALISM	to see and act realistically and practically
82. RESPONSIBILITY	to make and carry out responsible decisions
83. RISK	to take risks and chances
84. ROMANCE	to have intense, exciting love in my life
85. SAFETY	to be safe and secure
86. SELF-ACCEPTANCE	to accept myself as I am
87. SELF-CONTROL	to be disciplined in my own actions
88. SELF-ESTEEM	to feel good about myself
89. SELF-KNOWLEDGE	to have a deep and honest understanding of myself
90. SERVICE	to be helpful and of service to others
91. SEXUALITY	to have an active and satisfying sex life
92. SIMPLICITY	to live life simply, with minimal needs
93. SOLITUDE	to have time and space where I can be apart from others
94. SPIRITUALITY	to grow and mature spiritually
95. STABILITY	to have a life that stays fairly consistent
96. TOLERANCE	to accept and respect those who differ from me
97. TRADITION	to follow respected patterns of the past
98. VIRTUE	to live a morally pure and excellent life
99. WEALTH	to have plenty of money
100. WORLD PEACE	to work to promote peace in the world

Finally, interview the person about these core values. Some open questions that can be helpful here are:

- "Why did you choose this as a central value for you?"
- "In what ways is this important to you?"
- "How have you shown this core value in your daily life?"
- "In what ways could you be even more true to this value?"

Such a conversation about the client's five to 10 core values—asking open questions and following with reflective listening (Chapter 4)—can teach you much about the person's hopes, aspirations, and guiding principles for living. It also can strengthen your understanding and working alliance.

Having elicited a client's core values, it is further possible to ask how substance use affects the person's living out of each of these core values. Has it helped the person be consistent with this value?; has it hindered living out the value?; or is it irrelevant? You need not draw conclusions for the client; the answer is usually obvious, but asking about addictive behavior in relation to what the person holds dearest can sometimes crystallize motivation for change (Baumeister, 1994).

> What do your clients most want in life for themselves and those they love?

KEY POINTS

🔖 Spiritual/religious involvement is a consistent predictor of lower risk for SUDs.

🔖 People who develop behavioral dependence are often disconnected or even alienated from their spiritual/religious traditions and community (if they had one).

🔖 The program of AA and other 12-step groups is strongly spiritual but not affiliated with any religion, and welcomes all who desire sobriety regardless of belief.

🔖 Sudden transformational changes that release people from addictions are well documented, though most people change in a more gradual manner.

🔖 There has been a resurgence of research interest in psychedelics as a possible tool to facilitate recovery.

🔖 Exploring a person's core values can clarify what are often regarded as spiritual or meaning-in-life motivations for change.

Reflection Questions

Q How would you describe your own spirituality?

Q What role (if any) do you think spirituality has in recovery from addiction?

Q What would your own reaction be if psychedelics were confirmed in scientific research to facilitate recovery from addiction?

Q How do you understand the widely reported phenomenon of sudden transformational changes (like that of Bill W.) that release people from addiction?

CHAPTER 24

Professional Ethics

In Greek mythology, the Sphinx guarded the entrance to the city of Thebes and asked a riddle of those who wished to enter, devouring travelers who failed to answer correctly (Hamilton, 1999). One reported version of the riddle is "What creature goes on four feet in the morning, on two at noonday, and on three in the evening?" The correct answer was "humans," who early in life crawl on all fours, then learn to walk upright on two feet, and in later years walk with a stick. Francis Bacon (1619/1992) regarded this riddle as an allegory for the scientist's search for truth. In treating addictions, we are confronted daily with challenging riddles, fitting together the pieces of a puzzle to find what seems to be the best answer for the people we serve.

One of our goals in this book is to provide you with knowledge to solve some of these puzzles, but a different kind of riddle in clinical practice comes in the form of ethical questions to which there may not be black-and-white answers, yet which may need to be decided quickly. Getting one of these riddles wrong can indeed devour you in lawsuits, loss of license, or even criminal charges.

Sometimes an applicable law does mandate a clear answer. An example is found in longstanding laws that require professionals to break client confidentiality in order to protect people from clear and imminent danger, or to report child or elder abuse (Kalichman, 1999; Welfel, Danzinger, & Santoro, 2000). In many cases, however, the ethical dilemma falls within a legally permissive gray area where more than one answer could be argued to be the right one. Additional guidance may be provided by the code of ethics for your profession, although general ethical codes may not factor in the unique and specific circumstances that can muddle professional decision making (Pope & Vasquez, 2007). How then does one decide what is the right thing to do?

Ethics is the branch of philosophy that is concerned with values for defining what is right and wrong in human actions and decisions. Rarely do answers come from the memorization of facts. Ethics is a different sort of beast, a different kind of riddle. It is more about judgment and critical thinking than retrieval of information. The kind of riddle posed by the Sphinx was not one for which the answer could be retrieved from memory. It required thoughtful reflection to arrive at the right answer.

Ethical decision making is also not an appropriate arena for trial and error. It is not like scientific hypothesis testing. There isn't much room for "Oops! I guess that was the wrong decision. Oh well. I'll now know what to do differently in the future." Sometimes the ethical Sphinx gives us one chance to get it right, to make the best decision with the information that we have available at this particular moment, in a specific set of circumstances that we may never encounter again. Once this kind of decision has been made, we cannot take it back. Once done, a breach of confidentiality, misrepresentation, or a sexual boundary violation cannot be undone.

What It Means to Be a Professional

Why do we have to answer the Sphinx's questions at all? It is in part because we have unique access to the road on which they arise, and so we must decide how to respond when they do. Unlike a job, in which one may travel alone and operate independently, the nature of a profession is to do privileged work that interfaces with and impacts the lives of others. Ethical decision making is part of our duty as clinical professionals.

Differing standards exist for professions such as law, medicine, counseling, and clergy because particular values are attached to these professions, but there is also commonality. Professionals have unique specialized knowledge and thereby have significant influence over the lives of others. With this role and knowledge come respect, trust, and credibility to the public. Degrees and licenses are symbols that people can trust us even though they don't know us personally. Clients come to us in vulnerability, and expect competent professional treatment. They place in our hands their trust, sensitive private information, and significant influence. Though we work hard to have a collaborative partnership in our work with clients, a professional relationship is inherently one of uneven power.

> A professional relationship is inherently one of uneven power.

A Brief History of Ethics

Ethics have been debated for thousands of years. The professional oath for physicians that is attributed to Hippocrates dates from the fourth century B.C.E. and contains a variety of ethical principles including *primum non nocere*, translated as "First of all, to do no harm." Formal ethical standards of professional conduct, however, are surprisingly recent in origin. It was the Nazi medical experiments during World War II that prompted the development of formal safeguards to protect human participants in research. Principles of voluntary participation with informed consent arose from the Nuremberg trials in a 1948 code that required a balancing of the potential benefits of research against its risks. It took even longer to implement ethical principles systematically in clinical care.

A 1979 document known as the Belmont Report set forth three basic consensus principles as a moral basis for responsible conduct in research (U.S. National Commission for the Protection of Human Subjects of Biomedical and Behavioral Research, 2017). The first of these principles is autonomy, or respect for persons, meaning that individuals should be treated as self-determining agents and that people with diminished autonomy are entitled to additional protections. The second principle is beneficence, which means to maximize possible benefits and minimize possible risks. The third principle is justice, meaning that the benefits and risks of research should be distributed fairly. These principles provided a way of thinking about professional ethical responsibilities in terms of obligations and duties. A fourth principle of nonmaleficence (do no harm) has subsequently been differentiated from beneficence, leading to a practical four-principle approach for ethical decision making known as *principlism* (Beauchamp & Childress, 2001). These four basic principles represent a minimum consensus of what should guide providers' ethical decision making.

Nonmaleficence

The principle of nonmaleficence is that clinical providers should not cause harm. The Hippocratic Oath places this even before doing good. Unpleasant though it is to contemplate, what we do in our work with clients is not inert and so has the potential to harm people. Delivering an ineffective treatment may leave clients feeling hopeless, as though nothing will help them. A confrontational counseling style is particularly liable to do harm, especially with more vulnerable clients (Annis & Chan, 1983; Lieberman et al., 1973; MacDonough, 1976; White & Miller, 2007). Protecting confidentiality is an important part of preventing harm from disclosure of information.

It is also possible to do harm by *in*action. People who come into an emergency room or a trauma center with alcohol-related injuries are at substantially increased risk for future morbidity and mortality because of their drinking. It seems unethical, then, to do nothing to try to change the behavior that caused the injury. We are accountable to screen for addiction and do something about it rather than simply ignore it (see Chapter 5). There is increasing recognition of the obliga-

> It is possible to do harm by inaction.

tion to at least screen for SUDs in these opportunistic settings out of recognition that people are more likely to seek medical services than specialty treatment. Routine medical screening began earliest for tobacco smoking, then for excessive alcohol use, and most recently for illicit drug use. This idea of incorporating screening into general medical settings including emergency departments, primary care, and dental clinics has been promoted by the National Institute on Drug Abuse (Tai, Sparenborg, Ghitza, & Liu, 2014).

Beneficence

In addition to preventing harm, providers should actively promote clients' welfare. The treatment services that we provide should be those most likely to benefit and least likely to harm clients. This is a clear argument for offering the best evidence-based treatment methods at our disposal. It is what we expect of our own health care providers.

Autonomy

As much as possible, people should have choices, freedom, and adequate understanding when making decisions about treatment. The principle of autonomy is a reminder of our clients' inherent worth as human beings and the need to respect their own values and goals. Whatever clinicians may do, it is ultimately the client who decides whether, when, and how to change. In that sense, telling clients that they *can't* or *must* is not actually accurate. Honoring autonomy involves telling people the truth about their options, and having an open discussion about choices. These are fundamental to informed consent. It is also truth telling to acknowledge that only the client can decide whether or not to make changes.

> Honoring autonomy involves telling people the truth about their options, and having an open discussion about choices.

Justice

The principle of justice primarily has to do with an equal distribution of benefits and burdens. One important issue here is access to treatment. Ideally, effective treatment should be available on demand to anyone who wants and needs it, without regard to his or her personal characteristics or ability to pay. The perspective of "There but for fortune" is helpful here—that we don't deserve whatever advantages we may happen to have, and by the luck of the draw could be sitting in the client's chair instead (Rawls, 1971/1999).

Promoting justice of course includes ensuring that our services are fairly available and provided without discrimination. A sliding scale that adjusts fees to clients' ability to pay is one common approach in a fee-for-service context, as is providing pro bono work for those who can't afford treatment. Another example is taking appropriate caution when using assessment and treatment procedures with populations other than those with whom they have been developed and validated.

Ethical Balance

There are times when these four principles conflict with each other, and ethical navigation involves finding the right balance of considerations (Beauchamp & Childress, 2001). An ethical situation (see Box 24.1) may require giving greater weight to one of the principles while balancing with the others as much as possible given the particular dilemma under consideration.

BOX 24.1. An Ethical Puzzle

Consider what you might do in the following situation: You are treating a 30-year-old woman named Vanessa, who is on probation for a drug-related offense. She reenrolled in community college, maintained a B+ average in her first semester courses, earned a scholarship, and found a steady job working as a waitress. Vanessa knows that her probation officer, who referred her to treatment, requires regular updates from you regarding her progress, and specifically asked to be informed of any drug use. For the past 6 months she has been coming regularly for counseling, and all urine screens have been drug-free. Now with only a few weeks left in her second semester back in college, she is going into her finals with an A average. Vanessa arrives for this week's session on time and tearfully informs you that she made a terrible mistake and used cocaine once after receiving tragic news that her mother was diagnosed with pancreatic cancer and has only a few weeks to live. This is the first time Vanessa has used drugs since she was put on probation, and her urine drug screen was again clear. She is ashamed and tells you that she just wanted to be open and honest with you and work on the skills needed to maintain her sobriety and find alternative ways to cope with stress. She pleads with you to not tell her probation officer, knowing that she will not be able to complete the semester, will lose her job and scholarship, and could not spend the last few weeks with her mother if her probation is revoked and she is sent back to jail.

What do you do? How would you balance the four principles of nonmaleficence, benevolence, autonomy, and justice? What would affect your decision?

Two principles that often clash with each other are beneficience and nonmaleficence. In the process of trying to do good, there is a risk that some harm may be done. For example, the efficacy of some medications is directly related to the presence of risk and unpleasant side effects. To use a behavioral example, treating PTSD with exposure therapy necessarily causes the person to experience short-term distress.

Taleff (2009) recommended these steps as a process for evaluating ethical dilemmas:

1. Collect yourself and settle down. Take some deep breaths and get some emotional distance.
2. Clearly identify the ethical dilemma. Is there something wrong? An injustice done? A right violated? Someone harmed?
3. Start gathering your facts and evidence. What do you already know? What do you need to know, but don't? Who exactly is involved? How reliable are your facts?
4. Consult relevant guidelines, codes, or authorities. What do national and regional ethical guiding principles/codes have to say about the situation? With whom might you consult as reliable colleagues with good ethical judgment?
5. Look at the identified problem through various ethical perspectives. What are the issues from the perspective of nonmaleficence? Beneficence? Autonomy? Justice?
6. Look at the problem through critical thinking principles. If you could form an argument regarding this situation, what would be your premises and conclusions?
7. Weigh the arguments and evidence and make a first probable course of judgment and action. How would the judgment direct a course of action?
8. Rest and reflect. Focus on other things for a while (unless a decision needs to be made immediately).
9. Revisit your first judgment and first course of action by going through steps 1–7 again, and refine as necessary.
10. If your assessment reveals that your first judgment/decision seems to be the best thing to do, then it is time for action. Make a decision and act on it.

Practical Guidelines

With this background, we turn now to some specific practical issues, beginning with two common ones—informed consent and confidentiality—that illustrate how such issues may be complicated when treating addictions.

Informed Consent

Informed consent is a formal procedure that is required before people participate in research, and similar (though sometimes less formal) procedures are used in treatment. In primary care settings, this is often a generic consent to receive treatment, without specifying what treatment procedures will be used. More specific informed consent may be required with particular specialist procedures, such as surgery, and with experimental treatments.

Often consent is thought of as a one-time event occurring before treatment, but the consenting process can also be ongoing and revisited from time to time as needs, goals, and plans change. It may be necessary to obtain consent in formal written format, or in other circumstances it may be verbal and documented in case notes. In addiction treatment, the consent process can be compromised by short-term (intoxication or withdrawal) or long-term neurobiological changes related to drug use. This is another reason to revisit consent after the stabilization phase has been completed.

There are three primary elements of informed consent, the first of which is *competence*. The consenting person must have the ability to make a decision that is in his or her own best interest (Van Staden & Krüger, 2003). In court, this is a legal determination made by specified criteria. In practice, it is a judgment call whether the person is able to understand the situation and make an informed choice. When a person is legally incapable of giving informed consent, then permission is typically obtained from a legally authorized person except when immediate emergency care is required. As much as possible with clients who cannot themselves give consent (e.g., minors), still inform them of what is happening, consider their preferences and best interests, and seek their assent to treatment.

Comprehension, a second requirement for informed consent, implies the capacity to understand the information being presented. Information should be offered in language that the client can understand. Because of the possible acute and long-term effects of substance use, educational level is not itself a sufficient indicator of comprehension. It is wise therefore to check for comprehension of key points. With written consents, we have asked clients to read a key paragraph of the consent form in order to ensure reading ability. The person is always offered time to ask questions, and it is also reasonable to ask clients to tell you what they understood about key points, to make sure they comprehend. Some of the information commonly included in a consent process includes:

- A clear description of the treatment to be provided.
- A fair and balanced disclosure of what is known about the efficacy of the treatment, and of known risks and side effects.
- The expected duration of treatment and conditions for termination.

- Alternatives to the proposed treatment that are available, whether or not you yourself can provide them.
- The qualifications of staff to provide the treatment.
- The protections and limits of confidentiality.
- Financial aspects of treatment, such as fees and policies regarding missed or cancelled appointments.

A written and signed consent form offers some advantages. The original can be retained in the client's file, and the client can also be given a copy.

In addition to competence and comprehension, a third element that is necessary for informed consent is *freedom of choice*. The person should freely choose to participate in the research or treatment without any coercion or undue influence (such as excessive incentives). The consent must be clearly expressed, documented, witnessed, and maintained in the person's records.

Confidentiality and Its Limitations

Confidentiality implies an explicit contract or promise not to reveal anything about your client except under certain circumstances agreed to by both parties. Even the fact that a person is being treated is itself confidential information. This is both a standard component of professional ethics (not to discuss or disclose to anyone a client's private information without permission) and a stipulation of applicable laws. U.S. federal regulations require an even higher than normal level of confidentiality protection for client records of treatment for SUDs.

Privilege is a legal term describing certain specific types of relationships that enjoy protection from legal proceedings. In many jurisdictions, people don't have privilege unless they specifically ask for it in an explicit way. Therefore, it is wise in your consent form or elsewhere in client records to document that the person expects and requests confidentiality.

We advise our trainees to observe paranoid standards in protecting client confidentiality. Imagine that there are nosy people actively trying to find out private information about your client. There are some commonsense practical things to do. Close the door whenever you are discussing private information with or about a client. Keep client records in locked cabinets in a locked room with restricted access. Never discuss clients in a hallway or public place, even without using names or identifying information. If someone calls for information about a client, do not even acknowledge whether the person is in treatment without a written release of information. If you have such a release, ensure that you are talking to the appropriate person before disclosing any information.

People with SUDs are particularly stigmatized, so there are extra safeguards in place when working with this population. Inadvertent disclosure of treatment information could cause someone to lose a job, insurance, a security clearance, or a relationship, and to experience discrimination by other health care professionals. A U.S. federal rule (42 CFR, Part 2) provides special protection for the confidentiality of patients suffering from or seeking evaluation for SUDs. This rule applies to any treatment program receiving direct or indirect federal funding or a tax-exempt status and requires SUDs records to be kept separate from other health information and protected from subpoena or warrant if the records are requested. These special protections of data can pose challenges for research evaluating policies and practices to improve care for people with SUDs. There is ongoing ethical debate about how best to balance these special protections with scientific advancement of addiction treatment (Frakt & Bagley, 2015).

Addiction treatment is often mandated through a judicial system as an alternative to incarceration or as a condition of pretrial release, probation, or parole. Other offenders are advised by counsel to enter treatment as a proactive means to reduce legal consequences. The common practice of coerced treatment has been distinguished from rarer compulsory treatment of individuals who have committed no legal offense (Hall, Farrell, & Carter, 2014). *Coerced* treatment involves an ethical balancing of individual autonomy with protection of the public, whereas *compulsory* treatment of severely addicted people is mandated "for their own good" requiring a paternalistic judgment of what is in the person's best interest. Both practices have been controversial as human rights issues (Day, Tucker, & Howells, 2004; Hall et al., 2014). Recent meta-analyses reported little evidence that coerced treatment improves outcomes, with some studies showing detrimental effects relative to controls (Parhar, Wormith, Derkzen, & Beauregard, 2008; Werb et al., 2016). Few reliable data are currently available regarding the impact of compulsory treatment for nonoffenders.

A different question pertains to the ethics of denying access to treatment for incarcerated individuals. Medications for addiction (see Chapter 18) are becoming more available and accessible in U.S. prisons and jails, a decision largely driven by considerations of the ethics of restricting such access (Ludwig & Peters, 2014).

Working with clients who are mandated to treatment requires a clear mutual understanding of providers' reporting requirements. Clients who are coerced to treatment usually come with conditions for reporting of information. In most cases, disclosure is restricted to documenting treatment attendance and progress, so that it is possible to maintain trust with your client while still giving the courts the required information.

Group therapy (Chapter 22) presents some ethical complexities with regard to confidentiality because information is shared within the group. A standard way to address this issue is to establish the ethical ground rule that anything shared in the group remains within the group, and neither the group's membership nor its content are to be discussed with others. Each participant in the group should explicitly agree to this. A tradition in some 12-step groups is to recite this reminder at the end of each meeting: "Who you see here, what you hear here, stays here!" Clients, of course, are not bound by the same ethical and legal requirements that guide your professional practice, so you cannot guarantee the same level of anonymity and confidentiality as would apply in individual treatment.

What happens to confidentiality if your client is deceased? You might be asked, for example, for information that is relevant in settling a disputed estate or that would be helpful to an insurance company in determining whether the client's death was a suicide. However, a client's death does not negate confidentiality, nor can next of kin authorize release of information. You are not obliged to release information without a court ordering you to do so. Even in this case, federal law (described above) may protect your records from subpoena.

Duty to Report

There are important exceptions to confidentiality. Some issues are required by law to be reported, and addiction treatment confidentiality can be particularly tricky because illicit drug use is illegal. It is vital to be clear, with clients and with anyone to whom you report information, what you will and will not disclose.

Know your regional laws and contact your licensing or certification board for advice if you are unsure of requirements about breaking confidentiality. As we discussed earlier, any threats that are imminent, foreseeable, and dangerous (usually understood as suicide, homicide, or grave bodily harm to others) are reportable. For example, a client planning on running up his credit card bills and then declaring bankruptcy is not "dangerous" in this sense.

Professionals do have a duty to warn an intended victim or the police when a client divulges intent to kill (see Box 24.2). Even in this case, you can still protect the client's confidentiality by not revealing the fact that the person is being treated for a SUD or other unnecessary private information (Gendel, 2004).

Child or elder abuse is another reporting requirement that is an exception to confidentiality regulations. Regional laws typically require the reporting of disclosed abuse for the protection of the victim. State laws also mandate the reporting of certain infectious diseases, such as STDs and TB, to public health authorities. Again, to protect the welfare of your client or others, disclose only the necessary information. In the case of health care providers, it can be important to inform them of the patient's SUD diagnosis and prognosis. Health care providers may need this information to determine appropriate treatment and to avoid drug interactions. People with high tolerance for alcohol or other sedatives, for example, may require higher doses

---

BOX 24.2. The *Tarasoff* Case

Prosenjit Poddar came to the University of California Berkeley from India as a graduate student. There he met Tatiana Tarasoff. The two students had differing views of the relationship. Tarasoff felt that it was casual and she continued to date other men, while Poddar felt a serious monogamous relationship existed. Poddar was angered by her lack of commitment and began to stalk her. Poddar began to experience a severe mental crisis and eventually sought psychological help and told his psychologist of his intent to kill Tarasoff. The psychologist requested that the campus police detain Poddar and suggested that he be committed as a dangerous person. Rather than follow this suggestion, however, the campus police detained Poddar only briefly. A few months later, Poddar stopped treatment with the psychologist he had been seeing. Neither Tarasoff nor her parents had received any warning of the threat. Several months later, Poddar went through with the plan he had told his psychologist about and stabbed Tarasoff to death.

The question in the *Tarasoff* case was whether the psychologist had the responsibility to directly warn the intended victim. The original 1974 decision mandated warning the threatened individual, but a 1976 rehearing of the case by the California Supreme Court called for a "duty to protect" the intended victim. Therefore, this duty can be interpreted in several ways, including notifying police, warning the intended victim, and/or taking other reasonable steps to protect the threatened individual.

---

of anesthesia. Medical emergencies are another exception to confidentiality. For example, if a patient presents to the hospital with chest pain but without a history of heart problems, knowledge that the patient is a stimulant user would be important information for the medical team to have.

Identifying a pregnant woman as someone who uses substances does not generally imply an obligation to report to child protection or law enforcement agencies, although state laws may differ in this regard. There is, of course, good reason to work with pregnant women to abstain from alcohol, tobacco, and other psychoactive drugs, and the motivational approach described in Chapter 10 is a good option (Handmaker & Wilbourne, 2001). Pregnant women have a right to confidential or anonymous HIV counseling and testing, and also a right to refuse it. As long as a woman has custody of her infant, her consent is required for the infant to be tested.

Confidentiality When Working with Minors

When working with children or adolescents, confidentiality means something different because parents do have rights with regard to certain information. Children younger than a specific age (typically 14) cannot themselves agree to treatment without parental consent. Know your regional laws regarding the age at which the child's own assent or consent is required. Under most conditions, you have an option to deny parents access to treatment records if you believe that harm may come from it. It is wise, of course, to explain these conditions to both children and parents in advance before you begin treatment.

More generally, it is important to explain to your client and the family in their first session the standards of confidentiality. For example, make sure to inform adolescents that if they place themselves at risk of physical harm either deliberately or accidentally, you must let their parents know. It's helpful to give scenarios, but don't agree to tight limits such as "I will only tell if you are using these IV drugs" or "I will only tell if you are drinking and driving." If a need to inform parents arises, it is usually better to have the child inform the parent him- or herself (with you ensuring that it does happen) or for you to tell the parent with the child present.

Technology and Confidentiality

The growing use of smartphone technology and Internet-based applications (apps) offer novel options for treatment delivery, data collection, and record keeping; yet these innovations can also threaten confidentiality in new ways. Some apps may collect sensitive information such as alcohol and drug consumption, geo-location, physiological activity, self-reports of mood and cravings, and objective data on blood alcohol levels (You et al., 2017). Though these technologies offer unprecedented scope for real-time data collection and behavioral monitoring, these innovations challenge traditional confidentiality protections. Be particularly aware of how the use of electronic health records, apps, text messages, faxes, answering systems, e-mail, or portal messages may impact client confidentiality.

The growth of technology in the workplace brings both opportunities and dangers. If you use electronic means to communicate with clients, it is essential to ensure security at both sending and receiving points. If a consent form or other private information is to be e-mailed or faxed, who has access to the receiving machine? Electronic billing and other communication involves significant risk of inadvertent disclosure of sensitive information to unintended recipients. Electronic storage of client information in your office requires robust protection against hackers. If you audio-record sessions for later review or supervision purposes (which we encourage for continued feedback and professional development, and always with client knowledge and permission), written consent is advisable, and there should be a clear stated agreement about when and how such recordings will be used and destroyed.

Will you communicate with clients by e-mail or through portal messages? If you send text messages for scheduling or use portal messages to communicate, what happens if the client begins sending information that goes beyond logistics? Some providers will accept information from clients by e-mail, but do not send out messages to clients in this way in order to avoid unintended disclosure. It is wise to have clear policies and procedures for when e-mail is appropriate, who can read the e-mails, and who may respond to them. You should also inform your clients about what information and types of discussions are appropriate for e-mail and other forms of communication and those that are not (e.g., emergencies), how long a response might take, and why to avoid including identifying information. If particular forms of communication are used often in your practice, this should be in your informed consent form. It should also explain some of the risks of using this form of communication. For example, what if you receive your e-mail messages on your cell phone in addition to your firewalled computer? What if you happened to leave your cell phone at a restaurant or your computer on an airplane?

Boundary Issues

A professional relationship includes maintaining clear boundaries. *Boundary crossings* are less serious but nevertheless important infringements of professional courtesy (see Box 24.3). Some examples of inappropriate boundary crossings include arriving late for sessions, starting sessions late or ending them too early, having social contact with clients outside of sessions, or giving too much special attention to one of your clients. In contrast, *boundary violations* are major transgressions that exploit or harm the client. Examples include a dual relationship, such as any sexual contact with a client, or engaging in any business dealings with clients. Other boundary violations include giving or receiving significant gifts, or inappropriately violating confidentiality.

Self-Disclosure

How much personal information should you disclose to your client? When is it appropriate to disclose? Some professionals consider disclosing when the client's situation resonates with them personally. An important consideration here is *why* you would disclose. The normal rules of social reciprocity (you tell me something, and I tell you something) do not apply in professional relationships. You are not obliged to divulge personal information about yourself. If you choose to do so, be conscious of your intention. Here are some possibilities:

To Build Rapport

Perceived similarity is one source of alliance in relationships. In social conversation, it is common to look for points of shared experience and discuss them. Such "chat" is generally off-topic in professional service contexts,

BOX 24.3. Personal Reflection: An Ethical Choice

I had to look through my files to recover his research ID number, but I remembered him well, though I hadn't seen him for 3 months. Jack (whose name and identifying details have been changed to preserve anonymity) had been the second volunteer from AA to participate in a qualitative study on transformational change (Forcehimes, 2004).

The first question we had asked everyone who participated in the study was, "Tell me about your experience; how it was before, during, and after." There was an even divide between those who would delve right into the story with a succinct description and others who would go into copious detail. Jack was of the latter type; his story took 3 hours the first day and 90 minutes the second.

Jack had a troubled background, including sexual and physical abuse, exposure to gang violence, heavy drug and alcohol use, and financial struggles. He was a frequent drunk driver, but had never been arrested. His transforming experience was a dream, which to him was more real than any dream he had ever experienced. In his mind's eye, he saw himself driving on the freeway after a long night of drinking. His car hit the guard rail, then spun and collided head-on with another car. He got out of his car, uninjured, to examine the damages. In the other car, he saw the bloody wreckage of a family of four. The mother in the passenger seat was the only one breathing. Two small children had been thrown from the car, their small bodies distorted on the pavement, surrounded by pools of blood. The father had not been wearing his seatbelt and his head had gone through the windshield. He watched in horror as the dazed mother got out of the car to examine the remains of her family. His dream flashed forward and he saw himself in court, tortured by the agony of watching the mother sobbing. Then he saw himself in prison, unable to handle the misery he had inflicted on this family, hanging himself in his cell. Just as he was losing consciousness in his dream, he awoke in a cold sweat and vowed to never drink again. Ten years later he continued to keep that promise to himself.

Three months after I met with Jack, I was in an AA club recruiting volunteers for another study. In the meeting room, tables were arranged in a square formation and Jack was directly across from where I was sitting. In the tradition of AA, members each spoke for a few minutes about issues related to recovery as well as particular difficulties they were experiencing. When it was Jack's turn, his eyes filled with tears and he began explaining his present hardship. He expressed how alone he felt in the world and said that he felt like life wasn't worth living anymore.

After the meeting, I decided to forgo my recruiting efforts and instead talk with Jack. I told him that I was worried about him and that I thought it would be a good idea for him to talk to someone about his problems. I listened to the difficulties he was experiencing, and although he did not seem to be imminently suicidal, I gave him some local crisis numbers. As I turned to walk away, he said, "Hey, can you be my therapist?"

Ethical decision making is not always guided by absolute rules, and there are not always clear-cut answers. I began to think of the pros and cons: I knew about his history, he needed someone to talk with, and he obviously felt comfortable

(continued)

BOX 24.3. *(continued)*

talking to me. Also, he was feeling particularly rejected and my declining might feel like yet another abandonment, and I wanted to help him. On the other hand, I was just beginning the qualitative analyses of stories from our study, and the additional experience of being his therapist would clearly alter my interpretation of his story. There was also just something that felt not quite right about having these two different relationships with him: researcher and therapist. I've learned to pay attention to those "not quite right" feelings, even and especially when they conflict with something I want.

   As Jack detailed what he was struggling with, I told him that I would rather refer him to someone who had more experience in treating his particular issues, and that I would help him find the right therapist. He did begin therapy, and a few months later he called to say that he was doing much better.

—A. A. F.

but some professionals do choose modest self-disclosure in hopes of building rapport.

Solidarity in Recovery

If you are yourself in recovery from an SUD, there is a decision to make as to whether and when to disclose this. As mentioned previously, personal recovery status is unrelated to a professional's effectiveness in treating SUDs. Some clients do feel more understood if they know that their counselor is also in recovery, and clients may ask about your own recovery status. If you are in recovery and have not told your client, there is a risk of being inadvertently "outed" elsewhere, for example, at a mutual help meeting.

Answering Client Questions

Another reason to disclose is in answer to a client's question: "Are you in recovery?"; "Did you ever use drugs?" Again, the decision is yours, and you are not required to answer. With yes/no questions like these, one possibility is to say, "I'm willing to tell you, but first I'd like to understand what it will mean to you if the answer is 'Yes,' and what it will mean if the answer is 'No.'?" Discussing this first can address concerns or traps that underlie the question.

Desire to Be Genuine

In client-centered counseling, for example, such genuineness or congruence is a core therapeutic condition (Truax & Carkhuff, 1967). Congruence, however, typically has to do with one's immediate reaction to a client within the session, and not the recounting of your own past personal history.

A caution to keep in mind with any self-disclosure is to avoid identification with clients. A professional helping relationship is between unique individuals and not a mutual help group. Identifying with clients may impede your ability to see them as separate individuals and to help them without becoming overinvested in their choices. Identification is an appropriate issue to discuss in supervision.

Limits of Professional Expertise

Another standard aspect of professionalism is to practice within but not beyond your areas of expertise. A desire to be helpful and to have answers can lead to giving inadequate advice on issues outside your expertise (e.g., medical issues, legal issues, co-occurring disorders, case management problems). In other words, practicing outside one's expertise violates the precept to *first, do no harm*. It is common for clients to not understand the differences in training and expertise among various kinds of health professionals.

There are certainly times when needs for different professional expertise intersect. Clients in addiction treatment often bring significant medical and mental health issues as well. A client working with an addiction counselor might be taking a medication like buprenorphine for an opioid use disorder. Side effects or wondering if the dose is inadequate may come up in counseling. It is useful to have a team approach to treatment where possible, or at least to have in place a release to exchange information so that it is possible to communicate and discuss such concerns with professional colleagues.

The lines between addiction and other behavioral health problems also can be blurred. For example, a woman in treatment for substance use disorder may bring up feelings related to a history of child abuse and evidence symptoms of PTSD. Should you explore this? It depends on your professional training not just in addiction, but in the treatment of PTSD. Just talking about abuse and PTSD may be unhelpful, and runs the risk of reviving traumatic experiences without benefit. Professional practice should always remain within the bounds of one's expertise.

Professional Honesty

A related issue in most professional codes of ethics is truth telling and the avoidance of misleading statements. What if a client asks you about your "success rate" in treating a particular disorder? In one study, investigators called addiction treatment centers asking this very question, and the lowest estimate given was 80% (Miller & Hester, 1986). On further inquiry, none had any data to substantiate their claim. Representation of one's professional expertise, both verbally and in print and electronic media, should be an accurate description of training and experience. Avoid misleading or unsubstantiated statements, even and especially with the desire to impress and comfort clients.

Record Keeping

Client records are legal documents. Even when there are extra legal protections for addiction treatment records, you should not put anything in a client chart that you would not want to defend in court or to clients themselves. A good guideline is to keep client records factual based on what you have observed. Rather than writing, "The client used cocaine this week" (which you did not directly observe), it is better to write, "The client reported using cocaine this week." Discrete, objective documentation is particularly important in charting addiction treatment. Avoid judgmental comments or interpretations and embellishment that go beyond the facts. Be aware of any ways in which client records are flagged to indicate something about the client. For instance, electronic medical records are sometimes flagged to indicate patients who are frequent service users, "treatment resistant," or "drug seeking." While well intentioned, such icons and labels can create bias and influence treatment outcomes (Joy, Clement, & Sisti, 2016). Some clinicians maintain a "shadow chart," a separate set of notes on treatment, apart from the client's official medical record. These might be less formal notes on your thoughts and concerns, things you think of during a session or between sessions to raise on next meeting. Understand, however, that such records are equally subject to subpoena as the official treatment records.

Harm Reduction

The professional issue of gradualism, discussed in Chapter 19, has been a source of much debate in addiction treatment. To what extent should professionals try to protect clients from the adverse consequences of their own drug use? Although the prevention of harm is a common goal among treatment professionals; disagreements arise over specific methods for doing so (Miller, 2008).

The pragmatic question is this: If clients do not accept our own aspiration for their total abstention from all psychoactive drugs, is it ethical to do (or to not do?) whatever we can to at least prevent harm to themselves or others from their drug use? A parallel to this might be the medical question of whether a provider would refuse to treat a patient with hypertension who does not stop consuming salt, or a person with diabetes who continues to binge on sweets. If there is no negotiation on the goals and the message is "my way or the highway," people are unlikely to stay in treatment. We believe that an important goal is to keep clients engaged in the system of care and accept whatever incremental steps toward change they are willing to make.

Yet this topic of harm reduction is heavily debated and there are strong feelings from some people that efforts to prevent harm are problematic. What are some of the possible reasons why a professional might reject such attempts to prevent harm? Here are some arguments that have been expressed:

- Such harm reduction efforts only prolong the client's addiction by removing its natural negative consequences.
- It enables and implicitly condones illegal behavior.
- Anything but total abstinence from all psychoactive drugs will ultimately lead to deterioration and death.
- SUDs are self-inflicted, and people deserve whatever they get if they don't stop it.
- Harm reduction is just a foot in the door for the legalization of drugs.

Absolute opinions for or against harm reduction in general tend to be polemical, and in a way it comes down to what a provider, program, or system decides to do (or not do) in day-to-day practice with actual clients (see Box 19.1 in Chapter 19). For many clinicians, some measures to reduce risk of potential harm and suffering are reasonable (even if not comfortable), whereas others are unacceptable.

> Keep clients engaged and accept whatever steps toward change they are willing to make.

Less controversial than harm reduction approaches is screening for harm that has already occurred or is occurring. It is sensible to evaluate for common substance-related problems including infections (e.g., hepatitis, HIV, TB, STDs), domestic violence, child abuse/neglect, and suicide risk, and to provide appropriate treatment. What have been more controversial are proactive public health interventions to reduce harm from *future* substance use. One classic example is exchanging used needles for sterile ones to prevent the spread of blood-borne infections among intravenous drug users. Other examples are vaccinating intravenous drug users against hepatitis (Clark, 2005–2007) and offering supervised injection facilities where users can consume illicitly obtained drugs under supervision (Enns et al., 2016). Naloxone distribution is increasing as more states and nations allow pharmacists to dispense this life-saving medication without a prescription. Administering naloxone by injection or nasal spray can reverse an opiate overdose, and it is increasingly common to provide naloxone rescue kits prior to release from prison. Scotland's National Naloxone Programme yielded a 36% reduction in deaths related to opioids within 4 weeks of release from prison (Bird, McAuley, Perry, & Hunter, 2016). Harm reduction efforts incorporate a spectrum of strategies to meet people who use drugs where they are in the process of changing their use and preventing associated harm.

As with programs intended to prevent addiction problems, those claimed to reduce harm may or may not do so. For example, the use of electronic nicotine delivery systems (ENDS), though intended to be a harm reduction approach, could be doing more damage than good. Advocates claim that ENDS are far less dangerous than cigarettes, that any reduction in smoking is self-evidently harm reducing, and that they are significantly more effective than other pathways toward quitting smoking. Concerns include the dual use of tobacco and ENDS, potential health risks of flavorings in inhaled vapors, and the apparent targeting of a younger demographic that may promote smoking rather than reducing harm (S. Chapman & Daube, 2015). Much remains to be known about the health risks and benefits of e-cigarettes, and from a public health perspective there is currently insufficient evidence supporting ENDS as a harm reduction method.

Proponents of harm reduction measures regard them to be pragmatic and humanitarian efforts to prevent harm to users and to society. Opponents view them as condoning and facilitating continued drug use. People who use drugs' own motivations for accepting and using harm reduction strategies appear to be still more complex (Boucher et al., 2017).

Other Professional Practice Issues

Supervision

Some addiction treatment personnel are required by law or program policy to work under the supervision of a more highly trained licensed professional who reviews and approves their treatment plans and records. In this case, clients need to be informed about the supervisory arrangement and about who will have access to their case information. Other professionals are licensed for independent practice without ongoing supervision.

In either case, there is value in regular consultation with colleagues regarding clinical practice. These supervision or peer-consultation meetings can be thought of as a learning community and should not be focused primarily on administrative minutia but on the art and science of clinical care. They offer an important opportunity for continued professional learning, reflection, and practice improvement. Reviewing audio-recorded sessions (with clients' knowledge and permission, of course) together can be particularly valuable. Beyond case presentations and discussion, such regular meetings might also include a "journal club" discussing a clinically relevant article in a scientific or professional journal. There is growing evidence that therapists' effectiveness is enhanced by reflective and deliberate efforts to improve their own competence in practice (Chow et al., 2015; Goldberg et al., 2016).

It is particularly important and useful to discuss ethical quandaries with a supervisor or peers. Good ethical decision making involves deliberation, and not just fact retrieval. The sharing of this deliberation affords learning for all, and makes for better decision making.

Special Populations

The term "special populations" once referred to anyone other than white males, and more generally evokes the challenges of counseling people with demographics and cultural background different from one's own. A key justice issue here is equal access to treatment services (Miller, Villanueva, Tonigan, & Cuzmar, 2007). Discrimination in service delivery can occur simply through the way in which services are structured and provided. For example, offering treatment only during weekday work hours makes it more difficult for lower income working people to attend. Fees, child care, and location affect accessibility. Women who seek treatment for addiction tend to have fewer financial resources than men, are more likely to need child care, and tend to be more stigmatized (Lisansky, 1999). There are also comfort issues. Does the treatment setting feel safe? Do clients see other people like themselves on the staff, in pictures on the walls, or among other clients?

Another issue is how best to proceed when working with clients from a different ethnic or cultural background than your own. A key here is good listening, regarding clients as the experts on themselves (Miller, 2018). Rather than assuming that you understand, let your clients educate you regarding their own beliefs about addiction and its causes, as well as their hunches about what will work best for them. Assuming that you know how to work with someone because of their racial–ethnic background is risky in itself, because there is substantial variability within as well as across cultures.

It is not assured that treatment methods that work with one population will be effective with others. Nevertheless, evidence-based treatments from another population are a good place to start when considering options, and are arguably preferable to treatment methods with no scientific basis at all. It would, in fact, pose an ethical justice problem to deny delivery of an evidence-based treatment because a client came from a population other than the one in which the research had been done (Miller et al., 2007). Adaptations may be needed to make evidence-based treatments more accessible across cultures (Venner, Feldstein, & Tafoya, 2006; Venner et al., 2016).

Professional Development and Continuing Education

Staying current with the development of new and effective treatments is an ethical responsibility for addiction professionals, just as one expects this of one's own health care providers (Miller, Zweben, & Johnson, 2005). In North America and the United Kingdom, there is an increasing trend toward reimbursing only for treatments that have been scientifically validated.

This requires effort to keep up with emerging research. In a span of 5 years, literally hundreds of new studies are published that are relevant to practice in treating addictions. Few providers have the time and expertise to read this volume of scientific research critically. The usual way to keep up is through continuing professional education, a certain amount of which is normally required for licensed health professionals. However, there is rarely any requirement that the content of such materials or workshops reflect current scientific evidence. One can often fulfill the continuing education requirements of licensure without learning anything about evidence-based treatment or new research.

Various informational resources are available for keeping up with new developments. A remarkable source has been the public domain Treatment Improvement Protocol (TIP) series, with more than 60 volumes available online from the Center for Substance Abuse Treatment (*www.ncbi.nlm. nih.gov/books/NBK82999*). Another large and free resource is the Clinical Trials Network dissemination library (*ctndisseminationlibrary.org*). For keeping up to date on emerging addiction research that is relevant in health care, the online bimonthly newsletter *Alcohol, Other Drugs, and Health: Current Evidence* is an excellent and free resource (*www.bu.edu/aod-health*). There are practitioner-friendly journals presenting new research on addiction treatment, including the *Journal of Substance Abuse Treatment* and the *Brown University Digest of Addiction Theory and Application*. Other journals publish reviews that summarize a body of research for clinicians. Examples are *Drug and Alcohol Review* and *Clinical Psychology Review*. Such resources are available by subscription or may be accessible through a local university library. Google Scholar offers a free service providing regular alerts as new research appears on topics that you specify (*https://scholar.google.com*).

Simply reading about or even attending a workshop on an evidence-based treatment, however, is unlikely to be enough to change practice behavior significantly, although it may convince participants that they now understand and can use the new method (Miller et al., 2004). In this way, attending a workshop might even inoculate one against further learning because of the illusion that one has already mastered it (Miller & Mount, 2001). Learning any new complex skill typically requires deliberate practice over time with feedback and coaching. This is another way in which a learning community of peers can be helpful, working together to strengthen new skills and improve practice. Again we encourage listening to actual recordings (with client permission) of client sessions. This departs from a long tradition of closeted addiction treatment that occurs in secret behind closed doors (Miller, 2007), a tradition that deprives clinicians of feedback and opportunities to learn. Even listening to your own sessions can be instructive.

Counselor Impairment

Finally, as clinicians we have an ethical obligation to be sufficiently sound mentally and emotionally to be able to give clients our full and undistorted attention. The acute and cumulative effects of alcohol or other drugs represent only one potential source of professional impairment. Major life changes such as the loss of a loved one, a serious medical condition, or acute family distress can also distract, impairing clinical judgment and the ability to provide quality services for those who rely on us for help. It is important to recognize one's own limits and accept the need of a healing break from professional work. This requires a backup plan to ensure the care of clients currently in your care until you are able to resume work with them.

KEY POINTS

- Beyond the usual professional standards, addiction treatment requires additional ethical protections, particularly with regard to record keeping.

- Competence, comprehension, and freedom of choice are three key requirements for informed consent.

- Important ethical responsibilities include confidentiality, professional boundaries and honesty, duty to protect, and practicing within one's expertise.

- While supervision is a legal requirement for some providers, all professionals can benefit from ongoing consultation with knowledgeable colleagues.

- Professionals are responsible to be informed about emerging new knowledge and adjust treatment practices accordingly to provide effective care to clients.

Reflection Questions

Q Of the four ethical principles described (nonmaleficence, beneficence, autonomy, and justice), which one do you ponder most often in treating clients?

Q When you face a difficult ethical issue, what steps do you follow in deciding what to do?

Q What ethical issues regarding addiction treatment most concern you?

CHAPTER 25

Implementing Evidence-Based Practice

In his classic work *Diffusion of Innovation,* Everett Rogers (2003) described how a British sea captain had discovered in 1601 that citrus fruit could prevent scurvy, a major cause of death among sailors. Captain Lancaster commanded four sailing ships, and on one voyage he gave every sailor on one of his ships a daily tablespoon of lemon juice. The other three ships sailed on as usual. The results were dramatic. By halfway through the voyage, four of every 10 sailors on the three comparison ships were dead, which was not an unusual rate. Among the sailors given lemon juice, all remained healthy. It also became clear that citrus fruit could even reverse the deadly disease of scurvy. Despite this knowledge, it was 184 years before the British Navy implemented this practice by routinely providing citrus fruit to sailors, at which point scurvy was immediately eradicated.

Similarly, in 1846 the Hungarian physician Ignaz Semmelweis demonstrated that the frequent deaths of women from "childbed fever" following childbirth could be virtually eliminated if physicians would wash their hands with disinfectant before delivering a baby. His findings were vehemently rejected by the medical–scientific community, and he was committed by colleagues to an insane asylum where he died 2 weeks later. Decades passed and countless women perished needlessly before predelivery hand washing became routine (Broad & Wade, 1982).

The mere discovery of an effective treatment does not cause it to be used. There is notorious inertia in practice behavior; providers tend to continue doing what is familiar and comfortable unless they have a strong incentive to change. The resemblance to addictive behavior is noteworthy: it tends to persist until something interrupts it. Thankfully, in many domains of medicine this delay has been substantially curtailed. The publication of a clearly superior test or treatment for a major malady may influence practice within a few years, even becoming standard and expected procedure. Failure to provide clearly effective available treatment can constitute malpractice.

The picture has been much less clear in behavioral health. Providers of treatment for SUDs, for example, have been largely free to practice however they please behind closed doors. Even in systems that mandate the use of "evidence-based treatment," in the absence of any objective verification, the de facto requirement is merely to *say* that one is offering such treatment. Furthermore, providers can genuinely believe that they are competent in and providing an evidence-based approach when in fact they are not, or at least are not delivering with sufficient fidelity to make a difference in client outcomes (Miller & Mount, 2001; Miller & Rollnick, 2014). Auditing and quality assurance of behavioral treatments is no simple process.

Add to this a substantial confusion as to what constitutes evidence-based practice. How much and what quality of scientific evidence would suffice to designate a treatment to be effective? In pharmacotherapy the standards are somewhat clearer—a new medication must be shown in independent randomized trials to be reasonably safe and more effective than placebo, although not necessarily better than other available medications.

> Providers can genuinely believe they are competent in an evidence-based approach when in fact they are not.

In the United States, a National Registry of Evidence-Based Programs and Practices was developed to provide public information on the efficacy of treatments for SUDs. Unfortunately, the bar for scientific information of efficacy was set so low—essentially one positive clinical trial regardless of the number of negative trials—that more than 450 interventions were listed as evidence-based. Imagine having a life-threatening cancer and being told that there are over 450 effective treatments from which to choose.

From a scientific perspective, efficacy research in addiction treatment is rather well developed and sophisticated, with over 1,000 randomized clinical trials published. It is possible to compare the strength and quality of scientific evidence for various types of treatment (e.g., Miller & Wilbourne, 2002), and meta-analyses for specific methods are abundant. There has been less agreement about where to set the threshold line when constructing a list of "effective" treatments.

A different question is how to get effective methods into practice. It has been estimated that in the United States, only 10.5% of people with a serious alcohol use disorder actually receive an evidence-based treatment (Schmidt et al., 2012). A simple equation is

Effective treatment + Ineffective implementation = No benefit as captured in Dean Fixsen's witty aphorism that "People cannot benefit from a treatment to which they have not been exposed" (Fixsen, Naoom, Blase, Friedman, & Wallace, 2005). Pharmaceutical companies are quite sophisticated in how to promote the use of their products, including direct media marketing to potential consumers, but how do behavioral treatments come to be implemented in practice? There are two distinct but related dimensions when it comes to getting behavioral treatments into practice: dissemination and implementation.

Dissemination: Getting New Information to Practitioners

Some interventions are more likely than others to attract providers' interest in adopting and learning them. Through a lifetime of research, Everett Rogers (2003) identified five characteristics of innovations that favor their dissemination:

1. *Relative advantage.* Compared to current practice, does the innovation offer significant advantages? It may, for example, promise to solve a commonly encountered clinical problem. Perceived advantages might be in cost, convenience, effectiveness, prestige, or personal satisfaction.
2. *Compatibility.* How consistent is the innovation with current values, beliefs, practices, and needs?
3. *Simplicity.* How easy is the innovation to understand, learn, and use? Interventions that are perceived to be complicated, difficult, and confusing are less likely to be tried.
4. *Trialability.* Can the innovation be tried out on a tentative basis without large initial commitments of time, money, and effort?
5. *Observability.* Can you readily see the positive results of the innovation?

As in marketing, dissemination strategies that highlight these aspects of an innovation favor its adoption in everyday practice.

An innovation might be perceived as irrelevant (no advantage) for a particular population being served. For example, a new approach that is focused on working jointly with clients and their families may seem immaterial if those being served are largely estranged from their families (such as clients experiencing homelessness or severe drug problems). Peer support for an innovation may be lacking if it clashes with coworkers' values, beliefs, and current practices (Cunningham et al., 2012; Leeman, Birken, Powell, Rohweder, & Shea, 2017; Lundgren, Amodeo, Chassler, Krull, & Sullivan, 2013; Manual, Hagedorn, & Finney, 2011; Williams et al., 2016).

BOX 25.1. Personal Reflection: A Spectacular Implementation Failure

We placed a clinical psychology predoctoral student with a local private inpatient addiction treatment program, for the sole purpose of helping them develop and conduct research that would be of interest to their staff. In conversations with treatment providers there, the highest priority that emerged was getting help in motivating clients for change earlier in treatment. Their standard length of stay had been reduced from 28 to 21 days, and they lamented that just when their clients were becoming motivated it was time to discharge them. So we randomly assigned their clients at admission to receive or not receive an initial session of motivational enhancement therapy (MET), an approach unfamiliar to their staff. We provided the MET sessions soon after intake, and all clients then received treatment as usual. Although staff were not told which clients were in the intervention or control condition, they perceived a significant difference during treatment. Those who had received MET were rated by staff as more motivated, more punctual and engaged in treatment groups, and having neater appearance and better prognosis. Indeed, at 3-month follow-up, MET clients were twice as likely to be abstaining, with alcohol consumption reduced by 80%, as compared with 28% in the control group (Brown & Miller, 1993).

We were delighted to present the results to the program staff. The motivational intervention did exactly what they had hoped! In thanks for their participation we offered to return at their convenience to train their staff in MET free of charge.

The request never came. It was over 10 years later when I happened to encounter the woman who had directed the now-closed inpatient program. "Why did you never invite us back to train your staff?" I asked. She confided that their main corporate referral source had threatened to stop sending them clients unless they stuck with a strict 12-step approach and didn't water it down with university ideas.

—W. R. M.

Although drug companies can provide physicians with free samples of their products, efforts to disseminate behavioral interventions in addiction treatment have largely relied on transmitting information to providers, stakeholders, and educators. Major U.S. providers of such information have been the National Institute on Drug Abuse (NIDA), the National Institute on Alcohol Abuse and Alcoholism (NIAAA), and the Centers for Substance Abuse Treatment (CSAT) and Prevention (CSAP). Products have included monographs and treatment manuals, state-of-the-art assessment and evaluation materials, and treatment improvement protocols. These materials are often distributed after research has yielded encouraging findings, in hopes that the intervention will be adopted in clinical settings and tested in subsequent studies.

A further dissemination resource has been a network of Addiction Technology Transfer Centers (*http://attcnetwork.org/about/techtransfer.*

aspx) supported by the U.S. Substance Abuse and Mental Health Services Administration (SAMHSA). This network was created to promote the dissemination and implementation of evidence-based treatment methods by connecting front-line providers and agency administrators with the latest information on treatment research. Online education, conferences, and workshops are offered to enhance skill building among addiction treatment providers. NIDA and SAMHSA have also developed a "Blending Initiative" (*www.drugabuse.gov/nidamed-medical-health-professionals/ nidasamhsa-blending-initiative*) focused on accelerating the adoption of evidence-based treatment by transferring research into clinical practice. Meetings, conferences, and webinars have been offered to expose providers to cutting-edge treatments.

An innovative dissemination resource has also been established by NIAAA, termed the "Alcohol Treatment Navigator" (*https://alcoholtreatment.niaaa.nih.gov*). Its website mainly targets consumers rather than providers, to help them recognize and find quality care for alcohol use disorders. The "Navigator" educates consumers on the types of treatments available, provides access to online provider directories from SAMHSA, suggests important questions to ask potential providers, and gives step-by-step instructions on the search process.

Such dissemination strategies are intended to promote awareness, understanding, and (ideally) the use of new treatments. Feedback derived from these dissemination strategies can be used to refine and redistribute materials and strategies in the hope that providers, educators, and stakeholders will be motivated to make use of these new interventions. However, as illustrated at the beginning of this chapter, merely having access to such information does not guarantee that it will be adopted and used effectively (Ducharme, Chandler, & Harris, 2016). That is the domain of implementation science: how to promote not only the dissemination of information but also the effective implementation of treatment innovations, so that the gap between research and practice is reduced (Fixsen et al., 2005; Lash, Timko, Curran, McKay, & Burden, 2011).

Implementation: Facilitating Individual and Organizational Change

Implementation science focuses on strategies to address organizational and individual barriers to the practice of effective interventions. Whereas dissemination may convey information and (potentially) interest in an innovation, implementation involves getting it into sustainable practice.

An illustrative example is continuing professional education, frequently required in order to maintain professional licensure. A common strategy is to offer lectures or workshops for treatment providers, either live in a classroom setting or via digital media. Such events may increase knowledge about an intervention, but often have very little impact on practice behavior. For example, when a live 2-day workshop on motivational interviewing (MI) was evaluated by comparing pre- and posttraining audio practice samples, skill changes were small and transient, and there was no apparent change in client response (Miller & Mount, 2001). Of still greater concern, the workshop participants were confident that they had learned MI and were now using it effectively in practice, so they were significantly less interested in further MI training. A larger randomized trial of training strategies similarly found modest change in practice or client response after a 2-day MI workshop or self-guided training unless participants also received subsequent feedback and coaching based on observed practice (Miller et al., 2004). Didactic training alone seems to be similarly ineffective in developing competence in other evidence-based practices for treating SUDs (Miller et al., 2006), yet it remains a primary mode of continuing professional education.

This, in turn, highlights the importance of direct observation of practice when training and implementing a new treatment method. This is routine in medical education; residents in training are observed while learning a new surgical procedure. Indeed, much of medical care is witnessed by other staff rather than being solitary. In behavioral health, however, direct observation of practice has been less common once initial training is completed (Miller, 2007). With a complex treatment, there is really no way to know whether it is being learned or delivered with fidelity except by directly observing practice.

Some Barriers to Implementing Evidence-Based Treatments

A lack of adequate training is not the only barrier to effective implementation of evidence-based treatments. A common obstacle is the high demand of current workflow: "I already have too much to do." This has been a significant obstacle to implementing SBIRT (Screening, Brief Intervention and Referral to Treatment) in underfunded community health settings (Babor et al., 2007). Asking staff to do more with less discourages undertaking new tasks, and can fuel staff burn-out, fatigue, and turnover (Stanhope, Manuel, Jessell, & Halliday, 2018).

Nevertheless, treatment professionals are often willing to learn something new if it will significantly benefit their clients. Between-group differences in outcome are typically small to none when different bona fide treatments are compared (Imel et al., 2008; Miller & Moyers, 2015). With a large enough sample, even small differences can be *statistically* significant, but are they *clinically* meaningful? Highly experienced addiction treatment providers were asked to

> Treatment professionals are willing to learn something new if it will benefit their clients.

specify how much better the outcomes of a new intervention would have to be in order for them to (1) regard the difference as clinically important and (2) be interested in learning the new treatment themselves (Miller & Manuel, 2008). What they regarded to be a clinically meaningful advantage (e.g., abstinent days 11 percentage points higher) was larger than between-treatment differences often observed in clinical trials. However, if a new treatment did improve outcomes by that much, they would be interested in learning it. It also helps to have credible peer advocates or "champions" for implementing a new intervention (Gordon et al., 2011; Powell, Proctor, & Glass, 2014).

There can be organizational-level barriers to change as well (Hunter, Schwartz, & Friedmann, 2016). Resources for staff training are often limited, and funding priorities or institutional values may not favor new interventions (Williams et al., 2016). An organizational climate might be unfavorable for undertaking a new intervention if agency morale is low and there is mistrust between management and staff. It is also possible that an organization may simply not have the technical capacity to implement a new intervention. For example, implementing SBIRT may require an electronic record system for case finding and clinical reminders, and user-friendly computer programs for screening, intervention, referral, and follow-up.

Implementation Processes and Strategies

So what does help to overcome such barriers and implement change at an organizational level? We begin with a well-developed conceptual model for identifying strategies to implement and sustain new interventions in addiction treatment settings.

The Consolidated Framework for Implementation Research

The Consolidated Framework for Implementation Research (CFIR; Damschroder et al., 2009; Damschroder & Hagedorn, 2011) includes five broad domains that can facilitate or hinder effective implementation of new treatments. You may recognize overlap with the previously discussed characteristics that favor the dissemination of innovations (Rogers, 2003).

Characteristics of the Intervention

A first consideration is whether the intervention is adaptable (Lash et al., 2011). Can it be tailored to make it suitable in a particular clinical or cultural setting (Venner, Feldstein, & Tafoya, 2007)? Must it be adopted in its entirety as is, or can certain elements be dropped or modified while retaining effectiveness?

Outer Setting

What political/economic/social supports would be needed in order to implement the new treatment? Here are three examples of systemic changes that facilitated implementation of new SUD interventions in the United States:

- Congressional passage of the Affordable Care Act offered new opportunities for expanding and implementing SUD treatment in primary care and other medical settings (Humphreys & Frank, 2014).
- The National Institutes of Health and the Department of Veterans Affairs hospitals created investigator initiatives to pilot test behavioral health integration in health care settings (Ducharme et al., 2016).
- Foundational funding for SUD treatment enabled TANF (Temporary Assistance for Needy Families) women to receive intensive case management services for alcohol/drug problems along with financial aid (see Chapter 8).

Inner Setting

What changes would need to occur in the organizational climate and culture to implement a new treatment? Such issues include peer support or "champions" for a new approach, staff participation in decision making, information sharing, and training (Lash et al., 2011; Sorensen & Kosten, 2011). Will incentives be offered for staff who develop proficiency in the new method? An implementation team can be formed, engaging staff and managers in the planning, development, and adaptation of a new treatment. Pilot testing can be helpful before larger rollout (Lash et al., 2011; Lehman, Simpson, Knight, & Flynn, 2011; Sorensen & Kosten, 2011).

Characteristics of Individuals

How does the new treatment fit with the perceptions and values of those who would be learning and providing it (Lash et al., 2011)? Does it conflict with a prior ideological commitment? How will the new approach be reconciled with the importance of counselor–client relationship? Is it complementary to other currently used treatment methods?

Process of Implementation

How ready is the organization to develop, adapt, and execute an implementation plan? What new technology or technical assistance will be needed? How will clinicians' learning and the fidelity of treatment delivery be assessed in guiding implementation (Padwa et al., 2016)? In other words, are the systems and resources in place for carrying out the proposed implementation plan (Lash et al., 2011)?

Applying the CFIR in Practice Settings

An example of the CFIR framework is the implementation of alcohol screening and brief intervention in eight frontline programs in nine countries, involving 533,903 clients (Williams et al., 2011). From published reports, implementation strategies were categorized according to the five broad CFIR domains and then linked to actual rates of screening and brief intervention. Most of the programs used strategies associated with the five CFIR domains, albeit at different intensities. Here are some examples.

Characteristics of the Intervention

Adaptability of the intervention to the setting was most widely addressed. The World Health Organization settings were all encouraged to tailor implementation strategies to their nation's language and culture. Training activities were modified to accommodate the busy work schedules of providers.

Inner Setting

The World Health Organization offered continuing professional education credits for participating in training to advance the proficiency of staff, and the Department of Veterans Affairs hospital sites offered financial incentives for staff meeting performance standards.

Process of Implementation

All participating programs established planning committees to carry out implementation strategies. Some used opinion or implementation leaders to participate in planning committees and coordinate implementation plans. These committees met regularly to hone intervention procedures. The Veterans Health Administration had the most comprehensive and intensive implementation program. They used multiple implementation strategies associated with Inner Setting, Outer Setting, and Process of Implementation domains. These changes contributed to a 93% screening rate in primary care, which was higher than other programs in the study. Because the domains overlap and components were instigated together, it is not possible to determine which particular elements contributed most to successful implementation.

Other Research on Implementation Strategies

A meta-analysis of implementation studies in primary health care settings (Keurhorst et al., 2015) found that combining staff and organizational implementation strategies improved the uptake of screening and brief intervention activities more than single implementation strategies did alone. Staff implementation strategies included training and feedback in motivational interviewing and educational meetings on brief alcohol intervention with role-play exercises. Organizational implementation strategies included formally integrating medical and substance use services, web-based screening and intervention strategies, and changing the settings/sites of service delivery. Some studies also provided feedback to clients on their alcohol consumption practices and related problems, conducted outreach visits, and distributed educational materials on risky drinking. Studies that combined client, staff, and organization implementation strategies were generally more effective in reducing substance use problems than were studies that focused solely on staff implementation strategies.

Just as with medication, the intensity or "dose" level of an implementation strategy can matter. A potentially effective strategy may fail because its intensity was insufficient (e.g., Garner, Hunter, Funk, Griffin, & Godley, 2016; Harris et al., 2017; Ornstein et al., 2013; Rowe et al., 2013). As discussed earlier, for example, reaching proficiency in delivering a complex intervention is likely to require more than workshop or self-directed instruction.

In another multisite implementation trial (Schmidt et al., 2012), a coordinated range of strategies were applied simultaneously across multiple system levels to integrate evidence-based SUD treatment in diverse clinical settings (i.e., outpatient, withdrawal management, hospital, and mental health settings). This study was sponsored by the Robert Wood Johnson Foundation's Advanced Recovery program aimed at the adoption of evidence-based treatment for SUDs. An announcement was sent to Single-State Authorities inviting proposals to implement new interventions in three or four SUD treatment centers within their jurisdictions. Across 10 states, 12 sites were awarded grants to implement two promising new therapies based on encouraging findings from clinical trials: continuing care management (see Chapter 8) and medication-assisted treatment (see Chapter 18).

The sites were expected to use "top-down" and "bottom-up" implementation strategies similar those described in the CFIR. Such strategies included securing new or reallocating existing resources to cover the costs of the new therapies, providing education and feedback to providers to address philosophical differences among providers (e.g., on using medications), and identifying and involving policymakers who could be "champions" of the new treatment modalities. Along with the training activities, technical assistance was offered on the implementation of evidence-based practices.

The number and kinds of implementation strategies varied across sites, with most sites initiating strategies incrementally on a "trial-and-error" basis. There was overall progress in implementing both continuing care management (e.g., successful referrals to other programs for withdrawal management and outpatient treatment) and medication-assisted treatment (e.g., buprenorphine for opioid clients), with greater success in implementing the latter. In the four outpatient sites, rates of adoption of medication-assisted treatment doubled in the first 6 months. Other sites evidenced improvement in implementing continuing care, but not at the same level and pace as medication-assisted treatment.

BOX 25.2. Personal Reflection: The Challenge of Involving Significant Others in Treatment

It is clear from research that clients' outcomes are better when a supportive significant other (SSO) is involved in treatment (see Chapters 15 and 16), so the message is straightforward, right? Include SSOs in care rather than just treating individual clients. That's why, in designing the combined behavioral intervention (CBI) as a state-of-the-art treatment for the COMBINE trial, we advocated routine involvement of an SSO in sessions (Longabaugh, Zweben, LoCastro, & Miller, 2005). The SSO was to give constructive feedback about treatment plans, provide ongoing support to reduce drinking, and generally buttress the client's motivation for change. We anticipated that including an SSO in treatment would improve client outcomes, and once again in this study it did (Hunter-Reel, Witkiewitz, & Zweben, 2012).

Despite strong encouragement and prior research showing benefit, however, only about one-quarter of clients had an SSO attend even one CBI session. In fact, extensive SSO involvement occurred at only two of 11 sites. As chair of the behavioral intervention committee in COMBINE, I tried to find out why SSO involvement was disappointingly low. I contacted staff and investigators at other sites and learned that many therapists were accustomed to and comfortable with working mainly with individual clients, and not with family members or SSOs. Some were reluctant to add further difficulties to an already complex intervention such as CBI. In fact, most of the principal investigators were themselves inexperienced in working with SSOs.

So what was different about the two sites with high SSO involvement? At both sites, the principal investigators were primary developers of the SSO component of CBI, and thus "champions" of this process. Also, at those sites, therapists were intentionally hired who had competence in working with family members and SSOs, because that was one expectation for the position.

—A. Z.

Overall, successful implementation was attributed to using multifaceted, multilevel strategies for overcoming barriers in these settings. For example, settings that evidenced higher rates of adoption of medication-assisted treatment often included the amending of funding priorities to allow agencies to purchase medications for offenders, changing licensing and contracting agreements to support medications in treatment, and training in MI to encourage and assist clients in using medications. Once payment mechanisms were in place, training opportunities were offered to reduce ideological resistance to the use of medications.

In contrast, continuing care management strategies encountered unique challenges that were more difficult to overcome. The lack of available treatment slots for referral, high workflow, and staff turnover made adoption more difficult in these settings. At the same time, staff did not appear to sufficiently value this new treatment to embrace the additional demands involved. It seems that greater efforts might have been made to develop and support collaborations among stakeholders and providers to address these important issues.

Designing a Tailor-Made Implementation Plan

The implementation process often begins with brainstorming in focus groups with stakeholders and staff about problems encountered in delivering services. Such problems might entail low rates of successful referrals, high rates of no-shows and dropouts, frequent medication and treatment nonadherence, and general client and staff dissatisfaction with the quality of care being offered. Identify interventions that might address these problems and also have good empirical support (Leeman et al., 2017; Powell et al., 2017). Don't choose an intervention just because it is popular and has a training manual and curriculum (Ducharme et al., 2016). Ideally, choose an intervention that has demonstrated a causal link between the intervention and improved clinical outcomes (Lehman et al., 2011).

If you settle on a new treatment to implement, consider what CFIR factors might facilitate or interfere with delivering it, and how potential obstacles might be addressed (Powell et al., 2017). The CFIR model can help to match barriers that may arise with strategies to effectively overcome them. The CFIR can also help to prevent a mismatch between barriers and implementation strategies. For example, don't focus efforts on the "Characteristics of Individuals" domain if "Outer Setting" issues like funding priorities and reimbursement are the primary obstacles.

Above all, build consensus among staff and administrators by actively involving them in the implementation plan. Set realistic goals together and identify feasible strategies for successful implementation (Powell et al., 2017; Schmidt et al., 2012).

Issues Arising in the Implementation Process

The number and kinds of barriers arising when implementing a new intervention are often related to the complexity of the treatment. At the high end of complexity is a detailed, manualized, standardized approach with a fixed number of sessions and prescribed content over a specified time period. Adapting such a treatment in an ongoing clinical setting may require numerous modifications over time (Sorensen & Kosten, 2011). Such adaptations might include changing criteria for treatment eligibility, reformatting the delivery format from individual to group treatment, and reducing academic and proficiency standards for clinical staff (relative to those that were required in clinical trials). Of course, such modifications may alter fidelity of the intervention and lose "active ingredients," thereby impacting clinical outcomes. It is common for the effect size of a treatment to decrease when implemented in community practice, relative to original clinical trials.

For example, Lundgren and colleagues (2013) conducted a national study on implementing community-based SUD treatment for adolescents. They examined the relationship between the level of barriers experienced by staff in implementing new intervention programs and the level of modifications required to adapt the intervention in agency practice. The new interventions were comprised of MI and an adolescent community reinforcement approach (A-CRA), an intervention that entails learning new coping behaviors and involving a significant other in treatment (see Chapter 14). Staff who implemented A-CRA reported encountering a greater number of barriers in delivery, relative to those who implemented MI. A-CRA was a complex protocol where adolescents and parents were first seen separately followed by conjoint sessions. Major barriers in implementing A-CRA included insufficient staff training, clients who did not fit the criteria for the intervention, job stress, and having less experience in adopting new interventions. In contrast, staff implementing MI found the approach to be flexible, consistent with their skills and approach, and readily adaptable in their clinical setting. In sum, it is easier to implement an intervention that is less complex, and is more congruent with the organization's resources and approach (Lundgren et al., 2013).

Manual-Guided Treatment

A plethora of SUD treatment manuals have appeared as a byproduct of research, resulting particularly from the fact that it is difficult to get research funding for a clinical trial of a behavioral treatment without producing a manual that provides a high level of detail regarding the procedures to be used. Once a trial has been completed, the manual is often then made available for more general use. However, the prescribed level of session-by-session detail in such manuals tends to be unsuited to the ordinary flexibility and demands of community practice. Nevertheless, the advice to users, as it was to the original clinical trial therapists, is often to adhere precisely to the manual's instructions as a necessary condition for the treatment to "work."

We know of no scientific evidence that close adherence to a structured treatment manual improves client outcomes. A meta-analysis of clinical trials of MI found the opposite: that the effect size was substantially *reduced* in studies using a treatment manual. Clients receiving a highly structured and closely supervised manual-based SUD treatment often have outcomes that are little or no different from those of clients receiving unstructured treatment as usual within the same facilities (Miller & Moyers, 2015; Wells, Saxon, Calsyn, Jackson, & Donovan, 2010; Westerberg, Miller, & Tonigan, 2000). Precise adherence to manuals without adaptation can be particularly questionable when a treatment is being adapted for people from a different cultural background (Venner et al., 2007, 2016).

How, then, might manuals that come from clinical trials be useful later? The level of detail that they contain may be informative to students or new practitioners when learning a complex evidence-based treatment method such as contingency management (Chapter 13), the community reinforcement approach (Chapter 14), or behavioral couple therapy (Chapter 15). Counselors in training or those inexperienced in practice may find it helpful to have such detailed how-to guidelines to follow as they develop their skills. However, training should also emphasize appropriate flexibility and the importance of the therapeutic relationship (Miller & Moyers, 2015).

Evidence-Based Components

Manual-guided treatments are usually tested as a whole package, but often prescribe many specific details. Such protocols may contain some components that are effective, other details that are irrelevant, and some that may even be countertherapeutic. There may be effective components of complex

> Manual-guided treatments need to be used with a large dose of flexibility.

treatments that can be implemented as freestanding interventions. For example, the combined behavioral intervention (CBI; Longabaugh et al., 2005; Miller, 2004) offered a menu of evidence-based components that clinicians can apply flexibly according to the individual needs of clients without a prescribed number of sessions. Similarly, the community reinforcement approach on which CBI was based includes a set of well-defined procedures that counselors can draw upon depending on each client's situation (Azrin et al., 1982; Meyers & Miller, 2001; Meyers & Smith, 1995). CBI included a variety of "pull-out" procedures for responding to particular challenges in practice, such as resumed substance use or missed appointments (Miller, 2004).

Here are some examples of components from more complex methods that can be implemented in clinical practice. Such components might be less effective in isolation from the context of the larger parent approach. On the other hand, implementing one effective component may interest staff in learning more about the treatment approach from which it came.

Systematic Encouragement

Within a community reinforcement approach, Sisson and Mallams (1981) developed a procedure for encouraging clients to sample AA meetings, though it could be used to facilitate participation in many other treatment-relevant activities. As described in Chapter 17, 100% of clients receiving this procedure attended an AA meeting, whereas no one in the control condition (advised to attend and given a schedule of meetings) made it to a meeting.

Spouse-Monitored Medication

When disulfiram was added to the community reinforcement approach, so was a well-specified procedure described in Chapter 18 involving a regular daily event in which a client takes the medication in the presence of the spouse or a supportive significant other. The spouse's role is only to witness and lovingly encourage daily dosage. Adding this procedure to traditional treatment dramatically reduced drinking days, unemployment, and institutionalization (Azrin et al., 1982). Monitored disulfiram more generally increases medication adherence and abstinence (Brewer & Streel, 2018).

Sampling Pleasant Activities

Having clients sample and increase potentially enjoyable (and drug-free) activities has long been used as an effective component in the treatment of depression (Lewinsohn et al., 1992). It is also an important element of the community reinforcement approach, to render life in recovery more enjoyable and meaningful. A common procedure has been to have clients peruse a large menu of activities that they might enjoy, select one or more, and try them out between sessions. This moves beyond suppressing addictive behaviors, to render sober life more reinforcing.

Empathic Listening

The learnable interpersonal skill of empathic or reflective listening (see Chapter 4 and Miller, 2018) has a long track record of research in improving clinical outcomes in general (Truax & Carkhuff, 1967), and specifically in the treatment of SUDs (Miller & Moyers, 2015; Miller, Taylor, & West, 1980; Valle, 1981). Virtually all of the treatment methods described in this book can be delivered in an engaging, empathic style.

Implementation: Trying Something New

Experiments to improve treatment outcome need not be limited to well-funded research centers. When you consider adding a new procedure to your current treatment program, we recommend that you also take time to evaluate whether it actually does improve treatment acceptance, adherence, or outcome. What is the problem that you hope it will address? How would you know if it is working?

The basic structure of such an experiment can be relatively simple: to ask whether the benefit of adding this new element is worth the investment of time, training, and other resources (Miller, 1980). If you add a contingency management procedure (Chapter 13), for example, does it make a clinically meaningful difference (e.g., increase treatment attendance or the rate of drug-free urine samples)? A common approach is to assign clients randomly or arbitrarily to receive or not receive the additional intervention beyond treatment as usual. Alternatively, you can keep track of the outcome of interest for a few months with treatment as usual, then introduce the new intervention for a specific period of time (say, 2 months) and see whether you get the change you are hoping for. This can help you avoid continuing to add procedures that really don't make a difference. If a new component is not working, how might it be modified to be effective with your population? What level of staff proficiency is necessary to deliver the new procedure with fidelity? If it works, how could it be moved into routine use while maintaining quality and fidelity? How could you "scale up" (Fixsen, Blase, & Fixsen, 2017) the intervention so it can be used across a broader spectrum of clients and providers? Asking and addressing such questions can provide the building blocks of successful and sustainable implementation (Leeman et al., 2017; Powell et al., 2017, 2015).

SBIRT: An Implementation Case Example

Recent evidence on SBIRT (Screening, Brief Intervention, and Referral to specialty Treatment) raised serious questions about the utility of this approach in primary care settings (see Chapter 9). Findings indicated that SBIRT had not been effective in reducing illicit drug use, and a meta-analysis found that SBIRT clients with moderate and severe alcohol problems were no more likely to follow through on referrals to specialty care than those not receiving SBIRT. These deficiencies have been attributed to implementation problems such as lack of adequate staff training in the knowledge and skills necessary for delivering SBIRT in busy practice settings, or lack of sufficient resources to support such training. The requirements of effective training (e.g., workshops followed by coaching and feedback) may be too costly for these settings.

Guided by the principles of diffusion of innovation theory and the CFIR discussed earlier, an implementation demonstration project (Brooks et al., 2016) was conducted in three Federally Qualified Health Centers. Based on feedback from numerous focus groups, the investigators provided counselors with a toolkit comprised of 35 take-home cards containing tips and strategies for the cessation and maintenance of risky drinking or drug use. The toolkits included videos, pamphlets, and other material (e.g., a graphic novel) to guide changes in drinking and drug use.

After limited training, counselors introduced the toolkit in SBIRT sessions to show clients how they could flexibly and briefly use the tools to address problems encountered in everyday living to achieve and maintain sobriety. The messages were based on elements of cognitive-behavioral therapy, 12-step facilitation therapy, and motivational enhancement therapy—the three major elements of the aforementioned combined behavioral intervention (CBI). The toolkit was basically an add-on, take-away component to augment SBIRT.

Was it feasible in practice? As an experiment, 600 people with alcohol/drug problems were randomly assigned to receive a single session of SBIRT or an expanded SBIRT of two to five sessions using the toolkit. Counselors could use the cards in any order, and choose only those cards that were applicable to the particular needs of their clients. Clients receiving the SBIRT + Toolkit found the approach more helpful and satisfying than those given a single session of brief intervention. At the same time, providers reported that the simplicity and flexibility of the model were clearly compatible with routine methods of primary care treatment for SUD clients. At follow-up, both groups showed substantial reduction in alcohol and illicit drug use, with clients in the expanded SBIRT condition showing somewhat greater reduction in drinking and in use of their primary problem substance (Brooks et al., 2017). This study offers a number of important messages regarding implementation. The intervention was designed to fit in with SBIRT as delivered in primary health care settings. The innovation provided take-home materials for clients without substantially increasing the training or workload burden for providers. Counselors could use small or large portions of the model (i.e., cards and/or the graphic novel) flexibly, depending on the individual client's needs and preference. The study also demonstrated how specific components from more complex treatments can be used in routine clinical care. Finally, having an effective intervention to use reduced negative staff perceptions regarding SUD clients.

Attitudes in Implementing Evidence-Based Interventions

In this book we have discussed a wide variety of innovative and effective methods for treating SUDs. The field has moved away from a "one-size-fits-all" approach toward a menu of strategies to address the diverse capabilities, individual and social recovery resources of clients who are seen in medical, educational, workplace, family, criminal justice, and social service settings. With such a range of effective options it is possible to fit treatment to individual needs rather than expecting diverse people to fit into a unitary treatment model (see Chapter 7).

> We have moved away from a "one-size-fits-all" approach toward a menu of strategies.

We return here to the underlying mind-set and assumptions with which addiction treatment is provided (Chapter 4). Carl Rogers (1959, 1980) emphasized the fundamental role of *attitudes* in client care. Underlying attitudes have changed substantially in addiction treatment over recent decades, moving away from moralistic stereotypes of people with SUDs as difficult to treat, manipulative, and in denial. Rather than waiting for clients to "hit bottom," it is possible to shorten the length of time they spend in addiction. Treatment has shifted away from an expert and authoritarian stance toward a more empathic and collaborative approach. One factor in this change of treatment philosophy may be the widespread dissemination of MI and its underlying compassionate spirit (Hall, Staiger, Simpson, Best, & Lubman, 2016; Miller & Rollnick, 2013). Rather than installing insight, education, and corrective thinking, MI affirms client's strengths, evokes their own recovery resources, fosters optimism, and accepts imperfection (cf. Kurtz & Ketcham, 1992).

For example, medical management, a behavioral platform widely used in pharmacotherapy trials, was significantly improved by infusing MI in the intervention (Zweben et al., 2017). In line with the MI spirit, greater emphasis was placed on the benefits of change (e.g., improved relationships, enhanced quality of life) rather than on the risks of drinking. In the initial session, clients were encouraged to voice their own perspectives on the problem while practitioners demonstrated genuine acceptance of clients' views. This revised approach helped to engage and retain clients in treatment, with a medication adherence rate of 90%, an exceptionally high rate for an alcohol pharmacotherapy trial. A meta-analysis of 16 studies that included MI as a clinical intervention style found significantly improved medication adherence in chronic disease management with adults (Zomahoun et al., 2016).

In this sense, MI is not so much a separate intervention as a way of doing what else you do, a foundation for delivering other forms of treatment). MI has been integrated into many kinds of treatment including medication-assisted treatment (Pettinati & Mattson, 2010), cognitive-behavioral therapy (Naar & Safren, 2017), and SBIRT (Whittle, Buckelow, Satterfield, Lum, & O'Sullivan, 2015). These foundational attitudes of respect for autonomy, collaboration, acceptance, and exploring the client's own perspectives were inspired by Carl Rogers's emphasis on the healing qualities of empathic understanding and unconditional positive regard. They are also a solid foundation in treating addiction.

KEY POINTS

🕯 Clients cannot benefit from a treatment to which they are not exposed in sufficient "dose" or fidelity.

🕯 Analogous to marketing, dissemination focuses mainly on promoting awareness of a new treatment with the hope of motivating a target audience to adopt it in routine practice.

🕯 Implementation is an active process focused on identifying and overcoming barriers that interfere with the adoption, utilization, and sustainability of an intervention in practice.

🕯 The CFIR is a well-developed conceptual model that has been successfully applied in guiding the adoption of screening and intervention protocols in national and international health care programs.

🕯 The complexity of the intervention increases the number and kinds of barriers encountered in adopting, adapting, and sustaining a new intervention.

🕯 Higher levels of individual and organizational barriers often require more modifications to be made in the intervention to make it compatible in practice.

🕯 Modifications in turn may undermine the fidelity of an intervention and negatively affect clinical outcomes.

🕯 Implementing selected components of an intervention that have empirical support may be a flexible and feasible alternative to strictly following a treatment manual for a complex intervention.

Reflection Questions

◌ What are some important considerations in adopting or adapting an SUD intervention in specialty or nonspecialty settings to make it congruent with ongoing practice?

◌ How do you balance the implementation dilemma of modifying intervention components for ongoing practice while retaining integrity of the active ingredients of a treatment?

◌ If participating in online or live educational sessions have little or no effect on practice behavior, how might you modify continuing professional education?

◌ From what you have learned in this book, what interventions would you be most eager to implement where you work, and how would you begin?

References

Abbott, P. J., Moore, B., & Delaney, H. (2003). Community reinforcement approach and relapse prevention: 12- and 18-month follow-up. *Journal of Maintenance in the Addictions, 2*(3), 35–50.

Abbott, P. J., Quinn, D., & Knox, L. (1995). Ambulatory medical detoxification for alcohol. *American Journal of Drug and Alcohol Abuse, 21*(4), 549–563.

Abbott, P. J., Weller, S. B., Delaney, H. D., & Moore, B. A. (1998). Community reinforcement approach in the treatment of opiate addicts. *American Journal of Drug and Alcohol Abuse, 24,* 17–30.

Abellanas, L., & McLellan, A. T. (1993). "Stages of change" by drug problem in concurrent opioid, cocaine and cigarette users. *Journal of Psychoactive Drugs, 25,* 307–313.

Abraham, A., Rothrauff, T., & Roman, P. (2010). Implementation of alcohol pharmacotherapies in specialty aud treatment settings: How are programs using medications in routine treatment practice. *Alcoholism: Clinical and Experimental Research, 34*(6), 285A.

Advokat, C. D., Comaty, J. E., & Julian, R. M. (2019). *Julien's primer of drug action: A comprehensive guide to the actions, uses, and side effects of psychoactive drugs* (14th ed.). New York: Worth.

Agboola, S., McNeill, A., Coleman, T., & Leonardi Bee, J. (2010). A systematic review of the effectiveness of smoking relapse prevention interventions for abstinent smokers. *Addiction, 105*(8), 1362–1380.

Agosti, V., Nunes, E. V., & O'Shea, D. (2012). Do manualized psychosocial interventions help reduce relapse among alcohol-dependent adults treated with naltrexone or placebo?: A meta-analysis. *American Journal on Addictions, 21*(6), 501–507.

Ahmed, M. (2007). Towards evidence based emergency medicine: Best BETs from the Manchester Royal Infirmary. Is emergency department based brief intervention worthwhile in adults presenting with alcohol related events? *Journal of Emergency Medicine, 24*(11), 785–788.

Ait-Daoud, N., & Johnson, B. (2003). Medications for the treatment of alcoholism. In B. Johnson, P. Ruiz, & M. Galanter (Eds.), *Handbook of clinical alcoholism treatment* (pp. 119–130). Baltimore: Lippincott Williams & Wilkins.

Ajzen, I. (2002). Constructing a TPB questionnaire: Conceptual and methodological considerations Retrieved from *www.webcitation.org/66zom97zq*.

Al-Anon Family Group Headquarters. (1976). *Living with an alcoholic with the help of Al-Anon*. New York: Author.

Alcoholics Anonymous. (1976). *Alcoholics Anonymous: The story of how many thousands of men and women have recovered from alcoholism* (3rd ed.). New York: A.A. World Services.

Alcoholics Anonymous World Services. (1957). *Alcoholics Anonymous*. New York: Author.

Alcoholics Anonymous World Services. (2001). *Alcoholics Anonymous: The story of how many thousands of men and women have recovered from alcoholism* (4th ed.). New York: Author.

Alcoholics Anonymous World Services. (2015). *Alcoholics Anonymous 2014 membership survey*. New York: Author.

Aldridge, A., Dowd, W., & Bray, J. (2017). The relative impact of brief treatment versus brief intervention in primary health-care screening programs for substance use disorders. *Addiction, 112*, 54–64.

Aldridge, A., Linford, R., & Bray, J. (2017). Substance use outcomes of patients served by a large US implementation of Screening, Brief Intervention and Referral to Treatment (SBIRT). *Addiction, 112*(2), 43–53.

Aletraris, L., Shelton, J. S., & Roman, P. M. (2015). Counselor attitudes toward contingency management for substance use disorder: Effectiveness, acceptability, and endorsement of incentives for treatment attendance and abstinence. *Journal of Substance Abuse Treatment, 57*, 41–48.

Alexander, B. K. (2008). *The globalization of addiction: A study in poverty of the spirit*. New York: Oxford University Press.

Alexander, B. K., Beyerstein, B. L., Hadaway, P. F., & Coambs, R. B. (1981). Effect of early and later colony housing on oral ingestion of morphine in rats. *Pharmacology, Biochemistry, and Behavior, 15*(4), 571–576.

Alexander, B. K., Coambs, R. B., & Hadaway, P. F. (1978). The effect of housing and gender on morphine self-administration in rats. *Psychopharmacology, 58*(2), 175–179.

Alexander, J. A., Pollack, H., Nahra, T., Wells, R., & Lemak, C. H. (2007). Case management and client access to health and social services in outpatient substance abuse treatment. *Journal of Behavioral Health Services and Research, 34*(3), 221–236.

Alexander, J. F., Waldron, H. B., Robbins, M. S., & Neeb, A. A. (2013). *Functional family therapy for adolescent behavior problems*. Washington, DC: American Psychological Association.

Alterman, A. I., O'Brien, C. P., McLellan, A. T., August, D. S., Snider, E. C., Droba, M., . . . Schrade, F. X. (1994). Effectiveness and costs of inpatient versus day hospital cocaine rehabilitation. *Journal of Nervous and Mental Disease, 182*(3), 157–163.

Alterman, A., Snider, E., Caccioia, J., May, D., Parikh, G., Maany, I., & Rosenbaum, P. (1996). A quasi-experimental comparison of the effectiveness of 6- versus 12-hour per week outpatient treatments for cocaine dependence. *Journal of Nervous and Mental Disease, 184*, 54–56.

American Psychiatric Association. (1952). *Diagnostic and statistical manual of mental disorders*. Washington, DC: Author.

American Psychiatric Association. (1968). *Diagnostic and statistical manual of mental disorders* (2nd ed.). Washington, DC: Author.

American Psychiatric Association. (1980). *Diagnostic and statistical manual of mental disorders* (3rd ed.). Washington, DC: Author.

American Psychiatric Association. (1987). *Diagnostic and statistical manual of mental disorders* (3rd ed., rev.). Washington, DC: Author.

American Psychiatric Association. (1994). *Diagnostic and statistical manual of mental disorders* (4th ed.). Washington, DC: Author.

American Psychiatric Association. (2000). *Diagnostic and statistical manual of mental disorders* (4th ed., text rev.). Washington, DC.: Author.

American Psychiatric Association. (2013). *Diagnostic and statistical manual of mental disorders* (5th ed.). Arlington, VA: Author.

American Society of Addiction Medicine. (1996). *Patient placement criteria for the treatment of substance-related disorders* (2nd ed.). Chevy Chase, MD: Author.

American Society of Addiction Medicine. (2001). *Patient placement criteria for the treatment of substance-related disorders (PPC-2R).* Chevy Chase, MD: Author.

American Society of Addiction Medicine. (2013). *Advancing access to addiction medicine: Implications for opioid addiction treatment.* Rockville, MD: Author.

Andreas, J. B., Lauritzen, G., & Nordfjaern, T. (2015). Co-occurrence between mental distress and poly-drug use: A ten year prospective study of patients from substance abuse treatment. *Addictive Behaviors, 48,* 71–78.

Angarita, G. A., Reif, S., Pirard, S., Lee, S., Sharon, E., & Gastfriend, D. (2007). No-show for treatment in substance abuse patients with comorbid symptomatology: Validity results from a controlled trial of the ASAM patient placement criteria. *Journal of Addiction Medicine, 1,* 79–87.

Annis, H. M., & Chan, D. (1983). The differential treatment model: Empirical evidence from a personality typology of adult offenders. *Criminal Justice and Behavior, 10,* 159–73.

Annis, H. M., & Graham, J. M. (1988). *Situational Confidence Questionnaire (SCQ-329) user's guide.* Toronto, ON, Canada: Addiction Research Foundation.

Annis, H. M., & Graham, J. M. (1991). *Inventory of Drug-Taking Situations (IDT-SII): User's guide.* Toronto, ON, Canada: Addiction Research Foundation.

Annis, H. M., Graham, J. M., & Davis, C. D. (1987). *Inventory of Drinking Situations user's guide.* Toronto, ON, Canada: Addiction Research Foundation.

Anonymous. (1957). *The cloud of unknowing* (I. Progoff, Trans.). New York: Delta Books.

Anton, R. F., Lieber, C., Tabakoff, B., & CDTect Study Group. (2002). Carbohydrate-deficient transferrin and γ-glutamyltransferase for the detection and monitoring of alcohol use: Results from a multisite study. *Alcoholism: Clinical and Experimental Research, 26*(8), 1215–1222.

Anton, R. F., Litten, R. A., & Allen, J. P. (1995). Biological assessment of alcohol consumption. In J. P. Allen & M. Columbus (Eds.), *Assesssing alcohol problems: A guide for clinicians and researchers* (pp. 31–39). Rockville, MD: National Institute on Alcohol Abuse and Alcoholism.

Anton, R. F., Moak, D. H., Latham, P. K., Waid, L. R., Malcolm, R. J., Dias, J. K., & Roberts, J. S. (2001). Posttreatment results of combining naltrexone with cognitive-behavior therapy for the treatment of alcoholism. *Journal of Clinical Psychopharmacology, 21*(1), 72–77.

Anton, R. F., O'Malley, S. S., Ciraulo, D. A., Cisler, R. A., Couper, D., Donovan, D. M., . . . LoCastro, J. S. (2006). Combined pharmacotherapies and behavioral interventions for alcohol dependence: The COMBINE study: A randomized controlled trial. *JAMA, 295*(17), 2003–2017.

Apodaca, T. R., Magill, M., Longabaugh, R., Jackson, K. M., & Monti, P. M. (2013). Effect of a significant other on client change talk in motivational interviewing. *Journal of Consulting and Clinical Psychology, 81*(1), 35–46.

Apodaca, T. R., & Miller, W. R. (2003). A meta-analysis of the effectiveness of bibliotherapy for alcohol problems. *Journal of Clinical Psychology, 59,* 289–304.

Arlt, V. K. (2017). *Clinician mindfulness, motivational interviewing and treatment outcomes for substance-using adolescents.* Doctoral dissertation, Seattle Pacific University, Seattle, WA.

Aron, A., & Aron, E. N. (1980). The transcendental meditation program's effect on addictive behavior. *Addictive Behaviors, 5,* 3–12.

Ashe, M. L., Newman, M. G., & Wilson, S. J. (2015). Delay discounting and the use of mindful attention versus distraction in the treatment of drug addiction: A conceptual review. *Journal of the Experimental Analysis of Behavior, 103*(1), 234–248.

Aspinall, E. J., Nambiar, D., Goldberg, D. J., Hickman, M., Weir, A., Van Velzen, E., . . . Hutchinson, S. J. (2014). Are needle and syringe programmes associated with a reduction in HIV transmission among people who inject drugs?: A systematic review and meta-analysis. *International Journal of Epidemiology, 43*(1), 235–248.

Aubrey, L. L. (1998). *Motivational interviewing with adolescents presenting for outpatient substance abuse treatment.* Doctoral dissertation, University of New Mexico, Albuquerque, NM.

Aveyard, P., Begh, R., Parsons, A., & West, R. (2012). Brief opportunistic smoking cessation interventions: A systematic review and meta-analysis to compare advice to quit and offer of assistance. *Addiction, 107*(6), 1066–1073.

Azar, D., White, V., Coomber, K., Faulkner, A., Livingston, M., Chikritzhs, T., . . . Wakefield, M. (2015). The association between alcohol outlet density and alcohol use among urban and regional Australian adolescents. *Addiction, 111,* 65–72.

Azrin, N. H. (1976). Improvements in the community-reinforcement approach to alcoholism. *Behaviour Research and Therapy, 14*(5), 339–348.

Azrin, N. H., & Besalel, V. A. (1982). *Finding a job.* Berkeley, CA: Ten Speed Press.

Azrin, N. H., Sisson, R. W., Meyers, R. J., & Godley, M. (1982). Alcoholism treatment by disulfiram and community reinforcement therapy. *Journal of Behavior Therapy and Experimental Psychiatry, 13,* 105–112.

Babor, T. F. (2004). Brief treatments for cannabis dependence: Findings from a randomized multisite trial. *Journal of Consulting and Clinical Psychology, 72*(3), 455–466.

Babor, T. F. (2017). Does alcohol industry funding corrupt alcohol science?: A startling revelation about the early history of JSAD. *Journal of Studies on Alcohol and Drugs, 78*(2), 173–174.

Babor, T., Caetano, R., Casswell, S., Edwards, G., Giesbrecht, N., Graham, K., . . . Rossow, I. (2010). *Alcohol: No ordinary commodity* (2nd ed.). Oxford, UK: Oxford University Press.

Babor, T. F., & Del Boca, F. K. (Eds.). (2003). *Treatment matching in alcoholism.* Cambridge, UK: Cambridge University Press.

Babor, T. F., & Grant, M. (1989). From clinical research to secondary prevention: International collaboration in the development of the Alcohol Use Disorders Identification Test (AUDIT). *Alcohol Health and Research World, 13,* 371–374.

Babor, T. F., & Higgins-Biddle, J. C. (2000). Alcohol screening and brief intervention: Dissemination strategies for medical practice and public health. *Addiction, 95*(5), 677–686.

Babor, T. F., Higgins-Biddle, J. C., Saunders, J. B., & Monteiro, M. G. (2001). *The*

Alcohol Use Disorders Identification Test: Guidelines for use in primary health care (2nd ed.). Geneva, Switzerland: World Health Organization.

Babor, T. F., McRee, B. G., Kassebaum, P. A., Grimaldi, P. L., Ahmed, K., & Bray, J. (2007). Screening, Brief Intervention, and Referral to Treatment (SBIRT): Toward a public health approach to the management of substance abuse. *Substance Abuse, 28*(3), 7–30.

Bacon, F. (1619/1992). *The wisdom of the ancients*. London: Kessinger.

Baer, J. S., Kivlahan, D. R., Blume, A. W., McKnight, P., & Marlatt, G. A. (2001). Brief intervention for heavy-drinking college students: 4-year follow-up and natural history. *American Journal of Public Health, 91*(8), 1310–1316.

Baer, R. A. (2003). Mindfulness training as a clinical intervention: A conceptual and empirical review. *Clinical Psychology: Science and Practice, 10*(2), 125–143.

Baggio, S., Dupuis, M., Studer, J., Spilka, S., Daeppen, J. B., Simon, O., . . . Gmel, G. (2016). Reframing video gaming and Internet use addiction: Empirical cross-national comparison of heavy use over time and addiction scales among young users. *Addiction, 111*(3), 513–522.

Baingana, F., al'Absi, M., Becker, A. E., & Pringle, B. (2015). Global research challenges and opportunities for mental health and substance use disorders. *Nature, 527*(7578), S172–S177.

Baker, A., Heather, N., Wodak, A., Dixon, J., & Holt, P. (1993). Evaluation of a cognitive-behavioural intervention for HIV prevention among injecting drug users. *AIDS, 7*(2), 247–256.

Baker, A., Kochan, N., Dixon, F., Heather, N., & Wodak, A. (1994). Controlled evaluation of a brief intervention of HIV prevention among injecting drug users not in treatment. *AIDS Care, 6*(5), 559–570.

Baker, A., Turner, A., Kay-Lambkin, F. J., & Lewin, T. J. (2009). The long and the short of treatments for alcohol or cannabis misuse among people with severe mental disorders. *Addictive Behaviors, 34,* 852–858.

Baker, T. B., Piper, M. E., McCarthy, D. E., Bolt, D. M., Smith, S. S., Kim, S.-Y., . . . Hatsukami, D. (2007). Time to first cigarette in the morning as an index of ability to quit smoking: Implications for nicotine dependence. *Nicotine and Tobacco Research, 9*(Suppl. 4), S555–S570.

Bakken, K., Landheim, A. S., & Vaglum, P. (2007). Axis I and II disorders as long-term predictors of mental distress: A six-year prospective follow-up of substance-dependent patients. *BMC Psychiatry, 7,* 29–41.

Baldwin, S. A., Christian, S., Berkeljon, A., & Shadish, W. R. (2012). The effects of family therapies for adolescent delinquency and substance abuse: A meta-analysis. *Journal of Marital and Family Therapy, 38,* 281–304.

Ball, S. A., Martino, S., Nich, C., Frankforter, T. L., van Horn, D., Crits-Christoph, P., . . . Carroll, K. M. (2007). Site matters: Multisite randomized trial of motivational enhancement therapy in community drug abuse clinics. *Journal of Consulting and Clinical Psychology, 75,* 556–567.

Baltieri, D. A., Daró, F. R., Ribeiro, P. L., & De Andrade, A. G. (2008). Comparing topiramate with naltrexone in the treatment of alcohol dependence. *Addiction, 103*(12), 2035–2044.

Bamatter, W., Carroll, K. M., Añez, L. M., Paris, M. J., Ball, S. A., Nich, C., . . . Martino, S. (2010). Informal discussions in substance abuse treatment sessions with Spanish-speaking clients. *Journal of Substance Abuse Treatment, 39*(4), 353–363.

Bandura, A. (1997). *Self-efficacy: The exercise of control*. New York: W. H. Freeman.

Barber, J. G., & Crisp, B. R. (1995). Social support and prevention of relapse following treatment for alcohol abuse. *Research on Social Work Practice, 5*(3), 283–296.

Barber, W., & O'Brien, C. (1999). Pharmacotherapies. In B. S. McCrady & E. E. Epistein (Eds.), *Addictions: A comprehensive guidebook* (pp. 347–369). New York: Oxford University Press.

Barnett, E., Moyers, T. B., Sussman, S., Smith, C., Rohrbach, L. A., Sun, P., & Spruit-Metz, D. (2014). From counselor skill to decreased marijuana use: Does change talk matter? *Journal of Substance Abuse Treatment, 46*, 498–505.

Barnett, N. P., Apodaca, T. R., Magill, M., Colby, S. M., Gwaltney, C., Rohsenow, D. J., & Monti, P. M. (2010). Moderators and mediators of two brief interventions for alcohol in the emergency department. *Addiction, 105*(3), 452–465.

Barnett, N. P., Tidey, J., Murphy, J. G., Swift, R., & Colby, S. M. (2011). Contingency management for alcohol use reduction: A pilot study using a transdermal alcohol sensor. *Drug and Alcohol Dependence, 118*(2–3), 391–399.

Barnett, P. G., Trafton, J. A., & Humphreys, K. (2010). The cost of concordance with opiate substitution treatment guidelines. *Journal of Substance Abuse Treatment, 39*(2), 141–149.

Baros, A. M., Latham, P. K., Moak, D. H., Voronin, K., & Anton, R. F. (2007). What role does measuring medication compliance play in evaluating the efficacy of naltrexone? *Alcoholism: Clinical and Experimental Research, 31*(4), 596–603.

Barrison, I. G., Ruzek, J., & Murray-Lyons, I. M. (1987). Drinkwatchers: Description of subjects and evaluation of laboratory markers of heavy drinking. *Alcohol and Alcoholism, 22*(2), 147–154.

Barry, C. L., McGinty, E. E., Pescosolido, B. A., & Goldman, H. H. (2014). Stigma, discrimination, treatment effectiveness and policy: Public views about drug addiction and mental illness. *Psychiatric Services, 65*(10), 1269–1272.

Barry, D., Sullivan, B., & Petry, N. M. (2009). Comparable efficacy of contingency management for cocaine dependence among African American, Hispanic, and White methadone maintenance clients. *Psychology of Addictive Behaviors, 23*(1), 168–174.

Barry, M. J., & Edgman-Levitan, S. (2012). Shared decision making—Pinnacle of patient-centered care. *New England Journal of Medicine, 366*(9), 780–781.

Bartholow, B. D., & Heinz, A. (2006). Alcohol and aggression without consumption: Alcohol cues, aggressive thoughts, and hostile perception bias. *Psychological Science, 17*(1), 30–37.

Batki, S. L., Kauffman, J., Marion, I., Parrino, M., & Woody, G. (2005). *Medication-assisted treatment for opioid addiction in opioid treatment programs* (Vol. 43). Rockville, MD: Center for Substance Abuse Treatment.

Baumeister, R. F. (1994). The crystallization of discontent in the process of major life change. In T. F. Heatherton & J. L. Weinberger (Eds.), *Can personality change?* (pp. 281–297). Washington, DC: American Psychological Association.

Baumeister, R. F., Heatherton, T. F., & Tice, D. M. (1994). *Losing control: How and why people fail at self-regulation.* New York: Academic Press.

Beauchamp, T. L., & Childress, J. F. (2001). *Principles of biomedical ethics* (5th ed.). New York: Oxford University Press.

Beck, A. T., Wright, F. D., Newman, C. F., & Liese, B. S. (2001). *Cognitive therapy of substance abuse.* New York: Guilford Press.

Becker, H. C. (1998). Kindling in alcohol withdrawal. *Alcohol Health and Research World, 22*, 25–33.

Becker, H. C., & Hale, R. L. (1993). Repeated episodes of ethanol withdrawal potentiate the severity of subsequent withdrawal seizures: An animal model of alcohol withdrawal "kindling." *Alcoholism: Clinical and Experimental Research, 17,* 94–98.

Beckman, L. J. (1993). Alcoholics Anonymous and gender issues. In B. S. McCrady & W. R. Miller (Eds.), *Research on Alcoholics Anonymous: Opportunities and alternatives* (pp. 319–348). New Brunswick, NJ: Rutgers Center of Alcohol Studies.

Beckman, L. J., & Amarno, H. (1986). Personal and social difficulties faced by women and men entering alcoholism treatment. *Journal of Studies on Alcohol, 47,* 135–145.

Benishek, L. A., Dugosh, K. L., Kirby, K. C., Matejkowski, J., Clements, N. T., Seymour, B. L., & Festinger, D. S. (2014). Prize-based contingency management for the treatment of substance abusers: A meta-analysis. *Addiction, 109*(9), 1426–1436.

Benshoff, J. J., & Janikowski, T. P. (2000). *The rehabilitation model of substance abuse counseling.* Belmont, ON, Canada: Wadsworth.

Benson, H., & Klipper, M. Z. (2000). *The relaxation response.* New York: Quill.

Berglund, M., Thelander, S., Salaspuro, M., Franck, J., Andréasson, S., & Öjehagen, A. (2003). Treatment of alcohol abuse: An evidence-based review. *Alcoholism: Clinical and Experimental Research, 27*(10), 1645–1656.

Bergman, B. G., Greene, M. C., Slaymaker, V., Hoeppner, B. B., & Kelly, J. F. (2014). Young adults with co-occurring disorders: Substance use disorder treatment response and outcomes. *Journal of Substance Abuse Treatment, 46*(4), 420–428.

Berman, A. H., Bergman, H., Palmstierna, T., & Schlyter, F. (2005). Evaluation of the Drug Use Disorders Identification Test (DUDIT) in criminal justice and detoxification settings and in a Swedish population sample. *European Addiction Research, 11*(1), 22–31.

Bernstein, E., Bernstein, J., & Levenson, S. (1997). Project ASSERT: An ED-based intervention to increase access to primary care, preventive services and the substance abuse treatment system. *Annals of Emergency Medicine, 30,* 181–189.

Bernstein, E., Edwards, E., Dorfman, D., Heeren, T., Bliss, C., & Bernstein, J. (2009). Screening and brief intervention to reduce marijuana use among youth and young adults in a pediatric emergency department. *Academic Emergency Medicine, 16*(11), 1174–1185.

Bernstein, J., Bernstein, E., Tassiopoulos, K., Heeren, T., Levenson, S., & Hingson, R. (2005). Brief motivational intervention at a clinic visit reduces cocaine and heroin use. *Drug and Alcohol Dependence, 77*(1), 49–59.

Bernstein, S. L., D'Onofrio, G., Rosner, J., O'Malley, S., Makuch, R., Busch, S., . . . Toll, B. (2015). Successful tobacco dependence treatment in low-income emergency department patients: A randomized trial. *Annals of Emergency Medicine, 66*(2), 140–147.

Bertholet, N., Cunningham, J. A., Faouzi, M., Gaume, J., Gmel, G., Burnand, B., & Daeppen, J. B. (2015). Internet-based brief intervention for young men with unhealthy alcohol use: A randomized controlled trial in a general population sample. *Addiction, 110*(11), 1735–1743.

Bertrand, K., Roy, E., Vaillancourt, E., Vandermeerschen, J., Berbiche, D., & Boivin, J.-F. (2015). Randomized controlled trial of motivational interviewing for reducing injection risk behaviours among people who inject drugs. *Addiction, 110,* 832–841.

Beutler, L. E., Machado, P. P. P., & Neufeldt, S. A. (1994). Therapist variables. In A. E. Bergin & S. L. Garfield (Eds.), *Handbook of psychotherapy and behavior change* (4th ed., pp. 229–269). New York: Wiley.

Bickel, W. K., Amass, L., Higgins, S. T., Badger, G. J., & Esch, R. A. (1997). Effects of adding behavioral treatment to opioid detoxification with buprenorphine. *Journal of Consulting and Clinical Psychology, 65,* 803–810.

Bickel, W. K., Christensen, D. R., & Marsch, L. A. (2011). A review of computer-based interventions used in the assessment, treatment, and research of drug addiction. *Substance Use and Misuse, 46*(1), 4–9.

Bidney, M. (2004). Epiphany in autobiography: The quantum changes of Dostoevsky and Tolstoy. *Journal of Clinical Psychology, 60,* 471–480.

Bien, T. H. (2010). Paradise lost: Mindfulness and addictive behavior. In F. Didonna (Ed.), *Clinical handbook of mindfulness* (pp. 288–297). New York: Springer.

Bien, T. H., Miller, W. R., & Boroughs, J. M. (1993). Motivational interviewing with alcohol outpatients. *Behavioural and Cognitive Psychotherapy, 21,* 347–356.

Bien, T. H., Miller, W. R., & Tonigan, J. S. (1993). Brief interventions for alcohol problems: A review. *Addiction, 88*(3), 315–336.

Bird, S. M., McAuley, A., Perry, S., & Hunter, C. (2016). Effectiveness of Scotland's National Naloxone Programme for reducing opioid-related deaths: A before (2006–10) versus after (2011–13) comparison. *Addiction, 111*(5), 883–891.

Bird, V. J., Le Boutillier, C., Leamy, M., Larsen, J., Oades, L. G., Williams, J., & Slade, M. (2012). Assessing the strengths of mental health consumers: A systematic review. *Psychological Assessment, 24*(4), 1024–1033.

Bischof, G., Grothues, J. M., Reinhardt, S., Meyer, C., John, U., & Rumpf, H.-J. (2008). Evaluation of a telephone-based stepped care intervention for alcohol-related disorders: A randomized controlled trial. *Drug and Alcohol Dependence, 93*(3), 244–251.

Bischof, G., Iwen, J., Freyer-Adam, J., & Rumpf, H.-J. (2016). Efficacy of the community reinforcement and family training for concerned significant others of treatment-refusing individuals with alcohol dependence: A randomized controlled trial. *Drug and Alcohol Dependence, 163,* 179–185.

Blonigen, D. M., Timko, C., Finney, J. W., Moos, B. S., & Moos, R. H. (2011). Alcoholics Anonymous attendance, decreases in impulsivity and drinking and psychosocial outcomes over 16 years: Moderated-mediation from a developmental perspective. *Addiction, 106*(12), 2167–2177.

Blount, A. (1998). Introduction to integrated primary care. In A. Blount (Ed.), *Integrated primary care: The future of medical and mental health collaboration* (pp. 1–43). New York: Norton.

Blow, F. C., Barry, K. L., Walton, W. A., Maio, R. F., Chermack, S. T., Bingham, C. R., . . . Strecher, V. J. (2006). The efficacy of two brief intervention strategies among injured, at-risk drinkers in the emergency department: Impact of tailored messaging and brief advice. *Journal of Studies on Alcohol, 67*(4), 568–578.

Blow, F. C., Walton, M. A., Bohnert, A. S. B., Ignacio, R. V., Chermack, S., Cunningham, R. M., . . . Barry, K. L. (2017). A randomized controlled trial of brief interventions to reduce drug use among adults in a low-income urban emergency department: The HealthiER You study. *Addiction, 112*(8), 1395–1405.

Boß, L., Lehr, D., Schaub, M. P., Castro, R. P., Riper, H., Berking, M., & Ebert, D. D. (2018). Efficacy of a web-based intervention with and without guidance for employees with risky drinking: Results of a three-arm randomized controlled trial. *Addiction, 113*(4), 635–646.

Bobo, J. K., Mcilvain, H. E., Lando, H. A., Walker, R. D., & Leed-Kelly, A. (1998). Effect of smoking cessation counseling on recovery from alcoholism: Findings from a randomized community intervention trial. *Addiction, 93*(6), 877–887.

Bogenschutz, M. P. (2013). Studying the effects of classic hallucinogens in the treatment of alcoholism: Rationale, methodology, and current research with psilocybin. *Current Drug Abuse Reviews, 6*(1), 17–29.

Bogenschutz, M. P. (2017). It's time to take psilocybin seriously as a possible treatment for substance use disorders. *American Journal of Drug and Alcohol Abuse, 43*(1), 4–6.

Bogenschutz, M. P., Forcehimes, A. A., Pommy, J. A., Wilcox, C. E., Barbosa, P. C., & Strassman, R. J. (2015). Psilocybin-assisted treatment for alcohol dependence: A proof-of-concept study. *Journal of Psychopharmacology, 29*(3), 289–299.

Bogenschutz, M. P., Rice, S. L., Tonigan, J. S., Vogel, H. S., Nowinski, J., Hume, D., & Arenella, P. B. (2014). 12-step facilitation for the dually diagnosed: A randomized clinical trial. *Journal of Substance Abuse Treatment, 46*(4), 403–411.

Bohart, A. C., & Tallman, K. (1999). *How clients make therapy work: The process of active self-healing.* Washington, DC: American Psychological Association.

Bohnert, A. S., Bonar, E. E., Cunningham, R., Greenwald, M. K., Thomas, L., Chermack, S., . . . Walton, M. (2016). A pilot randomized clinical trial of an intervention to reduce overdose risk behaviors among emergency department patients at risk for prescription opioid overdose. *Drug and Alcohol Dependence, 163,* 40–47.

Bolton, J. M., Robinson, J., & Sareen, J. (2009). Self-medication of mood disorders with alcohol and drugs in the National Epidemiologic Survey on Alcohol and Related Conditions. *Journal of Affective Disorders, 115*(3), 367–375.

Bonelli, R. M., & Koenig, H. G. (2013). Mental disorders, religion and spirituality 1990 to 2010: A systematic evidence-based review. *Journal of Religion and Health, 52*(2), 657–673.

Borders, T. F., Curran, G. M., Mattox, R., & Booth, B. M. (2010). Religiousness among at-risk drinkers: Is it prospectively associated with the development or maintenance of an alcohol-use disorder? *Journal of Studies on Alcohol and Drugs, 71,* 136–142.

Bose, J., Hedden, S. L., Lipari, R. N., Park-Lee, E., Porter, J. D., Pemberton, M. R., . . . Hunter, D. (2016). *Key substance use and mental health indicators in the United States: Results from the 2015 National Survey on Drug Use and Health* (HHS Publication No. SMA 16-4984, NSDUH Series H-51). Rockville, MD: Substance Abuse and Mental Health Services Administration.

Boucher, L. M., Marshall, Z., Martin, A., Larose-Hebert, K., Flynn, J. V., Lalonde, C., . . . Kendall, C. (2017). Expanding conceptualizations of harm reduction: Results from a qualitative community-based participatory research study with people who inject drugs. *Harm Reduction Journal, 14*(1), 18.

Bowen, M. (1991). Alcoholism as viewed through family systems theory and family psychotherapy. *Family Dynamics of Addiction Quarterly, 1*(1), 94–102.

Bowen, S., Chawla, N., Collins, S. E., Witkiewitz, K., Hsu, S., Grow, J., . . . Marlatt, A. (2009). Mindfulness-based relapse prevention for substance use disorders: A pilot efficacy trial. *Substance Abuse, 30*(4), 295–305.

Bowen, S., Witkiewitz, K., Clifasefi, S. L., Grow, J., Chawla, N., Hsu, S. H., . . . Larimer, M. E. (2014). Relative efficacy of mindfulness-based relapse prevention, standard relapse prevention, and treatment as usual for substance use disorders: A randomized clinical trial. *JAMA Psychiatry, 71*(5), 547–556.

Bowen, S., Witkiewitz, K., Dillworth, T. M., & Marlatt, G. A. (2007). The role of thought suppression in the relationship between mindfulness meditation and alcohol use. *Addictive Behaviors, 32*(10), 2324–2328.

Bowman, K. M., & Jellinek, E. M. (1941). Alcohol addiction and its treatment. *Quarterly Journal of Studies on Alcohol, 2,* 98–176.

Boyer, E. W. (2012). Management of opioid analgesic overdose. *New England Journal of Medicine, 367*(2), 146–155.

Brady, J. V., & Lucas, S. E. (1984). *Testing drugs for physical dependence potential and abuse liability.* Washington, DC: U.S. Government Printing Office.

Brady, K. T., & Verduin, M. L. (2005). Pharmacotherapy of comorbid mood, anxiety, and substance use disorders. *Substance Use and Misuse, 40*(13–14), 1895–1897.

Brandsma, J. M., Maultsby, M., & Welsh, R. J. (1980). *The outpatient treatment of alcoholism: A review and comparative study.* Baltimore: University Park Press.

Bray, J. W., Del Boca, F. K., McRee, B. G., Hayashi, S. W., & Babor, T. F. (2017). Screening, Brief Intervention and Referral to Treatment (SBIRT): Rationale, program overview and cross-site evaluation. *Addiction, 112*, 3–11.

Brehm, S. S., & Brehm, J. W. (1981). *Psychological reactance: A theory of freedom and control.* New York: Academic Press.

Brewer, C. (1992). Controlled trials of antabuse in alcoholism: The importance of supervision and adequate dosage. *Acta Psychiatrica Scandinavica, 86*(S369), 51–58.

Brewer, C., & Streel, E. (2018). *Antabuse treatment for alcoholism.* North Charleston, SC: CreateSpace IPP.

Brewer, J. A., Bowen, S., Smith, J. T., Marlatt, G. A., & Potenza, M. N. (2010). Mindfulness-based treatments for co-occurring depression and substance use disorders: What can we learn from the brain? *Addiction, 105*(10), 1698–1706.

Brewer, J. A., Mallik, S., Babuscio, T. A., Nich, C., Johnson, H. E., Deleone, C. M., . . . Rounsaville, B. J. (2011). Mindfulness training for smoking cessation: Results from a randomized controlled trial. *Drug and Alcohol Dependence, 119*(1–2), 72–80.

Bride, B. E., & Humble, M. N. (2008). Increasing retention of African-American women on welfare in outpatient substance user treatment using low-magnitude incentives. *Substance Use and Misuse, 43*(8–9), 1016–1026.

Brigham, G. S., Slesnick, N., Winhusen, T. M., Lewis, D. F., Guo, X., & Somoza, E. (2014). A randomized pilot clinical trial to evaluate the efficacy of community reinforcement and family training for treatment retention (CRAFT-T) for improving outcomes for patients completing opioid detoxification. *Drug and Alcohol Dependence, 138*, 240–243.

Bringhurst, D. L., Watson, C. W., Miller, S. D., & Duncan, B. L. (2006). The reliability and validity of the Outcome Rating Scale: A replication study of a brief clinical measure. *Journal of Brief Therapy, 5*(1), 23–30.

Broad, W., & Wade, N. (1982). *Betrayers of the truth: Fraud and deceit in the halls of science.* New York: Simon & Schuster.

Brooks, A. C., Chambers, J. E., Lauby, J., Byrne, E., Carpenedo, C. M., Benishek, L. A., . . . Kirby, K. C. (2016). Implementation of a brief treatment counseling toolkit in federally qualified healthcare centers: Patient and clinician utilization and satisfaction. *Journal of Substance Abuse Treatment, 60*, 70–80.

Brooks, A. C., Ryder, D., Carise, D., & Kirby, K. C. (2010). Feasibility and effectiveness of computer-based therapy in community treatment. *Journal of Substance Abuse Treatment, 39*, 227–235.

Brooks, G. R. (1998). Group therapy for traditional men. In W. S. Pollack & R. F. Levant (Eds.), *New psychotherapy for men* (pp. 83–96). Hoboken, NJ: Wiley.

Brown, B. S., O'Grady, K., Battjes, R. J., & Farrell, E. V. (2004). Factors associated with treatment outcomes in an aftercare population. *American Journal on Addictions, 13*(5), 447–460.

Brown, H. P., Jr. (1990). Values and recovery from alcoholism through Alcoholics Anonymous. *Counseling and Values, 35*, 63–68.

Brown, J. M. (1998). Self-regulation and the addictive behaviors. In W. R. Miller & N. Heather (Eds.), *Treating addictive behaviors* (2nd ed., pp. 61–74). New York: Plenum Press.

Brown, J. M., & Miller, W. R. (1993). Impact of motivational interviewing on participation and outcome in residential alcoholism treatment. *Psychology of Addictive Behaviors, 7*(4), 211–218.

Brown, K. W., Ryan, R. M., & Creswell, J. D. (2007). Mindfulness: Theoretical foundations and evidence for its salutary effects. *Psychological Inquiry, 18*(4), 211–237.

Brown, R. L., & Rounds, L. A. (1995). Conjoint screening questionnaires for alcohol and drug abuse. *Wisconsin Medical Journal, 94*, 135–140.

Brown, S. A., Brumback, T., Tomlinson, K., Cummins, K., Thompson, W. K., Nagel, B. J., . . . Tapert, S. F. (2015). The National Consortium on Alcohol and NeuroDevelopment in Adolescence (NCANDA): A multisite study of adolescent development and substance use. *Journal of Studies on Alcohol and Drugs, 76*(6), 895–908.

Brown, S. A., Christiansen, B. A., & Goldman, M. S. (1987). The Alcohol Expectancy Questionnaire: An instrument for the assessment of adolescent and adult alcohol expectancies. *Journal of Studies on Alcohol, 48*(5), 483–491.

Brown, S. A., Goldman, M. S., Inn, A., & Anderson, L. R. (1980). Expectations of reinforcement from alcohol: Their domain and relation to drinking patterns. *Journal of Consulting and Clinical Psychology, 48*(4), 419–426.

Browne-Miller, A. (1993). *Gestalting addiction: The addiction-focused group therapy of Dr. Richard Louis Miller.* New York: Ablex.

Brownell, P. (2012). *Gestalt therapy for addictive and self-medicating behaviors.* New York: Springer.

Broyles, L. M., Binswanger, I. A., Jenkins, J. A., Finnell, D. S., Faseru, B., Cavaiola, A., . . . Gordon, A. J. (2014). Confronting inadvertent stigma and pejorative language in addiction scholarship: A recognition and response. *Substance Abuse, 35*(3), 217–221.

Buckland, P. R. (2008). Will we ever find the genes for addiction? *Addiction, 103,* 1768–1776.

Budney, A. J., Brown, P. C., & Stanger, C. (2013). Behavioral treatments. In B. S. McCrady & E. E. Epstein (Eds.), *Addictions: A comprehensive guidebook* (2nd ed., pp. 411–433). New York: Oxford University Press.

Budney, A. J., Roffman, R., Stephens, R. S., & Walker, D. (2007). Marijuana dependence and its treatment. *Addiction Science and Clinical Practice,* 4–16.

Budney, A. J., Sargent, J. D., & Lee, D. C. (2015). Vaping cannabis (marijuana): Parallel concerns to e-cigs? *Addiction, 110,* 1699–1704.

Burdzovic, A. J., Lauritzen, G., & Nordfjaern, T. (2015). Co-occurrence between mental distress and poly-drug use: A ten year prospective study of patients from substance abuse treatment. *Addictive Behaviors, 48,* 71–78.

Burke, B. L., Arkowitz, H., & Dunn, C. (2002). The efficacy of motivational interviewing and its adaptations: What we know so far. In W. R. Miller & S. Rollnick (Eds.), *Motivational interviewing: Preparing people for change* (2nd ed., pp. 217–250). New York: Guilford Press.

Burke, B. L., Dunn, C. W., Atkins, D. C., & Phelps, J. S. (2004). The emerging evidence base for motivational interviewing: A meta-analytic and qualitative inquiry. *Journal of Cognitive Psychotherapy, 18*(4), 309–322.

Burlingame, G. M., Fuhriman, A., & Johnson, J. E. (2002). Cohesion in group psychotherapy. In J. C. Norcross (Ed.), *Psychotherapy relationships that work: Therapist contributions and responsiveness to patients* (pp. 71–87). New York: Oxford University Press.

Burlingame, G. M., Seebeck, J. D., Janis, R. A., Whitcomb, K. R., Barkowski, S., Rosesndahl, J., & Strauss, B. (2016). Outcome difference between individual and group formats when identical and nonidentical treatments, patients, and doses are compared: A 25-year meta-analytic perspective. *Psychotherapy, 53*(4), 446–461.

Burnett, G., & Reading, H. (1970). The pharmacology of disulfiram in the treatment of alcoholism. *Addiction, 65*(4), 281–288.

Burns, L., & Teesson, M. (2002). Alcohol use disorders comorbid with anxiety, depression and drug use disorders: Findings from the Australian National Survey of Mental Health and Well Being. *Drug and Alcohol Dependence, 68*(3), 299–307.

Butler, S. F., Budman, S. H., Goldman, R. J., Newman, F. J., Beckley, K. E., Trottier, D., & Cacciola, J. S. (2001). Initial validation of a computer-administered Addiction Severity Index: The ASI–MV. *Psychology of Addictive Behaviors, 15*(1), 4–12.

Cahalan, D. (1970). *Problem drinkers*. San Francisco: Jossey-Bass.

Cahn, B. R., & Polich, J. (2006). Meditation states and traits: EEG, ERP, and neuroimaging studies. *Psychological Bulletin, 132*(2), 180–211.

Calabria, B., Clifford, A., Shakeshaft, A., Allan, J., Bliss, D., & Doran, C. (2013). The acceptability to Aboriginal Australians of a family-based intervention to reduce alcohol-related harms. *Drug and Alcohol Review, 32*(3), 328–332.

Calabria, B., Degenhardt, L., Briegleb, C., Vos, T., Hall, W., Lynskey, M., . . . McLaren, J. (2010). Systematic review of prospective studies investigating "remission" from amphetamine, cannabis, cocaine or opioid dependence. *Addictive Behaviors, 35*(8), 741–749.

Calsyn, D. A., Hatch-Maillette, M., Tross, S., Doyle, S. R., Crits-Christoph, P., Song, Y. S., . . . Berns, S. B. (2009). Motivational and skills training HIV/sexually transmitted infection sexual risk reduction groups for men. *Journal of Substance Abuse Treatment, 37*(2), 138–150.

Campbell, A. N. C., Nunes, E. V., Miele, G. M., Matthews, A., Polsky, D., Ghitza, U. E., . . . Crowell, A. R. (2012). Design and methodological considerations of an effectiveness trial of a computer-assisted intervention: An example from the NIDA Clinical Trials Network. *Contemporary Clinical Trials, 33*(2), 386–395.

Campbell, A. N. C., Turrigiano, E., Moore, M., Miele, G. M., Rieckmann, T., Hu, M.-C., . . . Nunes, E. V. (2015). Acceptability of a web-based community reinforcement approach for substance use disorders with treatment-seeking American Indians/Alaska Natives. *Community Mental Health Journal, 51*(4), 393–403.

Campbell, H. (1903). The study of inebriety: A retrospect and a forecast. *British Journal of Inebriety, 1*(1), 5–14.

Campbell, S. D., Adamson, S. J., & Carter, J. D. (2010). Client language during motivational enhancement therapy and alcohol use outcome. *Behavioural and Cognitive Psychotherapy, 38*(4), 39–415.

Campbell, T. C., Hoffmann, N. G., Madson, M. B., & Melchert, T. P. (2003). Performance of a brief assessment tool for identifying substance use disorders. *Addictive Disorders and Their Treatment, 2*(1), 13–17.

Campbell, W., Hester, R. K., Lenberg, K. L., & Delaney, H. D. (2016). Overcoming Addictions, a web-based application, and SMART Recovery, an online and in-person mutual help group for problem drinkers: Part 2. Six-month outcomes of a randomized controlled trial and qualitative feedback from participants. *Journal of Medical Internet Research, 18*(10).

Carbonari, J. P., & DiClemente, C. C. (2000). Using transtheoretical model profiles to differentiate levels of alcohol abstinence success. *Journal of Consulting and Clinical Psychology, 68*(5), 810–817.

Cardenas, H. L., & Ross, D. H. (1976). Calcium depletion of synaptosomes after morphine treatment. *British Journal of Pharmacology, 57*(4), 521–526.

Carr, S. (2011). *Scripting addiction: The politics of therapeutic talk and American sobriety.* Princeton, NJ: Princeton University Press.

Carroll, K. M. (1996). Relapse prevention as a psychosocial treatment: A review of controlled clinical trials. *Experimental and Clinical Psychopharmacology, 4,* 46–54.

Carroll, K. M. (1997a). *Improving compliance with alcoholism treatment* (Project MATCH Monograph Series Vol. 6). Rockville, MD: National Institute on Alcohol Abuse and Alcoholism.

Carroll, K. M. (1997b). Integrating psychotherapy and pharmacotherapy to improve drug abuse outcomes. *Addictive Behaviors, 22*(2), 233–245.

Carroll, K. M., Fenton, L. R., Ball, S. A., Nich, C., Frankforter, T. L., Shi, J., & Rounsaville, B. J. (2004). Efficacy of disulfiram and cognitive behavior therapy in cocaine-dependent outpatients: A randomized placebo-controlled trial. *Archives of General Psychiatry, 61*(3), 264–272.

Carroll, K. M., & Kiluk, B. D. (2012). Integrating psychotherapy and pharmacotherapy in substance abuse treatment. In S. Walters & F. Rotgers (Eds.), *Treating substance abuse: Theory and technique* (3rd ed., pp. 320–354). New York: Guilford Press.

Carroll, K. M., Nich, C., Ball, S. A., McCance, E., & Rounsavile, B. J. (1998). Treatment of cocaine and alcohol dependence with psychotherapy and disulfiram. *Addiction, 93*(5), 713–727.

Carroll, K. M., Nich, C., Lapaglia, D. M., Peters, E. N., Easton, C. J., & Petry, N. M. (2012). Combining cognitive behavioral therapy and contingency management to enhance their effects in treating cannabis dependence: Less can be more, more or less. *Addiction, 107*(9), 1650–1659.

Carroll, K. M., & Rounsaville, B. J. (2006). Behavioral therapies: The glass would be half full if only we had a glass. In W. R. Miller & K. M. Carroll (Eds.), *Rethinking substance abuse: What the science shows, and what we should do about it* (pp. 223–239). New York: Guilford Press.

Carroll, K. M., & Weiss, R. D. (2017). The role of behavioral interventions in buprenorphine maintenance treatment: A review. *American Journal of Psychiatry, 174*(8), 738–747.

Carruth, B. E., & Mendenhall, W. E. (Eds.). (1989). *Co-dependency: Issues in treatment and recovery.* New York: Haworth Press.

Carter, B. L., & Tiffany, S. T. (1999). Meta-analysis of cue-reactivity in addiction research. *Addiction, 94*(3), 327–340.

Casteneda, C. (1985). *The teachings of Don Juan: A Yaqui way of knowledge.* New York: Washington Square Press.

C'de Baca, J., Miller, W. R., & Lapham, S. C. (2001). A multiple risk factor approach to predicting DWI recidivism. *Journal of Substance Abuse Treatment, 21,* 207–215.

C'de Baca, J., & Wilbourne, P. (2004). Quantum change: Ten years later. *Journal of Clinical Psychology, 60,* 531–541.

Cermak, T. L. (1991). Co-addiction as a disease. *Psychiatric Annals, 21*(5), 266–272.

Chafetz, M. E. (1961). A procedure for establishing therapeutic contact with the alcoholic. *Quarterly Journal of Studies on Alcohol, 22,* 325–328.

Chafetz, M. E., Blane, H. T., Abram, H. S., Golner, J. H., Hastie, E. L., & Meyers, W. (1962). Establishing treatment relations with alcoholics. *Journal of Nervous and Mental Disease, 134,* 395–409.

Chapman, C., Burlingame, G., Rees, F., Gleave, R., Beecher, M., & Porter, G. (2012).

Clinical prediction in group psychotherapy. *Psychotherapy Research, 22*(6), 673–681.

Chapman, P. L. H., & Huygens, I. (1988). An evaluation of three treatment programmes for alcoholism: An experimental study with 6- and 18-month follow-ups. *Addiction, 83*(1), 67–81.

Chapman, S., & Daube, M. (2015). Ethical imperatives assuming ENDS effectiveness and safety are fragile. *Addiction, 110*(7), 1068–1069.

Chavez, L. J., Williams, E. C., Lapham, G., & Bradley, K. A. (2012). Association between alcohol screening scores and alcohol-related risks among female Veterans Affairs patients. *Journal of Studies on Alcohol and Drugs, 73*(3), 391–400.

Chebli, J. L., Blaszczynski, A., & Gainsbury, S. M. (2016). Internet-based interventions for addictive behaviours: A systematic review. *Journal of Gambling Studies, 32*(4), 1279–1304.

Cherpitel, C. J. (1995). Analysis of cut points for screening instruments for alcohol problems in the emergency room. *Journal of Studies on Alcohol and Drugs, 56*(6), 695–700.

Cherpitel, C. J. (2006). Screening for alcohol problems in the U.S. general population: Comparisons of the CAGE, RAPS4, and RAPS4-QF by gender, ethnicity, and service utilization. *Alcoholism: Clinical and Experimental Research, 26*(11), 1686–1691.

Chi, F. W., Kaskutas, L. A., Sterling, S., Campbell, C. I., & Weisner, C. (2009). Twelve-step affiliation and 3-year substance use outcomes among adolescents: Social support and religious service attendance as potential mediators. *Addiction, 104*(6), 927–939.

Chick, J., Anton, R., Checinski, K., Croop, R., Drummond, D. C., Farmer, R., . . . Ritson, B. (2000). A multicentre, randomized, double-blind, placebo-controlled trial of naltrexone in the treatment of alcohol dependence or abuse. *Alcohol and Alcoholism, 35*, 587–593.

Chick, J., Howlett, H., Morgan, M., & Ritson, B. (2000). United Kingdom multicentre acamprosate study (UKMAS): A 6-month prospective study of acamprosate versus placebo in preventing relapse after withdrawal from alcohol. *Alcohol and Alcoholism, 35*(2), 176–187.

Chiesa, A., & Serretti, A. (2010). A systematic review of neurobiological and clinical features of mindfulness meditations. *Psychological Medicine, 40*(8), 1239–1252.

Chiesa, A., & Serretti, A. (2014). Are mindfulness-based interventions effective for substance use disorders?: A systematic review of the evidence. *Substance Use and Misuse, 49*(5), 492–512.

Choi, S., Adams, S. M., Morse, S. A., & MacMaster, S. (2015). Gender differences in treatment retention among individuals with co-occurring substance abuse and mental health disorders. *Substance Use and Misuse, 50*(5), 653–663.

Chou, S. P., Goldstein, R. B., Smith, S. M., Huang, B., Ruan, W. J., Zhang, H., . . . Grant, B. F. (2016). The epidemiology of DSM-5 nicotine use disorder: Results from the National Epidemiologic Survey on Alcohol and Related Conditions–III. *Journal of Clinical Psychiatry, 77*(10), 1404–1412.

Chow, D. L., Miller, S. D., Seidel, J. A., Kane, R. T., Thornton, J. A., & Andrews, W. P. (2015). The role of deliberate practice in the development of highly effective psychotherapists. *Psychotherapy, 52*(3), 337–345.

Christian, E., Krall, V., Hulkower, S., & Stigleman, S. (2018). Primary care behavioral health integration: Promoting the quadruple aim. *North Carolina Medical Journal, 79*(4), 250–255.

Christo, G., & Franey, C. (1995). Drug users' spiritual beliefs, locus of control and the disease concept in relation to Narcotics Anonymous attendance and six-month outcomes. *Drug and Alcohol Dependence, 38,* 51–56.

Clark, H. W. (2005–2007). Center for Substance Abuse Treatment (CSAT), Substance Abuse and Mental Health Services Administration (SAMHSA): News from the Director, CSAT. *Journal of Maintenance in the Addictions, 3*(2/3/4), 13–16.

Cohen-Katz, J., Wiley, S. D., Capuano, T., Baker, D. M., Kimmel, S., & Shapiro, S. (2005). The effects of mindfulness-based stress reduction on nurse stress and burnout: Part II. A quantitative and qualitative study. *Holistic Nursing Practice, 19*(1), 26–35.

Collins, F. S., & Varmus, H. (2015). A new initiative on precision medicine. *New England Journal of Medicine, 372,* 793–795.

Compton, W. M., Blanco, C., & Wargo, E. M. (2015). Integrating addiction services into general medicine. *JAMA, 314*(22), 2401–2402.

Connors, G. J., & Dermen, K. H. (1996). Characteristics of participants in Secular Organizations for Sobriety (SOS). *American Journal of Drug and Alcohol Abuse, 22,* 281–295.

Connors, G. J., Donovan, D. M., & DiClemente, C. C. (2001). *Substance abuse treatment and the stages of change: Selecting and planning interventions.* New York: Guilford Press.

Connors, G. J., & Maisto, S. A. (1988). The alcohol expectancy construct: Overview and clinical applications. *Cognitive Therapy and Research, 12*(5), 487–504.

Connors, G. J., Tonigan, J. S., & Miller, W. R. (2001). Religiosity and responsiveness to alcoholism treatments. In R. Longabaugh & P. W. Wirtz (Eds.), *Project MATCH hypotheses: Results and causal chain analyses* (Vol. 8, pp. 166–175). Bethesda, MD: National Institute on Alcohol Abuse and Alcoholism.

Conrad, K. J., Hultman, C. I., Pope, A. R., Lyons, J. S., Baxter, W. C., Daghestani, A. N., . . . Manheim, L. M. (1998). Case managed residential care for homeless addicted veterans: Results of a true experiment. *Medical Care, 36*(1), 40–53.

Conway, K. P., Swendsen, J., Husky, M. M., He, J. P., & Merikangas, K. R. (2016). Association of lifetime mental disorders and subsequent alcohol and illicit drug use: Results from the National Comorbidity Survey–Adolescent Supplement. *Journal of the American Academy of Child and Adolescent Psychiatry, 55*(4), 280–288.

Cooney, J. L., Cooper, S., Grant, C., Sevarino, K., Krishnan-Sarin, S., Gutierrez, I. A., & Cooney, N. L. (2017). A randomized trial of contingency management for smoking cessation during intensive outpatient alcohol treatment. *Journal of Substance Abuse Treatment, 72,* 89–96.

Cooney, N. L., Zweben, A., & Fleming, M. F. (1995). Screening for alcohol problems and at-risk drinking in health-care settings. In R. K. Hester & W. R. Miller (Eds.), *Handbook of alcoholism treatment approaches: Effective alternatives* (2nd ed., pp. 45–60). New York: Allyn & Bacon.

Copeland, J. (1997). A qualitative study of barriers to formal treatment among women who self-managed change in addictive behaviours. *Journal of Substance Abuse Treatment, 14,* 183–190.

Corcoran, J. (2004). *Building strengths and skills: A collaborative approach to working with clients.* New York: Oxford University Press.

Cox, G. B. (1998). Outcome of a controlled trial of the effectiveness of intensive case management for chronic public inebriates. *Journal of Studies on Alcohol, 59*(5), 523–532.

Cranford, J. A. (2014). DSM-IV alcohol dependence and marital dissolution: Evidence from the National Epidemiologic Survey on Alcohol and Related Conditions. *Journal of Studies on Alcohol and Drugs, 75*(3), 520–529.

Crits-Christoph, P., Johnson, J. E., Connolly Gibbons, M. B., & Gallop, R. (2013). Process predictors of the outcome of group drug counseling. *Journal of Consulting and Clinical Psychology, 81*(1), 23–34.

Crits-Christoph, P., Siqueland, L., Blaine, J., Frank, A., Luborsky, L., Onken, L. S., . . . Beck, A. T. (1999). Psychosocial treatments for cocaine dependence: National Institute on Drug Abuse Collaborative Cocaine Treatment Study. *Archives of General Psychiatry, 56*(6), 493–502.

Croft, B., & Parish, S. L. (2013). Care integration in the Patient Protection and Affordable Care Act: Implications for behavioral health. *Administration and Policy in Mental Health and Mental Health Services Research, 40*(4), 258–263.

Cucciare, M. A., Weingardt, K. R., Ghaus, S., Boden, M. T., & Frayne, S. M. (2013). A randomized controlled trial of a web-delivered brief alcohol intervention in Veterans Affairs primary care. *Journal of Studies on Alcohol and Drugs, 74*, 428–436.

Culig, J., & Leppée, M. (2014). From Morisky to Hill-Bone: Self-report scales for measuring adherence to medication. *Collegium Antropologicum, 38*(1), 55–62.

Cummings, C. C., Gordon, J. R., & Marlatt, G. A. (1980). Relapse: Prevention and prediction. In W. R. Miller (Ed.), *The addictive behaviors: Treatment of alcoholism, drug abuses, smoking and obesity* (pp. 291–321). New York: Pergamon Press.

Cunningham, C. E., Henderson, J., Niccols, A., Dobbins, M., Sword, W., Chen, Y., . . . Schmidt, L. (2012). Preferences for evidence-based practice dissemination in addiction agencies serving women: A discrete-choice conjoint experiment. *Addiction, 107*(8), 1512–1524.

Cunningham, C., Stitzer, M., Campbell, A. N., Pavlicova, M., Hu, M. C., & Nunes, E. V. (2017). Contingency management abstinence incentives: Cost and implications for treatment tailoring. *Journal of Substance Abuse Treatment, 72*, 134–139.

Dalai Lama & Hopkins, J. (2017). *The heart of meditation: Discovering innermost awareness*. Boulder, CO: Shambala Books.

Daley, D. C., & Marlatt, G. A. (1999). *Managing your drug or alcohol problem: Client workbook*. New York: Academic Press.

D'Amico, E. J., Houck, J. M., Hunter, S. B., Miles, J. N., Osilla, K. C., & Ewing, B. A. (2015). Group motivational interviewing for adolescents: Change talk and alcohol and marijuana outcomes. *Journal of Consulting and Clinical Psychology, 83*(1), 68–80.

D'Amico, E. J., Osilla, K. C., & Hunter, S. B. (2010). Developing a group motivational interviewing intervention for adolescents at-risk for developing an alcohol or drug use disorder. *Alcoholism Treatment Quarterly, 28*(4), 417–436.

Damschroder, L. J., Aron, D. C., Keith, R. E., Kirsh, S. R., Alexander, J. A., & Lowery, J. C. (2009). Fostering implementation of health services research findings into practice: A consolidated framework for advancing implementation science. *Implementation Science, 4*(50).

Damschroder, L. J., & Hagedorn, H. J. (2011). A guiding framework and approach for implementation research in substance use disorders treatment. *Psychology of Addictive Behaviors, 25*(2), 194–205.

Dart, R. C., Suratt, H. L., Cicero, T. J., Parrino, M. W., Severtson, G., Bucher-Bertelson, B., & Green, J. L. (2015). Trends in opioid analgesic abuse and mortality in the United States. *New England Journal of Medicine, 372*, 241–248.

Datchi, C. C., & Sexton, T. L. (2013). Can family therapy have an effect on adult criminal conduct?: Initial evaluation of functional family therapy. *Couple and Family Psychology: Research and Practice, 2*(4), 278–293.

Dattilio, F. M. (2009). *Cognitive-behavioral therapy with couples and families: A comprehensive guide for clinicians.* New York: Guilford Press.

Daugherty, M., Love, C. T., James, W. H., & Miller, W. R. (2002). Substance abuse among displaced and indigenous peoples. In W. R. Miller & C. Weisner (Eds.), *Changing substance abuse through health and social systems* (pp. 225–239). New York: Kluwer/Plenum.

Daughters, S., Magidson, J. F., Anand, D., Seitz-Brown, C. J., Chen, Y., & Baker, S. (2018). The effect of a behavioral activation treatment for substance use on post-treatment abstinence: A randomized controlled trial. *Addiction, 113*(3), 535–544.

Davis, J. P., Berry, D., Dumas, T. M., Ritter, E., Smith, D. C., Menard, C., & Roberts, B. W. (2018). Substance use outcomes for mindfulness based relapse prevention are partially mediated by reductions in stress: Results from a randomized trial. *Journal of Substance Abuse Treatment, 91*, 37–48.

Dawson, D. A., Grant, B. F., Stinson, F. S., & Chou, P. S. (2006). Estimating the effect of help-seeking on achieving recovery from alcohol dependence. *Addiction, 101*(6), 824–834.

Day, A., Tucker, K., & Howells, K. (2004). Coerced offender rehabilitation: A defensible practice? *Psychology, Crime and Law, 10*(3), 259–269.

Day, E., & Strang, J. (2011). Outpatient versus inpatient opioid detoxification: A randomized controlled trial. *Journal of Substance Abuse Treatment, 40*(1), 56–66.

de Almeida Neto, A. C. (2017). Understanding motivational interviewing: An evolutionary perspective. *Evolutionary Psychological Science, 3*(4), 379–389.

de Jong, K., van Sluis, P., Nugter, M. A., Heiser, W. J., & Spinhoven, P. (2012). Understanding the differential impact of outcome monitoring: Therapist variables that moderate feedback effects in a randomized trial. *Psychotherapy Research, 22*, 464–474.

de Shazer, S., Dolan, Y., Korman, H., Trepper, T., McCollum, E., & Berg, I. K. (2007). *More than miracles: The state of the art of solution-focused brief therapy.* Binghamton, NY: Haworth Press.

Deci, E. L., Koestner, R., & Ryan, R. M. (1999). A meta-analytic review of experiments examining the effects of extrinsic rewards on intrinsic motivation. *Psychological Bulletin, 125*(6), 627–668.

Deci, E. L., & Ryan, R. M. (2008). Self-determination theory: A macrotheory of human motivation, development, and health. *Canadian Psychology, 49*(3), 182–185.

Decker, S. E., Kiluk, B. D., Frankforter, T., Babuscio, T., Nich, C., & Carroll, K. M. (2016). Just showing up is not enough: Homework adherence and outcome in cognitive–behavioral therapy for cocaine dependence. *Journal of Consulting and Clinical Psychology, 84*(10), 907–912.

DeFulio, A., & Silverman, K. (2011). Employment-based abstinence reinforcement as a maintenance intervention for the treatment of cocaine dependence: Post-intervention outcomes. *Addiction, 106*(5), 960–967.

Degenhardt, L., Charlson, F., Mathers, B., Hall, W. D., Flaxman, A. D., Johns, N., & Vos, T. (2014). The global epidemiology and burden of opioid dependence: Results from the global burden of disease 2010 study. *Addiction, 109*(8), 1320–1333.

Delaney, H. D., Miller, W. R., & Bisonó, A. M. (2007). Religiosity and spirituality among psychologists: A survey of clinician members of the American Psychological Association. *Professional Psychology: Research and Practice, 38*(5), 538–546.

DeMartini, K. S., & Carey, K. B. (2012). Optimizing the use of the AUDIT for alcohol screening in college students. *Psychological Assessment, 24*(4), 954–963.

Dench, S., & Bennett, G. (2000). The impact of brief motivational intervention at the start of an outpatient day programme for alcohol dependence *Behavioural and Cognitive Psychotherapy, 28*(2), 121–130.

Diaz, R. M., & Fruhauf, A. G. (1991). The origins and development of self-regulation: A developmental model on the risk for addictive behaviours. In N. Heather, W. R. Miller, & J. Greeley (Eds.), *Self-control and the addictive behaviours* (pp. 83–106). Sydney: Maxwell Macmillan Publishing Australia.

Dick, D. M., & Foroud, T. (2003). Candidate genes for alcohol dependence: A review of genetic evidence from human studies. *Alcoholism: Clinical and Experimental Research, 27*, 868–879.

DiClemente, C. (2010). Mindfulness: Specific or generic mechanisms of action? *Addiction, 105*, 1707–1708.

DiClemente, C. C., Carbonari, J. P., Montgomery, R., & Hughes, S. O. (1994). The Alcohol Abstinence Self-Efficacy Scale. *Journal of Studies on Alcohol, 55*(2), 141–148.

DiClemente, C. C., Doyle, S. R., & Donovan, D. M. (2009). Predicting treatment seekers' readiness to change their drinking behavior in the COMBINE Study. *Alcoholism: Clinical and Experimental Research, 33*(5), 879–892.

DiClemente, C. C., & Hughes, S. O. (1990). Stages of change profiles in outpatient alcoholism treatment. *Journal of Substance Abuse, 2*(2), 217–235.

DiClemente, C. C., & Velasquez, M. M. (2002). Motivational interviewing and the stages of change. In W. R. Miller & S. Rollnick, *Motivational interviewing: Preparing people for change* (2nd ed., pp. 201–216). New York: Guilford Press.

Dishion, T. J., McCord, J., & Poulin, F. (1999). When interventions harm: Peer groups and problem behavior. *American Psychologist, 54*(9), 755–764.

Ditman, K. S., Crawford, G. G., Forgy, E. W., Moskowitz, H., & MacAndrew, C. (1967). A controlled experiment on the use of court probation for drunk arrests. *American Journal of Psychiatry, 124*, 160–163.

Doblin, R. (1991). Pahnke's "Good Friday Experiment": A long-term follow-up and methodological critique. *Journal of Transpersonal Psychology, 23*(1), 1–25.

Dodge, K., Krantz, B., & Kenny, P. J. (2010). How can we begin to measure recovery? *Substance Abuse Treatment, Prevention and Policy, 5*(31).

Donohue, B., Azrin, N. H., Allen, D. N., Romero, V., Hill, H. H., Tracy, K., . . . Van Hasselt, V. B. (2009). Family behavior therapy for substance abuse and other associated problems: A review of its intervention components and applicability. *Behavior Modification, 33*(5), 495–519.

Donovan, D. (1995). Assessments to aid in the treatment planning process. In J. P. Allen & M. Columbus (Eds.), *Assessing alcohol problems: A guide for clinicians and researchers* (pp. 75–122). Rockville, MD: National Institute on Alcohol Abuse and Alcoholism.

Donovan, D. (2013). Evidence-based assessment strategies and measures in addictive behaviors. In B. S. McCrady & E. E. Epstein (Eds.), *Addictions: A comprehensive guidebook for practitioners* (2nd ed., pp. 311–351). New York: Oxford University Press.

Donovan, D. M., Anton, R. F., Miller, W. R., Longabaugh, R., Hosking, J. D., & Youngblood, M. (2008). Combined pharmacotherapies and behavioral interventions for alcohol dependence (The COMBINE Study): Examination of posttreatment drinking outcomes. *Journal of Studies on Alcohol and Drugs, 69*(1), 5–13.

Donovan, D. M., Hague, W. H., & O'Leary, M. R. (1975). Perceptual differentiation and defense mechanisms in alcoholics. *Journal of Clinical Psychology, 31,* 356–359.

Donovan, D. M., Ingalsbe, M. H., Benbow, J., & Daley, D. C. (2013). 12-step interventions and mutual support programs for substance use disorders: An overview. *Social Work in Public Health, 28*(3–4), 313–332.

Donovan, D., & Rosengren, D. B. (1999). Motivation for behavior change and treatment among substance abusers. In J. A. Tucker, D. M. Donovan, & G. A. Marlatt (Eds.), *Changing addictive behavior: Bridging clinical and public health strategies* (pp. 127–159). New York: Guilford Press.

Douaihy, A., & Driscoll, H. P. (2018). *Humanizing addiction practice: Blending science and personal transformation.* Cham, Switzerland: Springer.

Dougherty, D. M., Lake, S. L., Hill-Kapturczak, N., Liang, Y., Karns, T. E., Mullen, J., & Roache, J. D. (2015). Using contingency management procedures to reduce at-risk drinking in heavy drinkers. *Alcoholism: Clinical and Experimental Research, 39*(4), 743–751.

Doumas, D. M., Esp, S., Johnson, J., Trull, R., & Shearer, K. (2016). The eCHECKUP TO GO for High School: Impact on risk factors and protective behavioral strategies for alcohol use. *Addictive Behaviors, 64,* 93–100.

Dowell, D., Haegerich, T. M., & Chou, R. (2016). CDC guideline for prescribing opioids for chronic pain—United States 2016. *CDC Recommendations and Reports, 65*(1), 1–49.

Doyle, S. R., Donovan, D. M., & Simpson, T. L. (2011). Validation of a nine-dimensional measure of drinking motives for use in clinical applications: The Desired Effects of Drinking Scale. *Addictive Behaviors, 36*(11), 1052–1060.

Drake, R. E., Mueser, K. T., Brunette, M. F., & McHugo, G. J. (2004). A review of treatments for people with severe mental illnesses and co-occurring substance use disorders. *Psychiatric Rehabilitation Journal, 27,* 360–374.

Dubois, S., Mullen, N., Weaver, B., & Bédard, M. (2015). The combined effects of alcohol and cannabis on driving: Impact on crash risk. *Forensic Science International, 248,* 94–100.

Ducharme, L. J., Chandler, R. K., & Harris, A. H. (2016). Implementing effective substance abuse treatments in general medical settings: Mapping the research terrain. *Journal of Substance Abuse Treatment, 60,* 110–118.

Dunn, C., Deroo, L., & Rivara, F. P. (2001). The use of brief interventions adapted from motivational interviewing across behavioral domains: A systematic review. *Addiction, 96*(12), 1725–1742.

Dunn, C. W., & Ries, R. (1997). Linking substance abuse services with general medical care: Integrated, brief interventions with hospitalized patients. *American Journal of Drug and Alcohol Abuse, 23*(1), 1–13.

Durbeej, N., Berman, A. H., Gumpert, C. H., Palmstierna, T., Kristiansson, M., & Alm, C. (2010). Validation of the Alcohol Use Disorders Identification Test and the Drug Use Disorders Identification Test in a Swedish sample of suspected offenders with signs of mental health problems: Results from the mental disorder, substance abuse and crime study. *Journal of Substance Abuse Treatment, 39*(4), 364–377.

Dutcher, L. W., Anderson, R., Moore, M., Luna-Anderson, C., Meyers, R. J., Delaney, H. D., & Smith, J. E. (2009). Community Reinforcement And Family Therapy (CRAFT): An effectiveness study. *Journal of Behavior Analysis in Health, Sports, Fitness and Medicine, 2*(1), 80–90.

Dwyer, R., & Fraser, S. (2017). Engendering drug problems: Materialising gender in the

DUDIT and other screening and diagnostic "apparatuses." *International Journal of Drug Policy, 44,* 135–144.

Eack, S. M., Hogarty, S. S., Greenwald, D. P., Litschge, M. Y., McKnight, S. A., Bangalore, S. S., . . . Cornelius, J. R. (2015). Cognitive enhancement therapy in substance misusing schizophrenia: Results of an 18-month feasibility trial. *Schizophrenia Research, 161*(2–3), 478–483.

Edlund, M. J., Booth, B. M., & Han, X. (2012). Who seeks care where?: Utilization of mental health and substance use disorder treatment in two national samples of individuals with alcohol use disorders. *Journal of Studies on Alcohol and Drugs, 73*(4), 635–646.

Edwards, G. (1986). The alcohol dependence syndrome: A concept as stimulus to enquiry. *British Journal of Addiction, 81,* 171–183.

Edwards, G. (2006). Addiction: A journal and its invisible college. *Addiction, 101,* 629–637.

Edwards, G., & Gross, M. M. (1976). Alcohol dependence: Provisional description of a clinical syndrome. *British Medical Journal, 1,* 1058–1061.

Edwards, G., Orford, J., Egert, S., Guthrie, S., Hawker, A., Hensman, C., . . . Taylor, C. (1977). Alcoholism: A controlled trial of "treatment" and "advice." *Journal of Studies on Alcohol, 38*(5), 1004–1031.

Edwards, P., Harvey, C., & Whitehead, P. C. (1973). Wives of alcoholics: A critical review and analysis. *Quarterly Journal of Studies on Alcohol, 34*(1, Pt. A), 112–132.

Elliott, R., Bohart, A. C., Watson, J. C., & Greenberg, L. S. (2011). Empathy. *Psychotherapy, 48*(1), 43–49.

Ellis, A., & Velten, E. (1992). *Rational steps to quitting alcohol: When AA doesn't work for you.* New York: Barricade Books.

Elvy, G., Wells, J., & Baird, K. (1988). Attempted referral as intervention for problem drinking in the general hospital. *British Journal of Addiction, 83,* 83–89.

Elwafi, H. M., Witkiewitz, K., Mallik, S., Thornhill, T. A., 4th, & Brewer, J. A. (2013). Mindfulness training for smoking cessation: Moderation of the relationship between craving and cigarette use. *Drug and Alcohol Dependence, 130*(1–3), 222–229.

Elzerbi, C., Donoghue, K., & Drummond, C. (2015). A comparison of the efficacy of brief interventions to reduce hazardous and harmful alcohol consumption between European and non-European countries: A systematic review and meta-analysis of randomized controlled trials. *Addiction, 110*(7), 1082–1091.

Emmons, R. A. (2003). *The psychology of ultimate concerns: Motivation and spirituality in personality.* New York: Guilford Press.

Emrick, C. D., Tonigan, J. S., Montgomery, H., & Little, L. (1993). Alcoholics Anonymous: What is currently known? In B. S. McCrady & W. R. Miller (Eds.), *Research on Alcoholics Anonymous: Opportunities and alternatives* (pp. 41–76). New Brunswick, NJ: Rutgers Center of Alcohol Studies.

Ends, E. J., & Page, C. W. (1957). A study of three types of group psychotherapy with hospitalized inebriates. *Quarterly Journal of Studies on Alcohol, 18,* 263–277.

Enns, E. A., Zaric, G. S., Strike, C. J., Jairam, J. A., Kolla, G., & Bayoumi, A. M. (2016). Potential cost-effectiveness of supervised injection facilities in Toronto and Ottawa, Canada. *Addiction, 111*(3), 475–489.

Enser, B. J., Appleton, J. V., & Foxcroft, D. R. (2017). Alcohol-related collateral harm, the unseen dimension?: Survey of students aged 16–24 in Southern England. *Drugs: Education, Prevention and Policy, 24*(1), 40–48.

Epstein, E. E., & McCrady, B. (2009). *A cognitive-behavioral treatment program for overcoming alcohol problems: Therapist guide.* New York: Oxford University Press.

Epstein, E. E., McCrady, B. S., Hallgren, K. A., Gaba, A., Cook, S., Jensen, N., . . . Litt, M. D. (2018). Individual versus group female-specific cognitive behavior therapy for alcohol use disorder. *Journal of Substance Abuse Treatment, 88,* 27–43.

Ernst, D., Miller, W. R., & Rollnick, S. (2007). Treating substance abuse in primary care: A demonstration project. *International Journal of Integrated Care, 7*(4).

Erskine, H. E., Moffitt, T. E., Copeland, W. E., Costello, E. J., Ferrari, A. J., Patton, G., . . . Scott, J. G. (2015). A heavy burden on young minds: The global burden of mental and substance use disorders in children and youth. *Psychological Medicine, 45*(7), 1551–1563.

Evins, A. E., Cather, C., Pratt, S. A., Pachas, G. N., Hoeppner, S. S., Goff, D. C., . . . Schoenfeld, D. A. (2014). Maintenance treatment with varenicline for smoking cessation in patients with schizophrenia and bipolar disorder: A randomized clinical trial. *JAMA, 311*(2), 145–154.

Ewing, J. A. (1984). Detecting alcoholism: The CAGE Questionnaire. *Journal of the American Medical Association, 252*(14), 1905–1907.

Faigin, C. A., Pargament, K. I., & Hisham, R. (2014). Spiritual struggles as a possible risk factor for addictive behaviors: An initial empirical investigation. *International Journal for the Psychology of Religion, 24*(3), 201–214.

Fals-Stewart, W., & Kennedy, C. (2005). Addressing intimate partner violence in substance-abuse treatment. *Journal of Substance Abuse Treatment, 29*(1), 5–17.

Fals-Stewart, W., & Lam, W. K. K. (2008). Brief behavioral couples therapy for drug abuse: A randomized clinical trial examining clinical efficacy and cost-effectiveness. *Families, Systems, and Health, 26*(4), 377–392.

Fals-Stewart, W., & O'Farrell, T. J. (2003). Behavioral family counseling and naltrexone for male opioid-dependent patients. *Journal of Consulting and Clinical Psychology, 71*(3), 432–442.

Fals-Stewart, W., O'Farrell, T. J., & Birchler, G. R. (1997). Behavioral couples therapy for male substance-abusing patients: A cost outcomes analysis. *Journal of Consulting and Clinical Psychology, 65*(5), 789–802.

Farmer, K. C. (1999). Methods for measuring and monitoring medication regimen adherence in clinical trials and clinical practice. *Clinical Therapeutics, 21*(6), 1074–1090.

Farren, C. K., Snee, L., & McElroy, S. (2011). Gender differences in outcome at 2-year follow-up of treated bipolar and depressed alcoholics. *Journal of Studies on Alcohol and Drugs, 72*(5), 872–880.

Feighner, J. P., Robins, E., Guze, S. B., Woodruff, R. A., Winokur, G., & Munoz, R. (1972). Diagnostic criteria for use in psychiatric research. *Archives of General Psychiatry, 26,* 57–63.

Feingold, D., Fox, J., Rehm, J., & Lev-Ran, S. (2015). Natural outcome of cannabis use disorder: A 3-year longitudinal follow-up. *Addiction, 110*(12), 1963–1974.

Feldstein, S. W., & Miller, W. R. (2007). Does subtle screening for substance abuse work?: A review of the Substance Abuse Subtle Screening Inventory (SASSI). *Addiction, 102*(1), 41–50.

Feldstein Ewing, S. W., Walters, S., & Baer, J. S. (2013). Motivational interviewing groups for adolescents and emerging adults. In C. C. Wagner & K. S. Ingersoll (Eds.), *Motivational interviewing in groups* (pp. 387–406). New York: Guilford Press.

Field, M., & Rowe, A. (2017). Which leads to higher medication substitution treatment retention—methadone or buprenorphine?: A systematic literature review. Retrieved from *http://digitalcommons.usm.maine.edu/thinking_matters/111*.

Fingarette, H. (1988). *Heavy drinking: The myth of alcoholism as a disease*. Berkeley: University of California Press.

Finkelstein, N. B., & Mora, J. (2009). *Addressing the specific needs of women* (Vol. 51, Treatment Improvement Protocol Series). Rockville, MD: Center for Substance Abuse Treatment.

Fiorentine, R., Nakashima, J., & Anglin, M. D. (1999). Client engagement in drug treatment. *Journal of Substance Abuse Treatment, 17*(3), 199–206.

First, M. B., Williams, J., Karg, R. S., & Spitzer, R. L. (2015). *User's guide to the Structured Clinical Interview for DSM-5 Disorders (SCID-5-CV) Clinical Version*. Arlington, VA: American Psychiatric Press.

Fixsen, D. L., Blase, K. A., & Fixsen, A. A. M. (2017). Scaling effective innovations. *Criminology and Public Policy, 16*(2), 487–499.

Fixsen, D. L., Naoom, S. F., Blase, K. A., Friedman, R. M., & Wallace, F. (2005). *Implementation research: A synthesis of the literature*. Tampa: University of South Florida, National Implementation Research Network.

Fleming, M. F. (2002). Identification and treatment of alcohol use disorders in older adults. In A. M. Gurnack, R. Atkinson, & N. J. Osgood (Eds.), *Treating alcohol and drug abuse in the elderly* (pp. 85–108). New York: Springer.

Fleming, M. F., Lund, M. R., Wilton, G., Landry, M., & Scheets, D. (2008). The Healthy Moms Study: The efficacy of brief alcohol intervention in postpartum women. *Alcoholism: Clinical and Experimental Research, 32*(9), 1600–1606.

Fleming, M. F., & Manwell, L. B. (1999). Brief intervention in primary care settings. *Alcohol Research and Health, 23*(2), 128–137.

Fletcher, A. M. (2009). *Sober for good: New solutions for drinking problems—advice from those who have succeeded*. Boston: Houghton-Mifflin.

Fleury, M. J., Djouini, A., Huynh, C., Tremblay, J., Ferland, F., Menard, J. M., & Belleville, G. (2016). Remission from substance use disorders: A systematic review and meta-analysis. *Drug and Alcohol Dependence, 168*, 293–306.

Flórez, G., Saiz, P. A., García-Portilla, P., Álvarez, S., Nogueiras, L., & Bobes, J. (2011). Topiramate for the treatment of alcohol dependence: Comparison with naltrexone. *European Addiction Research, 17*(1), 29–36.

Forcehimes, A. A. (2004). De profundis: Spiritual transformations in Alcoholics Anonymous. *Journal of Clinical Psychology, 60*(5), 503–517.

Forcehimes, A. A., Tonigan, J. S., Miller, W. R., Kenna, G. A., & Baer, J. S. (2007). Psychometrics of the Drinker Inventory of Consequences (DrInC). *Addictive Behaviors, 32*(8), 1699–1704.

Fortney, J., Booth, B., Zhang, M., Humphrey, J., & Wiseman, E. (1998). Controlling for selection bias in the evaluation of Alcoholics Anonymous as aftercare treatment. *Journal of Studies on Alcohol, 59*, 690–697.

Frakt, A. B., & Bagley, N. (2015). Protection or harm?: Suppressing substance-use data. *New England Journal of Medicine, 372*(20), 1879–1881.

Frankl, V. E. (1969). *The will to meaning*. New York: World Publishing.

Franklin, B. (1904). Moral or prudential algebra: Letter to Joseph Priestly (September 19, 1772). In J. Bigelow (Ed.), *The works of Benjamin Franklin: Letters and misc. writings 1768–1772* (Vol. 5). New York: Putnam.

Frisman, L. K., Mueser, K. T., Covell, N. H., Lin, H.-J., Crocker, A., Drake, R. E., & Essock, S. M. (2009). Use of integrated dual disorder treatment via assertive community versus clinical case management for perons with co-occurring disorders and antisocial personality disorder. *Journal of Nervous and Mental Disease, 197,* 822–828.

Fromme, K., Stroot, E. A., & Kaplan, D. (1993). Comprehensive effects of alcohol: Development and psychometric assessment of a new expectancy questionnaire. *Psychological Assessment, 5*(1), 19–26.

Fuller, R. K., & Gordis, E. (2004). Does disulfiram have a role in alcoholism treatment today? *Addiction, 99*(1), 21–24.

Futterman, S. (1953). Personality trends in wives of alcoholics. *Journal of Psychiatric Social Work, 23,* 37–41.

Galante, J., Galante, I., Bekkers, M. J., & Gallacher, J. (2014). Effect of kindness-based meditation on health and well-being: A systematic review and meta-analysis. *Journal of Consulting and Clinical Psychology, 82*(6), 1101–1114.

Galanter, M., Dermatis, H., Post, S., & Santucci, C. (2013). Abstinence from drugs of abuse in community-based members of Narcotics Anonymous. *Journal of Studies on Alcohol and Drugs, 74*(2), 349–352.

Galanter, M., Egelko, S., & Edwards, H. (1993). Rational Recovery: Alternative to AA for addiction? *American Journal of Drug and Alcohol Abuse, 19,* 499–510.

Gallup, G. H., Jr. (2017). Religion. Retrieved September 11, 2017, from *www.gallup.com/poll/1690/religion.aspx.*

Garbutt, J. C. (2009). The state of pharmacotherapy for the treatment of alcohol dependence. *Journal of Substance Abuse Treatment, 36*(1), S1–S23.

Garbutt, J. C., Kranzler, H. R., O'Malley, S. S., Gastfriend, D. R., Pettinati, H. M., Silverman, B. L., . . . Group, V. S. (2005). Efficacy and tolerability of long-acting injectable naltrexone for alcohol dependence: A randomized controlled trial. *JAMA, 293*(13), 1617–1625.

Garbutt, J. C., West, S. L., Carey, T. S., Lohr, K. N., & Crews, F. T. (1999). Pharmacological treatment of alcohol dependence: A review of the evidence. *JAMA, 281*(14), 1318–1325.

Garcia-Rodriguez, O., Secades-Villa, R., Higgins, S. T., Fernandez-Hermida, J. R., Carballo, J. L., Errasti Perez, J. M., & Al-halabi Diaz, S. (2009). Effects of voucher-based intervention on abstinence and retention in an outpatient treatment for cocaine addiction: A randomized controlled trial. *Experimental and Clinical Psychopharmacology, 17*(3), 131–138.

Garland, E. L., Froeliger, B., & Howard, M. O. (2013). Mindfulness training targets neurocognitive mechanisms of addiction at the attention–appraisal–emotion interface. *Frontiers in Psychiatry, 4*(173).

Garland, E. L., Manusov, E. G., Froeliger, B., Kelly, A., Williams, J. M., & Howard, M. O. (2014). Mindfulness-oriented recovery enhancement for chronic pain and prescription opioid misuse: Results from an early-stage randomized controlled trial. *Journal of Consulting and Clinical Psychology, 82*(3), 448–459.

Garner, B. R. (2009). Research on the diffusion of evidence-based treatments within substance abuse treatment: A systematic review. *Journal of Substance Abuse Treatment, 36*(4), 376–399.

Garner, B. R., Hunter, S. B., Funk, R. R., Griffin, B. A., & Godley, S. H. (2016). Toward evidence-based measures of implementation: Examining the relationship between implementation and client outcomes. *Journal of Substance Abuse Treatment, 67,* 15–21.

Gartner, C. E., Carter, A., & Partridge, B. (2012). What are the public policy implications of a neurobiological view of addiction? *Addiction, 107*(7), 1199–1200.

Garvin, C. D., Reid, W., & Epstein, L. (1976). A task-centered approach. In R. W. Roberts & H. Northen (Eds.), *Theories of social work with groups* (pp. 238–267). New York: Columbia University Press.

Gastfriend, D. (2003). *Addiction treatment matching: Research foundations of the American Society of Addiction Medicine (ASAM) criteria.* Binghamton, NY: Haworth Medical Press.

Gaume, J., Bertholet, N., Faouzi, M., Gmel, G., & Daeppen, J. B. (2010). Counselor motivational interviewing skills and young adult change talk articulation during brief motivational interventions. *Journal of Substance Abuse Treatment, 39*(3), 272–281.

Gaume, J., Bertholet, N., Faouzi, M., Gmel, G., & Daeppen, J. B. (2013). Does change talk during brief motivational interventions with young men predict change in alcohol use? *Journal of Substance Abuse Treatment, 44*(2), 177–185.

Gendel, M. H. (2004). Forensic and medical legal issues in addiction psychiatry. *Psychiatric Clinics of North America, 27,* 611–626.

George, W. H., Frone, M. R., Cooper, M. L., Russell, M., Skinner, J. B., & Windle, M. (1995). A revised Alcohol Expectancy Questionnaire: Factor structure confirmation, and invariance in a general population sample. *Journal of Studies on Alcohol, 56,* 177–185.

Gilmore, S. K. (1973). *The counselor-in-training.* Englewood Cliffs, NJ: Prentice-Hall.

Glaser, F. B. (1993). Matchless?: Alcoholics Anonymous and the matching hypothesis. In B. S. McCrady & W. R. Miller (Eds.), *Research on Alcoholics Anonymous: Opportunities and alternatives* (pp. 379–395). New Brunswick, NJ: Rutgers Center of Alcohol Studies.

Glass, J. E., Andréasson, S., Bradley, K. A., Finn, S. W., Williams, E. C., Bakshi, A.-S., . . . Saitz, R. (2017). Rethinking alcohol interventions in health care: A thematic meeting of the International Network on Brief Interventions for Alcohol & Other Drugs (INEBRIA). *Addiction Science–Clinical Practice, 12*(14), 1–16.

Glass, J. E., Hamilton, A. M., Powell, B. J., Perron, B. E., Brown, R. T., & Ilgen, M. (2015). Specialty substance use disorder services following brief alcohol intervention: A meta-analysis of randomized controlled trials. *Addiction, 110*(9), 1404–1415.

Glass, J. E., Hamilton, A. M., Powell, B. J., Perron, B. E., Brown, R. T., & Ilgen, M. A. (2016). Revisiting our review of Screening, Brief Intervention and Referral to Treatment (SBIRT): Meta-analytical results still point to no efficacy in increasing the use of substance use disorder services. *Addiction, 111*(1), 181–183.

Glynn, L. H., & Moyers, T. B. (2010). Chasing change talk: The clinician's role in evoking client language about change. *Journal of Substance Abuse Treatment, 39*(1), 65–70.

Gmel, G., Gaume, J., Bertholet, N., Fluckiger, J., & Daeppen, J. B. (2013). Effectiveness of a brief integrative multiple substance use intervention among young men with and without booster sessions. *Journal of Substance Abuse Treatment, 44*(2), 231–240.

Godley, M. D., Godley, S. H., Dennis, M. L., Funk, R. R., Passetti, L. L., & Petry, N. M. (2014). A randomized trial of assertive continuing care and contingency management for adolescents with substance use disorders. *Journal of Consulting and Clinical Psychology, 82*(1), 40–51.

Godley, S. H., Hunter, B. D., Fernandez-Artamendi, S., Smith, J. E., Meyers, R. J., & Godley, M. D. (2014). A comparison of treatment outcomes for adolescent community reinforcement approach participants with and without co-occurring problems. *Journal of Substance Abuse Treatment, 46*(4), 463–471.

Godley, S. H., Smith, J. E., Passetti, L. L., & Subramaniam, G. (2014). The Adolescent Community Reinforcement Approach (A-CRA) as a model paradigm for the management of adolescents with substance use disorders and co-occurring psychiatric disorders. *Substance Abuse, 35*(4), 352–363.

Goldberg, L. R. (1970). Man versus model of man: A rationale plus evidence for a method of improving clinical inferences. *Psychological Bulletin, 73,* 422–432.

Goldberg, S. B., Babins-Wagner, R., Rousmaniere, T., Berzins, S., Hoyt, W. T., Whipple, J. L., . . . Wampold, B. E. (2016). Creating a climate for therapist improvement: A case study of an agency focused on outcomes and deliberate practice. *Psychotherapy, 53*(3), 367–375.

Goldman, M. S., Del Boca, F. K., & Darkes, J. (1999). Alcohol expectancy theory: The application of cognitive neuroscience. In K. E. Leonard & H. T. Blane (Eds.), *Psychological theories of drinking and alcoholism* (2nd ed., pp. 203–246). New York: Guilford Press.

Gonzalez, V. M., & Dulin, P. L. (2015). Comparison of a smartphone app for alcohol use disorders with an Internet-based intervention plus bibliotherapy: A pilot study. *Journal of Consulting and Clinical Psychology, 83*(2), 335–345.

Gordon, A. J., Kavanagh, G., Krumm, M., Ramgopal, R., Paidisetty, S., Aghevli, M., . . . Liberto, J. (2011). Facilitators and barriers in implementing buprenorphine in the Veterans Health Administration. *Psychology of Addictive Behaviors, 25*(2), 215–224.

Gordon, T. (1970). *Parent effectiveness training.* New York: Wyden.

Gordon, T., & Edwards, W. S. (1997). *Making the patient your partner: Communication skills for doctors and other caregivers.* New York: Auburn House Paperback.

Gorsuch, R. L. (1995). Religious aspects of substance abuse and recovery. *Journal of Social Issues, 51,* 65–83.

Gorsuch, R. L., & Butler, M. C. (1976). Initial drug abuse: A review of predisposing social psychological factors. *Psychological Bulletin, 83,* 120–137.

Gossop, M. (2015). The National Treatment Outcomes Research Study (NTORS) and its influence on addiction treatment policy in the United Kingdom. *Addiction, 110,* 50–53.

Gossop, M., Stewart, D., & Marsden, J. (2007). Attendance at Narcotics Anonymous and Alcoholics Anonymous meetings, frequency of attendance and substance use outcomes after residential treatment for drug dependence: A 5-year follow-up study. *Addiction, 103,* 119–125.

Gottheil, E., Sterling, R. C., & Weinstein, S. P. (1997a). Outreach engagement efforts: Are they worth the effort? *American Journal of Drug and Alcohol Abuse, 23*(1), 61–66.

Gottheil, E., Sterling, R. C., & Weinstein, S. P. (1997b). Pretreatment dropouts: Characteristics and outcomes. *Journal of Addictive Diseases, 16*(2), 1–14.

Gottman, J. M. (1994). *Why marriages succeed or fail.* New York: Simon & Schuster.

Gottman, J. M. (2014). *What predicts divorce?: The relationship between marital processes and marital outcomes.* New York: Psychology Press (Taylor & Francis).

Gottman, J. M., Gottman, J. S., & Declaire, J. (2007). *Ten lessons to transform your marriage: America's love lab experts share their strategies for strengthening your relationship.* New York: Three Rivers Press.

Gottman, J. M., & Silver, N. (2015). *The seven principles for making marriage work:*

A practical guide from the country's foremost relationship expert (rev. ed.). New York: Harmony.

Gowing, L. R., Ali, R. L., Allsop, S., Marsden, J., Turf, E. E., West, R., & Witton, J. (2015). Global statistics on addictive behaviours: 2014 status report. *Addiction, 110*(6), 904–919.

Graber, R. A., & Miller, W. R. (1988). Abstinence or controlled drinking goals for problem drinkers: A randomized clinical trial. *Psychology of Addictive Behaviors, 2*, 20–33.

Graham, K., Annis, H. M., Brett, P. J., & Venesoen, P. (1996). A controlled field trial of group versus individual cognitive-behavioural training for relapse prevention. *Addiction, 91*(8), 1127–1140.

Grant, B. F., Dawson, D. A., Stinson, F. S., Chou, P. S., Kay, W., & Pickering, R. (2003). The Alcohol Use Disorder and Associated Disabilities Interview Schedule–V (AUDADIS-IV): Reliability of alcohol consumption, tobacco use, family history of depression and psychiatric diagnostic modules in a general population sample. *Drug and Alcohol Dependence, 71*(1), 7–16.

Grant, B. F., Goldstein, R. B., Saha, T. D., Chou, S. P., Jung, J., Zhang, H., . . . Hasin, D. S. (2015). Epidemiology of DSM-5 alcohol use disorder: Results from the National Epidemiologic Survey on Alcohol and Related Conditions III. *JAMA Psychiatry, 72*(8), 757–766.

Grant, B. F., Goldstein, R. B., Smith, S. M., Jung, J., Zhang, H., Chou, S. P., . . . Saha, T. D. (2014). The Alcohol Use Disorder and Associated Disabilities Interview Schedule–5 (AUDADIS-5): Reliability of substance use and psychiatric disorder modules in a general population sample. *Drug and Alcohol Dependence, 148*, 27–33.

Grant, B. F., Saha, T. D., Ruan, W. J., Goldstein, R. B., Chou, S. P., Jung, J., . . . Hasin, D. S. (2016). Epidemiology of DSM-5 drug use disorder: Results from the National Epidemiologic Survey on Alcohol and Related Conditions–III. *JAMA Psychiatry, 73*(1), 39–47.

Gray, K. M., Carpenter, M. J., Baker, N. L., Hartwell, K. J., Lewis, A. L., Hiott, D. W., . . . Upadhyaya, H. P. (2011). Bupropion SR and contingency management for adolescent smoking cessation. *Journal of Substance Abuse Treatment, 40*(1), 77–86.

Gray, K. M., McClure, E. A., Baker, N. L., Hartwell, K. J., Carpenter, M. J., & Saladin, M. E. (2015). An exploratory short-term double-blind randomized trial of varenicline versus nicotine patch for smoking cessation in women. *Addiction, 110*(6), 1027–1034.

Greenfield, S. F., Brooks, A. J., Gordon, S. M., Green, C. A., Kropp, F., McHugh, R. K., . . . Miele, G. M. (2007). Substance abuse treatment entry, retention, and outcome in women: A review of the literature. *Drug and Alcohol Dependence, 86*(1), 1–21.

Greenfield, S. F., Cummings, A. M., Kuper, L. E., Wigderson, S. B., & Koro-Ljungberg, M. (2013). A qualitative analysis of women's experiences in single-gender versus mixed-gender substance abuse group therapy. *Substance Use and Misuse, 48*(9), 750–760.

Griffin, E. A., Jr., Melas, P. A., Zhou, R., Li, Y., Mercado, P., Kempadoo, K. A., . . . Kandel, D. B. (2017). Prior alcohol use enhances vulnerability to compulsive cocaine self-administration by promoting degradation of HDAC4 and HDAC5. *Science Advances, 3*, e1701682.

Griffiths, R. R., Richards, W. A., Johnson, M. W., McCann, U. D., & Jesse, R. (2008). Mystical-type experiences occasioned by psilocybin mediate the attribution of personal meaning and spiritual significance 14 months later. *Journal of Psychopharmacology, 22*, 621–632.

Gryczynski, J., Kelly, S. M., Mitchell, S. G., Kirk, A., O'Grady, K. E., & Schwartz, R. P. (2014). Validation and performance of the Alcohol, Smoking and Substance Involvement Screening Test (ASSIST) among adolescent primary care patients. *Addiction, 110*(2), 240–247.

Gryczynski, J., Mitchell, S. G., Gonzales, A., Moseley, A., Peterson, T. R., Ondersma, S. J., . . . Schwartz, R. P. (2015). A randomized trial of computerized vs. in-person brief intervention for illicit drug use in primary care: Outcomes through 12 months. *Journal of Substance Abuse Treatment, 50*, 3–10.

Gryczynski, J., Schwartz, R. P., Fishman, M. J., Nordeck, C. D., Grant, J., Nidich, S., . . . O'Grady, K. E. (2018). Integration of Transcendental Meditation (TM) into alcohol use disorder (AUD) treatment. *Journal of Substance Abuse Treatment, 87*, 23–30.

Gueorguieva, R., Wu, R., Krystal, J. H., Donovan, D., & O'Malley, S. S. (2013). Temporal patterns of adherence to medications and behavioral treatment and their relationship to patient characteristics and treatment response. *Addictive Behaviors, 38*(5), 2119–2127.

Hahn, J. A., Dobkin, L. M., Mayanja, B., Emenyonu, N. I., Kigozi, I. M., Shiboski, S., . . . Wurst, F. M. (2012). Phosphatidylethanol (PEth) as a biomarker of alcohol consumption in HIV-positive patients in sub-Saharan Africa. *Alcoholism: Clinical and Experimental Research, 36*(5), 854–862.

Hall, K., Staiger, P. K., Simpson, A., Best, D., & Lubman, D. I. (2016). After 30 years of dissemination, have we achieved sustained practice change in motivational interviewing? *Addiction, 111*(7), 1144–1150.

Hall, W., Farrell, M., & Carter, A. (2014). Compulsory treatment of addiction in the patient's best interests: More rigorous evaluations are essential. *Drug and Alcohol Review, 33*(3), 268–271.

Hallgren, K. A., & McCrady, B. S. (2016). We language and sustained reductions in drinking in couple-based treatment for alcohol use disorders. *Family Process, 55*(1), 62–78.

Halpern, S. D., French, B., Small, D. S., Saulsgiver, K., Harhay, M. O., Audrain-McGovern, J., . . . Volpp, K. G. (2015). Randomized trial of four financial-incentive programs for smoking cessation. *New England Journal of Medicine, 372*(22), 2108–2117.

Hamdi, N. R., Levy, M., Jaffee, W. B., Chisholm, S. M., & Weiss, R. D. (2011). Implementing an adapted version of the job seekers' workshop in a residential program for patients with substance use disorders. *Journal of Addiction Medicine, 5*(2), 148–152.

Hamilton, E. (1999). *Mythology: Timeless tales of gods and heroes.* New York: Warner Books.

Handelsman, L., Cochrane, K. J., Aronson, M. J., Ness, R., Rubenstein, K. J., & Kanof, P. D. (1987). Two new rating scales for opiate withdrawal. *American Journal of Drug and Alcohol Abuse, 13*, 293–308.

Handmaker, N. S., Miller, W. R., & Manicke, M. (1999). Findings of a pilot study of motivational interviewing with pregnant drinkers. *Journal of Studies on Alcohol, 60*, 285–287.

Handmaker, N. S., & Wilbourne, P. (2001). Motivational Interventions in prenatal clinics. *Alcohol Research and Health, 25*(3), 219–229.

Hanson, J., & Emrick, C. D. (1983). Whom are we calling "alcoholic"? *Bulletin of the Society of Psychologists in Addictive Behaviors, 2*, 164–178.

Hanson, T., Alessi, S. M., & Petry, N. M. (2008). Contingency management reduces drug-related human immunodeficiency virus risk behaviors in cocaine-abusing methadone patients. *Addiction, 103*(7), 1187–1197.

Harris, A. H. S., Brown, R., Dawes, M., Dieperink, E., Myrick, D. H., Gerould, H., . . . Hagedorn, H. J. (2017). Effects of a multifaceted implementation intervention to increase utilization of pharmacological treatments for alcohol use disorders in the US Veterans Health Administration. *Journal of Substance Abuse Treatment, 82*, 107–112.

Harris, J. S., Stewart, D. G., & Stanton, B. C. (2016). Urge surfing as aftercare in adolescent alcohol use: A randomized control trial. *Mindfulness, 8*(1), 144–149.

Hart, C. L., & Ksir, C. (2015). *Drugs, society and human behavior* (16th ed.). New York: McGraw Hill.

Hartman, R. L., Brown, T. L., Milavetz, G., Spurgin, A., Pierce, R. S., Gorelick, D. A., . . . Huestis, M. A. (2015). Cannabis effects on driving lateral control with and without alcohol. *Drug and Alcohol Dependence, 154*, 25–37.

Hartz, S. M., Pato, C. N., Medeiros, H., Cavazos-Rehg, P., Sobell, J. L., Knowles, J. A., . . . Pato, M. T. (2014). Comorbidity of severe psychotic disorders with measures of substance use. *JAMA Psychiatry, 71*(3), 248–254.

Hartzler, B., Beadnell, B., & Donovan, D. (2015). Predictive validity of addiction treatment clinicians' post-training contingency management skills for subsequent clinical outcomes. *Journal of Substance Abuse Treatment, 72*, 126–133.

Hartzler, B., Jackson, T. R., Jones, B. E., Beadnell, B., & Calsyn, D. A. (2014). Disseminating contingency management: Impacts of staff training and implementation at an opiate treatment program. *Journal of Substance Abuse Treatment, 46*(4), 429–438.

Hartzler, B., Lyon, A. R., Walker, D. D., Matthews, L., King, K. M., & McCollister, K. E. (2017). Implementing the teen marijuana check-up in schools: A study protocol. *Implementation Science, 12*, 103.

Hasin, D. S., & Grant, B. F. (2015). The National Epidemiologic Survey on Alcohol and Related Conditions (NESARC) waves 1 and 2: Review and summary of findings. *Social Psychiatry and Psychiatric Epidemiology, 50*(11), 1609–1640.

Hasin, D. S., Grant, B., & Endicott, J. (1990). The natural history of alcohol abuse: Implications for definitions of alcohol use disorders. *American Journal of Psychiatry, 147*(11), 1537–1541.

Hasin, D. S., O'Brien, C. P., Auriacombe, M., Borges, G., Bucholz, K., Budney, A., . . . Petry, N. M. (2013). DSM-5 criteria for substance use disorders: Recommendations and rationale. *American Journal of Psychiatry, 170*(8), 834–851.

Heather, N., Best, D., Kawalek, A., Field, M., Lewis, M., Rotgers, F., . . . Heim, D. (2018). Challenging the brain disease model of addiction: European launch of the Addiction Theory Network. *Addiction Research and Theory, 26*(4), 249–255.

Heather, N., & Hönekopp, J. (2013). Readiness to change and the transtheoretical model as applied to addictive disorders: A balanced appraisal. In L. R. Martin & M. R. DiMatteo (Eds.), *The Oxford handbook of health communication, behavior change, and treatment adherence* (pp. 214–250). Oxford, UK: Oxford University Press.

Heather, N., Hönekopp, J., Smailes, D., & UKATT Research Team. (2009). Progressive stage transition does mean getting better: A further test of the transtheoretical model in recovery from alcohol problems. *Addiction, 104*(6), 949–958.

Heather, N., & Robertson, I. (1984). *Controlled drinking.* London: Routledge.

Heatherton, T. F., Kozlowski, L. T., Frecker, R. C., & Fagerstrom, K. O. (1991). The

Fagerstrom Test for Nicotine Dependence: A revision of the Fagerstrom Tolerance Questionnaire. *British Journal of Addiction, 86*(9), 1119–1127.

Heckman, C. J., Egleston, B. L., & Hofmann, M. T. (2010). Efficacy of motivational interviewing for smoking cessation: A systematic review and meta-analysis. *Tobacco Control, 19*(5), 410–416.

Hedden, S. L., Kennet, J., Lipari, R., Medley, G., Tice, P., Copello, E. A. P., & Kroutil, L. A. (2015). *Behavioral health trends in the United States: Results from the 2014 National Survey on Drug Use and Health.* Rockville, MD: Substance Abuse and Mental Health Services Administration.

Heffner, J. L., Tran, G. Q., Johnson, C. S., Barrett, S. W., Blom, T. J., Thompson, R. D., & Anthenelli, R. M. (2010). Combining motivational interviewing with compliance enhancement therapy (MI-CET): Development and preliminary evaluation of a new, manual-guided psychosocial adjunct to alcohol-dependence pharmacotherapy. *Journal of Studies on Alcohol and Drugs, 71*(1), 61–70.

Heinälä, P., Alho, H., Kiianmaa, K., Lönnqvist, J., Kuoppasalmi, K., & Sinclair, J. D. (2001). Targeted use of naltrexone without prior detoxification in the treatment of alcohol dependence: A factorial double-blind, placebo-controlled trial. *Journal of Clinical Pharmacology, 21*(3), 287–292.

Heinz, A. J., Disney, E. R., Epstein, D. H., Glezen, L. A., Clark, P. I., & Preston, K. L. (2010). A focus-group study on spirituality and substance-user treatment. *Substance Use and Misuse, 45*(1–2), 134–153.

Hendershot, C. S., Witkiewitz, K., George, W. H., & Marlatt, G. A. (2011). Relapse prevention for addictive behaviors. *Substance Abuse Treatment, Prevention and Policy, 6,* 17.

Henderson, C. E., Wevodau, A. L., Henderson, S. E., Colbourn, S. L., Gharagozloo, L., North, L. W., & Lotts, V. A. (2016). An independent replication of the Adolescent-Community Reinforcement Approach with justice-involved youth. *American Journal on Addictions, 25*(3), 233–240.

Henggeler, S. W., Chapman, J. E., Rowland, M. D., Sheidow, A. J., & Cunningham, P. B. (2013). Evaluating training methods for transporting contingency management to therapists. *Journal of Substance Abuse Treatment, 45*(5), 466–474.

Henggeler, S. W., Melton, G. B., Brondino, M. J., & Scherer, D. G. (1997). Multisystemic therapy with violent and chronic juvenile offenders and their families: The role of treatment fidelity in successful dissemination. *Journal of Consulting and Clinical Psychology, 65,* 821–833.

Henggeler, S. W., Schoenwald, S. K., Letourneau, J. G., & Edwards, D. L. (2002). Transporting efficacious treatments to field settings: The link between supervisory practices and therapist fidelity in MST programs. *Journal of Clinical Child and Adolescent Psychology, 31,* 155–167.

Henggeler, S. W., Schoenwald, S. K., Rowland, M. D., & Cunningham, P. B. (2002). *Serious emotional disturbance in children and adolescents: Multisystemic therapy.* New York: Guilford Press.

Herrmann, E. S., Matusiewicz, A. K., Stitzer, M. L., Higgins, S. T., Sigmon, S. C., & Heil, S. H. (2017). Contingency management interventions for HIV, tuberculosis, and hepatitis control among individuals with substance use disorders: A systematized review. *Journal of Substance Abuse Treatment, 72,* 117–125.

Hersen, M., & Turner, S. M. (Eds.). (2003). *Diagnostic interviewing* (3rd ed.). New York: Springer.

Hesse, M., Vanderplasschen, W., Rapp, R., Broekaert, E., & Fridell, M. (2007). Case management for persons with substance use disorders. *Cochrane Database of Systematic Reviews, 17*(4), CD006265.

Hester, R. K. (2003). Behavioral self-control training. In R. K. Hester & W. R. Miller (Eds.), *Handbook of alcoholism treatment approaches: Effective alternatives* (3rd ed., pp. 152–164). Boston: Allyn & Bacon.

Hester, R. K., & Delaney, H. D. (1997). Behavioral self-control program for Windows: Results of a controlled clinical trial. *Journal of Consulting and Clinical Psychology, 65*, 686–693.

Hester, R. K., Delaney, H. D., & Campbell, W. (2011). *ModerateDrinking.com* and moderation management: Outcomes of a randomized clinical trial with non-dependent problem drinkers. *Journal of Consulting and Clinical Psychology, 79*(2), 215–224.

Hester, R. K., Delaney, H. D., Campbell, W., & Handmaker, N. (2009). A Web application for moderation training: Initial results of a randomized clinical trial. *Journal of Substance Abuse Treatment, 37*(3), 266–276.

Hester, R. K., Lenberg, K. L., Campbell, W., & Delaney, H. D. (2013). Overcoming Addictions, a web-based application, and SMART Recovery, an online and in-person mutual help group for problem drinkers: Part I. Three month outcomes of a randomized controlled trial. *Journal of Medical Internet Research, 15*(7).

Hester, R. K., Squires, D. D., & Delaney, H. D. (2005). The drinker's check-up: 12-month outcomes of a controlled clinical trial of a stand-alone software program for problem drinkers. *Journal of Substance Abuse, 28*, 159–169.

Hettema, J., Steele, J., & Miller, W. R. (2005). Motivational interviewing. *Annual Review of Clinical Psychology, 1*, 91–111.

Hibbert, L. J., & Best, D. W. (2011). Assessing recovery and functioning in former problem drinkers at different stages of their recovery journeys. *Drug and Alcohol Dependence, 30*(1), 12–20.

Higgins, S. T., & Abbott, P. J. (2001). CRA and treatment of cocaine and opioid dependence. In R. J. Meyers & W. R. Miller (Eds.), *A community reinforcement approach for addiction treatment* (pp. 123–146). Cambridge, UK: Cambridge University Press.

Higgins, S. T., Budney, A. J., Bickel, W. K., Foerg, F. E., Donham, R., & Badger, G. J. (1994). Incentives improve treatment retention and cocaine abstinence in ambulatory cocaine-dependent patients. *Archives of General Psychiatry, 51*, 568–576.

Higgins, S. T., Budney, A. J., Bickel, W. K., Foerg, F. E., Ogden, D., & Badger, G. J. (1995). Outpatient behavioral treatment for cocaine dependence: One-year outcome. *Experimental and Clinical Psychopharmacology, 3*, 205–212.

Higgins, S. T., Budney, A. J., Bickel, W. K., Hughes, J. R., Foerg, F., & Badger, G. (1993). Achieving cocaine abstinence with a behavioral approach. *American Journal of Psychiatry, 150*, 763–769.

Higgins, S. T., Delaney, D. D., Budney, A. J., Bickel, W. K., Hughes, J. R., Foerg, F., & Fenwick, J. W. (1991). A behavioral approach to achieving initial cocaine abstinence. *American Journal of Psychiatry, 148*, 1218–1224.

Higgins, S. T., Wong, C. J., Badger, G. J., Haug Ogden, D. E., & Dantona, R. L. (2000). Contingent reinforcement increases cocaine abstinence during outpatient treatment and one year of follow-up. *Journal of Consulting and Clinical Psychology, 68*, 64–72.

Hildebrand, M. (2015). The psychometric properties of the Drug Use Disorders Identification Test (DUDIT): A review of recent research. *Journal of Substance Abuse Treatment, 53*, 52–59.

Hill, P. C., & Hood, R. W., Jr. (1999). *Measures of religious behavior.* Birmingham, AL: Religious Education Press.

Hill, P. C., & Pargament, K. I. (2003). Advances in the conceptualization and measurement of religion and spirituality. *American Psychologist, 58,* 64–74.

Hill, P. C., Pargament, K. I., Hood, R. W., Jr., McCullough, M. E., Swyers, J. P., Larson, D. B., & Zinnbauer, B. J. (2000). Conceptualizing religion and spirituality: Points of communality, points of departure. *Journal for the Theory of Social Behavior, 30,* 51–77.

Hilton, M. E. (1991). The demographic distribution of drinking problems in 1984. In W. B. Clark & M. E. Hilton (Eds.), *Alcohol in America: Drinking practices and problems* (pp. 87–101). Albany: State University of New York Press.

Hilton, M. E., Maisto, S. A., Conigliaro, J., McNiel, M., Kraemer, K., Kelley, M. E., . . . Savetsky, J. (2001). Improving alcoholism treatment across the spectrum of services. *Alcoholism: Clinical and Experimental Research, 25*(1), 128–135.

Hingson, R., Heeren, T., Winter, M., & Wechsler, H. (2005). Magnitude of alcohol-related mortality and morbidity among U.S. college students aged 18–24: Changes from 1998 to 2001. *Annual Review of Public Health, 26,* 259–279.

Hodgins, D. C., Ching, L. E., & McEwen, J. (2009). Strength of commitment language in motivational interviewing and gambling outcomes. *Psychology of Addictive Behaviors, 23*(1), 122–130.

Hoffman, N. G., Halikas, J. A., & Mee-Lee, D. (1987). *The Cleveland admission, discharge and transfer criteria: Model for chemical dependence treatment programs.* Cleveland: Northern Ohio Chemical Dependency Treatment Directors Association.

Hoffman, N., Halikas, J., Mee-Lee, D., & Weedman, R. (1991). *American Society of Addiction Medicine placement criteria for the treatment of psychoactive substance use disorders.* Washington, DC: American Society of Addiction Medicine.

Holdstock, L., & de Wit, H. (1998). Individual differences in biphasic effects of ethanol. *Alcoholism: Clinical and Experimental Research, 22,* 1903–1911.

Hood, R. W., Jr., Hill, P. C., & Spilka, B. (2009). *The psychology of religion: An empirical approach* (4th ed.). New York: Guilford Press.

Horigan, V. E., Anderson, A. R., & Szapocznik, J. (2016). Taking brief strategic family therapy from bench to trench: Evidence generation across translational phases. *Family Process, 55,* 529–542.

Horigan, V. E., Foster, D. J., Brincks, A., Robbins, M. S., Perez, M. A., & Szapocznik, J. (2015). The effects of brief strategic family therapy (BSFT) on parent substance use and the association between parent and adolescent substance use. *Addictive Behaviors, 42,* 44–50.

Horsfall, J., Cleary, M., Hunt, G. E., & Walter, G. (2009). Psychosocial treatments for people with co-occurring severe mental illnesses and substance use disorders (dual diagnosis): A review of empirical evidence. *Harvard Review of Psychiatry, 17*(1), 24–34.

Horvath, A. T. (2000). SMART Recovery: Addiction recovery support from a cognitive-behavioral perspective. *Journal of Rational-Emotive and Cognitive Behavior Therapy, 18,* 181–191.

Horvath, A. T., & Yeterian, J. (2012). SMART Recovery: Self-empowering, science-based addiction recovery support. *Journal of Groups in Addiction and Recovery, 7*(2–4), 102–117.

Hser, Y.-I., Evans, E., Grella, C., Ling, W., & Anglin, D. (2015). Long-term course of opioid addiction. *Harvard Review of Psychiatry, 23*(2), 76–89.

Hughes, R. (1987). *The fatal shore: The epic of Australia's founding.* New York: Knopf.

Hulse, G. K., & Tait, R. J. (2003). Five-year outcomes of a brief alcohol intervention for adult in-patients with psychiatric disorders. *Addiction, 98*(8), 1061–1068.

Humphreys, K. (1993). Psychotherapy and the twelve step approach for substance abusers: The limits of integration. *Psychotherapy, 30,* 207–213.

Humphreys, K. (2003). Alcohol and drug abuse: A research-based analysis of the Moderation Management controversy. *Psychiatric Services, 54,* 621–622.

Humphreys, K., Blodgett, J. C., & Wagner, T. H. (2014). Estimating the efficacy of Alcoholics Anonymous without self-selection bias: An instrumental variables reanalysis of randomized clinical trials. *Alcoholism: Clinical and Experimental Research, 38*(11), 2688–2694.

Humphreys, K., & Frank, R. G. (2014). The Affordable Care Act will revolutionize care for substance use disorders in the United States. *Addiction, 109*(12), 1957–1958.

Humphreys, K., & Klaw, E. (2001). Can targeting nondependent problem drinkers and providing Internet-based services expand access to assistance for alcohol problems?: A study of the Moderation Management self-help/mutual aid organization. *Journal of Studies on Alcohol, 62,* 528–532.

Humphreys, K., & McLellan, A. T. (2011). A policy-oriented review of strategies for improving the outcomes of services for substance use disorder patients. *Addiction, 106*(12), 2058–2066.

Humphreys, K., & Moos, R. (2001). Can encouraging substance abuse patients to participate in self-help groups reduce demand for health care?: A quasi-experimental study. *Alcoholism: Clinical and Experimental Research, 25,* 711–716.

Humphreys, K., Wing, S., McCarty, D., Chappel, J., Gallant, L., Haberle, B., . . . Weiss, R. (2004). Self-help organizations for alcohol and drug problems: Toward evidence-based practice and policy. *Journal of Substance Abuse Treatment, 26,* 151–158.

Hunt, G. M., & Azrin, N. H. (1973). A community-reinforcement approach to alcoholism. *Behaviour Research and Therapy, 11,* 91–104.

Hunter, S. B., Schwartz, R. P., & Friedmann, P. D. (2016). Introduction to the special issue on the studies on the implementation of integrated models of alcohol, tobacco, and/or drug use interventions and medical care. *Journal of Substance Abuse Treatment, 60,* 1–5.

Hunter-Reel, D., McCrady, B., & Hildebrandt, T. (2009). Emphasizing interpersonal factors: An extension of the Witkiewitz and Marlatt relapse model. *Addiction, 104*(8), 1281–1290.

Hunter-Reel, D., Witkiewitz, K., & Zweben, A. (2012). Does session attendance by a supportive significant other predict outcomes in individual treatment for alcohol use disorders? *Alcoholism: Clinical and Experimental Research, 36*(6), 1237–1243.

Hurcom, C., Copello, A., & Orford, J. (2000). The family and alcohol: Effects of excessive drinking and conceptualizations of spouses over recent decades. *Substance Use and Misuse, 35*(4), 473–502.

Imel, Z. E., Wampold, B. E., Miller, S. D., & Fleming, R. R. (2008). Distinctions without a difference: Direct comparisons of psychotherapies for alcohol use disorders. *Psychology of Addictive Behaviors, 22*(4), 533–543.

Inciardi, J. A., Martin, S. S., & Scarpitti, F. R. (1996). Appropriateness of assertive case management for drug-involved prison releasees. *Journal of Case Management, 3*(4), 145–149.

Institute of Medicine. (1990). *Broadening the base of treatment for alcohol problems.* Washington, DC: National Academy Press.

Jackson, J. K. (1954). The adjustment of the family to the crisis of alcoholism. *Quarterly Journal of Studies on Alcohol, 15,* 562–586.

James, W. (1902/1994). *The varieties of religious experience*. New York: Modern Library Edition.

Janis, I. L., & Mann, L. (1977). *Decision making: A psychological analysis of conflict, choice and commitment*. New York: Free Press.

Jarusiewicz, B. (2000). Spirituality and addiction: Relationship to recovery and relapse. *Alcoholism Treatment Quarterly, 18*(4), 99–109.

Jarvis, B. P., Holtyn, A. F., Subramaniam, S., Tompkins, D. A., Oga, E. A., Bigelow, G. E., & Silverman, K. (2018). Extended-release injectable naltrexone for opioid use disorder: A systematic review. *Addiction, 113*(7), 1188–1209.

Jatlow, P., & O'Malley, S. S. (2010). Clinical (nonforensic) application of ethyl glucuronide measurement: Are we ready? *Alcoholism: Clinical and Experimental Research, 34*(6), 968–975.

Jellinek, E. M. (1960). *The disease concept of alcoholism*. Highland Park, NJ: Hillhouse Press.

Jensen, C. D., Cushing, C. C., Aylward, B. S., Craig, J. T., Sorell, D. M., & Steele, R. G. (2011). Effectiveness of motivational interviewing interventions for adolescent substance use behavior change: A meta-analytic review. *Journal of Consulting and Clinical Psychology, 79*(4), 433–440.

Jessor, R., & Jessor, S. L. (1977). *Problem behavior and psychosocial development: A longitudinal study of youth*. New York: Academic Press.

Jiménez-Murcia, S., Tremblay, J., Stinchfield, R., Granero, R., Fernández-Aranda, F., Mestre-Bach, G., . . . Menc, J. M. (2017). The involvement of a concerned significant other in gambling disorder treatment outcome. *Journal of Gambling Studies, 33*(3), 937–953.

Johnson, B. A., Ait-Daoud, N., Bowden, C. L., DiClemente, C. C., Roache, J. D., Lawson, K., . . . Ma, J. Z. (2003). Oral topiramate for treatment of alcohol dependence: A randomised controlled trial. *The Lancet, 361*(9370), 1677–1685.

Johnson, B. A., Rosenthal, N., Capece, J. A., Wiegand, F., Mao, L., Beyers, K., . . . Ciraulo, D. A. (2007). Topiramate for treating alcohol dependence: A randomized controlled trial. *JAMA, 298*(14), 1641–1651.

Johnson, E., & Herringer, L. G. (1993). A note on the utilization of common support activities and relapse following substance abuse treatment. *Journal of Psychology, 127,* 73–78.

Johnson, M. W., Garcia-Romeu, A., Cosimano, M. P., & Griffiths, R. R. (2014). Pilot study of the 5-HT2AR agonist psilocybin in the treatment of tobacco addiction. *Journal of Psychopharmacology, 28*(11), 983–992.

Johnson, V. E. (1986). *Intervention: How to help someone who doesn't want help*. Center City, MN: Hazelden.

Jonas, D. E., Garbutt, J. C., Amick, H. R., Brown, J. M., Brownley, K. A., Council, C. L., . . . Harris, R. P. (2012). Behavioral counseling after screening for alcohol misuse in primary care: A systematic review and meta-analysis for the U.S. Preventive Services Task Force. *Annals of Internal Medicine, 157*(9), 645–654.

Jones, A., Hayhurst, K. P., & Millar, T. (2017). Levels of motivation and readiness for treatment aligned with criminal justice referral and coercion among substance users in England. *Journal of Studies on Alcohol and Drugs, 78*(6), 884–888.

Jones, B. T., Corbin, W., & Fromme, K. (2001). A review of expectancy theory and alcohol consumption. *Addiction, 96*(1), 57–72.

Jones, M. C. (1968). Personality correlates and antecedents of drinking patterns in adult males. *Journal of Consulting and Clinical Psychology, 32,* 2–12.

Joslyn, G., Ravindranathan, A., Busch, G., Schuckit, M. A., & White, R. L. (2010).

Human variation in alcohol response is influenced by variation in neuronal signaling genes. *Alcoholism: Clinical and Experimental Research, 34,* 800–812.

Joy, M., Clement, T., & Sisti, D. (2016). The ethics of behavioral health information technology: Frequent flyer icons and implicit bias. *JAMA, 316*(15), 1539–1540.

Jung, C. G. (1961/1975). Letter to William G. Wilson, 30 January 1961. In G. Adler (Ed.), *Letters of Carl G. Jung* (Vol. 2, pp. 623–625). London: Routledge & Kegan Paul.

Kabat-Zinn, J. (2016). *Mindfulness for beginners: Reclaiming the present moment—and your life.* Boulder, CO: Sounds True.

Kadden, R., Carroll, K., Donovan, D. M., Cooney, N., Monti, P., Abrams, D. B., . . . Hester, R. (1992). *Cognitive-behavioral coping skills therapy manual* (Vol. 3). Rockville, MD: National Institute on Alcohol Abuse and Alcoholism.

Kalichman, S. C. (1999). Therapeutic jurisprudence and mandated reporting. In S. C. Kalichman (Ed.), *Mandated reporting of suspected child abuse: Ethics, law, and policy* (2nd ed., pp. 97–104). Washington, DC: American Psychological Association.

Kaminer, Y. (2001). Adolescent substance abuse treatment: Where do we go from here? *Psychiatric Services, 52*(2), 147–149.

Kampman, K. M., Dackis, C., Pettinati, H. M., Lynch, K. G., Sparkman, T., & O'Brien, C. P. (2011). A double-blind, placebo-controlled pilot trial of acamprosate for the treatment of cocaine dependence. *Addictive Behaviors, 36*(3), 217–221.

Kampman, K., & Jarvis, M. (2015). American Society of Addiction Medicine (ASAM) national practice guideline for the use of medications in the treatment of addiction involving opioid use. *Journal of Addiction Medicine, 9*(5), 358–367.

Kampman, K. M., Pettinati, H., Lynch, K. G., Dackis, C., Sparkman, T., Weigley, C., & O'Brien, C. P. (2004). A pilot trial of topiramate for the treatment of cocaine dependence. *Drug and Alcohol Dependence, 75*(3), 233–240.

Kampman, K. M., Volpicelli, J. R., McGinnis, D. E., Alterman, A. I., Weinrieb, R. M., D'Angelo, L., & Epperson, L. E. (1998). Reliability and validity of the Cocaine Selective Severity Assessment. *Addictive Behaviors, 23*(4), 449–461.

Karakurt, G., Whiting, K., VanEsch, C., Bolen, S., & Calabrese, J. (2016). Couple therapy for intimate partner violence: A systematic review and meta-analysis. *Journal of Marital and Family Therapy, 42,* 567–583.

Karno, M. P., & Longabaugh, R. (2003). Patient depressive symptoms and therapist focus on emotional material: A new look at Project MATCH. *Journal of Studies on Alcohol, 64,* 607–615.

Karno, M. P., & Longabaugh, R. (2005). An examination of how therapist directiveness interacts with patient anger and reactance to predict alcohol use. *Journal of Studies on Alcohol, 66,* 825–832.

Karyadi, K. A., VanderVeen, J. D., & Cyders, M. A. (2014). A meta-analysis of the relationship between trait mindfulness and substance use behaviors. *Drug and Alcohol Dependence, 143,* 1–10.

Kaskutas, L. A. (1994). What do women get out of self-help?: Their reasons for attending Women for Sobriety and Alcoholics Anonymous. *Journal of Substance Abuse Treatment, 11,* 185–195.

Kaskutas, L. A. (1996). Pathways to self-help among Women for Sobriety. *American Journal of Drug and Alcohol Abuse, 22,* 259–280.

Keating, T. (2009a). *Divine therapy and addiction: Centering prayer and the Twelve Steps.* Brooklyn, NY: Lantern Books.

Keating, T. (2009b). *Intimacy with God: An introduction to centering prayer.* New York: Crossroad.

Kelley, M. L., Bravo, A. J., Braitman, A. L., Lawless, A. K., & Lawrence, H. R. (2016). Behavioral couples treatment for substance use disorder: Secondary effects on the reduction of risk for child abuse. *Journal of Substance Abuse Treatment, 62,* 10–19.

Kellogg, S. H., & Kreek, M. J. (2005). Gradualism, identity, reinforcements, and change. *International Journal of Drug Policy, 16*(6), 369–375.

Kelly, J. F. (2017). Is Alcoholics Anonymous religious, spiritual, neither?: Findings from 25 years of mechanisms of behavior change research. *Addiction, 112*(6), 929–936.

Kelly, J. F., Bergman, B., Hoeppner, B. B., Vilsaint, C., & White, W. L. (2017). Prevalence and pathways of recovery from drug and alcohol problems in the United States population: Implications for practice, research, and policy. *Drug and Alcohol Dependence, 181,* 162–169.

Kelly, J. F., Dow, S. J., & Westerhoff, C. (2010). Does our choice of substance-related terms influence perceptions of treatment need?: An empirical investigation with two commonly used terms. *Journal of Drug Issues, 10*(4), 805–818.

Kelly, J. F., Finney, J. W., & Moos, R. (2005). Substance use disorder patients who are mandated to treatment: Characteristics, treatment process, and 1- and 5-year outcomes. *Journal of Substance Abuse Treatment, 28*(3), 213–223.

Kelly, J. F., & Greene, M. C. (2014). Beyond motivation: Initial validation of the Commitment to Sobriety Scale. *Journal of Substance Abuse Treatment, 46*(2), 257–263.

Kelly, J. F., & Hoeppner, B. (2015). A biaxial formulation of the recovery construct. *Addiction Research and Theory, 23*(1), 5–9.

Kelly, J. F., Hoeppner, B., Stout, R. L., & Pagano, M. (2012). Determining the relative importance of the mechanisms of behavior change within Alcoholics Anonymous: A multiple mediator analysis. *Addiction, 107*(2), 289–299.

Kelly, J. F., & Moos, R. (2003). Dropout from 12-step self-help groups: Prevalence, predictors, and counteracting treatment influences. *Journal of Substance Abuse Treatment, 24,* 241–250.

Kelly, J. F., Stout, R. L., Magill, M., Tonigan, J. S., & Pagano, M. E. (2010). Mechanisms of behavior change in Alcoholics Anonymous: Does Alcoholics Anonymous lead to better alcohol use outcomes by reducing depression symptoms? *Addiction, 105*(4), 626–636.

Kelly, J. F., Stout, R. L., Magill, M., Tonigan, J. S., & Pagano, M. E. (2011). Spirituality in recovery: A lagged mediational analysis of Alcoholics Anonymous' principal theoretical mechanism of behavior change. *Alcoholism: Clinical and Experimental Research, 35*(3), 454–463.

Kelly, J. F., Stout, R., Zywiak, W., & Schneider, R. (2006). A 3-year study of addiction mutual-help group participation following intensive outpatient treatment. *Alcoholism: Clinical and Experimental Research, 30,* 1381–1392.

Kelly, J. F., & Westerhoff, C. M. (2010). Does it matter how we refer to individuals with substance-related conditions?: A randomized study of two commonly used terms. *International Journal of Drug Policy, 21*(3), 202–207.

Keng, S. L., Smoski, M. J., & Robins, C. J. (2011). Effects of mindfulness on psychological health: A review of empirical studies. *Clinical Psychology Review, 31*(6), 1041–1056.

Kenney, S. R., Bailey, G. L., Anderson, B. J., & Stein, M. D. (2017). Heroin refusal self-efficacy and preference for medication-assisted treatment after inpatient detoxification. *Addictive Behaviors, 73,* 124–128.

Keoleian, V., Polcin, D., & Galloway, G. P. (2015). Text messaging for addiction: A review. *Journal of Psychoactive Drugs, 47*(2), 158–176.

Kessler, R. C. (1995). The National Comorbidity Survey: Preliminary results and future directions. *International Journal of Methods in Psychiatric Research, 5*(2), 139–151.

Keurhorst, M., van de Glind, I., Bitarello do Amaral-Sabadini, M., Anderson, P., Kaner, E., Newbury-Birch, D., . . . Laurant, M. (2015). Implementation strategies to enhance management of heavy alcohol consumption in primary health care: A meta-analysis. *Addiction, 110*(12), 1877–1900.

Khanna, S., & Greeson, J. M. (2013). A narrative review of yoga and mindfulness as complementary therapies for addiction. *Complementary Therapies in Medicine, 21*(3), 244–252.

Khantzian, E. J. (2012). Reflections on treating addictive disorders: A psychodynamic perspective. *American Journal on Addictions, 21,* 274–279.

Khantzian, E. J., Halliday, K. S., & McAuliffe, W. E. (1990). *Addiction and the vulnerable self: Modified dynamic group therapy for substance abusers.* New York: Guilford Press.

Kiefer, F., Jimenez-Arriero, M. A., Klein, O., Diehl, A., & Rubio, G. (2007). Cloninger's typology and treatment outcome in alcohol-dependent subjects during pharmacotherapy with naltrexone. *Addiction Biology, 13,* 124–129.

Kiluk, B. D., DeVito, E. E., Buck, M. B., Hunkele, K., Nich, C., & Carroll, K. M. (2017). Effect of computerized cognitive behavioral therapy on acquisition of coping skills among cocaine-dependent individuals enrolled in methadone maintenance. *Journal of Substance Abuse Treatment, 82,* 87–92.

Kiluk, B. D., Nich, C., Babuscio, T., & Carroll, K. M. (2010). Quality versus quantity: Acquisition of coping skills following computerized cognitive-behavioral therapy for substance use disorders. *Addiction, 105*(12), 2120–2127.

Kirby, K. C., Marlowe, D. B., Festinger, D. S., Garvey, K. A., & McMonaca, V. (1999). Community reinforcement training for family and significant others of drug abusers: A unilateral intervention to increase treatment entry of drug users. *Drug and Alcohol Dependence, 56*(1), 85–96.

Kirby, M. W., Braucht, G. N., Brown, E., Krane, S., McCann, M., & Vandemark, N. (1999). Dyadic case management as a strategy for prevention of homelessness among chronically debilitated men and women with alcohol and drug dependence. *Alcoholism Treatment Quarterly, 17*(1–2), 53–72.

Kirkpatrick, J. (1999). *Turnabout: New help for the woman alcoholic.* Fort Lee, NJ: Barricade Books.

Kirschenbaum, H. (2009). *The life and work of Carl Rogers.* Alexandria, VA: American Counseling Association.

Kirschenbaum, H. (2013). *Values clarification: Practical strategies for individual and group settings.* New York: Oxford University Press.

Kishline, A. (1994). *Moderate drinking: The Moderation Management guide for people who want to reduce their drinking.* New York: Crown.

Kishline, A., & Maloy, S. (2007). *Face to face.* New York: Meredith Books.

Kivlighan, D. M., 3rd, Goldberg, S. B., Abbas, M., Pace, B. T., Yulish, N. E., Thomas, J. G., . . . Wampold, B. E. (2015). The enduring effects of psychodynamic treatments vis-a-vis alternative treatments: A multilevel longitudinal meta-analysis. *Clinical Psychology Review, 40,* 1–14.

Klaw, E., Horst, D., & Humphreys, K. (2006). Inquirers, triers, and buyers of an alcohol harm reduction self-help organization. *Addiction Research and Theory, 14*(5), 527–535.

Kogan, L. S. (1957). The short-term case in a family agency: Part II. Results of a study. *Social Casework, 38*, 296–302.

Kohler, S., & Hofmann, A. (2015). Can motivational interviewing in emergency care reduce alcohol consumption in young people?: A systematic review and meta-analysis. *Alcohol and Alcoholism, 50*(2), 107–117.

Koob, G. F. (2005). The neurobiology of addiction: A hedonic Calvinist perspective. In W. R. Miller & K. M. Carroll (Eds.), *Rethinking substance abuse: What the science shows, and what we should do about it* (pp. 25–45). New York: Guilford Press.

Kosok, A. (2006). The Moderation Management programme in 2004: What type of drinker seeks controlled drinking? *International Journal of Drug Policy, 17*, 295–303.

Kosten, T. R., & O'Connor, P. G. (2003). Management of drug and alcohol withdrawal. *New England Journal of Medicine, 2003*(348), 1786–1795.

Kouimtsidis, C., Reynolds, M., Drummond, C., Davis, P., & Tarrier, N. (2007). *Cognitive-behavioral therapy in the treatment of addiction: A treatment planner for clinicians.* Chichester, UK: Wiley.

Koumans, A. J. R., & Muller, J. J. (1967). Use of letters to increase motivation for treatment in alcoholics. *Psychological Reports, 16*, 1152.

Koumans, A. J. R., Muller, J. J., & Miller, C. F. (1967). Use of telephone calls to increase motivation for treatment in alcoholics. *Psychological Reports, 21*, 327–328.

Kovanen, L., Basnet, S., Castren, S., Penkakoski, M., Saarikoski, S. T., Partonen, T., . . . Lahti, T. (2016). A randomised, double-blind, placebo-controlled trial of as-needed naltrexone in the treatment of pathological gambling. *European Addiction Research, 22*, 70–79.

Kranzler, H. R., & Kirk, J. (2001). Efficacy of naltrexone and acamprosate for alcoholism treatment: A meta-analysis. *Alcoholism: Clinical and Experimental Research, 25*(9), 1335–1341.

Krupitsky, E. M., Burakov, A. M., Dunaevsky, I. V., Romanova, T. N., Slavina, T. Y., & Grinenko, A. Y. (2007). Single versus repeated sessions of ketamine-assisted psychotherapy for people with heroin dependence. *Journal of Psychoactive Drugs, 39*(1), 13–19.

Krystal, J. H., Cramer, J. A., Krol, W. F., Kirk, G. F., & Rosenheck, R. A. (2001). Naltrexone in the treatment of alcohol dependence. *New England Journal of Medicine, 345*(24), 1734–1739.

Kuerbis, A. N., Neighbors, C. J., & Morgenstern, J. (2011). Depression's moderation of the effectiveness of intensive case management with substance-dependent women on temporary assistance for needy families: Outpatient substance use treatment utilization and outcomes. *Journal of Studies on Alcohol and Drugs, 72*(2), 297–307.

Kurtz, E. (1991). *Not-God: A history of Alcoholics Anonymous* (expanded ed.). Center City, MN: Hazelden.

Kurtz, E. (1999). Drugs and the spiritual: Bill W. takes LSD. In *The collected Ernie Kurtz* (pp. 39–50). Wheeling, WV: Bishop of Books.

Kurtz, E., & Ketcham, K. (1992). *The spirituality of imperfection: Storytelling and the journey to wholeness.* New York: Bantam Books.

Lai, H. M., Cleary, M., Sitharthan, T., & Hunt, G. E. (2015). Prevalence of comorbid substance use, anxiety and mood disorders in epidemiological surveys, 1990–2014: A systematic review and meta-analysis. *Drug and Alcohol Dependence, 154*, 1–13.

Lambert, M. J., Burlingame, G. M., Umphress, V., Hansen, N. B., Vermeersch, D. A., Clouse, G. C., & Yanchar, S. C. (1996). The reliability and validity of the Outcome Questionnaire. *Clinical Psychology and Psychotherapy, 3,* 249–258.

Lambert, M. J., Whipple, J., Smart, D., Vermeersch, D., Nielsen, S., & Hawkins, E. (2001). The effects of providing therapists with feedback on patient progress during psychotherapy: Are outcomes enhanced? *Psychotherapy Research, 11*(1), 49–68.

Lancaster, T., Stead, L., Silagy, C., & Sowden, A. (2000). Effectiveness of interventions to help people stop smoking: Findings from the Cochrane Library. *British Medical Journal, 321*(7257), 355–358.

Landy, M. S., Davey, C. J., Quintero, D., Pecora, A., & McShane, K. E. (2016). A systematic review on the effectiveness of brief interventions for alcohol misuse among adults in emergency departments. *Journal of Substance Abuse Treatment, 61,* 1–12.

Lapham, S., Forman, R., Alexander, M., Illeperuma, A., & Bohn, M. J. (2009). The effects of extended-release naltrexone on holiday drinking in alcohol-dependent patients. *Journal of Substance Abuse Treatment, 36*(1), 1–6.

Larson, D. B., & Wilson, W. P. (1980). Religious life of alcoholics. *Southern Medical Journal, 73,* 723–727.

Lash, S. J., Timko, C., Curran, G. M., McKay, J. R., & Burden, J. J. (2011). Implementation of evidence-based substance use disorder continuing care interventions. *Psychology of Addictive Behaviors, 25*(2), 238–251.

Laslett, A. M., Dietze, P., Matthews, S. M., & Clemens, S. (2004). *The Victorian alcohol statistics handbook: Vol. 6. Alcohol-related mortality.* Fitzroy, Australia: Turning Point Alcohol and Drug Centre.

Lawrence, E. C., & Sovik-Johnston, A. F. (2010). A competence approach to therapy with families with multiple problems. In D. A. Crenshaw (Ed.), *Reverence in healing: Honoring strengths without trivializing suffering* (pp. 137–149). Lanham, MD: Jason Aronson.

Leake, G. J., & King, A. S. (1977). Effect of counselor expectations on alcoholic recovery. *Alcohol Health and Research World, 1*(3), 16–22.

Lean, G. (1985). *Frank Buchman: A life.* London: Constable & Company.

Lee, C. S., Baird, J., Longabaugh, R., Nirenberg, T. D., Mello, M. J., & Woolard, R. (2010). Change plan as an active ingredient of brief motivational interventions for reducing negative consequences of drinking in hazardous drinking emergency-department patients. *Journal of Studies on Alcohol and Drugs, 71,* 726–733.

Lee, J. D., Friedmann, P. D., Kinlock, T. W., Nunes, E. V., Boney, T. Y., Hoskinson, R. A., Jr., . . . Gourevitch, M. N. (2016). Extended-release naltrexone to prevent opioid relapse in criminal justice offenders. *New England Journal of Medicine, 374*(13), 1232–1242.

Lee, J. D., Grossman, E., DiRocco, D., Truncali, A., Hanley, K., Stevens, D., . . . Gourevitch, M. N. (2010). Extended-release naltrexone for treatment of alcohol dependence in primary care. *Journal of Substance Abuse Treatment, 39*(1), 14–21.

Lee, J. D., Nunes, E. V., Jr., Novo, P., Bachrach, K., Bailey, G. L., Bhatt, S., . . . Hodgkins, C. C. (2018). Comparative effectiveness of extended-release naltrexone versus buprenorphine-naloxone for opioid relapse prevention (X: BOT): A multicentre, open-label, randomised controlled trial. *The Lancet, 391*(10118), 309–318.

Leeies, M., Pagura, J., Sareen, J., & Bolton, J. M. (2010). The use of alcohol and drugs to self-medicate symptoms of posttraumatic stress disorder. *Depression and Anxiety, 27*(8), 731–736.

Leeman, J., Birken, S. A., Powell, B. J., Rohweder, C., & Shea, C. M. (2017). Beyond "implementation strategies": Classifying the full range of strategies used in implementation science and practice. *Implementation Science, 12*(1), 125.

Lehman, W. E., Simpson, D. D., Knight, D. K., & Flynn, P. M. (2011). Integration of treatment innovation planning and implementation: Strategic process models and organizational challenges. *Psychology of Addictive Behaviors, 25*(2), 252–261.

Lembke, A. (2012). Time to abandon the self-medication hypothesis in patients with psychiatric disorders. *American Journal of Drug and Alcohol Abuse, 38*(6), 524–529.

Lembke, A., & Humphreys, K. (2012). Moderation Management: A mutual-help organization for problem drinkers who are not alcohol-dependent. *Journal of Groups in Addiction and Recovery, 7*(2–4), 130–141.

Levy, M. S. (2007). *Take control of your drinking . . . and you may not need to quit.* Baltimore: Johns Hopkins University Press.

Lewinsohn, P. M., Muñoz, R. F., Youngren, M. A., & Zeiss, A. M. (1992). *Control your depression* (rev. ed.). New York: Fireside.

Lhuintre, J., Moore, N., Tran, G., Steru, L., Langrenon, S., Daoust, S., . . . Boismare, F. (1990). Acamprosate appears to decrease alcohol intake in weaned alcoholics. *Alcohol and Alcoholism, 25*(6), 613–622.

Li, M., Chen, K., & Mo, Z. (2002). Use of qigong therapy in the detoxification of heroin addicts. *Alternative Therapies, 8*(1), 50–54, 56–59.

Liddle, H. A. (2016). Multidimensional family therapy: Evidence base for transdiagnostic treatment outcomes, change mechanisms, and implementation in community settings. *Family Process, 55*, 558–576.

Liddle, H. A., Dakof, G. A., Rowe, C. L., Henderson, C., Greenbaum, P., Wang, W., & Alberga, L. (2018). Multidimensional family therapy as a community-based alternative to residential treatment for adolescents with substance use and co-occurring mental health disorders. *Journal of Substance Abuse Treatment, 90*, 47–56.

Liddle, H. A., Dakof, G. A., Turner, R. M., Henderson, C. E., & Greenbaum, P. E. (2008). Treating adolescent drug abuse: A randomized trial comparing multidimensional family therapy and cognitive behavior therapy. *Addiction, 103*(10), 1660–1670.

Liddle, H. A., Rowe, C. L., Dakof, G. A., Henderson, C. E., & Greenbaum, P. E. (2009). Multidimensional family therapy for young adolescent substance abuse: Twelve-month outcomes of a randomized controlled trial. *Journal of Consulting and Clinical Psychology, 77*(1), 12–25.

Lieberman, M. A., Yalom, I. D., & Miles, M. D. (1973). *Encounter groups: First facts.* New York: Basic Books.

Liese, B. S., & Reis, D. J. (2016). Failing to diagnose and failing to treat an addicted client: Two potentially life-threatening clinical errors. *Psychotherapy, 53*(3), 342–346.

Lindson-Hawley, N., Thompson, T. P., & Begh, R. (2015). Motivational interviewing for smoking cessation. *Cochrane Database of Systematic Reviews, 3*, CD006936.

Lisansky, E. S. G. (1999). Women. In B. McCrady & E. E. Epstein (Eds.), *Addictions: A comprehensive guidebook* (pp. 527–541). London: Oxford University Press.

Litt, M. D., Kadden, R. M., Cooney, N. L., & Kabela, E. (2003). Coping skills and treatment outcomes in cognitive-behavioral and interactional group therapy for alcoholism. *Journal of Consulting and Clinical Psychology, 71*(1), 118–128.

Litten, R. Z., Ryan, M. L., Fertig, J. B., Falk, D. E., Johnson, B., Dunn, K. E., . . . Sarid-Segal, O. (2013). A double-blind, placebo-controlled trial assessing the efficacy of varenicline tartrate for alcohol dependence. *Journal of Addiction Medicine, 7*(4), 277–286.

Liu, S., Huang, J. L., & Wang, M. (2014). Effectiveness of job search interventions: A meta-analytic review. *Psychological Bulletin, 140*(4), 1009–1041.

Logan, D., & Marlatt, G. A. (2010). Harm reduction therapy: A practice-friendly review of research. *Journal of Clinical Psychology, 66,* 201–214.

Logan, F. A. (1993). Animal learning and motivation and addictive drugs. *Psychological Reports, 73,* 291–306.

Longabaugh, R., Beattie, M., Noel, N., Stout, R. L., & Malloy, P. (1993). The effect of social investment on treatment outcome. *Journal of Studies on Alcohol, 54,* 465–478.

Longabaugh, R., & Wirtz, P. W. (Eds.). (2001). *Project MATCH hypotheses: Results and causal chain analyses* (Project MATCH Monograph Series, Vol. 8). Bethesda, MD: National Institute on Alcohol Abuse and Alcoholism.

Longabaugh, R., Wirtz, P. W., Zweben, A., & Stout, R. L. (1998). Network support for drinking, Alcohol Anonymous, and long-term matching effects. *Addiction, 93,* 1313–1333.

Longabaugh, R., Wirtz, P. W., Zweben, A., & Stout, R. L. (2001). Network support for drinking. In R. Longabaugh & P. W. Wirtz (Eds.), *Project MATCH hypotheses: Results and casual chain analysis* (pp. 260–275). Bethesda, MD: National Institute on Alcohol Abuse and Alcoholism.

Longabaugh, R., Wirtz, P. W., Zywiak, W. H., & O'Malley, S. S. (2010). Network support as a prognostic indicator of drinking outcomes: The COMBINE study. *Journal of Studies on Alcohol and Drugs, 71*(6), 837–846.

Longabaugh, R., Zweben, A., LoCastro, J. S., & Miller, W. R. (2005). Origins, issues and options in the development of the combined behavioral intervention. *Journal of Studies on Alcohol, 66*(4), S179–S187.

Lozano, B. E., Stephens, R. S., & Roffman, R. A. (2006). Abstinence and moderate use goals in the treatment of marijuana dependence. *Addiction, 101,* 1589–1597.

Luborsky, L., McLellan, A. T., Woody, G. E., O'Brien, C. P., & Auerbach, A. (1985). Therapist success and its determinants. *Archives of General Psychiatry, 42,* 602–611.

Ludwig, A. S., & Peters, R. H. (2014). Medication-assisted treatment for opioid use disorders in correctional settings: An ethics review. *International Jurnal on Drug Policy, 25*(6), 1041–1046.

Lundahl, B. W., Kunz, C., Brownell, C., Tollefson, D., & Burke, B. L. (2010). A meta-analysis of motivational interviewing: Twenty-five years of empirical studies. *Research on Social Work Practice, 20*(2), 137–160.

Lundgren, L., Amodeo, M., Chassler, D., Krull, I., & Sullivan, L. (2013). Organizational readiness for change in community-based addiction treatment programs and adherence in implementing evidence-based practices: A national study. *Journal of Substance Abuse Treatment, 45*(5), 457–465.

MacDonough, T. S. (1976). Evaluation of the effectiveness of intensive confrontation in changing the behavior of alcohol and drug abusers. *Behavior Therapy, 7,* 408–409.

Maddock, J. E., Laforge, R., & Rossi, J. S. (2000). Short form of Situational Temptation Scale for heavy, episodic drinking. *Journal of Substance Abuse, 11*(3), 281–288.

Madras, B. K., Compton, W. M., Avula, D., Stegbauer, T., Stein, J. B., & Clark, H. W. (2009). Screening, Brief Interventions, Referral to Treatment (SBIRT) for illicit drug and alcohol use at multiple healthcare sites: Comparison at intake and 6 months later. *Drug and Alcohol Dependence, 99*(1–3), 280–295.

Madsen, W. (1974). *The American alcoholic: The nature–nurture controversy in alcoholic research and therapy.* Springfield, IL: Charles C Thomas.

Madson, M. B., Loignon, A. C., & Lane, C. (2009). Training in motivational interviewing: A systematic review. *Journal of Substance Abuse Treatment, 36*(1), 101–109.

Magill, M., Barnett, N. P., Apodaca, T. R., Rohsenow, D. J., & Monti, P. M. (2009). The role of marijuana use in brief motivational intervention with young adult drinkers treated in an emergency department. *Journal of Studies on Alcohol and Drugs, 70*(3), 409–413.

Magill, M., Colby, S. M., Orchowski, L., Murphy, J. G., Hoadley, A., Brazil, L. A., & Barnett, N. P. (2017). How does brief motivational intervention change heavy drinking and harm among underage young adult drinkers? *Journal of Consulting and Clinical Psychology, 85*(5), 447–458.

Magill, M., Mastroleo, N. R., Apodaca, T. R., Barnett, N. P., Colby, S. M., & Monti, P. M. (2010). Motivational interviewing with significant other participation: Assessing therapeutic alliance and patient satisfaction and engagement. *Journal of Substance Abuse Treatment, 39*(4), 391–398.

Magura, S. (2008). Effectiveness of dual focus mutual aid for co-occurring substance use and mental health disorders: A review and synthesis of the "double trouble" in recovery evaluation. *Substance Use and Misuse, 43*(12–13), 1904–1926.

Magura, S., Cleland, C. M., & Tonigan, J. S. (2013). Evaluating Alcoholics Anonymous's effect on drinking in Project MATCH using cross-lagged regression panel analysis. *Journal of Studies on Alcohol and Drugs, 74*(3), 378–385.

Magura, S., Rosenblum, A., Villano, C. L., Vogel, H. S., Fong, C., & Betzler, T. (2008). Dual-focus mutual aid for co-occurring disorders: A quasi-experimental outcome evaluation study. *American Journal of Drug and Alcohol Abuse, 34*(1), 61–74.

Magura, S., Staines, G., Kosanke, N., Rosenblum, A., Foote, J., DeLuca, A., & Bali, P. (2003). Predictive validity of the ASAM patient placement criteria for naturalistically matched vs. mismatched alcoholism patients. *American Journal on Addictions, 12,* 386–397.

Maisel, N. C., Blodgett, J. C., Wilbourne, P. L., Humphreys, K., & Finney, J. W. (2013). Meta-analysis of naltrexone and acamprosate for treating alcohol use disorders: When are these medications most helpful? *Addiction, 108*(2), 275–293.

Maisto, S. A., Krenek, M., Chung, T., Martin, C. S., Clark, D., & Cornelius, J. (2011). Comparison of the concurrent and predictive validity of three measures of readiness to change marijuana use in a clinical sample of adolescents. *Journal of Studies on Alcohol and Drugs, 72*(4), 592–601.

Maisto, S. A., & McKay, J. R. (1995). Diagnosis. In J. P. Allen & M. Columbus (Eds.), *Assessing alcohol problems: A guide for clinicians and researchers* (pp. 41–54). Rockville, MD: National Institute on Alcohol Abuse and Alcoholism.

Maisto, S. A., O'Farrell, T. J., Connors, G. J., & McKay, J. R. (1988). Alcoholics' attributions of factors affecting their relapse to drinking and reasons for terminating relapse episodes. *Addictive Behaviors, 13*(1), 79–82.

Maisto, S. A., Witkiewitz, K., Moskal, D., & Wilson, A. D. (2016). Is the construct of relapse heuristic, and does tt advance alcohol use disorder clinical practice? *Journal of Studies on Alcohol and Drugs, 77*(6), 849–858.

Majer, J. M., Jason, L. A., Ferrari, J. R., & Miller, S. A. (2011). A longitudinal analysis of categorical twelve-step involvement among a U.S. national sample of recovering substance abusers in residential treatment. *Journal of Substance Abuse Treatment, 41*(1), 37–44.

Mann, M. (1950). *Primer on alcoholism.* New York: Rinehart.

Mannelli, P., Peindl, K., Patkar, A. A., Wu, L. T., Tharwani, H. M., & Gorelick, D. A. (2011). Problem drinking and low-dose naltrexone-assisted opioid detoxification. *Journal of Studies on Alcohol and Drugs, 72*(3), 507–513.

Manohar, V. (1973). Training volunteers as alcoholism treatment counselors. *Quarterly Journal of Studies on Alcohol, 34,* 869–877.

Manuel, J. K., Austin, J. L., Miller, W. R., McCrady, B. S., Tonigan, J. S., Meyers, R. J., . . . Bogenschutz, M. P. (2012). Community reinforcement and family training: A pilot comparison of group and self-directed delivery. *Journal of Substance Abuse Treatment, 43*(1), 129–136.

Manuel, J. K., Hagedorn, H. J., & Finney, J. W. (2011). Implementing evidence-based psychosocial treatment in specialty substance use disorder care. *Psychology of Addictive Behaviors, 25*(2), 225–237.

Maraz, A., Griffiths, M. D., & Demetrovics, Z. (2016). The prevalence of compulsive buying: A meta-analysis. *Addiction, 111*(3), 408–419.

Maremmani, I., Balestri, C., Sbrana, A., & Tagliamonte, A. (2003). Substance (ab)use during methadone and naltrexone treatment: Interest of adequate methadone dosage. *Journal of Maintenance in the Addictions, 2*(1–2), 19–36.

Margolis, R. D., & Zweben, J. E. (1998). *Treating patients with alcohol and other drug problems: An integrated approach.* Washington, DC: American Psychological Association.

Markland, D., Ryan, R. M., Tobin, V., & Rollnick, S. (2005). Motivational interviewing and self-determination theory. *Journal of Social and Clinical Psychology, 24,* 811–831.

Marlatt, G. A. (1983). The controlled drinking controversy: A commentary. *American Psychologist, 38,* 1097–1110.

Marlatt, G. A. (1996). Taxonomy of high-risk situations for alcohol relapse: Evolution and development of a cognitive-behavioral model. *Addiction, 91*(Suppl.), S37–S49.

Marlatt, G. A., & Donovan, D. M. (Eds.). (2005). *Relapse prevention: Maintenance strategies in the treatment of addictive behaviors* (2nd ed.). New York: Guilford Press.

Marlatt, G. A., Witkiewitz, K., & Donovan, D. M. (2005). Relapse prevention for alcohol and drug problems. In G. A. Marlatt & D. M. Donovan (Eds.), *Relapse prevention: Maintenance strategies in the treatment of addictive behaviors* (2nd ed., pp. 1–44). New York: Guilford Press.

Marques, A. C. P. R., & Formigoni, M. L. O. S. (2001). Comparison of individual and group cognitive-behavioral therapy for alcohol and/or drug-dependent patients. *Addiction, 96*(6), 835–846.

Marsch, L. A., & Dallery, J. (2012). Advances in the psychosocial treatment of addiction: The role of technology in the delivery of evidence-based psychosocial treatment. *Psychiatric Clinics of North America, 35*(2), 481–493.

Marshall, E. J. (2015). Griffith Edwards' work on the life course of alcohol dependence. *Addiction, 110*(Suppl. 2), 12–15.

Martin, C. S., Chung, T., & Langenbucher, J. W. (2008). How should we revise diagnostic criteria for substance use disorders in the DSM-V? *Journal of Abnormal Psychology, 117*(3), 561–575.

Martin, G. W. (1995). The core-shell model: An institutional experiment. *Contemporary Drug Problems, 22,* 13–26.

Martin, G., Copeland, J., & Swift, W. (2005). The adolescent cannabis check-up: Feasibility of a brief intervention for young cannabis users. *Journal of Substance Abuse Treatment, 29,* 207–213.

Martin, J. (1980). Too few counselors effective. *U.S. Journal of Drug and Alcohol Dependence, 3*(12), 9.

Martino, D., Ball, S. A., Nich, C., Frankforter, T. C., & Carroll, K. M. (2009). Informal discussions in substance abuse treatment sessions. *Journal of Substance Abuse Treatment, 36,* 366–375.

Martins, S. S., Fenton, M. C., Keyes, K. M., Blanco, C., Zhu, H., & Storr, C. L. (2012). Mood and anxiety disorders and their association with non-medical prescription opioid use and prescription opioid-use disorder: Longitudinal evidence from the National Epidemiologic Study on Alcohol and Related Conditions. *Psychological Medicine, 42*(6), 1261–1272.

Maslow, A. H. (1943). A theory of human motivation. *Psychological Review, 50,* 370–396.

Maslow, A. H. (1970). *Motivation and personality* (2nd ed.). New York: Harper & Row.

Maslow, A. H. (1971). *The farther reaches of human nature.* New York: Viking Compass.

Mason, B., & Goodman, A. (1997). *Brief intervention and medication compliance procedures: Therapist's manual.* New York: Lipha Pharmaceuticals.

Mason, B. J., Goodman, A. M., Chabac, S., & Lehert, P. (2006). Effect of oral acamprosate on abstinence in patients with alcohol dependence in a double-blind, placebo-controlled trial: The role of patient motivation. *Journal of Psychiatric Research, 40*(5), 383–393.

Mason, B. J., & Ownby, R. L. (2000). Acamprosate for the treatment of alcohol dependence: A review of double-blind, placebo-controlled trials. *CNS Spectrums, 5*(2), 58–69.

Mason, M. J., Sabo, R., & Zaharakis, N. M. (2017). Peer network counseling as brief treatment for urban adolescent heavy cannabis users. *Journal of Studies on Alcohol and Drugs, 78*(1), 152–157.

McCambridge, J., & Cunningham, J. A. (2014). The early history of ideas on brief interventions for alcohol. *Addiction, 109*(4), 538–546.

McCambridge, J., & Rollnick, S. (2014). Should brief interventions in primary care address alcohol problems more strongly? *Addiction, 109*(7), 1054–1058.

McCollister, K. E., French, M. T., Freitas, D. M., Dennis, M. L., Scott, C. K., & Funk, R. R. (2013). Cost-effectiveness analysis of Recovery Management Checkups (RMC) for adults with chronic substance use disorders: Evidence from a 4-year randomized trial. *Addiction, 108*(12), 2166–2174.

McCollister, K. E., Scott, C. K., Dennis, M. L., Freitas, D. M., French, M. T., & Funk, R. R. (2014). Economic costs of a postrelease intervention for incarcerated female substance abusers: Recovery Management Checkups for women offenders (RMC-WO). *Journal of Offender Rehabilitation, 53*(7), 543–561.

McConnell, P. A., & Froeliger, B. (2015). Mindfulness, mechanisms and meaning: Perspectives from the cognitive neuroscience of addiction. *Psychological Inquiry, 26*(4), 349–357.

McCormack, R. P. (2017). Commentary on Blow et al. (2017): Leveraging technology may boost the effectiveness and adoption of interventions for drug use in emergency departments. *Addiction, 112*(8), 1406–1407.

McCrady, B. S. (2006). Family and other close relationships. In W. R. Miller & K. M. Carroll (Eds.), *Rethinking substance abuse: What the science shows, and what we should do about it* (pp. 166–181). New York: Guilford Press.

McCrady, B. S., & Epstein, E. E. (1996). Theoretical bases of family approaches to substance abuse treatment. In F. Rotgers, D. S. Keller, & J. Morgenstern (Eds.), *Treating substance abuse: Theory and technique* (pp. 117–142). New York: Guilford Press.

McCrady, B. S., & Epstein, E. E. (2008). *Overcoming alcohol problems: A couples-focused program—Therapist guide.* New York: Oxford University Press.

McCrady, B. S., & Epstein, E. E. (2009). *Overcoming alcohol problems: Workbook for couples.* New York: Oxford University Press.

McCrady, B. S., Epstein, E. E., Cook, S., Jensen, N., & Hildebrandt, T. (2009). A randomized trial of individual and couple behavioral alcohol treatment for women. *Journal of Consulting and Clinical Psychology, 77*(2), 243–256.

McCrady, B. S., Epstein, E. E., Hallgren, K. A., Cook, S., & Jensen, N. K. (2016). Women with alcohol dependence: A randomized trial of couple versus individual plus couple therapy. *Psychology of Addictive, 30*(3), 287–299.

McCrady, B. S., Epstein, E. E., & Kahler, C. W. (2004). Alcoholics Anonymous and relapse prevention as maintenance strategies after conjoint behavioral alcohol treatment for men: 18-month outcomes. *Journal of Consulting and Clinical Psychology, 72,* 870–878.

McDonald, H. P., Garg, A. X., & Haynes, R. B. (2002). Interventions to enhance patient adherence to medication prescriptions. *JAMA, 288*(22), 2868–2879.

McDonell, M. G., Kerbrat, A. H., Comtois, K. A., Russo, J., Lowe, J. M., & Ries, R. K. (2012). Validation of the co-occurring disorder quadrant model. *Journal of Psychoactive Drugs, 44*(3), 266–273.

McDonell, M. G., Leickly, E., McPherson, S., Skalisky, J., Srebnik, D., Angelo, F., . . . Ries, R. K. (2017). A randomized controlled trial of ethyl glucuronide-based contingency management for outpatients with co-occurring alcohol use disorders and serious mental illness. *American Journal of Psychiatry, 174*(4), 370–377.

McGarvey, E. L., Leon-Verdin, M., Bloomfield, K., Wood, S., Winters, E., & Smith, J. (2014). Effectiveness of A-CRA/ACC in treating adolescents with cannabis-use disorders. *Community Mental Health Journal, 50*(2), 150–157.

McGinty, E. E., Goldman, H. H., Pescosolido, B., & Barry, C. L. (2015). Portraying mental illness and drug addiction as treatable health conditions: Effects of a randomized experiment on stigma and discrimination. *Social Science and Medicine, 126,* 73–85.

McGovern, M. P., Clark, R. E., & Samnaliev, M. (2007). Co-occurring psychiatric and substance use disorders: A multistate feasibility study of the quadrant model. *Psychiatric Services, 58*(7), 949–954.

McGovern, M. P., Lambert-Harris, C., Xie, H., Meier, A., McLeman, B., & Saunders, E. (2015). A randomized controlled trial of treatments for co-occurring substance use disorders and post-traumatic stress disorder. *Addiction, 110*(7), 1194–1204.

McHugh, F., Lindsay, G. M., Hanlon, P., Hutton, I., Brown, M. R., Morrison, C., & Wheatley, D. J. (2001). Nurse led shared care for patients on the waiting list for coronary artery bypass surgery: A randomised controlled trial. *Heart, 86*(3), 317–323.

McKay, J. R. (2005). Is there a case for extended interventions for alcohol and drug use disorders? *Addiction, 100*(11), 1594–1610.

McKay, J. R., Alterman, A. I., McLellan, A. T., & Snider, E. C. (1994). Treatment goals, continuity of care, and outcome in a day hospital substance abuse rehabilitation program. *American Journal of Psychiatry, 151,* 254–259.

McKay, J. R., Cacciola, J. S., McLellan, A. T., Alterman, A. I., & Wirtz, P. W. (1997). An initial evaluation of the psychosocial dimensions of the American Society of

Addiction Medicine criteria for inpatient versus outpatient substance abuse rehabilitation. *Journal of Studies on Alcohol, 58,* 239–252.

McKay, J. R., McLellan, A. T., & Alterman, A. I. (1992). An evaluation of the Cleveland criteria for inpatient substance abuse treatment. *American Journal of Psychiatry, 149,* 1212–1218.

McKay, J. R., Van Horn, D., Oslin, D. W., Ivey, M., Drapkin, M. L., Coviello, D. M., . . . Lynch, K. G. (2011). Extended telephone-based continuing care for alcohol dependence: 24-month outcomes and subgroup analyses. *Addiction, 106*(10), 1760–1769.

McKay, J. R., Van Horn, D. H., Oslin, D. W., Lynch, K. G., Ivey, M., Ward, K., . . . Coviello, D. M. (2010). A randomized trial of extended telephone-based continuing care for alcohol dependence: Within-treatment substance use outcomes. *Journal of Consulting and Clinical Psychology, 78*(6), 912–923.

McKeganey, N., Russell, C., & Cockayne, L. (2013). Medically assisted recovery from opiate dependence within the context of the UK drug strategy: Methadone and suboxone (buprenorphine–naloxone) patients compared. *Journal of Substance Abuse Treatment, 44*(1), 97–102.

McKellar, J., Stewart, E., & Humphreys, K. (2003). Alcoholics Anonymous involvement and positive alcohol-related outcomes: Cause, consequence, or just a correlate?: A prospective 2-year study of 2,319 alcohol-dependent men. *Journal of Consulting and Clinical Psychology, 71,* 302–308.

McKetin, R., Hickey, K., Devlin, K., & Lawrence, K. (2010). The risk of psychotic symptoms associated with recreational methamphetamine use. *Drug and Alcohol Review, 29,* 358–363.

McLellan, A. T. (2006). What we need is a system: Creating a responsive and effective substance abuse treatment system. In W. R. Miller & K. M. Carroll (Eds.), *Rethinking substance abuse: What the science shows, and what we should do about it* (pp. 275–292). New York: Guilford Press.

McLellan, A. T., Grissom, G. R., Zanis, D., Randall, M., Brill, P., & O'Brien, C. P. (1997). Problem–service matching in addiction treatment. *Archives of General Psychiatry, 54*(8), 730–735.

McLellan, A. T., Hagan, T. A., Levine, M., Gould, F., Meyers, K., Bencivengo, M., & Durell, J. (1998). Supplemental social services improve outcomes in public addiction treatment. *Addiction, 93*(10), 1489–1499.

McLellan, A. T., Hagan, T. A., Levine, M., Meyers, K., Gould, F., Bencivengo, M., . . . Jaffe, J. (1999). Does clinical case management improve outpatient addiction treatment? *Drug and Alcohol Dependence, 55,* 91–103.

McLellan, A. T., Kushner, H., Metzger, D., Peters, R., Smith, I., Grissom, G., . . . Argeriou, M. (1992). The fifth edition of the Addiction Severity Index. *Journal of Substance Abuse Treatment, 9*(3), 199–213.

McLellan, A. T., Lewis, D. C., O'Brien, C. P., & Kleber, H. D. (2000). Drug dependence, a chronic medical illness: Implications for treatment, insurance, and outcomes evaluation. *JAMA, 284,* 1689–1695.

McLellan, A. T., McKay, J. R., Forman, R., Cacciola, J., & Kemp, J. (2010). Reconsidering the evaluation of addiction treatment: From retrospective follow-up to concurrent recovery monitoring. *Addiction, 100,* 447–458.

McLellan, A. T., Parikh, G., Bragg, A., Cacciola, J. S., Fureman, B., & Incmikofki, R. (1990). *Addiction Severity Index administration manual.* Philadelphia: VA Center for Studies of Addiction.

McLellan, A. T., Woody, G. E., Luborsky, L., & Goehl, L. (1988). Is the counselor an "active ingredient" in substance abuse rehabilitation?: An examination of treatment success among four counselors. *Journal of Nervous and Mental Disease, 176,* 423–430.

McNeely, J., Strauss, S. M., Rotrosen, J., Ramautar, A., & Gourevitch, M. N. (2016). Validation of an audio computer-assisted self-interview (ACASI) version of the alcohol, smoking and substance involvement screening test (ASSIST) in primary care patients. *Addiction, 111*(2), 233–244.

McNeely, J., Strauss, S. M., Wright, S., Rotrosen, J., Khan, R., Lee, J. D., & Gourevitch, M. N. (2014). Test–retest reliability of a self-administered Alcohol, Smoking and Substance Involvement Screening Test (ASSIST) in primary care patients. *Journal of Substance Abuse Treatment, 47*(1), 93–101.

McPherson, C., Boyne, H., & Willis, R. (2017). The role of family in residential treatment patient retention. *International Journal of Mental Health and Addiction, 15*(4), 933–941.

Mee-Lee, D., Shulman, G. D., Fishman, M. J., Gastfriend, D. R., & Miller, M. M. (2013). *The ASAM criteria: Treatment criteria for addictive, substance-related, and co-occurring conditions* (3rd ed.). Carson City, NV: Change Companies.

Mericle, A. A., Ta Park, V. M., Holck, P., & Arria, A. M. (2012). Prevalence, patterns, and correlates of co-occurring substance use and mental disorders in the United States: Variations by race/ethnicity. *Comprehensive Psychiatry, 53*(6), 657–665.

Merkx, M. J. M., Schippers, G. M., Koeter, M. W. J., De Wildt, A. J. M., Vedel, E., Goudriaan, A. E., & Van den Brink, W. (2014). Treatment outcome of alcohol use disorder outpatients with or without medically assisted detoxification. *Journal of Studies on Alcohol and Drugs, 7*(5), 993–998.

Merrall, E. L. C., Kariminia, A., Binswanger, I. A., Hobbs, M. S., Farrell, M., Marsden, J., . . . Bird, S. M. (2010). Meta-analysis of drug-related deaths soon after release from prison. *Addiction, 105*(9), 1545–1554.

Mewton, L., Slade, T., McBride, O., Grove, R., & Teesson, M. (2011). An evaluation of the proposed DSM-5 alcohol use disorder criteria using Australian national data. *Addiction, 106*(5), 941–950.

Meyers, R. J., & Miller, W. R. (Eds.). (2001). *A community reinforcement approach to addiction treatment.* Cambridge, UK: Cambridge University Press.

Meyers, R. J., Miller, W. R., Hill, D. E., & Tonigan, J. S. (1999). Community reinforcement and family training (CRAFT): Engaging unmotivated drug users in treatment. *Journal of Substance Abuse, 10*(3), 1–18.

Meyers, R. J., Miller, W. R., Smith, J. E., & Tonigan, J. S. (2002). A randomized trial of two methods for engaging treatment-refusing drug users through concerned significant others. *Journal of Consulting and Clinical Psychology, 70,* 1182–1185.

Meyers, R. J., & Smith, J. E. (1995). *Clinical guide to alcohol treatment: The community reinforcement approach.* New York: Guilford Press.

Meyers, R. J., & Wolfe, B. L. (2004). *Get your loved one sober: Alternatives to nagging, pleading and threatening.* Center City, MN: Hazelden Publishing and Educational Services.

Milam, J. R., & Ketcham, K. (1984). *Under the influence: A guide to the myths and realities of alcoholism.* New York: Bantam.

Miller, N. S., & Kipnis, S. S. (Eds.). (2006). *Detoxification and substance abuse treatment* (Treatment Improvement Protocol 45). Rockville, MD: Center for Substance Abuse Treatment.

Miller, S. D., Bargmann, S., Chow, D., Seidel, J., & Maeschalck, C. (2016). Feedback Informed Treatment (FIT): Improving the outcome of psychotherapy one person at a time. In W. O'Donohue & A. Maragakis (Eds.), *Quality improvement in behavioral health* (pp. 247–262). New York: Springer.

Miller, S. D., Duncan, B. L., Brown, J., Sorrell, R., & Chalk, M. B. (2006). Using formal client feedback to improve retention and outcome: Making ongoing real-time assessment feasible. *Journal of Brief Therapy, 5*(1), 5–22.

Miller, S. D., Duncan, B. L., Brown, J., Sparks, J., & Claud, D. (2003). The Outcome Rating Scale: A preliminary study of the reliability, validity, and feasibility of a brief visual analog measure. *Journal of Brief Therapy, 2*(2), 91–100.

Miller, S. D., Duncan, B. L., Sorrell, R., & Brown, G. S. (2005). The Partners for Change outcome management system. *Journal of Clinical Psychology, 61*(2), 199–208.

Miller, W. R. (1976). Alcoholism scales and objective assessment methods: A review. *Psychological Bulletin, 83*(4), 649–674.

Miller, W. R. (1978). Behavioral treatment of problem drinkers: A comparative outcome study of three controlled drinking therapies. *Journal of Consulting and Clinical Psychology, 46,* 74–86.

Miller, W. R. (1980). Maintenance of therapeutic change: A usable evaluation design. *Professional Psychology, 11,* 660–663.

Miller, W. R. (1983). Motivational interviewing with problem drinkers. *Behavioural Psychotherapy, 11,* 147–172.

Miller, W. R. (1985). Motivation for treatment: A review with special emphasis on alcoholism. *Psychological Bulletin, 98,* 84–107.

Miller, W. R. (1986). Haunted by the *zeitgeist*: Reflections on contrasting treatment goals and concepts of alcoholism in Europe and the United States. *Annals of the New York Academy of Sciences, 472,* 110–129.

Miller, W. R. (1996a). *Form 90: A structured assessment interview for drinking and related behaviors* (Vol. 5). Bethesda, MD: National Institute on Alcohol Abuse and Alcoholism.

Miller, W. R. (1996b). What is a relapse?: Fifty ways to leave the wagon. *Addiction, 91*(Suppl.), S15–S27.

Miller, W. R. (1998). Researching the spiritual dimensions of alcohol and other drug problems. *Addiction, 93,* 979–990.

Miller, W. R. (1999). Diversity training in spiritual and religious issues. In W. R. Miller (Ed.), *Integrating spirituality into treatment: Resources for practitioners* (pp. 253–263). Washington, DC: American Psychological Association.

Miller, W. R. (2000). Rediscovering fire: Small interventions, large effects. *Psychology of Addictive Behaviors, 14,* 6–18.

Miller, W. R. (2003). Spirituality, treatment and recovery. In M. Galanter (Ed.), *Recent developments in alcoholism* (pp. 391–404). New York: Plenum Press.

Miller, W. R. (Ed.). (2004). *Combined Behavioral Intervention manual: A clinical research guide for therapists treating people with alcohol abuse and dependence* (COMBINE Monograph Series, Vol. 1). Bethesda, MD: National Institute on Alcohol Abuse and Alcoholism.

Miller, W. R. (2007). Bring addiction treatment out of the closet. *Addiction, 102,* 863.

Miller, W. R. (2008). The ethics of harm reduction. In C. M. A. Geppert & L. W. Roberts (Eds.), *The book of ethics: Expert guidance for professionals who treat addiction* (pp. 41–53). Center City, MN: Hazelden.

Miller, W. R. (2014). Interactive journaling as a clinical tool. *Journal of Mental Health Counseling, 36*(1), 31–42.

Miller, W. R. (2015a). No more waiting lists! *Substance Use and Misuse, 50*(8–9), 1169–1170.

Miller, W. R. (2015b). Retire the concept of "relapse." *Substance Use and Misuse, 50*(8–9), 976–977.

Miller, W. R. (2017). *Lovingkindness: Realizing and practicing your true self.* Eugene, OR: Wipf & Stock.

Miller, W. R. (2018). *Listening well: The art of empathic understanding.* Eugene, OR: Wipf & Stock.

Miller, W. R., & Baca, L. M. (1983). Two-year follow-up of bibliotherapy and therapist-directed controlled drinking training for problem drinkers. *Behavior Therapy, 14,* 441–448.

Miller, W. R., Benefield, R. G., & Tonigan, J. S. (1993). Enhancing motivation for change in problem drinking: A controlled comparison of two therapist styles. *Journal of Consulting and Clinical Psychology, 61,* 455–461.

Miller, W. R., & Brown, J. M. (1991). Self-regulation as a conceptual basis for the prevention and treatment of addictive behaviours. In N. Heather, W. R. Miller, & J. Greeley (Eds.), *Self-control and the addictive behaviours* (pp. 3–79). Sydney: Maxwell Macmillan Publishing Australia.

Miller, W. R., & Brown, S. A. (1997). Why psychologists should treat alcohol and drug problems. *American Psychologist, 52,* 1269–1272.

Miller, W. R., & C'de Baca, J. (2001). *Quantum change: When epiphanies and sudden insights transform ordinary lives.* New York: Guilford Press.

Miller, W. R., & Carroll, K. M. (Eds.). (2006). *Rethinking substance abuse: What the science shows, and what we should do about it.* New York: Guilford Press.

Miller, W. R., & Cooney, N. L. (1994). Designing studies to investigate client/treatment matching. *Journal of Studies on Alcohol, Supplement No. 12,* 38–45.

Miller, W. R., Forcehimes, A. A., O'Leary, M., & LaNoue, M. (2008). Spiritual direction in addiction treatment: Two clinical trials. *Journal of Substance Abuse Treatment, 35,* 434–442.

Miller, W. R., Forcehimes, A. A., & Zweben, A. (2011). *Treating addiction: A guide for professionals.* New York: Guilford Press.

Miller, W. R., Gribskov, C. J., & Mortell, R. L. (1981). Effectiveness of a self-control manual for problem drinkers with and without therapist contact. *International Journal of the Addictions, 16,* 1247–1254.

Miller, W. R., Hedrick, K. E., & Taylor, C. A. (1983). Addictive behaviors and life problems before and after behavioral treatment of problem drinkers. *Addictive Behaviors, 8*(4), 403–412.

Miller, W. R., Hendrickson, S. M. L., Venner, K., Bisono, A., Daugherty, M., & Yahne, C. E. (2008). Cross-cultural training in motivational interviewing. *Journal of Teaching in the Addictions, 7,* 4–15.

Miller, W. R., & Hester, R. K. (1986). Inpatient alcoholism treatment: Who benefits? *American Psychologist, 41,* 794–805.

Miller, W. R., & Johnson, W. R. (2008). A natural language screening measure for motivation to change. *Addictive Behaviors, 33*(9), 1177–1182.

Miller, W. R., & Kurtz, E. (1994). Models of alcoholism used in treatment: Contrasting A.A. and other perspectives with which it is often confused. *Journal of Studies on Alcohol, 55,* 159–166.

Miller, W. R., Leckman, A. L., Delaney, H. D., & Tinkcom, M. (1992). Long-term follow-up of behavioral self-control training. *Journal of Studies on Alcohol, 53,* 249–261.

Miller, W. R., & Manuel, J. K. (2008). How large must a treatment effect be before it matters to practitioners?: An estimation method and demonstration. *Drug and Alcohol Review, 27,* 524–528.

Miller, W. R., & Mee-Lee, D. (2010). *Self-management: A guide to your feelings, motivations, and positive mental health* (addiction treatment ed.). Carson City, NV: The Change Companies.

Miller, W. R., & Mee-Lee, D. (2012). *Self-management: A guide to your feelings, motivations, and positive mental health.* Carson City, NV: The Change Companies.

Miller, W. R., Meyers, R. J., & Tonigan, J. S. (1999). Engaging the unmotivated in treatment for alcohol problems: A comparison of three strategies for intervention through family members. *Journal of Consulting and Clinical Psychology, 67,* 688–697.

Miller, W. R., Meyers, R. J., Tonigan, J. S., & Grant, K. A. (2001). Community reinforcement and traditional approaches: Findings of a controlled trial. In R. J. Meyers & W. R. Miller (Eds.), *A community reinforcement approach to addiction treatment* (pp. 79–103). Cambridge, UK: Cambridge University Press.

Miller, W. R., & Mount, K. A. (2001). A small study of training in motivational interviewing: Does one workshop change clinician and client behavior? *Behavioural and Cognitive Psychotherapy, 29,* 457–471.

Miller, W. R., & Moyers, T. B. (2015). The forest and the trees: Relational and specific factors in addiction treatment. *Addiction, 110*(3), 401–413.

Miller, W. R., & Moyers, T. B. (2017). Motivational interviewing and the clinical science of Carl Rogers. *Journal of Consulting and Clinical Psychology, 85*(8), 757–766.

Miller, W. R., Moyers, T. B., Arciniega, L., Ernst, D., & Forcehimes, A. (2005). Training, supervision and quality monitoring of the COMBINE study behavioral interventions. *Journal of Studies on Alcohol, 5,* 188–195.

Miller, W. R., & Muñoz, R. F. (2013). *Controlling your drinking* (2nd ed.). New York: Guilford Press.

Miller, W. R., & Page, A. (1991). Warm turkey: Other routes to abstinence. *Journal of Substance Abuse Treatment, 8,* 227–232.

Miller, W. R., & Pechacek, T. F. (1987). New roads: Assessing and treating psychological dependence. *Journal of Substance Abuse Treatment, 4*(2), 73–77.

Miller, W. R., & Rollnick, S. (2004). Talking oneself into change: Motivational interviewing, stages of change, and the therapeutic process. *Journal of Cognitive Psychotherapy, 18,* 299–308.

Miller, W. R., & Rollnick, S. (2013). *Motivational interviewing: Helping people change* (3rd ed.). New York: Guilford Press.

Miller, W. R., & Rollnick, S. (2014). The effectiveness and ineffectiveness of complex behavioral interventions: Impact of treatment fidelity. *Contemporary Clinical Trials, 37*(2), 234–241.

Miller, W. R., Rollnick, S., & Moyers, T. B. (2013). *Motivational interviewing: Helping people change* (DVD series). Carson City, NV: Change Companies.

Miller, W. R., & Rose, G. S. (2015). Motivational interviewing and decisional balance: Contrasting responses to client ambivalence. *Behavioural and Cognitive Psychotherapy, 43*(2), 129–141.

Miller, W. R., & Sanchez, V. C. (1994). Motivating young adults for treatment and lifestyle change. In G. Howard (Ed.), *Issues in alcohol use and misuse by young adults* (pp. 55–82). Notre Dame, IN: University of Notre Dame Press.

Miller, W. R., Sorensen, J., Selzer, J., & Brigham, G. (2006). Disseminating evidence-based practices in substance abuse treatment: A review with suggestions. *Journal of Substance Abuse Treatment, 31*(1), 25–39.

Miller, W. R., & Sovereign, R. G. (1989). The check-up: A model for early intervention in addictive behaviors. In T. Løberg, W. R. Miller, P. E. Nathan & G. A. Marlatt (Eds.), *Addictive behaviors: Prevention and early intervention* (pp. 219–231). Amsterdam: Swets & Zeitlinger.

Miller, W. R., Sovereign, R. G., & Krege, B. (1988). Motivational interviewing with problem drinkers: II. The Drinker's Check-Up as a preventive intervention. *Behavioural Psychotherapy, 16*, 251–268.

Miller, W. R., & Taylor, C. A. (1980). Relative effectiveness of bibliotherapy, individual and group self-control training in the treatment of problem drinkers. *Addictive Behaviors, 5*, 13–24.

Miller, W. R., Taylor, C. A., & West, J. (1980). Focused versus broad-spectrum behavior therapy for problem drinkers. *Journal of Consulting and Clinical Psychology, 48*(5), 590–601.

Miller, W. R., & Thoresen, C. E. (1999). Spirituality and health. In W. R. Miller (Ed.), *Integrating spirituality into treatment: Resources for practitioners* (pp. 3–18). Washington, DC: American Psychological Association.

Miller, W. R., & Thoresen, C. E. (2003). Spirituality, religion, and health: An emerging research field. *American Psychologist, 58*, 24–35.

Miller, W. R., & Tonigan, J. S. (1996). Assessing drinkers' motivation for change: The Stages of Change Readiness and Treatment Eagerness Scale (SOCRATES). *Psychology of Addictive Behaviors, 10*(2), 81–89.

Miller, W. R., Tonigan, J. S., & Longabaugh, R. (1995). *The Drinker Inventory of Consequences (DrInC): An instrument for assessing adverse consequences of alcohol abuse* (Vol. 4). Bethesda, MD: National Institute on Alcohol Abuse and Alcoholism.

Miller, W. R., Villanueva, M., Tonigan, J. S., & Cuzmar, I. (2007). Are special treatments needed for special populations? *Alcoholism Treatment Quarterly, 25*(4), 63–78.

Miller, W. R., Walters, S. T., & Bennett, M. E. (2001). How effective is alcoholism treatment in the United States? *Journal of Studies on Alcohol, 62*, 211–220.

Miller, W. R., & Weisner, C. (Eds.). (2002). *Changing substance abuse through health and social systems.* New York: Kluwer/Plenum.

Miller, W. R., & Weisner, C. (2002). Integrated care: The need for evidence-based policy. In W. R. Miller & C. Weisner (Eds.), *Changing substance abuse through health and social systems* (pp. 243–253). New York: Kluwer/Plenum.

Miller, W. R., Westerberg, V. S., Harris, R. J., & Tonigan, J. S. (1996). What predicts relapse?: Prospective testing of antecedent models. *Addiction, 9*(Suppl.), S155–S171.

Miller, W. R., Westerberg, V. S., & Waldron, H. B. (2003). Evaluating alcohol problems in adults and adolescents. In R. K. Hester & W. R. Miller (Eds.), *Handbook of alcoholism treatment approaches: Effective alternatives* (3rd ed., pp. 78–112). Boston: Allyn & Bacon.

Miller, W. R., & Wilbourne, P. L. (2002). Mesa Grande: A methodological analysis of clinical trials of treatment for alcohol use disorders. *Addiction, 97*(3), 265–277.

Miller, W. R., Wilbourne, P. L., & Hettema, J. E. (2003). What works?: A summary of alcohol treatment outcome research. In R. K. Hester & W. R. Miller (Eds.), *Handbook of alcoholism treatment approaches: Effective alternatives* (3rd ed., pp. 13–63). Boston: Allyn & Bacon.

Miller, W. R., Yahne, C. E., Moyers, T. B., Martinez, J., & Pirritano, M. (2004). A randomized trial of methods to help clinicians learn motivational interviewing. *Journal of Consulting and Clinical Psychology, 72*(6), 1050–1062.

Miller, W. R., Yahne, C. E., & Tonigan, J. S. (2003). Motivational interviewing in drug abuse services: A randomized trial. *Journal of Consulting and Clinical Psychology, 71,* 754–763.

Miller, W. R., Zweben, A., DiClemente, C. C., & Rychtarik, R. G. (1992). *Motivational Enhancement Therapy manual: A clinical research guide for therapists treating individuals with alcohol abuse and dependence* (Project MATCH Monograph Series, Vol. 2). Rockville, MD: National Institute on Alcohol Abuse and Alcoholism.

Miller, W. R., Zweben, J. E., & Johnson, W. (2005). Evidence-based treatment: Why, what, where, when, and how? *Journal of Substance Abuse Treatment, 29,* 267–276.

Milmoe, S., Rosenthal, R., Blane, H. T., Chafetz, M. E., & Wolf, I. (1967). The doctor's voice: Postdictor of successful referral of alcoholic patients. *Journal of Abnormal Psychology, 72,* 78–84.

Miranda, R., Meyerson, L. A., Myers, R. R., & Lovallo, W. R. (2003). Altered affective modulation of the startle reflex in alcoholics with antisocial personality disorder. *Alcoholism: Clinical and Experimental Research, 27,* 1901–1911.

Mirijello, A., D'Angelo, C., Ferrulli, A., Vassallo, G., Antonelli, M., Caputo, F., . . . Addolorato, G. (2015). Identification and management of alcohol withdrawal syndrome. *Drugs, 75*(4), 353–365.

Mitcheson, L., Bhavsar, K., & McCambridge, J. (2009). Randomized trial of training and supervision in motivational interviewing with adolescent drug treatment providers. *Journal of Substance Abuse Treatment, 37,* 73–78.

Moffitt, T. E., Arseneault, L., Belsky, D., Dickson, N., Hancox, R. J., Harrington, H., . . . Caspi, A. (2011). A gradient of childhood self-control predicts health, wealth, and public safety. *Proceedings of the National Academy of Sciences of the USA, 108*(7), 2693–2698.

Montgomery, H. A., Miller, W. R., & Tonigan, J. S. (1993). Differences among AA groups: Implications for research. *Journal of Studies on Alcohol, 54,* 502–504.

Montgomery, H. A., Miller, W. R., & Tonigan, J. S. (1995). Does Alcoholics Anonymous involvement predict treatment outcome? *Journal of Substance Abuse Treatment, 12,* 241–246.

Montgomery, L., Carroll, K. M., & Petry, N. M. (2015). Initial abstinence status and contingency management treatment outcomes: Does race matter? *Journal of Consulting and Clinical Psychology, 83*(3), 473–481.

Monti, P. M., Abrams, D. B., Kadden, R. M., & Cooney, N. L. (1989). *Treating alcohol dependence: A coping skills training guide.* New York: Guilford Press.

Monti, P. M., Colby, S. M., Mastroleo, N. R., Barnett, N. P., Gwaltney, C. J., Apodaca, T. R., . . . Cioffi, W. G. (2014). Individual versus significant-other-enhanced brief motivational intervention for alcohol in emergency care. *Journal of Consulting and Clinical Psychology, 82*(6), 936–948.

Monti, P. M., Colby, S. M., & O'Leary, T. A. (2001). *Adolescents, alcohol, and substance abuse: Reaching teens through brief interventions.* New York: Guilford Press.

Monti, P. M., Kadden, R., Rohsenow, D. J., Cooney, N. L., & Abrams, D. B. (2002). *Treating alcohol dependence: A coping skills training guide* (2nd ed.). New York: Guilford Press.

Moore, B. A., Buono, F. D., Printz, D. M. B., Lloyd, D. P., Fiellin, D. A., Cutter, C. J.,

. . . Barry, D. T. (2017). Customized recommendations and reminder text messages for automated, computer-based treatment during methadone. *Experimental and Clinical Psychopharmacology, 25*(6), 485–495.

Moore, S. E., Norman, R. E., Sly, P. D., Whitehouse, A. J. O., Zubrick, S. R., & Scott, J. (2014). Adolescent peer aggression and its association with mental health and substance use in an Australian cohort. *Journal of Adolescence, 37*(1), 11–21.

Moos, R. H. (1993). *Coping Responses Inventory (CRI): Adult form manual.* Odessa, FL: Psychological Assessment Resources.

Moos, R. H., Finney, J. W., & Cronkite, R. C. (1990). *Alcoholism treatment: Context, process, and outcome.* New York: Oxford University Press.

Moos, R. H., Finney, J., & Maude-Griffin, P. (1993). The social climate of self-help and mutual support groups: Assessing group implementation, process, and outcome. In B. S. McCrady & W. R. Miller (Eds.), *Research on Alcoholics Anonymous: Opportunities and alternatives* (pp. 251–274). Piscataway, NJ: Rutgers Center of Alcohol Studies.

Moos, R. H., & Moos, B. S. (2005). Paths of entry into Alcoholics Anonymous: Consequences for participation and remission. *Alcoholism: Clinical and Experimental Research, 29,* 1858–1868.

Moos, R. H., & Moos, B. S. (2006). Participation in treatment and Alcoholics Anonymous: A 16-year follow-up of initially untreated individuals. *Journal of Clinical Psychology, 62,* 735–750.

Morandi, S., Silva, B., Golay, P., & Bonsack, C. (2017). Intensive case management for addiction to promote engagement with care of people with severe mental and substance use disorders: An observational study. *Substance Abuse Treatment, Prevention, and Policy, 12*(1), 26.

Morgenstern, J., Blanchard, K. A., Kahler, C., Barbosa, K. M., McCrady, B. S., & McVeigh, K. H. (2008). Testing mechanisms of action for intensive case management. *Addiction, 103*(3), 469–477.

Morgenstern, J., Hogue, A., Dauber, S., Dasaro, C., & McKay, J. R. (2009). A practical clinical trial of coordinated care management to treat substance use disorders among public assistance beneficiaries. *Journal of Consulting and Clinical Psychology, 77*(2), 257–269.

Morgenstern, J., Kahler, C., Frey, R. M., & Lavouvie, E. (1996). Modeling therapeutic response to 12-step treatment: Optimal responders, nonresponders and partial responders. *Journal of Substance Abuse, 8,* 45–59.

Morgenstern, J., Kuerbis, A., Amrhein, P., Hail, L., Lynch, K., & McKay, J. R. (2012). Motivational interviewing: A pilot test of active ingredients and mechanisms of change. *Psychology of Addictive Behaviors, 26*(4), 859–869.

Morgenstern, J., & Longabaugh, R. (2000). Cognitive-behavioral treatment for alcohol dependence: A review of evidence for its hypothesized mechanisms of action. *Addiction, 95,* 1475–1490.

Morini, L., & Polettini, A. (2009). Ethyl glucuronide in hair: A sensitive and specific marker of chronic heavy drinking. *Addiction, 104*(6), 915–920.

Morisky, D. E., Green, L. W., & Levine, D. M. (1986). Concurrent and predictive validity of a self-reported measure of medication adherence. *Medical Care, 24,* 67–74.

Morrill, M. I., Eubanks-Fleming, C. J., Harp, A. G., Sollenberger, J. W., Darling, E. V., & Cordova, J. V. (2011). The marriage check-up: Increasing access to marital health care. *Family Process, 50,* 471–485.

Moyer, A., Finney, J. W., Swearingen, C. E., & Vergun, P. (2002). Brief interventions for alcohol problems: A meta-analytic review of controlled investigations in treatment-seeking and non-treatment-seeking populations. *Addiction, 97*(3), 279–292.

Moyers, T. B., Houck, J. M., Glynn, L. H., Hallgren, K. A., & Manual, J. K. (2017). A randomized controlled trial to influence client language in substance use disorder treatment. *Drug and Alcohol Dependence, 172,* 43–50.

Moyers, T. B., Houck, J. M., Glynn, L. H., & Manuel, J. K. (2011). Can specialized training teach clinicians to recognize, reinforce, and elicit client language in motivational interviewing? *Alcoholism: Clinical and Experimental Research, 335*(S1), 296.

Moyers, T. B., Houck, J. M., Rice, S. L., Longabaugh, R., & Miller, W. R. (2016). Therapist empathy, Combined Behavioral Intervention, and alcohol outcomes in the COMBINE research project. *Journal of Consulting and Clinical Psychology, 84*(3), 221–229.

Moyers, T. B., Martin, T., Houck, J. M., Christopher, P. J., & Tonigan, J. S. (2009). From in-session behaviors to drinking outcomes: A causal chain for motivational interviewing. *Journal of Consulting and Clinical Psychology, 77*(6), 1113–1124.

Moyers, T. B., & Miller, W. R. (2013). Is low therapist empathy toxic? *Psychology of Addictive Behaviors, 27*(3), 878–884.

Moyers, T. B., & Rollnick, S. (2002). A motivational interviewing perspective on resistance in psychotherapy. *Journal of Clinical Psychology, 58*(2), 185–193.

Mueser, K. T., & Drake, R. E. (2007). Comorbidity: What have we learned and where are we going? *Clinical Psychology: Science and Practice, 14*(1), 64–69.

Mueser, K. T., Drake, R. E., Turner, W., & McGovern, M. (2006). Comorbid substance use disorders and psychiatric disorders. In W. R. Miller & K. M. Carroll (Eds.), *Rethinking substance abuse: What the science shows, and what we should do about it* (pp. 115–133). New York: Guilford Press.

Mueser, K. T., & Gingerich, S. (2013). Treatment of co-occurring psychotic and substance use disorders. *Social Work in Public Health, 28,* 424–439.

Mulligan, D. H. (Ed.). (1995). *The tuberculosis epidemic: Legal and ethical issues for alcohol and other drug abuse treatment providers.* Rockville, MD: Center for Substance Abuse Treatment.

Muñoz, R. F., Bunge, E. L., Chen, K., Schueller, S. M., Bravin, J. I., Shaughnessy, E. A., & Pérez-Stable, E. J. (2016). Massive open online interventions: A novel model for delivering behavioral-health services worldwide. *Clinical Psychological Science, 4*(2), 194–205.

Muñoz, R. F., Le, H.-N., Clarke, G. N., Barrera, A. Z., & Torres, L. D. (2009). Preventing first onset and recurrence of major depressive episodes. In I. H. Gotlib & C. L. Hammen (Eds.), *Handbook of depression* (2nd ed., pp. 533–553). New York: Guilford Press.

Muñoz, R. F., Lenert, L. L., Delucchi, K., Stoddard, J., Perez, J. E., Penilla, C., & Perez-Stable, E. J. (2006). Toward evidence-based Internet interventions: A Spanish/English web site for international smoking cessation trials. *Nicotine and Tobacco Research, 8*(1), 77–87.

Murphy, A., Rhodes, A. G., & Taxman, F. S. (2012). Adaptability of contingency management in justice settings: Survey findings on attitudes towards using rewards. *Journal of Substance Abuse Treatment, 43*(2), 168–177.

Naar, S., & Safren, S. A. (2017). *Motivational interviewing and CBT: Combining strategies for maximum effectiveness.* New York: Guilford Press.

Naar-King, S., & Suarez, M. (Eds.). (2011). *Motivational interviewing with adolescents and young adults.* New York: Guilford Press.

Najavits, L. M. (2002). *Seeking safety: A treatment manual for PTSD and substance abuse.* New York: Guilford Press.

Najavits, L. M., Crits-Christoph, P., & Dierberger, A. (2000). Clinicians' impact on the quality of substance use disorder treatment. *Substance Use and Misuse, 35*(12–14), 2161–2190.

Najavits, L. M., & Weiss, R. D. (1994). Variations in therapist effectiveness in the treatment of patients with substance use disorders: An empirical review. *Addiction, 89,* 679–688.

Najavits, L. M., Weiss, R. D., Shaw, S. R., & Muenz, L. R. (1998). Seeking Safety: Outcome of a new cognitive-behavioral psychotherapy for women with posttraumatic stress disorder and substance dependence. *Journal of Traumatic Stress, 11*(3), 437–456.

National Institute on Alcohol Abuse and Alcoholism. (1996, May 28). How to cut down on your drinking. Retrieved from *http://pubs.niaaa.nih.gov/publications/handout.htm.*

National Institute on Alcohol Abuse and Alcoholism. (2005). Helping patients who drink too much: A clinician's guide. Retrieved from *http://pubs.niaaa.nih.gov/publications/Practitioner/CliniciansGuide2005/clinicians_guide.htm.*

National Institute on Drug Abuse. (2010). Screening for drug use in general medical settings: Resource guide. Retrieved from *www.drugabuse.gov/sites/default/files/resource_guide.pdf.*

Navidian, A., Kermansaravi, F., Tabas, E. E., & Saeedinezhad, F. (2016). Efficacy of group motivational interviewing in the degree of drug craving in the addicts under the methadone maintenance treatment (MMT) in South East of Iran. *Archives of Psychiatric Nursing, 30*(2), 144–149.

Nay, W. R. (2012). *Taking charge of anger: Six steps to asserting yourself without losing control* (2nd ed.). New York: Guilford Press.

Nay, W. R. (2014). *The anger management workbook: Use the STOP method to replace destructive responses with constructive behavior.* New York: Guilford Press.

Neighbors, C., Lewis, M. A., Atkins, D. C., Jensen, M. M., Walter, T., Fossos, N., . . . Larimer, M. E. (2010). Efficacy of Web-based personalized normative feedback: A two-year randomized controlled trial. *Journal of Consulting and Clinical Psychology, 78*(6), 898–911.

Nesvåg, R., Knudsen, G. P., Bakken, I. J., Høye, A., Ystrom, E., Suren, P., . . . Reichborn-Kjennerud, T. (2015). Substance use disorders in schizophrenia, bipolar disorder, and depressive illness: A registry-based study. *Social Psychiatry and Psychiatric Epidemiology, 50*(8), 1267–1276.

Nguyen Anh-Huong, & Thich Nhat Hanh. (2006). *Walking meditation: Peace is every step.* Boulder, CO: Sounds True.

Nicolaus, M. (2012). Empowering your sober self: The LifeRing approach to addiction recovery. *Journal of Groups in Addiction and Recovery, 7*(2–4), 118–129.

Nielsen, S., Hillhouse, M., Mooney, L., Ang, A., & Ling, W. (2015). Buprenorphine pharmacotherapy and behavioral treatment: Comparison of outcomes among prescription opioid users, heroin users and combination users. *Journal of Substance Abuse Treatment, 48*(1), 70–76.

Nilsen, P. (2010). Brief alcohol intervention—where to from here?: Challenges remain for research and practice. *Addiction, 105*(6), 954–959.

Nirenberg, T. D., Sobell, L. C., & Sobell, M. B. (1980). Effective and inexpensive procedures for decreasing client attrition in an outpatient alcohol treatment program. *Journal of Drug and Alcohol Abuse, 7,* 73–82.

Noel, N. E., & McCrady, B. S. (1993). Alcohol-focused spouse involvement with behavioral marital therapy. In T. J. O'Farrell (Ed.), *Treating alcohol problems: Marital and family interventions* (pp. 210–235). New York: Guilford Press.

Noel, P. E. (2006). The impact of therapeutic case management on participation in adolescent substance abuse treatment. *American Journal of Drug and Alcohol Abuse, 32*(3), 311–327.

Norcross, J. C., Krebs, P. M., & Prochaska, J. O. (2011). Stage of change. In J. C. Norcross (Ed.), *Psychotherapy relationships that work: Evidence-based responsiveness* (2nd ed., pp. 279–300). New York: Oxford University Press.

Nowinski, J. (1999). Self-help groups for addictions. In B. McCrady & B. Epstein (Eds.), *Addictions: A comprehensive guidebook* (pp. 328–346). New York: Oxford University Press.

Nowinski, J. (2003). Facilitating 12-step recovery from substance abuse and addiction. In F. Rotgers, J. Morgenstern & S. Walters (Eds.), *Treating substance abuse* (pp. 31–66). New York: Guilford Press.

Nowinski, J., & Baker, S. (1998). *The twelve-step facilitation handbook: A systematic approach to early recovery from alcoholism and addiction.* San Francisco: Jossey Bass.

Nowinski, J., Baker, S., & Carroll, K. M. (1992). *Twelve step facilitation therapy manual: A clinical research guide for therapists treating individuals with alcohol abuse and dependence.* Rockville, MD: National Institute on Alcohol Abuse and Alcoholism.

O'Farrell, T. J., & Fals-Stewart, W. (2006). *Behavioral couples therapy for alcoholism and drug abuse.* New York: Guilford Press.

O'Farrell, T. J., Murphy, C. M., Stephan, S. H., Fals-Stewart, W., & Murphy, M. (2004). Partner violence before and after couples-based alcoholism treatment for male alcoholic patients: The role of treatment involvement and abstinence. *Journal of Consulting and Clinical Psychology, 72*(2), 202–217.

O'Farrell, T. J., Murphy, M., Alter, J., & Fals-Stewart, W. (2010). Behavioral family counseling for substance abuse: A treatment development pilot study. *Addictive Behaviors, 35*(1), 1–6.

O'Farrell, T. J., Schumm, J. A., Murphy, M. M., & Muchowski, P. M. (2017). A randomized clinical trial of behavioral couples therapy versus individually-based treatment for drug-abusing women. *Journal of Consulting and Clinical Psychology, 85*(4), 309–322.

Office of the Surgeon General. (2016). *Facing addiction in America: The Surgeon General's report on alcohol, drugs, and health.* Washington, DC: U.S. Department of Health and Human Services.

Ogle, R. L., & Miller, W. R. (2004). The effects of alcohol intoxication and gender on the social information processing of hostile provocations involving male and female provocateurs. *Journal of Studies on Alcohol, 65,* 54–62.

Oliveto, A., Poling, J., Mancino, M. J., Feldman, Z., Cubells, J. F., Pruzinsky, R., . . . Chopra, M. P. (2011). Randomized, double blind, placebo-controlled trial of disulfiram for the treatment of cocaine dependence in methadone-stabilized patients. *Drug and Alcohol Dependence, 113*(2–3), 184–191.

O'Malley, S. S., Corbin, W. R., Leeman, R. F., DeMartini, K. S., Fucito, L. M., Ikomi, J., . . . Kranzler, H. R. (2015). Reduction of alcohol drinking in young adults by naltrexone: A double-blind, placebo-controlled, randomized clinical trial of efficacy and safety. *Journal of Clinical Psychiatry, 76*(2), e207–e213.

O'Malley, S. S., & Kosten, T. R. (2006). Pharmacotherapy of addictive disorders. In

W. R. Miller & K. Carroll (Eds.), *Rethinking substance abuse: What the science shows, and what we should do about it* (pp. 240–256). New York: Guilford Press.

O'Malley, S. S., Rounsaville, B. J., Farren, C., Namkoong, K., Wu, R., Robinson, J., & O'Connor, P. G. (2003). Initial and maintenance naltrexone treatment for alcohol dependence using primary care vs specialty care: A nested sequence of 3 randomized trials. *Archives of Internal Medicine, 163*(14), 1695–1704.

O'Malley, S. S., Zweben, A., Fucito, L. M., Wu, R., Piepmeier, M. E., Ockert, D. M., . . . Jatlow, P. (2018). Effect of varenicline combined with medical management on alcohol use disorder with comorbid cigarette smoking: A randomized clinical trial. *JAMA Psychiatry, 75*(2), 129–138.

Ondersma, S. J., Svikis, D. S., Thacker, L. R., Beatty, J. R., & Lockhart, N. (2014). Computer-delivered screening and brief intervention (e-SBI) for postpartum drug use: A randomized trial. *Journal of Substance Abuse Treament, 46*(1), 52–59.

Orford, J. (2017). How does the common core to the harm experienced by affected family members vary by relationship, social and cultural factors? *Drugs: Education, Prevention and Policy, 24*(1), 9–16.

Orford, J., Velleman, R., Natera, G., Templeton, L., & Copello, A. (2013). Addiction in the family is a major but neglected contributor to the global burden of adult ill-health. *Social Science and Medicine, 78*, 70–77.

Ornstein, S. M., Miller, P. M., Wessell, A. M., Jenkins, R. G., Nemeth, L. S., & Nietert, P. J. (2013). Integration and sustainability of alcohol screening, brief intervention, and pharmacotherapy in primary care settings. *Journal of Studies on Alcohol and Drugs, 74*(4), 598–604.

Oslin, D. W., Lynch, K. G., Pettinati, H. M., Kampman, K. M., Gariti, P., Gelfand, L., . . . Dackis, C. (2008). A placebo-controlled randomized clinical trial of naltrexone in the context of different levels of psychosocial intervention. *Alcoholism: Clinical and Experimental Research, 32*(7), 1299–1308.

Ouimette, P. C., Finney, J. W., & Moos, R. H. (1997). Twelve-step and cognitive-behavioral treatment for substance abuse: A comparison of treatment effectiveness. *Journal of Consulting and Clinical Psychology, 65*, 230–240.

Owens, M. D., & McCrady, B. S. (2014). The role of the social environment in alcohol or drug relapse of probationers recently released from jail. *Addictive Disorders and Their Treatment, 13*(4), 179–189.

Padwa, H., Teruya, C., Tran, E., Lovinger, K., Antonini, V. P., Overholt, C., & Urada, D. (2016). The implementation of integrated behavioral health protocols in primary care settings in Project Care. *Journal of Substance Abuse Treatment, 62*, 74–83.

Pagano, M. E., White, W. L., Kelly, J. F., Stout, R. L., & Tonigan, J. S. (2013). The 10-year course of Alcoholics Anonymous participation and long-term outcomes: A follow-up study of outpatient subjects in Project MATCH. *Substance Abuse, 34*(1), 51–59.

Palpacuer, C., Duprez, R., Huneau, A., Locher, C., Boussageon, R., Laviolle, B., & Naudet, F. (2017). Pharmacologically controlled drinking in the treatment of alcohol dependence or alcohol use disorders: A systematic review with direct and network meta-analyses on nalmefene, naltrexone, acamprosate, baclofen, and topiramate. *Addiction, 113*(2), 220–237.

Panepinto, W. C., & Higgins, M. J. (1969). Keeping alcoholics in treatment: Effective follow-through procedures. *Quarterly Journal of Studies on Alcohol, 30*, 414–419.

Paolino, T. J., McCrady, B. S., & Kogan, K. B. (1978). Alcoholic marriages: A longitudinal empirical assessment of alternative theories. *British Journal of Addiction, 73*(2), 129–138.

Parhar, K. K., Wormith, J. S., Derkzen, D. M., & Beauregard, A. M. (2008). Offender coercion in treatment: A meta-analysis of effectiveness. *Criminal Justice and Behavior, 35*(9), 1109–1135.

Peele, S. (2000). What addiction is and is not: The impact of mistaken notions of addiction. *Addiction Research, 8*(6), 599–607.

Pemberton, M. R., Williams, J., Herman-Stahl, M., Calvin, S. L., Bradshaw, M. R., Bray, R. M., . . . Mitchell, G. M. (2011). Evaluation of two Web-based alcohol interventions in the U.S. military. *Journal of Studies on Alcohol and Drugs, 72*, 480–489.

Pérez-Mañá, C., Castells, X., Vidal, X., Casas, M., & Capellà, D. (2011). Efficacy of indirect dopamine agonists for psychostimulant dependence: A systematic review and meta-analysis of randomized controlled trials. *Journal of Substance Abuse Treatment, 40*(2), 109–122.

Peteet, J. R. (1993). A closer look at the role of a spiritual approach in the addictions treatment. *Journal of Substance Abuse Treatment, 10*, 263–267.

Peterson, C., & Seligman, M. E. P. (2004). *Character strengths and virtues: A handbook and classification.* New York: Oxford University Press.

Petry, N. M. (2012). *Contingency management for substance abuse treatment: A guide to implementing this evidence-based practice.* New York: Routledge.

Petry, N. M., Alessi, S. M., Barry, D., & Carroll, K. M. (2015). Standard magnitude prize reinforcers can be as efficacious as larger magnitude reinforcers in cocaine-dependent methadone patients. *Journal of Consulting and Clinical Psychology, 83*(3), 464–472.

Petry, N. M., Alessi, S. M., & Hanson, T. (2007). Contingency management improves abstinence and quality of life in cocaine abusers. *Journal of Consulting and Clinical Psychology, 75*(2), 307–315.

Petry, N. M., Alessi, S. M., & Rash, C. J. (2013). Contingency management treatments decrease psychiatric symptoms. *Journal of Consulting and Clinical Psychology, 81*(5), 926–931.

Petry, N. M., & Armentano, C. (1999). Prevalence, assessment, and treatment of pathological gambling: A review. *Psychiatric Services, 50*(8), 1021–1027.

Petry, N. M., Barry, D., Alessi, S. M., Rounsaville, B. J., & Carroll, K. M. (2012). A randomized trial adapting contingency management targets based on initial abstinence status of cocaine-dependent patients. *Journal of Consulting and Clinical Psychology, 80*(2), 276–285.

Petry, N. M., DePhilippis, D., Rash, C. J., Drapkin, M., & McKay, J. R. (2014). Nationwide dissemination of contingency management: The Veterans Administration initiative. *American Journal on Addictions, 23*(3), 205–210.

Petry, N. M., & Martin, B. (2002). Low-cost contingency management for treating cocaine- and opioid-abusing methadone patients. *Journal of Consulting and Clinical Psychology, 70*(2), 398–405.

Petry, N. M., Peirce, J. M., Stitzer, M. L., Blaine, J., Roll, J. M., Cohen, A., . . . Li, R. (2005). Effect of prize-based incentives on outcomes in stimulant abusers in outpatient psychosocial treatment programs. *Archives of General Psychiatry, 62*, 1148–1156.

Petry, N. M., Weinstock, J., & Alessi, S. M. (2011). A randomized trial of contingency management delivered in the context of group counseling. *Journal of Consulting and Clinical Psychology, 79*(5), 686–696.

Petry, N. M., Weinstock, J., Alessi, S. M., Lewis, M. W., & Dieckhaus, K. (2010). Group-based randomized trial of contingencies for health and abstinence in HIV patients. *Journal of Consulting and Clinical Psychology, 78*(1), 89–97.

Petry, N. M., Weinstock, J., Ledgerwood, D. M., & Morasco, B. (2008). A randomized trial of brief interventions for problem and pathological gamblers. *Journal of Consulting and Clinical Psychology, 76*(2), 318–328.

Pettinati, H. M. (2006). Improving medication adherence in alcohol dependence. *Journal of Clinical Psychiatry, 67*(Suppl. 14), 23–29.

Pettinati, H. M., & Mattson, M. E. (2010). *Medical Management treatment manual: A clinical guide for researchers and clinicians providing pharmacotherapy for alcohol dependence* (rev. ed.). Rockville, MD: National Institute on Alcohol Abuse and Alcoholism.

Pettinati, H. M., Volpicelli, J. R., Pierce, J. D., Jr., & O'Brien, C. P. (2000). Improving naltrexone response: An intervention for medical practitioners to enhance medication compliance in alcohol dependent patients. *Journal of Addictive Diseases, 19*(1), 71–83.

Pettinati, H. M., Weiss, R. D., Dundon, W., Miller, W. R., Donovan, D., Ernst, D. B., & Rounsaville, B. J. (2005). A structured approach to medical management: A psychosocial intervention to support pharmacotherapy in the treatment of alcohol dependence. *Journal of Studies on Alcohol* (Suppl. 15), 170–178, discussion 168–169.

Pettinati, H. M., Weiss, R. D., Miller, W. R., Donovan, D., Ernst, D. B., Rounsaville, B. J., & Mattson, M. E. (2004). *Medical management treatment manual: A clinical research guide for medically trained clinicians providing pharmacotherapy as part of the treatment for alcohol dependence* (Vol. 2; DHHS Publication No. 04-5289). Bethesda, MD: Department of Health and Human Services,.

Phillips, D. P., & Brewer, K. M. (2011). The relationship between serious injury and blood alcohol concentration (BAC) in fatal motor vehicle accidents: BAC = 0.01% is associated with significantly more dangerous accidents than BAC = 0.00%. *Addiction, 106*(9), 1614–1622.

Pinto, H., Maskrey, V., Swift, L., Rumball, D., Wagle, A., & Holland, R. (2010). The SUMMIT trial: A field comparison of buprenorphine versus methadone maintenance treatment. *Journal of Substance Abuse Treatment, 39*(4), 340–352.

Pirlott, A. G., Kisbu-Sakarya, Y., Defrancesco, C. A., Elliot, D. L., & Mackinnon, D. P. (2012). Mechanisms of motivational interviewing in health promotion: A Bayesian mediation analysis. *International Journal of Behavioral Nutrition and Physical Activity, 9*(1), 69.

Pope, K. S., & Vasquez, M. J. T. (2007). *Ethics in psychotherapy and counseling: A practical guide* (3rd ed.). San Francisco: Jossey-Bass.

Poston, J. M., & Hanson, W. E. (2010). Meta-analysis of psychological assessment as a therapeutic intervention. *Psychological Assessment, 22*(2), 203–212.

Powell, B. J., Beidas, R. S., Lewis, C. C., Aarons, G. A., McMillen, J. C., Proctor, E. K., & Mandell, D. S. (2017). Methods to improve the selection and tailoring of implementation strategies. *Journal of Behavioral Health Services and Research, 44*(2), 177–194.

Powell, B. J., Proctor, E. K., & Glass, J. E. (2014). A systematic review of strategies for implementing empirically supported mental health interventions. *Research on Social Work Practice, 24*(2), 192–212.

Powell, B. J., Waltz, T. J., Chinman, M. J., Damschroder, L. J., Smith, J. L., Matthieu, M. M., . . . Kirchner, J. E. (2015). A refined compilation of implementation strategies: Results from the Expert Recommendations for Implementing Change (ERIC) project. *Implementation Science, 10*(1).

Powers, M. B., Vedel, E., & Emmelkamp, P. M. G. (2008). Behavioral couples therapy

(BCT) for alcohol and drug use disorders: A meta-analysis. *Clinical Psychology Review, 28*(6), 952–962.

Prescott, D. S., Maeschalck, C. L., & Miller, S. D. (Eds.). (2017). *Feedback informed treatment in clinical practice: Reaching for excellence.* Washington, DC: American Psychological Association.

President's Commission on Combating Drug Addiction and the Opioid Crisis. (2017). *Final report.* Washington, DC: Office of National Drug Control Policy.

Preston, J., & Johnson, J. (2016). *Clinical psychopharmacology made ridiculously simple* (8th ed.). Miami, FL: Medmaster.

Prochaska, J. O., & DiClemente, C. C. (1992). Stage of change in the modification of problem behaviors. In M. Hersen, R. M. Eisler, & W. R. Miller (Eds.), *Progress in behavior modification* (pp. 184–212). Sycamore, IL: Sycamore.

Prochaska, J. O., & Norcross, J. C. (2013). *Systems of psychotherapy: A transtheoretical analysis* (8th ed.). Stamford, CT: Cenage Learning.

Prochaska, J. O., & Velicer, W. F. (1997). The transtheoretical model of health behavior change. *American Journal of Health Promotion, 12*(1), 38–48.

Proctor, S. L., Hoffman, N. G., & Allison, S. (2012). The effectiveness of interactive journaling in reducing recidivism among substance dependent jail inmates. *International Journal of Offender Therapy and Comparative Criminology, 56*(2), 317–332.

Project MATCH Research Group. (1993). Project MATCH: Rationale and methods for a multisite clinical trial matching patients to alcoholism treatment. *Alcoholism: Clinical and Experimental Research, 17,* 1130–1145.

Project MATCH Research Group. (1997a). Matching alcoholism treatments to client heterogeneity: Project MATCH posttreatment drinking outcomes. *Journal of Studies on Alcohol, 58*(1), 7–29.

Project MATCH Research Group. (1997b). Project MATCH secondary *a priori* hypotheses. *Addiction, 92,* 1671–1698.

Project MATCH Research Group. (1998a). Matching alcoholism treatments to client heterogeneity: Project MATCH three-year drinking outcomes. *Alcoholism: Clinical and Experimental Research, 22*(6), 1300–1311.

Project MATCH Research Group. (1998b). Matching patients with alcohol disorders to treatments: Clinical implications from Project MATCH. *Journal of Mental Health, 7*(6), 589–602.

Project MATCH Research Group. (1998c). Matching alcoholism treatments to client heterogeneity: Treatment main effects and matching effects on drinking during treatment. *Journal of Studies on Alcohol, 59,* 631–639.

Project MATCH Research Group. (1998d). Therapist effects in three treatments for alcohol problems. *Psychotherapy Research, 8,* 455–474.

Project MATCH Research Group. (1998e). Therapist effects in three treatments for alcohol problems. *Psychotherapy Research, 8,* 455–474.

Prue, D. M., Keane, T. M., Cornell, J. E., & Foy, D. W. (1979). An analysis of distance variables that affect aftercare attendance. *Community Mental Health Journal, 15,* 149–154.

Pruyser, P. W. (1976). *The minister as diagnostician: Personal problems in pastoral perspective.* Philadelphia: Westminster Press.

Quisenberry, A., Eddy, C. R., Patterson, D. L., Franck, C. T., & Bickel, W. K. (2015). Regret expression and social learning increases delay to sexual gratification. *PLOS ONE, 10*(8), e0135977.

Quisenberry, A., Koffarnus, M. N., Franck, C., & Bickel, W. K. (2015). Strength from recovery: Former drug-dependent individuals discount the future less than current users and controls. *Drug and Alcohol Dependence, 156,* e183.

Rachman, A. W. (1990). Judicious self-disclosure in group analysis. *Group, 14*(3), 132–144.

Rapp, C. A., & Goscha, R. J. (2006). *The strengths model: Case management with people with psychiatric disabilities* (2nd ed.). New York: Oxford University Press.

Rapp, R. C. (2002). Strengths-based case management: Enhancing treatment for persons with substance abuse problems. In D. Saleebey (Ed.), *The strengths perspective in social work practice* (3rd ed., pp. 124–142). New York: Allyn & Bacon.

Rapp, R. C., Kelliher, C. W., Fisher, J. H., & Hall, F. J. (1994). Strengths-based case management: A role in addressing denial in substance abuse treatment. *Journal of Case Management, 3,* 139–144.

Rapp, R. C., Kelliher, C. W., Fisher, J. H., & Hall, F. J. (1996). Strengths-based case management: A role in addressing denial in substance abuse treatment. In H. A. Siegal & R. C. Rapp (Eds.), *Case management and substance abuse treatment: Practice and experience* (pp. 21–36). New York: Springer.

Rapp, R. C., Otto, A. L., Lane, D. T., Redko, C., McGatha, S., & Carlson, R. G. (2008). Improving linkage with substance abuse treatment using brief case management and motivational interviewing. *Drug and Alcohol Dependence, 94*(1–3), 172–182.

Rapp, R. C., Van Den Noortgate, W., Broekaert, E., & Vanderplasschen, W. (2014). The efficacy of case management with persons who have substance abuse problems: A three-level meta-analysis of outcomes. *Journal of Consulting and Clinical Psychology, 82*(4), 605–618.

Rapp, R. C., Xu, J., Carr, C. A., Lane, D. T., Wang, J., & Carlson, R. (2006). Treatment barriers identified by substance abusers assessed at a centralized intake unit. *Journal of Substance Abuse Treatment, 30*(3), 227–235.

Rash, C. J., Stitzer, M., & Weinstock, J. (2017). Contingency management: New directions and remaining challenges for an evidence-based intervention. *Journal of Substance Abuse Treatment, 72,* 10–18.

Rawls, J. (1971/1999). *A theory of justice.* Boston: Belknap Press of Harvard University Press.

Reback, C. J., Peck, J. A., Dierst-Davies, R., Nuno, M., Kamien, J. B., & Amass, L. (2010). Contingency management among homeless, out-of-treatment men who have sex with men. *Journal of Substance Abuse Treatment, 39*(3), 255–263.

Rehm, J., Baliunas, D., Borges, G. L., Graham, K., Irving, H., Kehoe, T., . . . Taylor, B. (2010). The relation between different dimensions of alcohol consumption and burden of disease: An overview. *Addiction, 105*(5), 817–843.

Rentscher, K. E., Soriano, E. C., Rohrbaugh, M. J., Shoham, V., & Mehl, M. R. (2017). Partner pronoun use, communal coping, and abstinence during couple-focused intervention for problematic alcohol use. *Family Process, 56*(2), 348–363.

Richards, W. A. (2008). The phenomenology and potential religious import of states of consciousness facilitated by psilocybin. *Archive for the Psychology of Religion, 30*(1), 189–199.

Richter, K. P., & Ellerbeck, E. F. (2015). It's time to change the default for tobacco treatment. *Addiction, 110*(3), 381–386.

Ridgely, M. (1994). Practical issues in the application of case management to substance abuse treatment. *Journal of Case Management, 3*(4), 132–138.

Ries, R. K., Dyck, D. G., Short, R., Srebnik, D., Fisher, A., & Comtois, K. A. (2004). Outcomes of managing disability benefits among patients with substance dependence and severe mental illness. *Psychiatric Services, 55*(4), 445–447.

Rinker, D. V., & Neighbors, C. (2015). Latent class analysis of DSM-5 alcohol use disorder criteria among heavy-drinking college students. *Journal of Substance Abuse Treatment, 57,* 81–88.

Riordan, B. C., Conner, T. S., Flett, J. A. M., & Scarf, D. (2015). A brief orientation week ecological momentary intervention to reduce university student alcohol consumption. *Journal of Studies on Alcohol and Drugs, 76,* 525–529.

Roback, H. B. (2000). Adverse outcomes in group psychotherapy: Risk factors, prevention, and research directions. *Journal of Psychotherapy Practice and Research, 9*(3), 113–122.

Robbins, M. S., Feaster, D. J., Horigian, V. E., Rohrbaugh, M., Shoham, V., Bachrach, K., . . . Szapocznik, J. (2011). Brief strategic family therapy versus treatment as usual: Results of a multisite randomized trial for substance using adolescents. *Journal of Consulting and Clinical Psychology, 79*(6), 713–727.

Robbins, M. S., Szapocznik, J., & Horigian, V. E. (2009). Brief strategic family therapy for adolescents with behavior problems. In J. H. Bray & M. Stanton (Eds.), *The Wiley–Blackwell handbook of family psychology* (pp. 416–430). Chistester, UK: Wiley–Blackwell.

Roberts, M. (2001). *Horse sense for people.* Toronto, ON, Canada: Knopf.

Robertson, A. G., & Swartz, M. S. (2018). Extended-release naltrexone and drug treatment courts: Policy and evidence for implementing an evidence-based treatment. *Journal of Substance Abuse Treatment, 85,* 101–104.

Robins, L. N., Cottler, L. B., Bucholz, K. K., Compton, W. M., North, C. S., & Rourke, K. M. (2000). *Diagnostic Interview Schedule for the DSM-IV (DIS-IV).* St. Louis, MO: Washington University School of Medicine.

Robins, L. N., Helzer, J. E., & Davis, D. H. (1975). Narcotic use in Southeast Asia and afterward: An interview study of 898 Vietnam veterans. *Archives of General Psychiatry, 32,* 955–961.

Robinson, E. A., Cranford, J. A., Webb, J. R., & Brower, K. J. (2007). Six-month changes in spirituality, religiousness, and heavy drinking in a treatment-seeking sample. *Journal of Studies on Alcohol and Drugs, 68*(2), 282–290.

Robinson, E. A., Krentzman, A. R., Webb, J. R., & Brower, K. J. (2011). Six-month changes in spirituality and religiousness in alcoholics predict drinking outcomes at nine months. *Journal of Studies on Alcohol and Drugs, 72*(4), 660–668.

Robinson, J., Sareen, J., Cox, B. J., & Boulton, J. M. (2011). Role of self-medication in the development of comorbid anxiety and substance use disorders: A longitudinal investigation. *Archives of General Psychiatry, 68*(8), 800–807.

Robles, R. R., Reyes, J. C., Colón, H. M., Sahai, H., Marrero, C. A., Matos, T. D., . . . Shepard, E. W. (2004). Effects of combined counseling and case management to reduce HIV risk behaviors among Hispanic drug injectors in Puerto Rico: A randomized controlled study. *Journal of Substance Abuse Treatment, 27*(2), 145–152.

Roerecke, M., & Rehm, J. (2013). Alcohol use disorders and mortality: A systematic review and meta-analysis. *Addiction, 108,* 1562–1578.

Rogers, C. R. (1959). A theory of therapy, personality, and interpersonal relationships as developed in the client-centered framework. In S. Koch (Ed.), *Psychology: The study of a science: Vol. 3. Formulations of the person and the social contexts* (pp. 184–256). New York: McGraw-Hill.

Rogers, C. R. (1980). *A way of being.* Boston: Houghton Mifflin.

Rogers, E. M. (2003). *Diffusion of innovations* (5th ed.). New York: Free Press.

Rohr, R. (2011). *Breathing under water: Spirituality and the twelve steps.* Cincinnati, OH: St. Anthony Messenger Press.

Rohsenow, D. J. (1983). Drinking habits and expectancies about alcohol's effects for self versus others. *Journal of Consulting and Clinical Psychology, 51*(5), 752–756.

Rohsenow, D. J., Colby, S. M., Monti, P. M., Swift, R. M., Martin, R. A., Mueller, T. I., . . . Eaton, C. A. (2000). Predictors of compliance with naltrexone among alcoholics. *Alcoholism, Clinical and Experimental Research, 24*(10), 1542–1549.

Rohsenow, D. J., Tidey, J. W., Martin, R. A., Colby, S. M., Sirota, A. D., Swift, R. M., & Monti, P. M. (2015). Contingent vouchers and motivational interviewing for cigarette smokers in residential substance abuse treatment. *Journal of Substance Abuse Treatment, 55,* 29–38.

Rokeach, M. (1973). *The nature of human values.* New York: Free Press.

Rollnick, S. (1998). Readiness, importance, and confidence: Critical conditions of change in treatment. In W. R. Miller & N. Heather (Eds.), *Treating addictive behaviors* (2nd ed., pp. 49–60). New York: Plenum Press.

Rollnick, S., Heather, N., Gold, R., & Hall, W. (1992). Development of a short "readiness to change" questionnaire for use in brief, opportunistic interventions among excessive drinkers. *British Journal of Addiction, 87*(5), 743–754.

Rollnick, S., Miller, W. R., & Butler, C. (2008). *Motivational interviewing in health care: Helping patients change behavior.* New York: Guilford Press.

Room, R., & Greenfield, T. (1993). Alcoholics Anonymous, other 12-step movements and psychotherapy in the US population, 1990. *Addiction, 88,* 555–562.

Roos, C. R., & Witkiewitz, K. (2016). Adding tools to the toolbox: The role of coping repertoire in alcohol treatment. *Journal of Consulting and Clinical Psychology, 84*(7), 599–601.

Roozen, H. G. (2010). Community reinforcement and family training: An effective option to engage treatment-resistant substance-abusing individuals in treatment. *Addiction, 105*(10), 1729–1738.

Rose, S., & Zweben, A. (2003). Interrelationship of substance abuse and social problems. In W. R. Miller & C. Weisner (Eds.), *Addressing addictions through health and social systems* (pp. 145–156). New York: Plenum Press.

Rose, S., Zweben, A., Ockert, D., & Baier, A. (2014). Interface between substance abuse treatment and other health and social systems. In B. McCrady & E. Epstein (Eds.), *Addition: A comprehensive guidebook for practitioners* (2nd ed., pp. 421–438). New York: Guilford Press.

Rose, S., Zweben, A., & Stoffel, V. (1999). Interfaces between substance abuse treatment and other health and social systems. In B. S. McCrady & E. E. Epstein (Eds.), *Addiction: A comprehensive guidebook for practitioners* (pp. 421–436). New York: Guilford Press.

Rosenberg, M. B. (2015). *Nonviolent communication: A language of life.* Encinitas, CA: Puddle Dancer Press.

Rosenblum, A. (2012). Computer-based interventions: Development, implementation and outcomes. *Journal of Substance Abuse Treatment, 43*(3), e4.

Rosengren, D. B. (2009). *Building motivational interviewing skills: A practiitioner workbook.* New York: Guilford Press.

Rosengren, D. B. (2018). *Building motivational interviewing skills: A practitioner workbook* (2nd ed.). New York: Guilford Press.

Rothman, J. (2003). An overview of case management. In A. R. Roberts & G. J. Greene (Eds.), *Social worker's desk reference* (pp. 467–480). Washington, DC: National Association of Social Workers.

Rotunda, R. J., West, L., & O'Farrell, T. J. (2004). Enabling behavior in a clinical sample of alcohol-dependent clients and their partners. *Journal of Substance Abuse Treatment, 26*(4), 269–276.

Rowe, C. L. (2012). Family therapy for drug abuse: Review and updates 2003–2010. *Journal of Marital and Family Therapy, 38,* 59–81.

Rowe, C., Rigter, H., Henderson, C., Gantner, A., Mos, K., Nielsen, P., & Phan, O. (2013). Implementation fidelity of multidimensional family therapy in an international trial. *Journal of Substance Abuse Treatment, 44*(4), 391–399.

Rudd, R. A., Aleshire, N., Zibbell, J. E., & Gladden, R. M. (2016). Increases in drug and opioid overdose deaths—United States, 2000–2014. *Morbidity and Mortality Weekly Report, 64*(50–51), 1378–1382.

Ruether, R. R. (1998). *Women and redemption: A theological history.* Minneapolis, MN: Augsburg Fortress.

Russell, M., Martier, S. S., Sokol, R. J., Mudar, P., Bottoms, S., Jacobson, S., & Jacobson, J. (1994). Screening for pregnancy risk-drinking. *Alcoholism: Clinical and Experimental Research, 18*(5), 1156–1161.

Rutan, J. S., Stone, W. N., & Shay, J. J. (2014). *Psychodynamic group psychotherapy* (5th ed.). New York: Guilford Press.

Ryan, R. M., & Deci, E. L. (2008). A self-determination theory approach to psychotherapy: The motivational basis for effective change. *Canadian Psychology, 49,* 186–193.

Rychtarik, R. G., Connors, G. J., Dermen, K. H., & Stasiewicz, P. R. (2000). Alcoholics Anonymous and the use of medications to prevent relapse: An anonymous survey of member attitudes. *Journal of Studies on Alcohol, 61,* 134–138.

Sacks, S., & Ries, R. K. (Eds.). (2005). *Substance abuse treatment for persons with co-occurring disorders* (Treatment Improvement Protocol 42). Rockville, MD: Center for Substance Abuse Treatment.

Safren, S. A., Sprich, S., Perlman, C. A., & Otto, M. W. (2005). *Mastering your adult ADHD: A cognitive-behavioral treatment program client workbook.* New York: Oxford University Press.

Saitz, R. (2005). Unhealthy alcohol use. *New England Journal of Medicine, 352*(6), 596–607.

Saitz, R., Cheng, D. M., Allensworth-Davies, D., Winter, M. R., & Smith, P. C. (2014). The ability of single screening questions for unhealthy alcohol and other drug use to identify substance dependence in primary care. *Journal of Studies on Alcohol and Drugs, 75*(1), 153–157.

Saitz, R., Horton, N. J., Larson, M. J., Winter, M., & Samet, J. H. (2005). Primary medical care and reductions in addiction severity: A prospective cohort study. *Addiction, 100*(1), 70–78.

Saitz, R., Larson, M. J., LaBelle, C., Richardson, J., & Samet, J. H. (2008). The case for chronic disease management for addiction. *Journal of Addiction Medicine, 2*(2), 55–65.

Saitz, R., Palfai, T. P., Cheng, D. M., Alford, D. P., Bernstein, J. A., Lloyd-Travaglini, C. A., . . . Samet, J. H. (2014). Screening and brief intervention for drug use in primary care: The ASPIRE randomized clinical trial. *JAMA, 312*(5), 502–513.

Salas-Wright, C. P., Vaughn, M. G., Maynard, B. R., Clark, T. T., & Snyder, S. (2017). Public or private religiosity: Which is protective for adolescent substance use and by what pathways? *Youth and Society, 49*(2), 228–253.

Salvendy, J. T. (1999). Ethnocultural considerations in group psychotherapy. *International Journal of Group Psychotherapy, 49,* 429–464.

Salzberg, S. (2010). *Real happiness: The power of meditation.* New York: Workman.

Samaha, A.-N. (2014). Can antipsychotic treatment contribute to drug addiction in schizophrenia? *Progress in Neuro-Psychopharmacology and Biological Psychiatry, 52,* 9–16.

Samet, J. H., & Fiellin, D. A. (2015). Opioid substitution therapy—Time to replace the term. *The Lancet, 385*(9977), 1508–1509.

Samet, J. H., Friedmann, P., & Saitz, R. (2001). Benefits of linking primary medical care and substance abuse services: Patient, provider, and societal perspectives. *Archives of Internal Medicine, 161*(1), 85–91.

SAMHSA Office of Applied Studies. (2010). *National Survey of Substance Abuse Treatment Services (N-SSATS): Data on substance abuse treatment facilities* (DASIS Series: S-54, HHS Publication No. 10-4579). Rockville, MD: Substance Abuse and Mental Health Services Administration.

Samson, J. E., & Tanner-Smith, E. E. (2015). Single-session alcohol interventions for heavy drinking college students: A systematic review and meta-analysis. *Journal of Studies on Alcohol and Drugs, 76*(4), 530–543.

Sanchez-Craig, M. (1980). Random assignment to abstinence or controlled drinking in a cognitive-behavioral program: Short-term effects on drinking behavior. *Addictive Behaviors, 5,* 35–39.

Sanchez-Craig, M. (1995). *Drink Wise: How to quit drinking or cut down* (2nd ed.). Toronto, ON, Canada: Centre for Addiction and Mental Health.

Sanchez-Craig, M. (1996). *A therapist's manual: Secondary prevention of alcohol problems.* Toronto, ON, Canada: Addiction Research Foundation.

Sanchez-Craig, M., Davila, R., & Cooper, G. (1996). A self-help approach for high-risk drinking: Effect of an initial assessment. *Journal of Consulting and Clinical Psychology, 64,* 694–700.

Santa Ana, E. J., LaRowe, S. D., Armeson, K., Lamb, K. E., & Hartwell, K. (2016). Impact of group motivational interviewing on enhancing treatment engagement for homeless veterans with nicotine dependence and other substance use disorders: A pilot investigation. *American Journal on Addictions, 25*(7), 533–541.

Santisteban, D. A., Perez-Vidal, A., Coatsworth, J. D., Kurtines, W. M., Schwartz, S. J., LaPerriere, A., & Szapocznik, J. (2003). Efficacy of brief strategic family therapy in modifying Hispanic adolescent behavior problems and substance use. *Journal of Family Psychology, 17*(1), 121–133.

Sarkola, T., Dahl, H., Eriksson, C. P., & Helander, A. (2003). Urinary ethyl glucuronide and 5-hydroxytryptophol levels during repeated ethanol ingestion in healthy human subjects. *Alcohol and Alcoholism, 38*(4), 347–351.

Sartor, C. E., Lynskey, M. T., Heath, A. C., Jacob, T., & True, W. (2007). The role of childhood risk factors in initiation of alcohol use and progression to alcohol dependence. *Addiction, 102*(2), 216–225.

Sass, H., Soyka, M., Mann, K., & Zieglgänsberger, W. (1996). Relapse prevention by acamprosate: Results from a placebo-controlled study on alcohol dependence. *Archives of General Psychiatry, 53*(8), 673–680.

Saunders, B., Wilkinson, C., & Phillips, M. (1995). The impact of a brief motivational intervention with opiate users attending a methadone programme. *Addiction, 90*(3), 415–424.

Sawangjit, R., Khan, T. M., & Chaiyakunapruk, N. (2017). Effectiveness of pharmacy-based needle/syringe exchange programme for people who inject drugs: A systematic review and meta-analysis. *Addiction, 112*(2), 236–247.

Sawyer, A. M., & Borduin, C. M. (2011). Effects of multisystemic therapy through midlife: A 21.9-year follow-up to a randomized clinical trial with serious and violent juvenile offenders. *Journal of Consulting and Clinical Psychology, 79*(5), 643–652.

Sayegh, C. S., Huey, S. J., Zara, E. J., & Jhaveri, K. (2017). Follow-up treatment effects of contingency management and motivational interviewing on substance use: A meta-analysis. *Psychology of Addictive Behaviors, 31*(4), 403–414.

Sayers, S. L., Kohn, C. S., & Heavey, C. (1998). Prevention of marital dysfunction: Behavioral approaches and beyond. *Clinical Psychology Review, 18*(6), 713–744.

Schaef, A. W. (1992). *Co-dependence: Misunderstood—mistreated.* San Francisco: Harper.

Schmidt, E. A., Carns, A., & Chandler, C. (2001). Assessing the efficacy of Rational Recovery in the treatment of alcohol/drug dependency. *Alcoholism Treatment Quarterly, 19,* 97–106.

Schmidt, L. K., Bojesen, A. B., Nielsen, A. S., & Andersen, K. (2018). Duration of therapy—Does it matter?: A systematic review and meta-regression of the duration of psychosocial treatments for alcohol use disorder. *Journal of Substance Abuse Treatment, 84,* 57–67.

Schmidt, L. A., Rieckmann, T., Abraham, A., Molfenter, T., Capoccia, V., Roman, P., . . . McCarty, D. (2012). Advancing recovery: Implementing evidence-based treatment for substance use disorders at the systems level. *Journal of Studies on Alcohol and Drugs, 73*(3), 413–422.

Schoenthaler, S. J., Blum, K., Braverman, E. R., Giordano, J., Thompson, B., Oscar-Berman, M., . . . Gold, M. S. (2015). NIDA-Drug Addiction Treatment Outcome Study (DATOS) relapse as a function of spirituality/religiosity. *Journal of Reward Deficiency Syndrome, 1*(1), 36–45.

Schomerus, G., Corrigan, P. W., Klauer, T., Kuwert, P., Freyberger, H. J., & Lucht, M. (2011). Self-stigma in alcohol dependence: Consequences for drinking-refusal self-efficacy. *Drug and Alcohol Dependence, 114*(1), 12–17.

Schomerus, G., Lucht, M., Holzinger, A., Matschinger, H., Carta, M. G., & Anger-meyer, M. C. (2011). The stigma of alcohol dependence compared with other mental disorders: A review of population studies. *Alcohol and Alcoholism, 46*(2), 105–112.

Schuckard, E., Miller, S. D., & Hubble, M. A. (2017). Feedback informed treatment: Historical and empirical foundations. In D. S. Prescott, C. L. Maeschalck, & S. D. Miller (Eds.), *Feedback informed treatment in clinical practice: Reaching for excellence.* Washington, DC: American Psychological Association.

Schuckit, M. A. (2009). An overview of genetic influences in alcoholism. *Journal of Substance Abuse Treatment, 36*(1), S1–S14.

Schuckit, M. A., Mazzanti, C., Smith, T. L., Ahmed, U., Radel, M., Iwata, N., & Goldman, D. (1999). Selective genotyping for the role of 5-HT 2A, 5-HT 2C, and GABA α6 receptors and the serotonin transporter in the level of response to alcohol: A pilot study. *Biological Psychiatry, 45*(5), 647–651.

Schuckit, M. A., & Smith, T. L. (2010). Onset and course of alcoholism over 25 years in middle class men. *Drug and Alcohol Dependence, 113*(1), 21–28.

Schumm, J. A., O'Farrell, T. J., Kahler, C. W., Murphy, M. M., & Muchowski, P. (2014). A randomized clinical trial of behavioral couples therapy versus individually based treatment for women with alcohol dependence. *Journal of Consulting and Clinical Psychology, 82*(6), 993–1004.

Schumm, J. A., O'Farrell, T. J., Murphy, C. M., & Fals-Stewart, W. (2009). Partner violence before and after couples-based alcoholism treatment for female alcoholic patients. *Journal of Consulting and Clinical Psychology, 77*(6), 1136–1146.

Schunk, D. H. (1991). Self-efficacy and academic motivation. *Educational Psychologist, 26,* 207–231.

Schwalbe, C. S., Oh, H. Y., & Zweben, A. (2014). Sustaining motivational interviewing: A meta-analysis of training studies. *Addiction, 109*(8), 1287–1294.

Schwartz, R. P., Gryczynski, J., Mitchell, S. G., Gonzales, A., Moseley, A., Peterson, T. R., . . . O'Grady, K. E. (2014). Computerized versus in-person brief intervention for drug misuse: A randomized clinical trial. *Addiction, 109*(7), 1091–1098.

Schwartz, R. P., Kelly, S. M., O'Grady, K. E., Gandhi, D., & Jaffe, J. H. (2011). Interim methadone treatment compared to standard methadone treatment: 4-month findings. *Journal of Substance Abuse Treatment, 41*(1), 21–29.

Scott, C. K., & Dennis, M. L. (2009). Results from two randomized clinical trials evaluating the impact of quarterly recovery management checkups with adult chronic substance users. *Addiction, 104*(6), 959–971.

Secades-Villa, R., Garcia-Fernandez, G., Pena-Suarez, E., Garcia-Rodriguez, O., Sanchez-Hervas, E., & Fernandez-Hermida, J. R. (2013). Contingency management is effective across cocaine-dependent outpatients with different socioeconomic status. *Journal of Substance Abuse Treatment, 44*(3), 349–354.

Secades-Villa, R., Garcia-Rodriguez, O., Lopez-Nunez, C., Alonso-Perez, F., & Fernandez-Hermida, J. R. (2014). Contingency management for smoking cessation among treatment-seeking patients in a community setting. *Drug and Alcohol Dependence, 140,* 63–68.

Sellman, J. D., Sullivan, P. F., Dore, G. M., Adamson, S. J., & MacEwan, I. (2001). A randomized controlled trial of motivational enhancement therapy (MET) for mild to moderate alcohol dependence. *Journal of Studies on Alcohol, 62,* 389–396.

Semaan, S., Neumann, M. S., Hutchins, K., D'Anna, L. H., & Kamb, M. L. (2010). Brief counseling for reducing sexual risk and bacterial STIs among drug users— Results from project RESPECT. *Drug and Alcohol Dependence, 106*(1), 7–15.

Serebruany, V. L., Oshrine, B. R., Malinin, A. I., Atar, D., Michelson, A. D., & Ferguson, J. J., 3rd. (2005). Noncompliance in cardiovascular clinical trials. *American Heart Journal, 150*(5), 882–886.

Shafil, M., Lavely, R., & Jaffe, R. (1975). Meditation and the prevention of alcohol abuse. *American Journal of Psychiatry, 132*(9), 942–945.

Shaner, A., Eckman, T. A., Roberts, L. J., Wilkins, J. N., Tucker, D. E., Tsuang, J. W., & Mintz, J. (1995). Disability income, cocaine use, and repeated hospitalization among schizophrenic cocaine abusers: A government-sponsored revolving door? *New England Journal of Medicine, 333,* 777–783.

Shapiro, S. L., Astin, J. A., Bishop, S. R., & Cordova, M. (2005). Mindfulness-based stress reduction for health care professionals: Results from a randomized trial. *International Journal of Stress Management, 12*(2), 164–176.

Shapiro, S. L., Brown, K. W., Thoresen, C., & Plante, T. G. (2011). The moderation of mindfulness-based stress reduction effects by trait mindfulness: Results from a randomized controlled trial. *Journal of Clinical Psychology, 67*(3), 267–277.

Sharon, E., Krebs, C., Turner, W., Desai, N., Binus, G., & Penk, W. (2004). Predictive validity of the ASAM patient placement criteria for hospital utilization. *Journal of Addictive Diseases, 22,* 79–93.

Shavelson, L. (2001). *Hooked: Five addicts challenge our misguided drug rehab system.* New York: Norton.

Shepard, D. S., Lwin, A. K., Barnett, N. P., Mastroleo, N., Colby, S. M., Gwaltney, C., & Monti, P. M. (2016). Cost-effectiveness of motiational intervention with significant others for patients with alcohol abuse. *Addiction, 111*, 832–839.

Shevlov, D. V., Suchday, S., & Friedberg, J. P. (2009). A pilot study measuring the impact of yoga on the trait of mindfulness. *Behavioural and Cognitive Psychotherapy, 37*(5), 595–598.

Shorey, R. C., Martino, S., Lamb, K. E., LaRowe, S. D., & Santa Ana, E. J. (2015). Change talk and relatedness in group motivational interviewing: A pilot study. *Journal of Substance Abuse Treatment, 51*, 75–81.

Shorkey, C. T., & Rosen, W. (1993). Alcohol addiction and codependency. In E. M. Freeman (Ed.), *Substance abuse treatment: A family systems perspective* (pp. 100–122). Thousand Oaks, CA: SAGE.

Siegal, H. A., Fisher, J. H., Rapp, R. C., Kelliher, C. W., Wagner, J. H., O'Brien, W. F., & Cole, P. A. (1996). Enhancing substance abuse treatment with case management: Its impact on employment. *Journal of Substance Abuse Treatment, 13*(2), 93–98.

Siegal, H. A., Li, L., & Rapp, R. C. (2002). Case management as a therapeutic enhancement: Impact on post-treatment criminality. *Journal of Addictive Diseases, 21*(4), 37–46.

Siegal, H. A., Rapp, R. C., Kelliher, C. W., Fisher, J. H., Wagner, J. H., & Cole, P. A. (1995). The strengths perspective of case management: A promising inpatient substance abuse treatment enhancement. *Journal of Psychoactive Drugs, 27*(1), 67–72.

Siegal, H. A., Rapp, R. C., Li, L., Saha, P., & Kirk, K. D. (1997). The role of case management in retaining clients in substance abuse treatment: An exploratory analysis. *Journal of Drug Issues, 27*(4), 821–832.

Simioni, N., Rolland, B., & Cottencin, O. (2015). Interventions for increasing alcohol treatment utilization among patients with alcohol use disorders from emergency departments: A systematic review. *Journal of Substance Abuse Treatment, 58*, 6–15.

Simpson, T. L., & Miller, W. R. (2002). Concomitance between childhood sexual and physical abuse and substance use disorders. *Clinical Psychology Review, 22*, 27–77.

Sinadinovic, K., Wennberg, P., & Berman, A. H. (2014). Internet-based screening and brief intervention for illicit drug users: A randomized controlled trial with 12-month follow-up. *Journal of Studies on Alcohol and Drugs, 75*, 428–436.

Sinclair, J. D. (2001). Evidence about the use of naltrexone and for different ways of using it in the treatment of alcoholism. *Alcohol and Alcoholism, 36*(1), 2–10.

Singleton, C. K., & Martin, P. R. (2001). Molecular mechanisms of thiamine utilization. *Current Molecular Medicine, 1*(2), 197–207.

Sisson, R. W., & Azrin, N. H. (1986). Family-member involvement to initiate and promote treatment of problem drinkers. *Journal of Behavior Therapy and Experimental Psychiatry, 17*, 15–21.

Sisson, R. W., & Azrin, N. H. (1993). Community reinforcement training for families: A method to get alcoholics into treatment. In T. J. O'Farrell (Ed.), *Treating alcohol problems: Marital and family interventions* (pp. 242–258). New York: Guilford Press.

Sisson, R. W., & Mallams, J. H. (1981). The use of systematic encouragement and community access procedures to increase attendance at Alcoholics Anonymous and Al-Anon meetings. *American Journal of Drug and Alcohol Abuse, 8*, 371–376.

Skoglund, C., Hermansson, U., & Beck, O. (2015). Clinical trial of a new technique for drugs of abuse testing: A new possible sampling technique. *Journal of Substance Abuse Treatment, 48*(1), 132–136.

Slesnick, N., Guo, X., Brakenhoff, B., & Bantchevska, D. (2015). A comparison of three interventions for homeless youth evidencing substance use disorders: Results of a randomized clinical trial. *Journal of Substance Abuse Treatment, 54,* 1–13.

Slesnick, N., Kang, M. J., Bonomi, A. E., & Prestopnik, J. L. (2008). Six- and twelve-month outcomes among homeless youth accessing therapy and case management services through an urban drop-in center. *Health Services Research, 43*(1), 211–229.

Slesnick, N., Meyers, R. J., Mead, M., & Segelken, D. H. (2000). Bleak and hopeless no more: Engagement of runaway substance abusing youth and their families. *Journal of Substance Abuse Treatment, 19,* 215–222.

Slesnick, N., & Prestopnik, J. L. (2009). Comparison of family therapy outcome with alcohol-abusing, runaway adolescents. *Journal of Marital and Family Therapy, 35*(3), 255–277.

Slesnick, N., Prestopnik, J. L., Meyers, R. J., & Glassman, M. (2007). Treatment outcome for street-living, homeless youth. *Addictive Behaviors, 32,* 1237–1251.

Smeerdijk, M., Keet, R., Dekker, N., van Raaij, B., Krikke, M., Koeter, M., . . . Linszen, D. (2012). Motivational interviewing and interaction skills training for parents to change cannabis use in young adults with recent-onset schizophrenia: A randomized controlled trial. *Psychological Medicine, 42*(8), 1627–1636.

Smeerdijk, M., Keet, R., van Raaij, B., Koeter, M., Linszen, D., de Haan, L., & Schippers, G. (2015). Motivational interviewing and interaction skills training for parents of young adults with recent-onset schizophrenia and co-occurring cannabis use: 15-month follow-up. *Psychological Medicine, 45*(13), 2839–2848.

Smith, D. C., Davis, J. P., Ureche, D. J., & Dumas, T. M. (2016). Six month outcomes of a peer-enhanced community reinforcement approach for emerging adults with substance misuse: A preliminary study. *Journal of Substance Abuse Treatment, 61,* 66–73.

Smith, J. E., Gianini, L. M., Garner, B. R., Malek, K. L., & Godley, S. H. (2014). A behaviorally-anchored rating system to monitor treatment integrity for community clinicians using the adolescent community reinforcement approach. *Journal of Child and Adolescent Substance Abuse, 23*(3), 185–199.

Smith, J. E., & Meyers, R. J. (2004). *Motivating substance abusers to enter treatment: Working with family members.* New York: Guilford Press.

Smith, J. E., Meyers, R. J., & Delaney, H. D. (1998). The community reinforcement approach with homeless alcohol-dependent individuals. *Journal of Consulting and Clinical Psychology, 66,* 541–548.

Smith, J. P., & Randall, C. L. (2012). Anxiety and alcohol use disorders: Comorbidity and treatment considerations. *Alcohol Research: Current Reviews, 34*(4), 414–431.

Smith, P. C., Schmidt, S. M., Allensworth-Davies, D., & Saitz, R. (2010). A single-question screening test for drug use in primary care. *Archives of Internal Medicine, 170*(13), 1155–1160.

Smith, P. F., & Darlington, C. L. (1996). The development of psychosis in epilepsy: A re-examination of the kindling hypothesis. *Behavioural Brain Research, 75*(1–2), 59–66.

Smith, R. C., Lein, C., Collins, C., Lyles, J. S., Given, B., Dwamena, F. C., . . . Given, C. W. (2003). Treating patients with medically unexplained symptoms in primary care. *Journal of General Internal Medicine, 18*(6), 478–489.

Smith, S. S., Jorenby, D. E., Fiore, M. C., Anderson, J. E., Mielke, M. M., Beach, K. E., . . . Baker, T. B. (2001). Strike while the iron is hot: Can stepped-care treatments resurrect relapsing smokers? *Journal of Consulting and Clinical Psychology, 69*(3), 429–439.

Sobell, L. C., & Sobell, M. B. (1992). Timeline follow-back: A technique for assessing self-reported alcohol consumption. In R. A. Litten & J. P. Allen (Eds.), *Measuring alcohol consumption: Psychosocial and biological methods* (pp. 41–72). Totowa, NJ: Humana Press.

Sobell, L. C., & Sobell, M. B. (1996). *Timeline follow back: A calendar method for assessing alcohol and drug use (user's guide)*. Toronto, ON, Canada: Addiction Research Foundation.

Sobell, L. C., & Sobell, M. B. (2011). *Group therapy for substance use disorders.* New York: Guilford Press.

Sobell, M. B., & Sobell, L. C. (2000). Stepped care as a heuristic approach to the treatment of alcohol problems. *Journal of Consulting and Clinical Psychology, 68*(4), 573–579.

Solomon, K. E., & Annis, H. M. (1990). Outcome and efficacy expectancy in the prediction of post-treatment drinking behaviour. *British Journal of Addiction, 85*(5), 659–665.

Sorensen, J. L., & Kosten, T. (2011). Developing the tools of implementation science in substance use disorders treatment: Applications of the consolidated framework for implementation research. *Psychology of Addictive Behaviors, 25*(2), 262–268.

Sournia, J. C. (1990). *A history of alcoholism.* Cambridge, MA: Basil Blackwell.

Spears, C. A., Hedeker, D., Li, L., Wu, C., Anderson, N. K., Houchins, S. C., . . . Wetter, D. W. (2017). Mechanisms underlying mindfulness-based addiction treatment versus cognitive behavioral therapy and usual care for smoking cessation. *Journal of Consulting and Clinical Psychology, 85*(11), 1029–1040.

Srebnik, D., Sugar, A., Coblentz, P., McDonell, M. G., Angelo, F., Lowe, J. M., . . . Roll, J. (2013). Acceptability of contingency management among clinicians and clients within a co-occurring mental health and substance use treatment program. *American Journal on Addictions, 22*(5), 432–436.

SRNT Subcommittee on Biochemical Verification of Tobacco Use And Cessation. (2002). Biochemical verification of tobacco use and cessation. *Nicotine and Tobacco Research, 4*(2), 149–159.

Stahl, S. M. (2017). *Prescriber's guide: Stahl's essential psychopharmacology* (6th ed.). New York: Cambridge University Press.

Stallvik, M., Gastfriend, D. R., & Nordahl, H. M. (2015). Matching patients with substance use disorder to optimal level of care with the ASAM criteria software. *Journal of Substance Use, 20*(6), 389–398.

Stallvik, M., & Nordahl, H. M. (2014). Convergent validity of the ASAM criteria in co-occurring disorders. *Journal of Dual Diagnosis, 10*(2), 68–78.

Stanhope, V., Manuel, J. I., Jessell, L., & Halliday, T. M. (2018). Implementing SBIRT for adolescents within community mental health organizations: A mixed methods study. *Journal of Substance Abuse Treatment, 90*, 38–46.

Stecker, T., McGovern, M. P., & Herr, B. (2012). An intervention to increase alcohol treatment engagement: A pilot trial. *Journal of Substance Abuse Treatment, 43*(2), 161–167.

Stein, M. D., Flori, J. N., Blevins, C. E., Conti, M. T., Anderson, B. J., & Bailey, G. L. (2017). Knowledge, past use, and willingness to start medication-assisted treatment among persons undergoing alcohol detoxification. *American Journal of Addictions, 26*, 118–121.

Stein, M. D., Risi, M. M., Flori, J. N., Conti, M. T., Anderson, B. J., & Bailey, G. L.

(2016). Gender differences in the life concerns of persons seeking alcohol detoxification. *Journal of Substance Abuse Treatment, 53*, 34–38.

Steinberg, M. P., & Miller, W. R. (2015). *Motivational interviewing in diabetes care.* New York: Guilford Press.

Steiner, C. M. (1984). *Games alcoholics play.* New York: Ballantine Books.

Stephens, R. S., Roffman, R. A., Fearer, S. A., Williams, C., & Burke, R. S. (2007). The marijuana check-up: Promoting change in ambivalent marijuana users. *Addiction, 102*(6), 947–957.

Sterling, S., Kline-Simon, A. H., Jones, A., Satre, D. D., Parthasarathy, S., & Weisner, C. (2017). Specialty addiction and psychiatry treatment initiation and engagement: Results from an SBIRT randomized trial in pediatrics. *Journal of Substance Abuse Treatment, 82*, 48–54.

Stevens, S., Arbiter, N., & Glider, P. (1989). Women residents: Expanding their role to increase treatment effectiveness in substance abuse programs. *International Journal of the Addictions, 24*(5), 425–434.

Stinson, F. S., & DeBakey, S. F. (1992). Alcohol-related mortality in the United States: 1979–1988. *British Journal of Addiction, 87*, 777–783.

Stormshak, E. A., Connell, A. M., Véronneau, M.-H., Myers, M. W., Dishion, T. J., Kavanagh, K., & Caruthers, A. S. (2011). An ecological approach to promoting early adolescent mental health and social adaptation: Family-centered intervention in public middle schools. *Child Development, 82*, 209–225.

Stout, R. L., Rubin, A., Zwick, W., Zywiak, W., & Bellino, L. (1999). Optimizing the cost-effectiveness of alcohol treatment: A rationale for extended case monitoring. *Addictive Behaviors, 24*(1), 17–35.

Strain, E. C. (2009). *Incorporating alcohol pharmacotherapies into medical practice: A treatment improvement protocol* (Vol. 27). Rockville, MD: U.S. Department of Health and Human Services.

Substance Abuse and Mental Health Services Administration. (1998). *Comprehensive case management for substance abuse treatment* (Vol. 27). Rockville, MD: U.S. Department of Health and Human Services.

Substance Abuse and Mental Health Services Administration. (2009). *Results from the 2008 national survey on drug use and health: National findings.* Rockville, MD: U.S. Department of Health and Human Services.

Substance Abuse and Mental Health Services Administration. (2012). *Results from the 2011 national survey on drug use and health: Sumary of national findings.* Rockville, MD: Author.

Substance Abuse and Mental Health Services Administration. (2017). *National Survey of Substance Abuse Treatment Services (N-SSATS): 2016.* Rockville, MD: Author.

Sugarman, D. E., Campbell, A. N. C., Iles, B. R., & Greenfield, S. F. (2017). Technology-based interventions for substance use and comorbid disorders: An examination of the emerging literature. *Harvard Review of Psychiatry, 25*(3), 123–134.

Suitt, K. G., Castro, Y., Caetano, R., & Field, C. A. (2015). Predictive utility of alcohol use disorder symptoms across race/ethnicity. *Journal of Substance Abuse Treatment, 56*, 61–67.

Sullivan, J. T., Sykora, K., Schneiderman, J., Naranjo, C. A., & Sellers, E. M. (1989). Assessment of alcohol withdrawal: The Revised Clinical Institute Withdrawal Assessment for Alcohol scale (CIWA-Ar). *British Journal of Addiction, 84*, 1353–1357.

Sullivan, W. P. (2003). Case management with substance-abusing clients. In A. R.

Roberts & G. J. Greene (Eds.), *Social worker's desk reference* (pp. 492–496). Washington, DC: National Association of Social Workers.

Sullivan, W. P., Wolk, J. L., & Hartmann, D. J. (1992). Case management in alcohol and drug treatment: Improving client outcomes. *Families in Society, 73,* 195–203.

Svikis, D. S., Keyser-Marcus, L., Stitzer, M., Rieckmann, T., Safford, L., Loeb, P., . . . Zweben, J. (2012). Randomized multi-site trial of the Job Seekers' Workshop in patients with substance use disorders. *Drug and Alcohol Dependence, 120*(1–3), 55–64.

Swann, A. C. (2010). The strong relationship between bipolar and substance-use disorder. *Annals of the New York Academy of Sciences, 1187,* 276–293.

Swift, J. K., & Callahan, J. L. (2010). A comparison of client preferences for intervention empirical support versus common therapy variables. *Journal of Clinical Psychology, 66*(12), 1217–1231.

Swift, J. K., Callahan, J. L., & Vollmer, B. M. (2011). Preferences. *Journal of Clinical Psychology: In Session, 67*(2), 155–165.

Swift, R. M. (2003). Topiramate for the treatment of alcohol dependence: Initiating abstinence. *The Lancet, 361*(9370), 1666–1667.

Szapocznik, J., Hervis, O., & Schwartz, S. (2003). *Brief strategic family therapy for adolescent drug abuse.* Bethesda, MD: National Institute on Drug Abuse.

Szapocznik, J., Kurtines, W. M., Foote, F. H., Perez-Vidal, A., & Hervis, O. (1983). Conjoint versus one-person family therapy: Some evidence for the effectiveness of conducting family therapy through one person. *Journal of Consulting and Clinical Psychology, 51*(6), 889–899.

Szapocznik, J., Kurtines, W. M., Foote, F. H., Perez-Vidal, A., & Hervis, O. (1986). Conjoint versus one-person family therapy: Further evidence for the effectiveness of conducting family therapy through one person with drug-abusing adolescents. *Journal of Consulting and Clinical Psychology, 54*(3), 395–397.

Szapocznik, J., Muir, J. A., Duff, J. H., Schwartz, S. J., & Brown, C. H. (2015). Brief strategic family therapy: Implementing evidence-based models in community settings. *Psychotherapy Research, 25*(1), 121–133.

Szapocznik, J., Schwartz, S. J., Muir, J. A., & Brown, C. H. (2012). Brief strategic family therapy: An intervention to reduce adolescent risk behavior. *Couple and Family Psychology: Research and Practice, 1*(2), 134–145.

Szapocznik, J., & Williams, R. A. (2000). Brief Strategic Family Therapy: Twenty-five years of interplay among theory, research and practice in adolescent behavior problems and drug abuse. *Clinical Child and Family Psychology Review, 3*(2), 117–134.

Tai, B., Sparenborg, S., Ghitza, U. E., & Liu, D. (2014). Expanding the National Drug Abuse Treatment Clinical Trials Network to address the management of substance use disorders in general medical settings. *Substance Abuse and Rehabilitation, 5,* 75–80.

Takamatsu, S. K., Martens, M. P., & Arterberry, B. J. (2016). Depressive symptoms and gambling behavior: Mediating role of coping motivation and gambling refusal self-efficacy. *Journal of Gambling Studies, 32*(2), 535–546.

Taleff, M. J. (2009). *Advanced ethics for addiction professionals.* New York: Springer.

Tang, Y. Y., Holzel, B. K., & Posner, M. I. (2015). The neuroscience of mindfulness meditation. *Nature Review: Neuroscience, 16*(4), 213–225.

Tanum, L., Solli, K. K., Benth, J. Š., Opheim, A., Sharma-Haase, K., Krajci, P., & Kunøe, N. (2017). Effectiveness of injectable extended-release naltrexone vs daily buprenorphine-naloxone for opioid dependence: A randomized clinical noninferiority trial. *JAMA Psychiatry, 74*(12), 1197–1205.

Tarter, R. E., Kirisci, L., Mezzich, A., Cornelius, J. R., Pajer, K., Vanyukov, M., . . . Clark, D. (2003). Neurobehavioral disinhibition in childhood predicts early age at onset of substance use disorder. *American Journal of Psychiatry, 160*(6), 1078–1085.

Tatarsky, A., & Marlatt, G. A. (2010). State of the art in harm reduction psychotherapy: An emerging treatment for substance misuse. *Journal of Clinical Psychology, 66*, 117–122.

Taxman, F. S. (2012). Justice steps: Implementing contingency management in criminal justice settings. *Journal of Substance Abuse Treatment, 43*(3), e3.

Taylor, M., Leonardi-Bee, J., Agboola, S., McNeill, A., & Coleman, T. (2011). Cost effectiveness of interventions to reduce relapse to smoking following smoking cessation. *Addiction, 106*(10), 1819–1826.

Teesson, M., Marel, C., Darke, S., Ross, J., Slade, T., Burns, L., . . . Mills, K. L. (2015). Long-term mortality, remission, criminality and psychiatric comorbidity of heroin dependence: 11-year findings from the Australian Treatment Outcome Study. *Addiction, 110*(6), 986–993.

Test, M. A. (2003). Guidelines for assertive community treatment teams. In A. R. Roberts & G. J. Greene (Eds.), *Social worker's desk reference* (pp. 511–513). Washington, DC: National Association of Social Workers.

Thich Nhat Hanh. (2015). *The miracle of mindfulness: An introduction to the practice of meditation* (Mobi Ho, Trans.). Boston: Beacon Press.

Thomas, E., Adams, K. B., Yoshioka, M. R., & Ager, R. D. (1990). Unilateral relationship enhancement in the treatment of spouses for uncooperative alcohol abusers. *American Journal of Family Therapy, 18*, 334–344.

Thomas, E., & Santa, C. (1982). Unilateral family therapy for alcohol abuse: A working conception. *American Journal of Family Therapy, 10*, 49–52.

Thomas, E. J., Santa, C., Bronson, D., & Oyserman, D. (1987). Unilateral familly therapy with spouses of alcoholics. *Journal of Social Service Research, 10*, 145–163.

Tiderington, E., Stanhope, V., & Henwood, B. F. (2013). A qualitative analysis of case managers' use of harm reduction in practice. *Journal of Substance Abuse Treatment, 44*(1), 71–77.

Tillich, P. (1973). *Systematic theology* (Vol. 1). Chicago: University of Chicago Press.

Timko, C., Moos, R. H., Finney, J. W., & Lesar, M. D. (2000). Long-term outcomes of alcohol use disorders: Comparing untreated individuals with those in Alcoholics Anonymous and formal treatment. *Journal of Studies on Alcohol, 61*, 529–540.

Tomlin, K. M., & Richardson, H. (2004). *Motivational interviewing and stages of change: Integrating best practices for substance abuse professionals.* Center City, MN: Hazelden.

Toneatto, T., Vettese, L., & Nguyen, L. (2007). The role of mindfulness in the cognitive-behavioural treatment of problem gambling. *Journal of Gambling Issues, 19*, 91–100.

Tonigan, J. S. (2001). Benefits of Alcoholics Anonymous attendance: Replication of findings between clinical research sites in Project MATCH. *Alcoholism Treatment Quarterly, 19*(1), 67–77.

Tonigan, J. S. (2003). Spirituality and AA practices three and ten years after Project MATCH. *Alcoholism: Clinical and Experimental Research, 26*(5), 660A.

Tonigan, J. S., Ashcroft, F., & Miller, W. R. (1995). A.A. group dynamics and 12-step activity. *Journal of Studies on Alcohol, 56*, 616–621.

Tonigan, J. S., Connors, G. J., & Miller, W. R. (1996). The Alcoholics Anonymous

Involvement Scale (AAI): Reliability and norms. *Psychology of Addictive Behaviors, 10,* 75–80.

Tonigan, J. S., Connors, G. J., & Miller, W. R. (2003). Participation and involvement in Alcoholics Anonymous. In T. F. Babor & F. K. D. Boca (Eds.), *Treatment matching in alcoholism* (pp. 184–204). Cambridge, UK: Cambridge University Press.

Tonigan, J. S., & Kelly, J. F. (2004). Beliefs about AA and the use of medications: A comparison of three groups of AA-exposed alcohol dependent persons. *Alcoholism Treatment Quarterly, 22,* 67–78.

Tonigan, J. S., & Miller, W. R. (2002). The Inventory of Drug Use Consequences (InDUC): Test–retest stability and sensitivity to detect change. *Psychology of Addictive Behaviors, 16*(2), 165–168.

Tonigan, J. S., Miller, W. R., & Brown, J. M. (1994). The reliability of Form 90: An instrument for assessing alcohol treatment outcome. *Journal of Studies on Alcohol, 58*(4), 358–364.

Tonigan, J. S., Miller, W. R., & Connors, G. J. (2001). The search for meaning in life as a predictor of alcoholism treatment outcome. In R. Longabaugh & P. W. Wirtz (Eds.), *Project MATCH hypotheses: Results and causal chain analyses* (Vol. 8, pp. 154–165). Bethesda, MD: National Institute on Alcohol Abuse and Alcoholism.

Tonigan, J. S., Miller, W. R., & Schermer, C. (2002). Atheists, agnostics and Alcoholics Anonymous. *Journal of Studies on Alcohol, 63,* 534–541.

Tonigan, J. S., & Rice, S. L. (2010). Is it beneficial to have an AA sponsor? *Psychology of Addictive Behaviors, 24*(3), 397–403.

Tonigan, J. S., Rynes, K., Toscova, R., & Hagler, K. (2013). Do changes in selfishness explain 12-step benefit?: A prospective lagged analysis. *Substance Abuse, 34*(1), 13–19.

Tonstad, S. (2006). Smoking cessation efficacy and safety of varenicline, an α4β2 nicotinic receptor partial agonist. *Journal of Cardiovascular Nursing, 21*(6), 433–436.

Toumbourou, J. W., Hamilton, M., U'Ren, A., Stevens-Jones, P., & Storey, G. (2002). Narcotics Anonymous participation and changes in substance use and social support. *Journal of Substance Abuse Treatment, 23,* 61–66.

Trimpey, J., Velten, E., & Dain, R. (1993). Rational recovery from addictions. In W. Dryden & L. K. Hill (Eds.), *Innovations in rational–emotive therapy* (pp. 253–271). Thousand Oaks, CA: SAGE.

Tross, S., Campbell, A. N. C., Cohen, L. R., Calsyn, D., Pavlicova, M., Miele, G., . . . Nunes, E. V. (2008). Effectiveness of HIV-STD sexual risk reduction groups for women in substance abuse treatment programs: Results of a NIDA Clinical Trials Network trial. *Journal of Acquired Immune Deficiency Syndrome, 48*(5), 581–589.

Truax, C. B., & Carkhuff, R. R. (1967). *Toward effective counseling and psychotherapy.* Chicago: Aldine.

Turner, B. J., McCann, B. S., Dunn, C. W., Darnell, D. A., Beam, C. R., Kleiber, B., . . . Fukunaga, R. (2017). Examining the reach of a brief alcohol intervention service in routine practice at a level 1 trauma center. *Journal of Substance Abuse Treatment, 79,* 29–33.

Tuten, M., DeFulio, A., Jones, H. E., & Stitzer, M. (2012). Abstinence-contingent recovery housing and reinforcement-based treatment following opioid detoxification. *Addiction, 107*(5), 973–982.

U.S. National Commission for the Protection of Human Subjects of Biomedical and

Behavioral Research. (2017). *The Belmont Report: Ethical principles and guidelines for the protection of human subjects of research.* London: Forgotten Books.

UKATT Research Team. (2005). Effectiveness of treatment for alcohol problems: Findings of the randomized UK alcohol treatment trial (UKATT). *British Medical Journal, 331*(7516), 541–544.

Urbanoski, K., Kenaszchuk, C., Inglis, D., Rotondi, N. K., & Rush, B. (2018). A system-level study of initiation, engagement, and equity in outpatient substance use treatment. *Journal of Substance Abuse Treatment, 90,* 19–28.

Urbanoski, K., Veldhuizen, S., Krausz, M., Schutz, C., Somers, J. M., Kirst, M., . . . Goering, P. (2018). Effects of comorbid substance use disorders on outcomes in a Housing First intervention for homeless people with mental illness. *Addiction, 113*(1), 137–145.

Vader, A. M., Walters, S. T., Prabhu, G. C., Houck, J. M., & Field, C. A. (2010). The language of motivational interviewing and feedback: Counselor language, client language, and client drinking outcomes. *Psychology of Addictive Behaviors, 24*(2), 190–197.

Valle, S. K. (1981). Interpersonal functioning of alcoholism counselors and treatment outcome. *Journal of Studies on Alcohol, 42,* 783–790.

Van der Stouwe, T., & Asscher, J. J. (2014). The effectiveness of multisystemic therapy (MST): A meta-analysis. *Clinical Psychology Review, 34*(6), 468–481.

Van Ryzin, M. J., Stormshak, E. A., & Dishion, T. J. (2012). Engaging parents in the family check-up in middle school: Longitudinal effects on family conflict and problem behavior through the high school transition. *Journal of Adolescent Health, 50*(6), 627–633.

Van Staden, C. W., & Krüger, C. (2003). Incapacity to give informed consent owing to mental disorder. *Journal of Medical Ethics, 29,* 41–43.

Vanderplasschen, W., Rapp, R. C., Wolf, J. R., & Broekaert, E. (2004). The development and implementation of case management for substance use disorders in North America and Europe. *Psychiatric Services, 55*(8), 913–922.

Vanderplasschen, W., Wolf, J., Rapp, R. C., & Broekaert, E. (2007). Effectiveness of different models of case management for substance-abusing populations. *Journal of Psychoactive Drugs, 39*(1), 81–95.

Velasquez, M., Maurer, G. G., Crouch, C., & DiClemente, C. C. (2001). *Group treatment for substance abuse: A stages-of-change therapy manual.* New York: Guilford Press.

Velasquez, M. M., Stephens, N. S., & Ingersoll, K. S. (2006). Motivational interviewing in groups. *Journal of Groups in Addiction and Recovery, 1,* 27–50.

Velasquez, M. M., von Sternberg, K., & Parrish, D. E. (2013). CHOICES: An integrated behavioral intervention to prevent alcohol-exposed pregnancies among high-risk women in community settings. *Social Work in Public Health, 28,* 224–233.

Venner, K. L., Feldstein, S. W., & Tafoya, N. (2006). *Adapting helpful treatments for Native Americans: A manual for using motivational interviewing with Native Americans.* Albuquerque: University of New Mexico, Center on Alcoholism, Substance Abuse and Addictions.

Venner, K. L., Feldstein, S. W., & Tafoya, N. (2007). Helping clients feel welcome: Principles of adapting treatment cross culturally. *Alcoholism Treatment Quarterly, 25,* 11–20.

Venner, K. L., Greenfield, B. L., Hagler, K. J., Simmons, J., Lupee, D., Homer, E., . . . Smith, J. E. (2016). Pilot outcome results of culturally adapted evidence-based substance use disorder treatment with a Southwest tribe. *Addictive Behaviors Reports, 3*, 21–27.

Venner, K. L., & Miller, W. R. (2001). Progression of alcohol problems in a Navajo sample. *Journal of Studies on Alcohol, 62*, 158–165.

Vidrine, J. I., Spears, C. A., Heppner, W. L., Reitzel, L. R., Marcus, M. T., Cinciripini, P. M., . . . Wetter, D. W. (2016). Efficacy of mindfulness-based addiction treatment (MBAT) for smoking cessation and lapse recovery: A randomized clinical trial. *Journal of Consulting and Clinical Psychology, 84*(9), 824–838.

Villanti, A. C., Feirman, S. P., Niaura, R. S., Pearson, J. L., Glasser, A. M., Collins, L. K., & Abrams, D. B. (2018). How do we determine the impact of e-cigarettes on cigarette smoking cessation or reduction?: Review and recommendations for answering the research question with scientific rigor. *Addiction, 113*(3), 391–404.

Villanueva, M., Tonigan, J. S., & Miller, W. R. (2007). Response of Native American clients to three treatment methods for alcohol dependence. *Journal of Ethnicity in Substance Abuse, 6*(2), 41–48.

Viner, R. M., Christie, D., Taylor, V., & Hey, S. (2003). Motivational/solution-focused intervention improves HbA1cin adolescents with Type 1 diabetes: A pilot study. *Diabetic Medicine, 20*(9), 739–742.

Vlasova, N., Schumacher, J. E., Oryschhuk, O., Dumchev, K. V., Slobodyanyuk, P., Moroz, V. M., . . . Houser, S. (2011). STEPS outpatient program improves alcohol treatment outcomes in Ukranian regional narcologic dispensary. *Addictive Disorders and Their Treatment, 10*(1), 6–13.

Voegtlin, W. L., & Lemere, F. (1942). The treatment of alcohol addiction: A review of the literature. *Quarterly Journal of Studies on Alcohol, 2*, 717–803.

Vohs, K. D., & Baumeister, R. F. (Eds.). (2011). *Handbook of self-regulation: Research, theory, and applications* (2nd ed.). New York: Guilford Press.

Volkow, N. D. (2017). Medications for opioid use disorder: Bridging the gap in care. *The Lancet, 391*(10118), 285–287.

Volkow, N. D., Koob, G. F., & McLellan, T. (2016). Neurobiologic advances from the brain disease model of addiction. *New England Journal of Medicine, 374*, 363–371.

Volkow, N. D., Swanson, J. M., Evins, A. E., DeLisi, L. E., Meier, M. H., Gonzalez, R., . . . Baler, R. (2016). Effects of cannabis use on human behavior, including cognition, motivation, and psychosis: A review. *JAMA Psychiatry, 73*(3), 292–297.

Volpicelli, J., Pettinati, H., McLellan, A. T., & O'Brien, C. P. (2001). *Combining medication and psychosocial treatments for addictions: The BRENDA approach.* New York: Guilford Press.

Vuchinich, R. E., & Heather, N. (Eds.). (2003). *Choice, behavioural economics and addiction.* New York: Pergamon Press.

Wagner, C. C., & Ingersoll, K. S. (2013). *Motivational interviewing in groups.* New York: Guilford Press.

Waldron, H. B., Kern-Jones, S., Turner, C. W., Peterson, T. R., & Ozechowski, T. J. (2007). Engaging resistant adolescents in drug abuse treatment. *Journal of Substance Abuse Treatment, 32*, 133–142.

Waldron, H. B., Miller, W. R., & Tonigan, J. S. (2001). Client anger as a predictor of differential response to treatment. In R. Longabaugh & P. W. Wirtz (Eds.), *Project MATCH hypotheses: Results and causal chain analyses* (Vol. 8, pp. 134–148). Bethesda, MD: National Institute on Alcohol Abuse and Alcoholism.

Waldron, H. B., & Turner, C. W. (2008). Evidence-based psychosocial treatments for adolescent substance abuse. *Journal of Clinical Child and Adolescent Psychology, 37*(1), 238–261.

Walitzer, K. S., Dermen, K. H., & Connors, G. J. (1999). Strategies for preparing clients for treatment: A review. *Behavior Modification, 23*(1), 129–151.

Walker, D., Stephens, R., Rowland, J., & Roffman, R. (2011). The influence of client behavior during motivational interviewing on marijuana treatment outcome. *Addictive Behaviors, 36*(6), 669–673.

Walker, D. D., Stephens, R. S., Towe, S., Banes, K., & Roffman, R. (2015). Maintenance check-ups following treatment for cannabis dependence. *Journal of Substance Abuse Treatment, 56,* 11–15.

Walker, E. R., & Druss, B. G. (2017). Cumulative burden of comorbid mental disorders, substance use disorders, chronic medical conditions, and poverty on health among adults in the U.S.A. *Psychology, Health and Medicine, 22*(6), 727–735.

Walker, E. R., Pratt, L. A., Schoenborn, C. A., & Druss, B. G. (2017). Excess mortality among people who report lifetime use of illegal drugs in the United States: A 20-year follow-up of a nationally representative survey. *Drug and Alcohol Dependence, 171,* 31–38.

Walker, R., Rosvall, T., Field, C. A., Allen, S., McDonald, D., Salim, Z., . . . Adinoff, B. (2010). Disseminating contingency management to increase attendance in two community substance abuse treatment centers: Lessons learned. *Journal of Substance Abuse Treatment, 39*(3), 202–209.

Wallace, C. J., Lecomte, T., Wilde, J., & Liberman, R. P. (2001). CASIG: A consumer-centered assessment for planning individualized treatment and evaluating program outcomes. *Schizophrenic Research, 50,* 105–119.

Walsh, D. C., Hingson, R. W., Merrigan, D. M., Morelock Levenson, S., Cupples, A., Heeren, T., . . . Kelly, C. A. (1991). A randomized trial of treatment options for alcohol-abusing workers. *New England Journal of Medicine, 325,* 775–782.

Walsh, J. (2003). Clinical case management. In A. R. Roberts & G. J. Greene (Eds.), *Social worker's desk reference* (pp. 472–476). Washington, DC: National Association of Social Workers.

Walters, O. S. (1957). The religious background of 50 alcoholics. *Quarterly Journal of Studies on Alcohol, 18,* 405–413.

Walters, S. T., Bennett, M. E., & Miller, J. H. (2000). Reducing alcohol use in college students: A controlled trial of two brief interventions. *Journal of Drug Education, 30*(3), 361–372.

Wampold, B. E. (2015). How important are the common factors in psychotherapy?: An update. *World Psychiatry, 14*(3), 270–277.

Wampold, B. E., & Imel, Z. E. (2015). *The great psychotherapy debate: The evidence for what makes psychotherapy work* (2nd ed.). New York: Routledge.

Watkins, S. L., Glantz, S. A., & Chaffee, B. W. (2018). Association of noncigarette tobacco product use with future cigarette smoking among youth in the Population Assessment of Tobacco and Health (PATH) study, 2013–2015. *JAMA Pediatrics, 172*(2), 181–187.

Webb, J. R., & Trautman, R. P. (2010). Forgiveness and alcohol use: Applying a specific spiritual principle to substance abuse problems. *Addictive Disorders and Their Treatment, 9*(1), 8–17.

Wegscheider-Cruse, S. (1990). Co-dependency and dysfunctional family systems. In R. C. Engs (Ed.), *Women: Alcohol and other drugs* (pp. 157–163). Dubuque, IA: Kendall/Hunt.

Weisner, C. (1995). The core-shell model: Implications for treatment assessment and community work. The emergence of assessment/referral programs in Ontario: An experiment in changing treatment systems through community development. *Contemporary Drug Problems, 22,* 151–158.

Weisner, C. (2002). What is the scope of the problem and its impact on health and social systems? In W. R. Miller & C. Weisner (Eds.), *Changing substance abuse through health and social systems* (pp. 3–14). New York: Kluwer Academic/Plenum Press.

Weisner, C., Mertens, J., Parthasarathy, S., Moore, C., & Lu, Y. (2001). Integrating primary medical care with addiction treatment: A randomized controlled trial. *JAMA, 286*(14), 1715–1723.

Weiss, B., Caron, A., Ball, S., Tapp, J., Johnson, M., & Weisz, J. R. (2005). Iatrogenic effects of group treatment for antisocial youths. *Journal of Consulting and Clinical Psychology, 73*(6), 1036–1044.

Weiss, R. D. (2004). Adherence to pharmacotherapy in patients with alcohol and opioid dependence. *Addiction, 99*(11), 1382–1392.

Weiss, R. D., & Connery, H. S. (2011). *Integrated group therapy for bipolar disorder and substance abuse.* New York: Guilford Press.

Weiss, R. D., Griffin, M. L., Potter, J. S., Dodd, D. R., Dreifuss, J. A., Connery, H. S., & Carroll, K. M. (2014). Who benefits from additional drug counseling among prescription opioid-dependent patients receiving buprenorphine–naloxone and standard medical management? *Drug and Alcohol Dependence, 140,* 118–122.

Weissman, M. M., Markowitz, J. C., & Klerman, G. (2000). *Comprehensive guide to interpersonal psychotherapy.* New York: Basic Books.

Welfel, E. R., Danzinger, P. R., & Santoro, S. (2000). Mandated reporting of abuse/maltreatment of older adults: A primer for counselors. *Journal of Counseling and Development, 78*(3), 284–292.

Wells, E. A., Donovan, D. M., Daley, D. C., Doyle, S. R., Brigham, G., Garrett, S. B., . . . Walker, R. (2014). Is level of exposure to a 12-step facilitation therapy associated with treatment outcome? *Journal of Substance Abuse Treatment, 47*(4), 265–274.

Wells, E. A., Peterson, P. L., Gainey, R. R., Hawkins, J. D., & Catalano, R. F. (1994). Outpatient treatment for cocaine abuse: A controlled comparison of relapse prevention and twelve-step approaches. *American Journal of Drug and Alcohol Abuse, 20,* 1–17.

Wells, E. A., Saxon, A. J., Calsyn, D. A., Jackson, T. R., & Donovan, D. M. (2010). Study results from the Clinical Trials Network's first 10 years: Where do they lead? *Journal of Substance Abuse Treatment, 38*(Suppl. 1), S14–S30.

Wendt, D. C., & Gone, J. P. (2017). Group therapy for substance use disorders: A survey of clinician practices. *Journal of Groups in Addiction and Recovery, 12,* 243–259.

Wendt, D. C., & Gone, J. P. (2018). Complexities with group therapy facilitation in substance use disorder specialty treatment settings. *Journal of Substance Abuse Treatment, 88,* 9–17.

Werb, D., Kamarulzaman, A., Meacham, M. C., Rafful, C., Fischer, B., Strathdee, S. A., & Wood, E. (2016). The effectiveness of compulsory drug treatment: A systematic review. *International Journal on Drug Policy, 28,* 1–9.

Wesson, D. R., & Ling, W. (2003). The Clinical Opiate Withdrawal Scale (COWS). *Journal of Psychoactive Drugs, 35*(2), 253–259.

Westerberg, V. S., Miller, W. R., & Tonigan, J. S. (2000). Comparison of outcomes for clients in randomized versus open trials of treatment for alcohol use disorders. *Journal of Studies on Alcohol, 61,* 720–727.

Westerberg, V. S., Tonigan, J. S., & Miller, W. R. (1998). Reliability of Form 90D: An instrument for quantifying drug use. *Substance Abuse, 19*(4), 179–189.

Whipple, J. L., Lambert, M. J., Vermeersch, D. A., Smart, D. W., Nielsen, S. L., & Hawkins, E. J. (2003). Improving the effects of psychotherapy: The use of early identification of treatment and problem-solving strategies in routine practice. *Journal of Counseling Psychology, 50*(1), 59–68.

White, A., Kavanagh, D., Stallman, H., Klein, B., Kay-Lambkin, F., Proudfoot, J., . . . Young, R. (2010). Online alcohol interventions: A systematic review. *Journal of Medical Internet Research, 12*(5), e62.

White, W. L. (2004). Transformational change: A historical review. *Journal of Clinical Psychology, 60,* 461–470.

White, W. L., & Miller, W. R. (2007). The use of confrontation in addiction treatment: History, science, and time for a change. *The Counselor, 8*(4), 12–30.

Whiteford, H. A., Ferrari, A., Degenhardt, L., Feigin, V. L., & Vos, T. (2015). The global burden of mental, neurological and substance use disorders: An analysis of the Global Burden of Disease Study 2010. *PLOS ONE, 10*(2), e0116820.

Whitfield, J. B., Heath, A. C., Madden, P. A. F., Landers, J. G., & Martin, N. G. (2018). Effects of high alcohol intake, alcohol-related symptoms and smoking on mortality. *Addiction, 113*(1), 158–166.

Whittle, A. E., Buckelow, S. M., Satterfield, J. M., Lum, P. J., & O'Sullivan, P. (2015). Addressing adolescent substance use: Teaching screening, brief intervention, and referral to treatment (SBIRT) and motivational interviewing (MI) to residents. *Substance Abuse, 36*(3), 325–331.

Whitworth, A. B., Oberbauer, H., Fleischhacker, W., Lesch, O., Walter, H., Nimmerrichter, A., . . . Potgieter, A. (1996). Comparison of acamprosate and placebo in long-term treatment of alcohol dependence. *The Lancet, 347*(9013), 1438–1442.

WHO ASSIST Working Group. (2002). The Alcohol, Smoking and Substance Involvement Screening Test (ASSIST): Development, reliability and feasibility. *Addiction, 97*(9), 1183–1194.

Wiggins, J. S. (1973). *Personality and prediction.* Reading, MA: Addison-Wesley.

Wilcox, C., & Bogenschutz, M. P. (2014). Pharmacotherapies for alcohol and drug use disorders. In B. McCrady & E. Epstein (Eds.), *Addiction: A comprehensive guidebook for practitioners* (2nd ed., pp. 526–550). New York: Guilford Press.

Willenbring, M. L. (1994). Case management applications in substance use disorders. *Journal of Case Management, 3*(4), 150–157.

Willenbring, M. L. (1996). Case management applications in substance use disorders. In H. A. Siegal & R. C. Rapp (Eds.), *Case management and substance abuse treatment: Practice and experience* (pp. 51–76). New York: Springer.

Willenbring, M. L., & Olson, D. H. (1999). A randomized trial of integrated outpatient treatment for medically ill alcoholic men. *Archives of Internal Medicine, 159*(16), 1946–1952.

Williams, E. C., Achtmeyer, C. E., Young, J. P., Rittmueller, S. E., Ludman, E. J., Lapham, G. T., . . . Bradley, K. A. (2016). Local implementation of alcohol screening and brief intervention at five Veterans Health Administration primary care clinics: Perspectives of clinical and administrative staff. *Journal of Substance Abuse Treatment, 60,* 27–35.

Williams, E. C., Johnson, M. L., Lapham, G. T., Caldeiro, R. M., Chew, L., Fletcher, G. S., . . . Bradley, K. A. (2011). Strategies to implement alcohol screening and brief intervention in primary care settings: A structured literature review. *Psychology of Addictive Behaviors, 25*(2), 206–214.

Williams, R., & Vinson, D. C. (2001). Validation of a single screening question for problem drinking. *Journal of Family Practice, 50,* 307–312.

Wilsnack, S. (1973). The needs of the female drinker: Dependency, power or what? In M. E. Chafetz (Ed.), *Proceedings of the second annual alcoholism conference of the National Institute on Alcohol Abuse and Alcoholism* (pp. 65–83). Washington, DC: U.S. Government Printing Office.

Winhusen, T. M., Kropp, F., Babcock, D., Hague, D., Erickson, S. J., Renz, C., . . . Somoza, E. C. (2008). Motivational enhancement therapy to improve treatment utilization and outcome in pregnant substance users. *Journal of Substance Abuse Treatment, 35*(2), 161–173.

Winters, A. (1978). Review and rationale of the Drinkwatchers International program. *American Journal of Drug and Alcohol Abuse, 5*(3), 321–326.

Witbrodt, J., Kaskutas, L. A., Bond, J., & Delucchi, K. (2012). Does sponsorship improve outcomes above Alcoholics Anonymous attendance?: A latent class growth curve analyses. *Addiction, 107*(2), 301–311.

Witbrodt, J., Ye, Y., Bond, J., Chi, F., Weisner, C., & Mertens, J. (2014). Alcohol and drug treatment involvement, 12-step attendance and abstinence: 9-year cross-lagged analysis of adults in an integrated health plan. *Journal of Substance Abuse Treatment, 46*(4), 412–419.

Witkiewitz, K., & Bowen, S. (2010). Depression, craving, and substance use following a randomized trial of mindfulness-based relapse prevention. *Journal of Consulting and Clinical Psychology, 78*(3), 362–374.

Witkiewitz, K., Bowen, S., Douglas, H., & Hsu, S. H. (2013). Mindfulness-based relapse prevention for substance craving. *Addictive Behaviors, 38*(2), 1563–1571.

Witkiewitz, K., Bowen, S., Harrop, E. N., Douglas, H., Enkema, M., & Sedgwick, C. (2014). Mindfulness-based treatment to prevent addictive behavior relapse: Theoretical models and hypothesized mechanisms of change. *Substance Use and Misuse, 49*(5), 513–524.

Witkiewitz, K., Donovan, D. M., & Hartzler, B. (2012). Drink refusal training as part of a combined behavioral intervention: Effectiveness and mechanisms of change. *Journal of Consulting and Clinical Psychology, 80*(3), 440–449.

Witkiewitz, K., Hartzler, B., & Donovan, D. (2010). Matching motivation enhancement treatment to client motivation: Re-examining the Project MATCH motivation matching hypothesis. *Addiction, 105,* 1403–1413.

Witkiewitz, K., Hallgren, K. A., Kranzler, H. R., Mann, K. F., Hasin, D. S., Falk, D. E., . . . Anton, R. F. (2017). Clinical validation of reduced alcohol consumption after treatment for alcohol dependence using the World Health Organization risk drinking levels. *Alcoholism: Clinical and Experimental Research, 41*(1), 179–186.

Witkiewitz, K., Lustyk, M. K., & Bowen, S. (2013). Retraining the addicted brain: A review of hypothesized neurobiological mechanisms of mindfulness-based relapse prevention. *Psychology of Addictive Behaviors, 27*(2), 351–365.

Witkiewitz, K., Maisto, S. A., & Donovan, D. M. (2010). A comparison of methods for estimating change in drinking following alcohol treatment. *Alcoholism: Clinical and Experimental Research, 34*(12), 2116–2125.

Witkiewitz, K., & Marlatt, G. A. (2004). Relapse prevention for alcohol and drug problems: That was Zen, this is Tao. *American Psychologist, 59*(4), 224–235.

Witkiewitz, K., Hallgren, K. A., Kranzler, H. R., Mann, K. F., Hasin, D. S., Falk, D. E., . . . Anton, R. F. (2017). Clinical validation of reduced alcohol consumption after treatment for alcohol dependence using the World Health Organization risk drinking levels. *Alcoholism: Clinical and Experimental Research, 41*(1), 179–186.

Witkiewitz, K., Roos, C. R., Pearson, M. R., Hallgren, K. A., Maisto, S. A., Kirouac, M., . . . Heather, N. (2017). How much is too much?: Patterns of drinking during alcohol treatment and associations with post-treatment outcomes across three alcohol clinical trials. *Journal of Studies on Alcohol and Drugs, 78*(1), 59–69.

Witkiewitz, K., Vowles, K. E., McCallion, E., Frohe, T., Kirouac, M., & Maisto, S. A. (2015). Pain as a predictor of heavy drinking and any drinking lapses in the COMBINE study and the UK Alcohol Treatment Trial. *Addiction, 110,* 1262–1271.

Witkiewitz, K., Warner, K., Sully, B., Barricks, A., Stauffer, C., Thompson, B. L., & Luoma, J. B. (2014). Randomized trial comparing mindfulness-based relapse prevention with relapse prevention for women offenders at a residential addiction treatment center. *Substance Use and Misuse, 49*(5), 536–546.

Woititz, J. G. (1984). Adult children of alcoholics. *Alcoholism Treatment Quarterly, 1*(1), 71–99.

Wolff, J. L., & Roter, D. L. (2008). Hidden in plain sight: Medical visit companions as a resource for vulnerable older adults. *Archives of Internal Medicine, 168*(13), 1409–1415.

Wolff, N., & Shi, J. (2015). Screening for substance use disorder among incarcerated men with the Alcohol, Smoking, Substance Involvement Screening Test (ASSIST): A comparative analysis of computer-administered and interviewer-administered modalities. *Journal of Substance Abuse Treatment, 53,* 22–32.

Wurst, F. M., Dresen, S., Allen, J. P., Wiesbeck, G., Graf, M., & Weinmann, W. (2006). Ethyl sulphate: A direct ethanol metabolite reflecting recent alcohol consumption. *Addiction, 101*(2), 204–211.

Wurst, F. M., Wiesbeck, G. A., Metzger, J. W., & Weinmann, W. (2004). On sensitivity, specificity, and the influence of various parameters on ethyl glucuronide levels in urine—Results from the WHO/ISBRA study. *Alcoholism: Clinical and Experimental Research, 28*(8), 1220–1228.

Xie, H., Drake, R. E., McHugo, G. J., Xie, L., & Mohandas, A. (2010). The 10-year course of remission, abstinence, and recovery in dual diagnosis. *Journal of Substance Abuse Treatment, 39*(2), 132–140.

Yablonsky, L. (1965). *Synanon: The tunnel back.* Baltimore: Penguin Books.

Yablonsky, L. (1989). *The therapeutic community: A successful approach for treating substance abusers.* New York: Gardner Press.

Yahne, C. E., & Miller, W. R. (1999). Evoking hope. In W. R. Miller (Ed.), *Integrating spirituality into treatment: Resources for practitioners* (pp. 217–233). Washington, DC: American Psychological Association.

Yalom, I. D., & Leszcz, M. (2008). *The theory and practice of group psychotherapy* (5th ed.). New York: Basic Books.

You, C. W., Chen, Y. C., Chen, C. H., Lee, C. H., Kuo, P. H., Huang, M. C., & Chu, H. H. (2017). Smartphone-based support system (SoberDiary) coupled with a bluetooth breathalyser for treatment-seeking alcohol-dependent patients. *Addictive Behaviors, 65,* 174–178.

Zarkin, G., Bravy, J., Hinde, J., & Saitz, R. (2015). Costs of screening and brief intervention for illicit drug use in primary care settings. *Journal of Studies on Alcohol and Drugs, 76*(2), 222–228.

Zemore, S. E., & Ajzen, I. (2014). Predicting substance abuse treatment completion using a new scale based on the theory of planned behavior. *Journal of Substance Abuse Treatment, 46*(2), 174–182.

Zemore, S. E., Kaskutas, L. A., Mericle, A., & Hemberg, J. (2017). Comparison of 12-step groups to mutual help alternatives for AUD in a large, national study:

Differences in membership characteristics and group participation, cohesion, and satisfaction. *Journal of Substance Abuse Treatment, 73,* 16–26.

Zemore, S. E., Lui, C., Mericle, A., Hemberg, J., & Kaskutas, L. A. (2018). A longitudinal study of the comparative efficacy of Women for Sobriety, LifeRing, SMART Recovery, and 12-step groups for those with AUD. *Journal of Substance Abuse Treatment, 88,* 18–26.

Zemore, S. E., Murphy, R. D., Mulia, N., Gilbert, P. A., Martinez, P., Bond, J., & Polcin, D. L. (2014). A moderating role for gender in racial/ethnic disparities in alcohol services utilization: Results from the 2000 to 2010 national alcohol surveys. *Alcoholism, Clinical and Experimental Research, 38*(8), 2286–2296.

Zgierska, A., Rabago, D., Zuelsdorff, M., Coe, C., Miller, M., & Fleming, M. (2008). Mindfulness meditation for alcohol relapse prevention: A feasibility pilot study. *Journal of Addiction Medicine, 2*(3), 165–173.

Zinberg, N. E. (1984). *Drug, set, and setting: The basis for controlled intoxicant use.* New Haven, CT: Yale University Press.

Zomahoun, H. T. V., Guénette, L., Grégoire, J.-P., Lauzier, S., Lawani, A. M., Ferdynus, C., . . . Moisan, J. (2016). Effectiveness of motivational interviewing interventions on medication adherence in adults with chronic diseases: A systematic review and meta-analysis. *International Journal of Epidemiology, 46*(2), 589–602.

Zuroff, D. C., Kelly, A. C., Leybman, M. J., Blatt, S. J., & Wampold, B. E. (2010). Between-therapist and within-therapist differences in the quality of the therapeutic relationship: Effects on maladjustment and self-critical perfectionism. *Journal of Clinical Psychology, 66*(7), 681–697.

Zweben, A. (2012). Case management in substance abuse treatment. In S. Walters (Ed.), *Treating substance abuse* (3rd ed., pp. 402–421). New York: Guilford Press.

Zweben, A., & Barrett, D. (1997). Facilitating compliance in alcoholism treatment. In B. Blackwell (Ed.), *Compliance and treatment alliance in serious mental illness* (pp. 277–293). Newark, NJ: Gordon & Breach.

Zweben, A., Bonner, M., Chaim, G., & Santon, P. (1988). Facilitative strategies for retaining the alcohol-dependent client in outpatient treatment. *Alcoholism Treatment Quarterly, 5*(1–2), 3–24.

Zweben, A., Pettinati, H. M., Weiss, R. D., Youngblood, M., Cox, C. E., Mattson, M. E., . . . Ciraulo, D. (2008). Relationship between medication adherence and treatment outcomes: The COMBINE study. *Alcoholism: Clinical and Experimental Research, 32*(9), 1661–1669.

Zweben, A., Piepmeier, M. E., Fucito, L., & O'Malley, S. S. (2017). The clinical utility of the Medication Adherence Questionnaire (MAQ) in an alcohol pharmacotherapy trial. *Journal of Substance Abuse Treatment, 77,* 72–78.

Zweben, A., Rose, S., Stout, R. L., & Zywiak, W. H. (2003). Case monitoring and motivational style brief interventions. In R. K. Hester & W. R. Miller (Eds.), *Handbook of alcoholism treatment approaches: Effective alternatives* (3rd ed., pp. 113–130). Boston: Allyn & Bacon.

Zweben, A., & Zuckoff, A. (2002). Motivational interviewing and treatment adherence. In W. R. Miller & S. Rollnick, *Motivational interviewing: Preparing people for change* (2nd ed., pp. 299–319). New York: Guilford Press.

Index

Note. *b* following a page number indicates boxed text.